ORTHOPEDIC NURSING

ORTHOPEDIC NURSING

Carroll B. Larson, M.D., F.A.C.S.

Professor Emeritus of Orthopedic Surgery and
formerly Chairman of the Department of Orthopedic
Surgery, The University of Iowa, Iowa City, Iowa

Marjorie Gould, R.N., B.S., M.S.

Associate Professor, College of Nursing,
The University of Iowa, Iowa City, Iowa

NINTH EDITION

with 466 figures

The C. V. Mosby Company

St. Louis   1978

NINTH EDITION

Copyright © 1978 by The C. V. Mosby Company

Previous editions copyrighted 1943, 1949, 1953, 1957, 1961, 1965, 1970, 1974

Printed in the United States of America

The C. V. Mosby Company
11830 Westline Industrial Drive
St. Louis, Missouri 63141

Library of Congress Cataloging in Publication Data

Larson, Carroll Bernard, 1909-
    Orthopedic nursing.

    Includes bibliographies and index.
    1. Orthopedic nursing. I. Gould, Marjorie,
joint author.
RD753.L36 1978   610.73′677   78-3429
ISBN 0-8016-2866-0

CB/CB/B 9 8 7 6 5 4 3 2 1

Preface

Each year the rate of change accelerates in health care delivery. The health care consumer is increasingly sophisticated in his knowledge of health and displays a growing interest in health maintenance and illness prevention. New technology and close cooperation of medicine and engineering have provided a variety of new techniques and materials for more effective treatment of health problems. Advances in surgical concepts and practice have broadened the knowledge base for all health professionals. Greater attention is being focused on proper utilization of facilities, assurance of quality care, and cost containment, resulting in fewer hospital admissions, shorter hospital stays, and interdisciplinary care of acute and complex health problems. To evaluate care, medical and nursing audits have been implemented and standards of care established. These quality control procedures have indicated the need for careful documentation of patient problems to ensure continuity of care.

In the midst of continuous and rapid change, the fundamental aspects of quality nursing care remain constant: concern and respect for the patient and his rights, recognition of and providing for the patient's physical and psychosocial needs, and the necessity for teaching health maintenance and disease prevention. This ninth edition reemphasizes these established fundamentals and updates the core of basic knowledge upon which the progress of orthopedic surgery and orthopedic nursing depends. We hope that the information in this book will provide direction for the nurse in assessment of the orthopedic patient's needs, help develop the skills needed to plan and implement holistic nursing care, and enhance the nurse's ability to evaluate the care given.

This ninth edition includes a new chapter entitled "Emergency nursing on the orthopedic patient unit" by Dolores J. Whitehead, R.N., M.S. Particular credit is due her for this substantial contribution. The entire text has been revised and expanded when appropriate in keeping with current knowledge and practice, and ninety new illustrations (photographs, roentgenograms, and drawings) have been included. Special appreciation is extended to the artist, Pamela Luther, for her work.

Further credit is recognized for the helpful updating of information on amputations by Donald Shurr, R.P.T., on care of the cerebrovascular patient by Karen Kirkman, R.P.T., and on bone tumors by Michael Bonfiglio, M.D. We are especially grateful to the instructors, students, and practitioners who continue to offer their comments and suggestions, thus increasing the usefulness of each edition.

C. B. L.
M. L. G.

Contents

ORTHOPEDIC NURSING

1 Introduction

HISTORICAL BACKGROUND

Orthopedics is a medical speciality that includes investigation, preservation, restoration, and development of the form and function of the extremities, spine, and associated structures by medical, surgical, and physical methods. Normal reactions of the musculoskeletal system to events of daily living, such as standing, sitting, walking, running, and manipulative tasks of the arms and hands, constitute the major concern of orthopedics. To relieve musculoskeletal disabilities, and thus enable the individual to carry out normal tasks, necessitates an insight into the behavior of living bones and muscles. A clear concept of bone structure, physiologic response of bone to stresses of gravity, and activities of daily living is the special contribution orthopedics has to offer toward the knowledge of musculoskeletal abnormalities that afflict mankind.

The term *orthopaedia* (from the Greek *orthos*, straight; *paides*, child) was coined in 1741 by Nicholas Andrey as the title for his book devoted to a discussion of the deformities of the child. Orthopedics was practiced by "strap-and-buckle" doctors for nearly 120 years before surgery was applied to the art. Dr. Virgil P. Gibney, Surgeon-in-Chief of the New York Hospital for the Ruptured and Crippled, advocated surgery for the correction of certain deformities, and this was looked upon by many of his contemporaries as meddlesome. His persistence produced results superior to those obtained from other mechanical means, and in 1887 the American Orthopaedic Association was organized as a forum for orthopedic surgeons. The transactions of the Association were pub-

lished annually and included reports on an ever-increasing number of case studies, surgical operations, and investigations. Their publication continues today as *The Journal of Bone and Joint Surgery*.

World War I and the years following saw the organization of hospital orthopedic services as well as sections or departments of orthopedics in medical schools. In increasing numbers the graduates joined the general medical communities. In 1922 the Shriners Hospitals for Crippled Children (currently twenty-one) came into being, since only 400 orthopedic surgeons were available in the entire United States, and some remote areas had none except those who worked in the Shriners Hospitals. In 1932 the American Academy of Orthopaedic Surgeons was organized for the purpose of providing continuing education. In 1934 the American Board of Orthopaedic Surgery was formed to establish standards of training for orthopedic surgeons, and examinations have been held yearly for candidates who wish to become certified in the practice of orthopedic surgery. By 1977, more than 8,000 orthopedic surgeons had been certified by the Board.

Although orthopedic surgery as a specialty is relatively new, medical problems that involve bones have existed for half a million years, as evidenced in the Java man. Skeletons preserved from antiquity have yielded evidence by which anthropologists and archeologists have determined the state of industrial, social, and recreational activities of ancient people. Defects found in the skull rank trephining (removal of a circular disk of bone from the skull) as the earliest of operations sub-

1

stantiated by writings in the Egyptian papyri in 1600 B.C. The translations of Hippocrates by Galen (131-201 A.D.) provide classic descriptions of clubfeet and congenital dislocations of the hip. In the fifteen century Leonardo da Vinci made anatomic drawings from human dissections, but not until the seventeenth century, after the invention of the microscope by Leeuwenhoek, did Klopton Havers provide the histology of bone which is recognized to this day as the haversian system in cortical bone.

In the eighteenth century, John Hunter offered insight into the capability of bones to produce longitudinal and directional growth that later led Wolff (1836-1902) to develop his famous law: "Bones in their external and internal architecture conform with the intensity and direction of the stresses to which they are habitually subjected." The Wolff concept—that bone is formed through the tension of muscles and the pressure of body weight coupled with gravitational pull—constitutes the major thesis of present-day authorities on skeletal development.

History reveals that from earliest times man has had the problem of caring for crippling conditions and broken bones. Hippocrates in his book entitled *On Surgery* described numerous deformities. History also reveals that in centuries past crippled persons were not always treated kindly but were ridiculed, ignored, and abused. During primitive times, they were abandoned to die. The philosophy prevailed that only the fit should survive. Thus, through the centuries, the crippled/deformed individual, unable to work, resorted to begging. In the seventeenth century (1601) The Poor Relief Act was passed in England. This was a beginning, an attempt to provide help for the crippled individual as well as the poor person.

Treatment of muscles, ligaments, bones, and joints has taken many forms. One of the earliest devices used for the treatment of fractures was the wooden splint. Hippocrates used bandages stiffened with gums and waxes for splinting. In India the fractured limb was enclosed in a mold of clay. By 850 A.D. egg white splints were commonly used. Cloth soaked with a mixture of egg white and flour or lead was wrapped about the extremity. Later, liquid plaster of Paris was used for immobilization. The injured limb was placed in a box and the liquid plaster poured around it. The use of the plaster-of-Paris bandages with which we are familiar today was first described in 1852. The bandages were used on the battlefront by a Dutch army officer named Matthysen. Finely powdered plaster was rubbed into coarse-meshed cotton material, which was then rolled into bandages. By 1872 plaster of Paris was being used extensively in the treatment of orthopedic conditions. However, reports of paralysis of limbs or of sudden deaths following the application of plaster caused many objections to its use.[3]

The use of crutches is not new. Crutches have been used throughout history. Down through the ages the typical crutch was the shoulder-high stick with a crosspiece for the axillary bar. In the eighteenth century, with the invention of the saw, the crutch made with two sticks, an axillary bar, and a hand bar came into use.

The use of traction in the treatment of bone conditions was described in 1856 by Henry G. Davis (1807-1896) in an article entitled "The use of weights and pulleys and other traction devices for the treatment of fractures" published in the *American Medical Monthly*, May, 1856. Gurdon Buck is credited with having been the first surgeon successfully to apply the principle of "continued elastic extension to the treatment of fractures of the femur."[15] Thus, the term *Buck's extension* is used today to describe a particular type of traction.

From earliest recorded time, makeshift substitutes such as forked sticks, peg legs, and crutches have been utilized to help the individual who lost a limb. At best, these crude devices were poor substitutes for the missing limb, and many such individuals became beggars or peddlers. During the sixteenth century, Ambroise Paré, a surgeon in the French army, improved the surgical procedure for amputation by revitalizing the use of ligatures. Because of his interest and ability in devising artificial limbs with movable joints, he has been called the founder of "modern principles of amputation."[1] Limbs designed by Paré were made of heavy metals.

In the nineteenth century, James Potts

of London began to construct wooden artificial limbs with steel joints. Also during the nineteenth century, due to the large number of industrial accidents, the demand for prostheses increased. At that time, the trained prosthetist became the limb maker. Previously, artificial limbs were made by carpenters and blacksmiths.

The twentieth century, with two world wars, fostered much interest and great progress in prosthetics. Many centers have been established, and prosthetic research today is extensive. In these centers, physicians work closely with certified prosthetists in devising and fitting artificial limbs.

Orthopedic conditions were prevalent during the eighteenth and nineteenth centuries. Poverty, malnutrition, and low standards of living existed. Tuberculosis was a common cause of illness. Polluted milk and crowded living conditions were conducive to the spread of the tubercle bacilli, and tuberculous involvement of bones and joints frequently followed pulmonary infection, resulting in bone destruction and severe crippling conditions. Other kinds of bone and joint infections were common. The sequelae of repeated attacks of osteomyelitis were deformity and disability. Rickets due to malnutrition involved infants and small children and caused bending and bowing of bones.[12] The deformities that developed in the young child remained, of course, throughout his life. Poliomyelitis (infantile paralysis) was prevalent, and survivors of the disease were plagued with varying degrees of muscle weakness and paralysis. During this time, treatment for the orthopedic patient consisted primarily of supportive care, good nutrition, rest, exercise, fresh air, and sunshine. The lack of funds and facilities made treatment unavailable to many. Along with the supportive care, braces and splints were devised to help the individual to be ambulatory—thus the term "strap-and-buckle" was applied to the early orthopedic doctor.

The foregoing description contrasts sharply with today's treatment and care of the orthopedic patient. The use of anesthetics, antibiotics, vaccines, and blood transfusions, plus the knowledge of asepsis, the perfection of many orthopedic surgical procedures, and provision for early diagnosis, treatment, and follow-up care, provide a different kind of prognosis and hope for the disabled person.

During the nineteenth century, orthopedics became a specialty. As the specialty developed, wards and hospitals were established for the care of the crippled person. Buckminister Brown (1819-1891) was the first American surgeon to devote his practice to the treatment of orthopedic conditions. In 1862 he established the first ward for crippled children at the House of the Good Samaritan in Boston.[7]

In 1863 the Hospital for the Ruptured and Crippled was founded in New York City by James Knight (1810-1887). In 1940 the name was changed to the Hospital for Special Surgery. At this hospital, Virgil Pendleton Gibney (1847-1927) established the first residency training program in orthopedic surgery.[15]

Edward Hickling Bradford (1848-1926) established an orthopedic ward at the Boston City Hospital. The Bradford frame, which has been used during the past century in the care of the orthopedic patient, was designed and used by him.[7]

John Ball Brown (1784-1862) founded the "Orthopaedique Infirmary for the treatment of spinal distortions, club feet, etc." in 1838 in Boston.[7]

In Great Britian, the Royal Orthopaedic Infirmary was established in 1840 by William John Little (1819-1894). Little, who had infantile paralysis as a child, devoted much time to the care of the child with spastic paralysis. Because of his writings dealing with this condition, it became known as "Little's disease."[9]

In Liverpool, Hugh Owen Thomas (1834-1891), a qualified physician, was well known for his ability to set broken bones and to reduce dislocated joints. A number of appliances in use today bear his name—Thomas heel, Thomas splint, and the Thomas collar. His nephew, Sir Robert Jones (1857-1933), became an orthopedic surgeon and was influential in helping to establish orthopedic surgery as a specialty.[12]

In 1900, on the first day of October, an old and derelict farmhouse at Oswestry in Shropshire near the border of Wales became the "Baschurch Home." In less than forty years, this home was to become an orthopedic hospital of more than 300 beds, with a staff of aftercare nurses and orthopedic clinics stretching through eight counties, and a training clinic for cripples with the nucleus of a village settlement. Agnes Hunt[8] (1862-1948), who has been referred to as the Florence Nightingale of orthopaedic nursing,[17] was the founder of this home. Agnes Hunt was herself a cripple. At the age of 10 years, because of a blister on her heel, her "apprentice to crippledom had begun, and also the great education of pain."[8]

In 1904, Sir Robert Jones of Liverpool became the consulting orthopedic surgeon. He made monthly visits and performed operations at the Baschurch Home. In 1908 Agnes Hunt started a training school to prepare nurses for "this branch of their profession."[8] In 1933, following the death of Sir Robert Jones, the hospital's name was changed to the Robert Jones and Agnes Hunt Orthopaedic Hospital.[8]

It is interesting to note that during the early part of the twentieth century, articles describing the care of the child with an orthopedic condition appeared in the first issues of the *American Journal of Nursing*. The following excerpts are indicative of the nursing needs of the crippled child at that time. It will be apparent to the reader that some of the instructions and advice given the nurse in these writings are still applicable today.

"Pressure applied by the point of the finger should be rapidly followed by a restoration of the normal color. If the part becomes dark and bluish, the venous circulation is interfered with and swelling will result; if white and cold, the arterial supply is cut off indicating deep and dangerous pressure. Numbness is the sign of pressure on a nerve. In every case, the tension must be relieved. In the case of plaster splints, they must be cut through and opened sufficiently to remove the symptoms, and then fixed by a bandage."*

"If the caretakers of children and those who are working in their midst were more on the alert in watching their progress and growth, their discernment would enable them to adopt effective prophylactic mea-

sures against the development of these diseases."*

"In congenital club-foot much can be accomplished by mechanical correction . . . it is frequently treated by fixation in a plaster-of-Paris bandage; and watchfulness must be exerted to guard against injuries to the circulation. If a brace has been worn, and the deformity corrected sufficiently to do away with the brace, the walk of the child must be carefully watched and care taken to have the shoe of proper shape and size."*

Other writings stated that the Children's Aid Society of New York City "has provided not only a teacher but a nurse trained in orthopaedic work, who understands the children and their limitations and who is fitted to give the daily attention which is absolutely necessary in many cases. After the morning exercises, the braces are looked to, abscesses dressed, straps changed, etc., and each child is made as comfortable as skilled care can make him."†

In 1939 Jessie L. Stevenson wrote, "Every nurse, institutional, private duty or public health, who gives bedside care or teaches the art of nursing to student nurses or to families, is responsible for making or preventing crippling . . . Orthopedic nursing must be a part of all good nursing but the reverse is equally true, all good nursing is a part of orthopedic nursing."‡

Carmelita Calderwood referred to orthopedic nursing "as the application of the principles of body mechanics to all nursing." She further stated that the definition "sometimes presents an unfamiliar concept to nurses . . . but [that] analysis of any [well-selected] equipment or apparatus used in the care of the orthopedic patient will reveal that its fundamental purpose is maintenance or restoration of good body mechanics."§

---

*From Wood, E. W.: The nursing care of orthopaedic surgical cases, Am J Nurs **2**:425-429, Mar 1902.

†From Curtis, A.: The crippled children's school, Am J Nurs **1**:427-428, Mar 1901.

‡From Stevenson, J. L.: What is orthopedic nursing? Am J Nurs **39**:11-17, Jan 1939.

§From Funsten, R. V., and Calderwood, C.: Orthopedic nursing, ed. 2, St. Louis, 1949, The C. V. Mosby Co.

---

*From Ashton, E.: The application of splints to growing children, Am J Nurs **2**:32-36, Oct 1901.

The twentieth century has seen a great increase in society's willingness to accept the responsibility of providing treatment and help for the disabled individual. Two world wars have helped the nation focus on the importance of helping the disabled civilian, as well as the disabled veteran, to live an independent productive life.

In some instances, private agencies have led the way in providing facilities for the care of the handicapped, as well as providing for research and for the preparation of needed personnel. The list is long and increases each year— Easter Seal Society for Crippled Children and Adults, National Foundation-March of Dimes, and the Shriners Hospitals for Crippled Children are examples. Also, since the beginning of the present century, much legislation has been passed in an attempt to meet the needs of the disabled. In 1935, Congress passed the Social Security Act. The purpose of this act was ". . . to provide for the general welfare by establishing a system of Federal old-age benefits, and by enabling the several states to make more adequate provision for aged persons, blind persons, dependent and crippled children, maternal and child welfare, public health, and the administration of their unemployment compensation laws; to establish a Social Security Board; to raise revenue; and for other purposes."*

The Children's Bureau, which was established in 1921, was given the responsibility of planning the programs concerned with maternal and child health, crippled children, and child welfare services provided for by the Social Security Act of 1935. The aspect of this Act that had particular significance for orthopedic nursing was the provision for locating and securing care for crippled children. To provide this service, increased numbers of public health nurses with orthopedic preparation were needed in the late 1930's.

"Before the passage of the act, a variety of services for the care of crippled children had been developed. Some of the large visiting nurse associations, for example, had well developed orthopedic services staffed by nurses who were also trained physical therapists. But there was no generally recognized standards for the preparation of nurses who were to practice orthopedic nursing. Realizing that the number of orthopedic nurses was far too small to meet the needs of the new program for crippled children, the Children's Bureau sought information and advice from the profession. There were no postgraduate courses in that field. The problem was then taken to the NOPHN. That organization which had been receiving requests for assistance from various quarters acted promptly. A new orthopedic council proceeded to set up tentative standards for courses for graduate nurses. Universities were encouraged to offer advanced courses in orthopedic nursing, and also basic courses for public health nursing supervisors who had not had good undergraduate preparation for that field. Within a short time plans were underway for courses at Harvard, Western Reserve, and Teachers College."*

"The Children's Bureau program for the care of crippled children had already been launched, under provision of the Social Security Act, when the National Foundation for Infantile Paralysis was organized in 1938. . . . A grant from the foundation to the NOPHN in 1939 made possible the appointment of a nurse consultant. Jessie L. Stevenson, a public health nurse equipped with knowledge and experience in both orthopedic nursing and physical therapy, accepted the position. The service modestly begun by one nurse became a stimulating force in the improvement of many nursing services. In caring for those already crippled, Miss Stevenson pointed out, the nurse 'must see beyond the orthopedic defect to the patient as a person.' The Joint Orthopedic Nursing Advisory Service, financed by the National Foundation for Infantile Paralysis and administered by the NOPHN, was organized in 1941, and a consultant, Carmelita Calderwood, was engaged by the NLNE to work in cooperation with Miss Stevenson. JONAS provided consultant service to individuals, hospitals, schools of nursing, universities, and nursing service agencies. For several years, it administered scholarship funds

---

*From Public Law No. 271, 74th Congress, H. R. 7260.

*From Roberts, M. M.: American nursing, New York, 1954, The Macmillan Co., p. 275.

provided by the foundation. The service was so successful that, fortunately, it was continued in the postwar period with its mounting incidence of polio. . . . The preparation of handbooks and other publications, of annotated lists of publications, and of visual aids was an important feature of the JONAS service which after the reorganization of 1952 became the Nursing Advisory Service for Orthopedics and Poliomyelitis of the National League for Nursing (NLN)."*

Discovery of the Salk vaccine in 1955 drastically changed the face of orthopedic nursing. The National Foundation for Infantile Paralysis redirected its efforts to prevention and treatment of birth defects and changed its name accordingly. Increased attention was focused on such orthopedic problems as spina bifida, clubfoot, and rheumatoid arthritis. Concurrent changes in nursing and throughout the entire health care delivery system began to emphasize health maintenance, rehabilitation, and care of the patient within his total environment. The American Nurses' Association began to develop standards of practice, both general and specific, and nursing evidenced a growing sense of accountability and advocacy in patient care.

In July, 1972, the Orthopedic Nurses' Association was founded in Atlanta, Georgia, with a membership of twenty-four nurses. As of May, 1977, the number of local chapters had increased to seventy-four, and members may be found in each of the states and in several foreign countries. This organization has assumed leadership in facilitating continuing education for orthopedic nurses. The first edition of the *ONA Journal*, a monthly publication, was published in August, 1974. Previous to this, the *ONA Newsletter* provided a means of communicating with nurses in the local chapters.

The Annual Congress of the Association provides opportunities for learning and the valuable exchange of ideas. Standards of orthopedic nursing practice have been established to provide assurance that service of a high quality will be maintained, and teaching aids have been made available.

*From Roberts, M. M.: American nursing, New York, 1954, The Macmillan Co., pp. 434 and 435.

ORTHOPEDIC NURSING AND THE NURSING PROCESS

In orthopedic nursing, as in other areas of nursing, utilization of the nursing process is helping nurses to provide comprehensive and individualized care for their patients. The nursing process involves the problem-solving approach and provides for the assessment of patient data, identification of nursing needs, planning and implementation of nursing care, and evaluation of the care given.

The first phase of the process consists of patient assessment and the identification of the nursing needs. Establishment of the patient's nursing needs must be based on an analysis and synthesis of significant patient information. This information provides the nurse with an understanding of the patient's perception of his illness and hospitalization, adjustments he and his family have been able to make, methods used to cope with pain and physical disability, the social and economic implications for the family, and many details such as dietary needs, presence of urinary and bowel problems, sleeping difficulties, self-care abilities, etc. This initial assessment may be facilitated by the use of a health history or admissions interview which, when carefully completed, provides a systematic method of securing essential information and also an opportunity to involve the patient and/or family in planning the needed care. However, it is important for the nurse to remember that the identification and analysis of patient information is not a one-time function but a continuous process. Each patient-nurse contact provides the nurse with an opportunity to gain a better understanding of the patient's strengths and weaknesses, to become aware of changing needs, and to evaluate the nursing care being given.

Assessment also must include specific orthopedic needs that deal primarily with functional abilities of the extremities and postural problems. This involves an understanding of the normal neuromusculoskeletal system and knowledge of the existing orthopedic disorder, the medical care and treatment planned, and the complications that may be encountered. Early detection of a scoliotic condition is dependent upon an understanding of normal posture and the ability to recognize symptoms indicative of a beginning spinal curvature. Neurovascular checks are vital aspects of the assessment needs of the patient in traction or a cast. Assessing and determining the need for active and/or passive range of motion and change of body positions are necessary aspects of the care needed by the immobilized patient.

Musculoskeletal difficulties affect all age groups (each with its own problems) and include both acute and life-long crippling conditions. Orthopedic nursing involves caring for the person hoping and working to overcome a disability or injury as well as the individual confronted with a terminal illness. The patient coping with a physical disability and body image change is also making emotional adjustments. Nursing care involves helping the patient adjust to the psychologic difficulties as well as the physiologic problems.

In the *Standards of Orthopedic Nursing Practice,*[30] "**orthopedic nursing practice** is defined as the nursing care of individuals with known and/or predicted neuro-musculo-skeletal alterations. In planning nursing interventions, nurses who engage in orthopedic nursing practice must take into account related physiological, social and behavioral problems resulting from or affecting the individual's response and/or adjustment to the neuro-musculo-skeletal alteration. The practice of orthopedic nursing is carried out in those settings which deliver primary, acute and long term care and nursing prevention of potential neuro-musculo-skeletal problems.

"The scope of orthopedic nursing practice encompasses those nursing activities which assist the individual to modify his life style and environment so that he can attain optimum neuro-musculo-skeletal function compatible with his life goals. The nursing activities are directed toward providing continuity of care through assessment, intervention and evaluation, and revision of the nursing care plan."*

The second phase of the nursing process involves the identification of the nursing intervention(s) needed to solve or minimize the problem. This phase involves the use of a nursing care plan. For example, the elderly person recovering from a femoral neck fracture must not develop pressure sores. Assessment is concerned with the patient's general health, circulatory problems, skin condition, fluid and dietary needs, mental status, and bowel and bladder problems, as well as the restrictions related to activity and position changes. Based on the assessment findings, a nursing care plan is devised with the intent of maintaining an intact integument. Priorities are established and the needed care is carefully outlined with and communicated to the patient, unit personnel, and other authorized persons.

The third phase of the nursing process involves implementation of the nursing care. In this phase, all aspects of nursing are involved—planning, consulting, communicating, teaching, and supervising as well as giving direct nursing care.

The fourth stage deals with evaluation and recording. Evaluation must be concerned with the care given and the meeting of the patient's nursing needs. Since this aspect of the process is based on the previous phases, the evaluation will reflect the effectiveness of the complete process. Methods of evaluating the quality of nursing care rendered vary widely. The nursing audit, peer review, and the establishment of standards of care are the methods used most frequently.

In summary, it might be well to state that the phases of the nursing process rarely follow one another in an orderly sequence. Assessment and evaluation are going on continuously and consequently lead to the setting of new goals and revision of the care plan and care given—the phases overlap and may be in process concurrently.

Many facets of orthopedic nursing will be discussed throughout this book, and each assumes varying degrees of importance depending on the patient's needs at a particular time. Two aspects of care that may be neglected in a busy situation are discharge planning and teaching. Both of these have particular significance for the orthopedic patient and should start at the time of ad-

---

*From Orthopedic Nurses' Association and American Nurses' Association, Division on Medical-Surgical Nursing Practice: Standards of orthopedic nursing practice, Kansas City Mo., 1975, American Nurses' Association, p. 5.

mission or shortly thereafter. Knowledge of the environment to which the patient is returning and the available family and community resources are of vital concern. To provide the needed follow-up care, early planning with the patient and with other health workers is essential. Likewise, teaching the patient (or responsible person) in relation to his nursing needs must be an ongoing process during hospitalization and not a last-minute task done just prior to discharge. If teaching and planning for home care are slighted or omitted, the quality of care rendered also is changed.

REFERENCES

Historical background

1 American Academy of Orthopaedic Surgeons: Orthopaedic appliances atlas. Vol 2. Artificial limbs: a consideration of aids employed in the practice of orthopaedic surgery, Ann. Arbor, Mich., 1960, J. W. Edwards.
2 Ashton, E.: The application of splints to growing children, Am J Nurs 2:32-36, Oct 1901.
3 Atkinson, E.: Plaster casts—their preparation in the hospital, Walpole, Mass., 1937, Lewis Manufacturing Co.
4 Curtis, A.: The crippled children's school, Am J Nurs 1:427-428, Mar 1901.
5 Fliegel, O., and Feuer, S. G.: Historical development of lower-extremity prostheses, Arch Phys Med Rehabil 47:275-285, May 1966.
6 Funsten, R. V., and Calderwood, C.: Orthopedic nursing, ed. 2, St. Louis, 1949, The C. V. Mosby Co.
7 Hilt, N. E., and Schmitt, E. W. Jr.: Pediatric orthopedic nursing, St. Louis, 1975, The C. V. Mosby Co.
8 Hunt, A.: This is my life, New York, 1942, G. P. Putnam's Sons.
9 Jones, A. R.: William John Little, J Bone Joint Surg [Br] 31:123-126, Feb 1949.
10 Knocke, F. J., and Knocke, L. S.: Orthopaedic nursing, Philadelphia, 1951, F. A. Davis Co.
11 Public Law No. 271, 74th Congress, H. R. 7260.
12 Roaf, R., and Hodkinson, L. J.: Textbook of orthopaedic nursing, Philadelphia, 1971, F. A. Davis Co.
13 Roberts, M. M.: American nursing: history and interpretation, New York, 1954, The Macmillan Co.
14 Sarmiento, A., editor: Symposium on amputation surgery and prosthetics, Orthop Clin North Am 3:265-494, Jul 1972.
15 Shands, A. R., Jr.: The early orthopaedic surgeons of America, St. Louis, 1970, The C. V. Mosby Co.
16 Stevenson, J L.: What is orthopedic nursing? Am J Nurs 39:11-17, Jan 1939.
17 Watson-Jones, R.: Dame Agnes Hunt, J Bone Joint Surg [Br] 30:709-713, Nov 1948.
18 Wilson, A. B., Jr.: Limb prosthetics—1970, Artif Limbs 14:1-52, Spring 1970.
19 Wood, E. W.: The nursing care of orthopaedic surgical cases, Am J Nurs 2:425-429, Mar 1902.

Orthopedic nursing and the nursing process

20 Bailit, H., Lewis, J., Hochheiser, L., and Bush, N.: Assessing the quality of care, Nurs Outlook 23:153-159, Mar 1975.
21 Bloch, D.: Some crucial terms in nursing: what do they really mean? Nurs Outlook 22:689-694, Nov 1974.
22 Bower, F. L.: The process of planning nursing care, ed. 2, St. Louis, 1977, The C. V. Mosby Co.
23 Brown, S.: Orthopedic nursing action, ONA J 2:279-281, Nov 1975.
24 Carrieri, V. K., and Sitzman, J.: Components of the nursing process, Nurs Clin North Am 6:115-124, Mar 1971.
25 Daubenmire, M. J., and King, I. M.: Nursing process models: a systems approach, Nurs Outlook 21:512-517, Aug 1973.
26 Davis, A. I.: Measuring quality, Superv Nurse 8:17-22, 25-26, Feb 1977.
27 Lewis, L.: This I believe . . . about the nursing process—key to care, Nurs Outlook 16:26-29, May 1968.
28 Marriner, A.: The nursing process, St. Louis, 1975, The C. V. Mosby Co.
29 Nowlin, O. B.: Guidelines for pediatric-orthopedic nursing history, ONA J 2:119, May 1975.
30 Orthopedic Nurses' Association and American Nurses' Association Division on Medical-Surgical Nursing Practice: Standards of orthopedic nursing practice, Kansas City, Mo., 1975, American Nurses' Association.
31 Wiener, C. L.: Pain assessment on an orthopedic ward, Nurs Outlook 23:508-516, Aug 1975.
32 Yura, H., and Walsh, M. B.: The nursing process: assessing, planning, implementing, evaluating, ed. 2, New York, 1973, Appleton-Century-Crofts.
33 Zimmerman, D. S., and Gohrke, C.: The goal-directed nursing approach: it does work, Am J Nurs 70:306-310, Feb 1970.

Unit I
GENERAL CONSIDERATIONS IN ORTHOPEDIC NURSING

2 Structure and function of bone and joints

BONE

The sciences of biology, chemistry, physiology, and physics are interrelated in a molecular concept relating to function and structure. To study bone structure and function, one should examine whole bones and all structures attached to them (anatomy), the parts or types of tissue found in bone (histology), the cells that form these tissues (interrelated sciences), and the matrix material separating these cells (interrelated sciences).

Many consider bone to be an inactive mechanical framework, nearly inert. This is not the case, however. Bone is alive and a dynamic tissue in the body with a unique chemical and physical construction that serves important functions. Its amazing organization, from gross shape to molecular grouping, makes for tensile strength nearly as great as that of cast iron but with relatively little weight. In many respects bone is similar to living, reinforced concrete, with collagen fibers acting as tie rods and calcium salt forming the cement. Cellular components and a blood supply maintain this structure, and materials continually undergo alteration and replacement.

Long bones, such as the femur, contain four major types of connective tissue: fibrous, bone, cartilage, and blood-forming elements of marrow.

Functions

Bones perform the following important functions:

1 Provide a framework for the body
2 Serve as a storage site for minerals (calcium, phosphorus, magnesium) used by all body organs
3 Form a system of levers to help convert force generated by muscles into motion and locomotion
4 Protect internal organs (brain, heart, etc.)
5 Produce blood
6 Are capable of growth while continuing other functions

Bone growth—anatomic remodeling

A growing long bone consists of the following parts (Fig. 1):

1 Epiphysis—the secondary center of ossification of any bone (located at the ends of long bones)
2 Diaphysis—the shaft of a long bone
3 Metaphysis or epiphyseal plate—the growth zone between the epiphysis and the diaphysis

The two types of bone, intramembranous and endochondral (intracartilaginous), grow in the following manner.

Intramembranous bone (bone growth between membranes) generally forms flat bones such as those of the skull. Bone forms between two layers of fibrous connective tissue or periosteum through cellular secretion of collagen matrix that then mineralizes (Fig. 2). Appositional growth continues as new cells continue to lay down more of the mineralized matrix. At the same time, other specialized cells remodel bone by tearing it down in appropriate locations. This process allows growth yet maintains correct size and shape.

Endochondral bone (bone growth within cartilage) forms the long bones in the limbs, most tubular bones, and the spine. By the eighth week of embryonic life, cartilage models of most bones have formed, but they have not mineralized (ossified). Three different processes of ossification occur in this cartilage model:

1 A *primary center of ossification* develops in the central shaft region of the

cartilage model (Fig. 3). As blood vessels enter this region, carltiage is destroyed and replaced by mineralized bone matrix. As growth proceeds, this region of ossification enlarges toward the ends of the bone, accounting for most of the increase in bone length.

2 Bone increases in diameter as it lengthens. This growth in diameter, called *periosteal bone formation*, is identical to intramembranous ossification. New bone is formed by the periosteal covering along its shaft (Fig. 4).

3 Many bones have *secondary centers of ossification* that develop as blood vessels enter the cartilage model in regions separate from the primary center. The epiphysis or mineralized region at the ends of the growing long bone is a secondary center of ossification (Fig. 4).

In a long bone the secondary center of ossification or epiphysis is separated from the primary center by the epiphyseal plate. Cartilage cells of the epiphyseal plate are highly specialized and organized in rows. A bone lengthens as ossification occurs in and along these rows of cartilage with simultaneous replacement of this cartilage by cell divisions within the epiphyseal plate. When bone reaches its adult state and growth stops, the epiphyseal plate

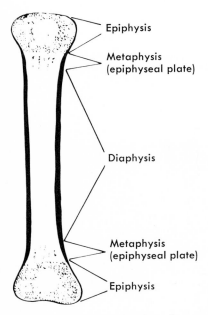

Fig. 1 Parts of a growing long bone.

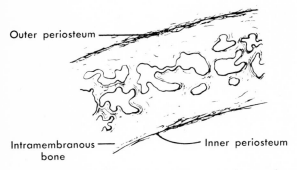

Fig. 2 Diagram showing the periosteal growth zones on the surfaces of a flat intramembranous bone. The central blood-filled cavities enlarge as the bone matures.

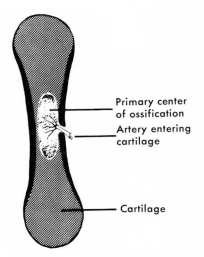

Fig. 3 Diagram showing cartilage model of a long bone. As the blood vessels enter the shaft (diaphyseal) region, cartilage is destroyed and replaced by bone.

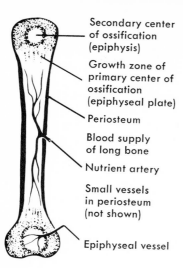

Secondary center of ossification (epiphysis)

Growth zone of primary center of ossification (epiphyseal plate)

Periosteum

Blood supply of long bone

Nutrient artery

Small vessels in periosteum (not shown)

Epiphyseal vessel

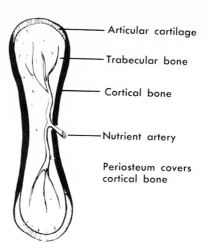

Articular cartilage

Trabecular bone

Cortical bone

Nutrient artery

Periosteum covers cortical bone

Fig. 4 Diagram illustrating the centers of ossification in an endochondral (intracartilaginous) bone (see text). Note that each region of ossification has a well-developed blood supply.

Fig. 5 Diagram of an adult endochondral bone in which the epiphyseal plate cartilage has been replaced by bone.

Fig. 6 Roentgenograms of a boy's foot at ages 8 months, **A**, 2½ years, **B**, and 13 years, **C**. At 8 months of age, only the primary centers of ossification are visible. At 2½ years of age, small epiphyseal centers are forming near the end of the bones. (In the foot, epiphyseal centers develop only at one end of the bones.) At 18 years of age, epiphyseal centers are well developed and about to fuse with the diaphysis.

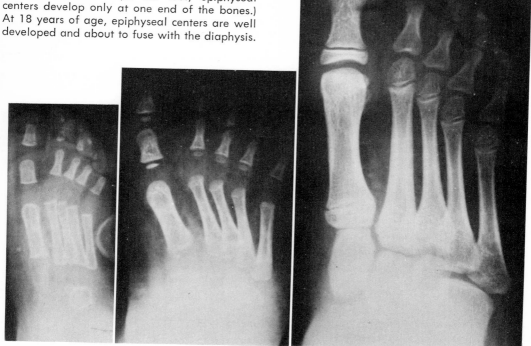

A   B   C

becomes completely resorbed and replaced by bone (Fig. 5).

The primary and secondary centers of ossification are seen in roentgenograms of endochondral bones (Fig. 6). Prior to ossification, the cartilage bone model is not visible. Then, as ossification progresses, the primary center develops and enlarges, followed by development of epiphyseal centers. These centers of ossification eventually fuse in the adult.

Bone turnover—histologic remodeling

Throughout life there is constant replacement of older bone elements. This takes place by the eating away (resorption) of bone in some areas together with the formation of new bone in other areas. This normally amounts to a state of constant remodeling in which the losses equal the gains, and the total amount is not changed. It is assumed that by this phenomenon the skeleton can respond to changes in strength requirements by redistribution of more bone in areas needed. It is also by alterations in the resorption and formation process that calcium can be replaced or stored according to the needs of the body.

Types of ossified connective tissue— bone. The dense region of the periphery of a bone, the cortex, is composed of very compact *cortical bone.* Bone in the central marrow space thins out to resemble a sponge and is called spongy, trabecular, or cancellous bone. The dense cortex gives bone its major strength. The arrangement of trabecular bone along lines of stress also adds considerable strength with very little addition of weight and allows room for blood-forming elements of the marrow.

At a cellular level there are two patterns of organization, the lamellar and the woven. Woven bone is initially laid down during growth or remodeling. It is disorganized and appears woven at the microscopic level—hence the term *woven bone.* A normal mature bone is highly organized into the basic pattern shown in Fig. 7. This architecture is described as being a *lamellar* pattern. In many pathologic conditions, and especially in fracture healing, large amounts of woven bone are produced.

Neurovascular supply. Bone, like any other living tissue, is supplied with blood and has an extensive vascular network. In

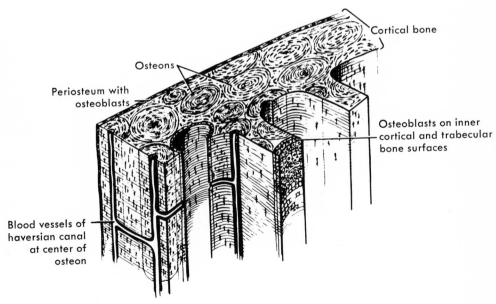

Fig. 7 Three-dimensional diagram illustrating both the longitudinal and cross sections of various components in the shaft (diaphysis) of a long bone. Osteons run lengthwise in the bone along lines of stress and are the basic structure of both the cortex and the central trabeculae. Osteons are formed around central canals that offer a supply of nutrients to all parts of the bone.

fact, about 8% of the blood in each heart-beat goes to supply bone. Blood vessels in the periosteum penetrate the bone and supply the outer one-third of the cortex. Nutrient arteries course through the bone cortex to supply the bone marrow, trabecular bone, and inner two-thirds of the cortex. Epiphyseal centers are supplied with blood via epiphyseal vessels.

Nerves have been observed along the course of these vessels and even within the microscopic blood vascular canals (haversian canals) within cortical and trabecular bone. Exact function of these small nerves is not known. Studies suggest that they transmit deep bone pain, regulate blood flow, regulate growth, and control bone repair.

Structural unit of bone—the osteon. The basic structural unit of bone is called an *osteon.* An osteon includes a central neurovascular supply (the haversian canal) and the tube of cells and bone matrix surrounding this central canal (Fig. 7). The osteons, which are the basic structure in trabecular and cortical lamellar bone, line up along the lines of force through the bone. The diameter of any one osteon is limited by the distance bone cells can live away from their central blood supply, up to about twenty cell layers. Length is not critical, and the osteons are very often very long. It is the parallel arrangement of many osteons—like a bundle of sticks—that gives bone its great strength at the cellular level.

Bone cells. Cells of bone, like those of all living tissues, have three basic functions:

1 Reproduction—cells divide, forming new cells.
2 Transformation of energy—bone cells take nutrients and oxygen supplied by the blood and convert them to substances the cell can use for energy.
3 Production of new substances—the new substances are usually proteins, most significantly collagen, the tie rod of the bone matrix.

Three main types of bone cells are osteoblasts, osteocytes, and osteoclasts.

Osteoblasts are bone-forming cells that cover all growing surface of bone and initially lay down woven bone. These cells originate from undifferentiated cells located near blood vessels, then begin to form bone, and eventually are surrounded by bone.

An *osteocyte* is an osteoblast that has become completely surrounded by bone matrix. Osteocytes are the mature bone cells that maintain living bone but do not form new bone.

Cells that tear down bone are called *osteoclasts.* These cells form by the fusion of osteoblasts or osteocytes into multinucleated giant cells. These giant cells usually contain about 20 nuclei, but 150 or more have been found in a single osteoclast. An osteocyte itself may be capable of bone destruction, which makes it in essence a single-celled osteoclast. The mechanisms by which these cells destroy bone are not clear.

Bone matrix and bone mineral. Matrix material surrounding osteocytes contains organic material (protein, carbohydrate, and small amounts of fat) and minerals (calcium salt crystals).

Organic bone matrix. With mineral removed, 90% of bone matrix consists of fibrous collagen proteins. Collagen is the same protein found in all fibrous connective tissue and the supporting structure on which the calcium salt crystals form. Vitamin C has an important role in collagen formation. The role of carbohydrate and fat in bone matrix is not clear, but they may play some role in the mineralization process.

Bone mineral. Blood calcium concentration remains one of the most critically regulated factors in the human body. This vitally important chemical regulates nerve impulses, muscle contractions, including heart muscle, and transport of materials into and out of all cells. The control of the blood calcium level is vital for life itself. This calcium control depends on at least three factors:

1 *Bone matrix,* acting as a reservoir for calcium (99% of total body calcium is stored as bone)
2 *Hormones,* especially parathyroid hormone, which carefully control blood calcium levels
3 *Vitamins,* especially vitamins D, C, and A, which promote absorption of calcium from the intestine and help regulate bone matrix mineralization

The higher magnification obtained with the electron microscope has added greatly to the study of bone. The structures within each cell, the formation of collagen fibers, and the laying down of needlelike calcium salt crystals around collagen fibers have been studied. Research into the integration of bone metabolism with molecular structure has just begun and will hopefully clarify more aspects of normal bone function and structure.

Bone metabolism

Metabolic bone disease describes any general disease state that stems from a disturbance of the body's normal metabolism and affects the skeleton. Affected bone often represents a response to an altered calcium metabolism. The persistent skeletal involvement seen in abnormal states of calcium balance illustrates its importance in maintaining proper amounts of this mineral in the bloodstream.

Bone contains 99% of all the body calcium. Together with structural support, its most important function is to serve as a calcium reservoir for the bloodstream.

When calcium is needed to sustain life, bone and the small intestinal tract increase or decrease their supply while the kidney and the large bowel control the excretion. Calcium is also present in perspiration, but its contribution to the total excretion picture and the mechanism of its control are not yet known.

The proper supply of calcium and phosphorus is vital to every tissue in the body. Calcium is involved in most cellular systems; i.e., muscle contraction, nerve conduction, blood clotting, etc. Phosphorus has multiple roles in metabolism). Paramount is its integral role in energy-producing compounds (i.e., adenosine triphosphate and adenosine diphosphate). This complex system, designed to maintain a constant blood level of these divalent ions, appears to be marginally capable of passively sustaining itself as long as no outside influence attempts to upset its balance. Therefore, traffic-controlling features are

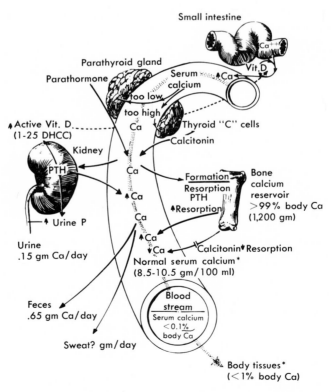

Fig. 8 Diagram of calcium homeostasis. The control features maintain the proper serum calcium needed for the body tissues. A low serum calcium stimulates absorption of calcium from the intestine, retention of calcium by the kidney, and release of calcium from the bone. A high serum calcium stimulates release of calcitonin, which inhibits calcium resorption from the bone.

essential to the system (Fig. 8). These features are capable of opening and shutting the appropriate flood gates in a homeostatic response to its major and minor needs. The index of these features is lengthy and their execution complex incompletely understood. Three of the more important ones will be discussed.

Parathyroid hormone

The parathyroid gland, which produces parathyroid hormone, is located in and around the thyroid gland and is probably the main traffic controller for calcium metabolism. It monitors the calcium content of the bloodstream by constantly testing for its ionized form (free Ca^{++}). When the serum level is too low, it releases stored parathormone (PTH) and manufactures more to replace the original supply. Like most hormones, PTH is carried to different sites via the bloodstream. It operates to increase the blood calcium levels. In the intestine, parathormone interacts with vitamin D to increase the absorption of calcium by stimulating what is, in effect, a biologic pump mechanism.

In the bone, its main affect is a release of the mineral. This is accomplished through (1) stimulation of the cells (osteoclasts and osteocytes) to eat away or dissolve the bone and (2) some similar but direct resorptive chemical effect. Interestingly, the rate of new bone formation is also moderately increased. In the kidney, PTH creates an increased excretion of phosphorus into the urine and a retention of calcium in the blood. Also reported is a conversion of vitamin D to its most active form by this hormone. This may account for the intestinal action of PTH. In the laboratory, several factors have been found to increase or decrease the bone's response to parathormone. These include oxygen, the degree of acidity, vitamin C, vitamin D, fluoride, heparin, etc. However, the presence of PTH is necessary for any of these to produce an effect.

Calcitonin

In the same general location near the thyroid gland are cells that produce another hormone, calcitonin. This hormone is released in response to high serum calcium levels (hypercalcemia). It appears to act chiefly on bone, causing a cessation of bone resorption and an abrupt drop in the serum calcium concentration.

Vitamin D

Vitamins are organic substances essential to the body's normal metabolism, which must be supplied by diet. Although vitamin D is called a vitamin, it behaves more like a hormone. (A hormone is a chemical substance formed by a gland or organ in one part of the body and carried through the bloodstream to another part of the body which it stimulates to functional activity.) Vitamin D is synthesized from a cholesterol compound in the skin in the presence of sunlight. It is then transported to the intestines and bone where it has a specific action. The original label *vitamin D* stemmed from the fact that most of this compound can be and is supplied through the diet, either from plant food stuffs or meat. Initial forms either manufactured in the skin or absorbed through the intestine can be converted by the liver or kidney into metabolites significantly more potent in stimulating their target organs. The most active vitamin D metabolite (1-25 dihydrochlecalciferol or 1-25 DHCC) is produced in the kidney in the presence of parathyroid hormone. This compound is much more potent than vitamin D, which is produced by the skin. Vitamin D metabolites act principally on the intestine, and their role is one of increased calcium absorption. This appears to be by activation of a biologic "pump," which responds to (1) a change in the resistance of the intestinal cell wall to the flow of calcium ions and (2) the production of the calcium transport protein that actively guides the mineral across the intestinal cell into the bloodstream.

In bone, the effect of vitamin D is problematic. Certainly, in the laboratory its action is similar to parathyroid hormone in that it mobilizes more mineral for the bloodstream. Since this requires the presence of PTH, it may be simply enhancement of the latter's effectiveness.

Common laboratory tests

Blood tests. Blood tests for mineral metabolism include serum calcium, serum phosphorus, and serum alkaline phosphatase determinations.

Serum calcium. Determination of the

serum calcium values is a standard and valuable test. Often, disease states can be placed in a broad range or category on the basis of these results alone. The range of normal values must be known for each laboratory but usually lies somewhere between 8.5 and 10.5 mg calcium per each 100 ml of serum. Newer methods, such as atomic absorption spectroscopy (ATM; ABS), now used in many places, offer greater precision and a smaller range of normal values. All of these values measure the *total* calcium concentration. However, about 50% of the total calcium in the blood is bound to protein molecules and not readily available for use. The parathyroid gland apparently responds to the concentration of ionized or free calcium. Presently this measurement is done in research laboratories along with the total calcium values. A low albumin concentration tends to give a false low total calcium value. Thus, the protein content should be known when a specimen is sent for calcium analysis.

Blood content values fluctuate rapidly, and repeated tests may be needed to determine normal trends. Because of the powerful homeostatic mechanisms described previously, serum calcium values can be normal despite the presence of active metabolic bone disease. For example, serum calcium may be normal in a child with bowed legs and obvious rickets caused by a diet poor in calcium or vitamin D. This situation can exist because of the sacrifice the skeleton is making to maintain the proper supply to the rest of the body. High calcium levels may be found in hyperparathyroidism, vitamin D overdose, terminal cancer patients, hyperthyroidism, and patients on prolonged bed rest. Low calcium values may be seen in rickets and hypoparathyroidism.

Serum phosphorus. Phosphorus values change in a predictable pattern throughout each day. Hence, blood for the serum phosphorus test should be drawn about the same time every day. The time before breakfast is acceptable because food intake can falsely elevate this value. The normal range must be known for each hospital, but averages are 2.5-4.5 mg for each 100 ml. High phosphorus values can occur along with low calcium levels in kidney failure

and hypoparathyroidism. High phosphorus and calcium levels are seen in normal patients on bed rest. Low values are commonly seen in rickets, salt-losing kidney conditions (renal tubular defects), and malabsorption syndromes from intestinal disease or after surgical removal of the upper portion of the intestinal tract. Hyperparathyroidism is suspected when a calcium rise accompanies a phosphorus decline.

Serum alkaline phosphatase. Serum alkaline phosphatase is an enzyme produced in the bone, liver, and intestine. The contribution of each can be determined if necessary. The value is usually reported as the total and in the absence of active liver disease is felt to represent some aspect of active new bone formation. Testing methods and resulting values vary considerably. Most commonly used are Bodansky (2-4.5 units), King-Armstrong (5-10 units), and Bessey-Lowry-Brock (30-85 units). These values tend to become higher during fracture healing and during normal active growth periods. The maximal normal value is reached at infancy and rises again at the age of 16 or 17 years. High values (hyperphosphatasia) indicate that a skeletal disorder is present. The highest value is seen in Paget's disease (200-3,000 IU), and this test can be used as a sign of disease activity. Situations causing excessive parathyroid hormone activity or osteomalacia (rickets) are also accompanied by high alkaline phosphatase levels. Since active liver disease can markedly alter this test, other liver function tests should be obtained when a high value is present. Low levels are seen in a rare enzyme deficiency state named hypophosphatasia. The patients have symptoms similar to rickets but low alkaline phosphatase levels and poor ability to heal their fractures.

Serum parathyroid hormone. A number of medical centers are now equipped to directly evaluate the blood concentrations of parathormone. This is done by assay tests in which antibodies are collected from laboratory animals previously injected with an extract of the human hormone. This antiparathyroid hormone serum is then labeled with an isotope for easy detection and reacted with the blood of the patient. This test will be used routinely as it becomes standardized and available.

Urine tests. Urine tests include urine calcium and urine phosphorus determinations.

Urine calcium. Collection of urine for calcium is often used for diagnosis, imbalance studies, and as a monitor of treatment programs. It is usually collected for a twenty-four hour period to avoid any misleading momentary fluctuations. All else being equal, the amount of calcium released in the urine reflects the concentration in the bloodstream. Thus, changes in oral intake, vitamin D level, parathormone levels etc. will be reflected in this test. Since renal disease will decrease the ability to excrete calcium, initial kidney function tests are necessary; e.g., creatinine clearance.

Urine phosphorus. Excretion of phosphorus remains a constant proportion (about 70%) of the dietary intake regardless of a disease state. It is of value to obtain this test for reflection of dietary intake and because the urine calcium is inversely related to the phosphorus content.

Radiographic evaluation

Many metabolic disease states have typical roentgenographic patterns that help to identify them. Roentgenographic examination of patients receiving therapy often shows recognizable indications of success or failure. Quantitative density methods are also widely used for sensitively monitoring the effects of treatment.

Bone biopsy

Often the initial diagnosis of bone disease is best made by analysis of the bone itself. Subsequently, the success or failure of treatment in many bone diseases can be most accurately followed by repeating the biopsy after the establishment of a treatment program for six to twelve months. Research techniques in which bone is studied without its being decalcified will allow quantitation of the state of bone turnover. These techniques are becoming widely used because they allow a very sensitive assessment of response to therapy.

Metabolic bone diseases
Rickets

Rickets is a disease of childhood causing soft, deformed bones as a result of a deficiency of vitamin D. Microscopically,

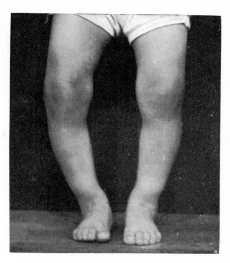

Fig. 9 Bowlegs (genu varum) resulting from active rickets. If the rickets is brought under control, the bowlegs will correct themselves during further growth.

wide areas of unmineralized bone indicate a lack of adequate calcium content. Clinically, there is marked bowing of the legs (Fig. 9) and arms, along with muscle weakness and bone tenderness. Roentgenograms classically display wide growth plates; long bones flare at the ends. Two basic classes of rickets can be distinguished according to their response to vitamin D replacement: nutritional rickets and resistant rickets.

Nutritional rickets. Nutritional rickets is a result of an actual deficiency state, either from poor diet or lack of sunlight. It is no longer common in the United States because milk and food are fortified with vitamin D. The minimum daily vitamin D requirement is about 400 IU.

Resistant rickets. Resistant rickets is not corrected with replacement of a normal intake of vitamin D and may even require from fifty to a thousand times this dose for an effect. Various causes can produce resistant rickets, the most common including hereditary hypophosphatemia, kidney salt-wasting defects, and malabsorption syndromes of childhood (Fig. 10).

Hereditary hypophosphatemic rickets. In hereditary hypophosphatemic rickets, the most common form in the United States today, there is a persistently low serum phosphorus level. Genetically, the disease

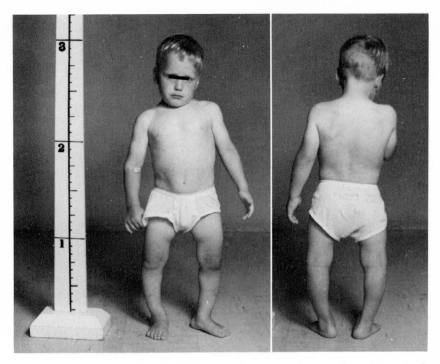

Fig. 10 Vitamin D—resistant rickets. The patient is 5 years of age, of average weight, and mildly dwarfed in height and shows the bowleg deformities that improve with proper high dosage of vitamin D intake.

is transmitted as a sex-linked dominant trait. Affected women transmit the trait to one-half their sons and/or daughters. Affected men transmit it to all their daughters but none of their sons. The serum calcium level is usually normal, and the alkaline phosphatase level is high. Urine calcium and calcium balance studies are usually below normal. Urine phosphorus level is often higher than normal. The actual metabolic defect is not yet known. Treatment may be successful with near-toxic levels of vitamin D.

Renal tubular rickets. Many individual salt-wasting kidney defects produce renal tubular rickets that is also "resistant" to vitamin D and mineral replacement.

Malabsorption syndromes. Studies in England show that many patients with rickets have intestinal diseases (e.g., celiac disease) in which absorption of dietary vitamin D is poor.

Osteomalacia

Osteomalacia is essentially the adult corollary to rickets in a child. The differ-

ence is that the mechanisms of bone growth are no longer vulnerable and only bone turnover mechanisms are affected. Thus, shortness of stature and marked bowing of extremities are not found in osteomalacia. The same factors that cause rickets are known to cause osteomalacia. Patients with colitis, postgastrectomy syndromes, cirrhosis, etc., as well as vegetarians and patients taking anticonvulsive drugs, develop osteomalacia. Usually there is a history of bone or spinal pain from crush fractures. The radiographic changes and clinical symptoms are often difficult to distinguish from osteoporosis. Serum calcium, urine calcium, and serum phosphorus values may be slightly lower than normal.

Azotemic renal osteodystrophy

Most patients with uremia from chronic kidney failure also have distinct bone pathology. The skeletal changes manifest varying combinations of two pathologic processes: (1) inadequate mineralization (i.e., rickets or osteomalacia) and (2) hyperparathyroidism. As the renal disease

progresses, the bone changes become increasingly severe and lead to more frequent orthopedic consultations. Renal dialysis causes further deterioration, but successful renal transplant corrects the bone problems. The serum phosphorus and urea nitrogen levels are usually very high in this category. The total calcium and ionized calcium values are usually low. Parathyroid hormone levels are extremely high. Treatment modalities include correction of calcium balance, vitamin D supplements, correction of acid-base balance, and sometimes parathyroidectomy. The only absolute way to arrest and reverse the skeletal deterioration is by successful renal transplantation.

Hyperparathyroidism

Excessive production of parathyroid hormone (PTH) eventually causes predictable effects on the entire body. The high serum calcium levels cause soft tissue calcifications, alterations in muscle contractility, renal stones, and marked bone destruction. The excessive resorption of the skeleton is referred to as osteitis fibrosa. Fractures are frequent and can result in deformities. Roentgenographic examination reveals a general decrease in bone mass with frequent cystic areas notable. Under the microscope, marked resorptive activity is obvious. There are three distinct forms of parathyroid hyperactivity: primary, secondary, and tertiary.

Primary hyperparathyroidism. Primary hyperparathyroidism is usually associated with a tumor (adenoma) that produces parathyroid hormone. Surgery is required to correct the problem.

Secondary hyperparathyroidism. A chronic state of inadequate serum calcium levels can cause an enlargement of the gland and an abnormally high production of parathyroid hormone. The condition is encountered most often in patients with intestinal malabsorption and chronic renal failure. Its treatment involves correction of the low calcium levels, if possible.

Tertiary hyperparathyroidism. The term tertiary hyperparathyroidism refers to the rare situation in which a patient with a long-standing secondary hyperparathyroidism develops a gland that appears to "run wild." The clinical picture is then similar to that of primary hyperparathyroidism with hypercalcemia and high levels of circulating parathyroid hormone. This condition may be caused by an adenoma or an overproduction of normal-appearing glandular tissue. Again, the treatment is surgical removal.

Paget's disease (osteitis deformans)

Paget's disease is a disease of the bone in which there is overactivity of osteoblasts and osteoclasts, building and destroying bone in an unaltered chemical pattern. High levels of phosphatase occur and are an index to the rapidity and amount of new bone being formed. The cause of this disease is entirely unknown, and the treatment is limited to the correction of deformities that occur. Persons afflicted are usually past middle age, and the bones involved may be few or many.

The bones become broader and weaker than normal and are easily fractured. The fractures heal readily. In the generalized form of the disease, the patient becomes shorter and, because the skull expands, may require a larger hat. In rare instances, the involved bone may show malignant changes.

Osteoporosis

Osteoporosis (porous bone) is presently defined as a clinical condition in which there is a decrease in the total amount of bone to the point that fractures occur with minor trauma. As opposed to osteomalacia, the bone in this instance appears normal under the microscope and is well mineralized, but there is simply not enough of it. Osteoporosis is a very common end result of many different causes.

Primary osteoporosis. As the term primary indicates, in this type of osteoporosis there is no identifiable cause. Senile osteoporosis is the most common type. Many of the patients are postmenopausal women (over 50 years old) or even older men. They are usually seen because of back pain that is out of proportion to any history of trauma. If there have been old vertebral body crush fractures, loss of height and a round back posture are detected. Whereas a moderate loss of bone mass is normal with aging, persons with osteoporosis show a

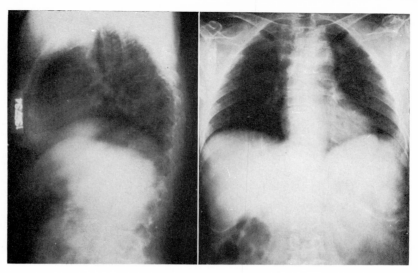

Fig. 11 Osteoporosis, a metabolic disorder of older persons (especially women) in which calcium in the bone is depleted and the bone matrix fails to produce replacement bone, resulting in a weakening of the involved structure.

much greater loss than others of the same age. As a result, they have a twofold chance of incurring fractures of the wrist, hip, humerus, and vertebral body (usually thoracic spine). As many as 70% of the patients with hip fractures are diagnosed as having osteoporosis. Laboratory values are usually normal. Roentgenograms reveal a diffuse wash-out of bone (radiolucency) and often a loss of trabecular patterns and thin cortices (Fig. 11). A bone biopsy reveals thin and porous but otherwise normal-appearing bone. By measurement, the osteoclastic resorption is often slightly increased. No light has yet been shed on the cause, but many factors are suspected, such as poor diet, estrogen deficiency, and lack of exercise. No adequate prevention or treatment is yet proved. Presently it is common to attempt improvement in the protein, calcium, and vitamin D intake. Also, an exercise program is frequently prescribed. Estrogen replacement and high fluoride and calcium doses may have some merit. Back pain and fractures are treated as discussed in subsequent chapters.

Secondary osteoporosis. In secondary osteoporosis there is an identifiable cause of the condition. The list of causes is long, but only three will be noted here: nutritional, endocrine, and disuse.

Nutritional osteoporosis. Various abnormal nutritional states are known to cause osteoporosis, such as vitamin C deficiency (scurvy), milk malabsorption syndromes (lactose intolerance and others), acid diets, and calcium deficient diets.

Endocrine osteoporosis. Abnormal function of many different endocrine glands—e.g., hyperthyroidism, hyperparathyroidism (mild), Cushing's syndrome, acromegaly, and hypogonadism—will produce an osteoporosis.

Disuse osteoporosis. Bed rest and inactivity are well-known causes of osteoporosis. Lack of gravity or normal stresses and strains appears to be the main factor here since astronauts have developed the same problems despite their exercise programs while in space. On the other hand, stressing a bone by exercise is known to increase the bone mass and strengthen it.

Nursing implications. The patient who has been inactive or confined to bed rest for an extended period of time may have very fragile bones because of the demineralization process resulting from disuse. Fractures of the long bones, vertebral bodies, or pelvis may occur with little or no trauma. Turning in bed may be sufficient stress to cause a fracture. Usually the patient experiences pain, and the "snap" may be audible. However, in some instances, because of pain already present or because

of absence of normal sensation, the patient is not aware of any increased pain or discomfort. The fractures become apparent because of a deformed position of the extremity. Needless to say, extreme care and gentleness should be exercised when turning or ambulating this type of patient.

When collapse of the vertebral bodies occurs, an increase in the anteroposterior curves of the spine develop. This is particularly apparent in the thoracic region, and the result is a rounded back or kyphosis. With compression fracture of the vertebrae, the patient experiences severe back pain. The altered alignment of the spine places strain on the supporting ligaments and muscles and can cause pressure on nerve roots. The patient is uncomfortable when standing or walking and consequently is inclined to spend more time in the horizontal position, thus becoming less active. This, in turn, increases disuse demineralization of bone.

To overcome osteoporosis, new bone formation must exceed the process of bone resorption. Treatment consists of exercise, frequent rest periods, and avoidance of severe fatigue. For rest periods and sleep, the patients should have a firm supporting mattress. Exercise in the form of walking is encouraged. Wearing a spinal support such as a corset or light brace when in the upright position usually helps to decrease the back discomfort. The support serves to immobilize and protect the spine, enabling the patient to be up and about safely. It also helps the patient to use correct body mechanics—e.g., flexing the knees as opposed to rounding the back when stooping. Incorrect methods of stooping or sitting cause increased pain and fatigue in the back area. In addition, the patient should be cautioned to avoid lifting or engaging in activities that cause twisting of the spine. Analgesics and muscle relaxants are frequently prescribed, and attention to dietary intake to ensure adequate intake of protein, vitamin D, and calcium is an essential part of the treatment. Estrogen therapy tends to slow the process of osteoporosis.

Extensive laboratory studies are made on patients with osteoporosis. Careful instruction of nursing personnel is necessary to prevent loss of specimens and to ensure collection of specimens at specified times.

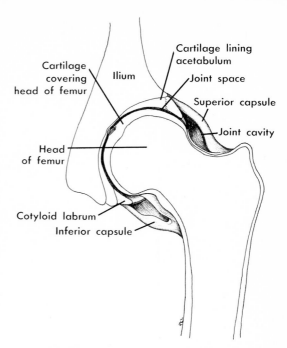

Fig. 12 Anterior view of the hip joint.

JOINTS
Anatomy and function

The bony skeleton of the body is rigid and supports all body organs in the upright position. If the bones were rigidly connected, change from one position to another would not be possible. However, nature has endowed the body with hinges between bones to allow for changes in position. These hinges are called joints, and all joints have certain properties in common: (1) a certain flexibility or range in which the hinge can open and close, (2) stability furnished by ligaments that permit the joint to move in one plane while movement in another plane is prevented, and (3) muscles that control the movements of the joint.

Joints are classified by the functions each will perform. The hip joint is a ball-and-socket type that permits motion ·in any direction and is stable since the socket (acetabulum) plus the cotyloid labrum (fibrocartilaginous thickening of the capsule) envelop nearly the entire head of the femur (Fig. 12). The shoulder joint also is classified as a ball-and-socket type; however, the socket (glenoid) is shallow so that stability must be provided by the cap-

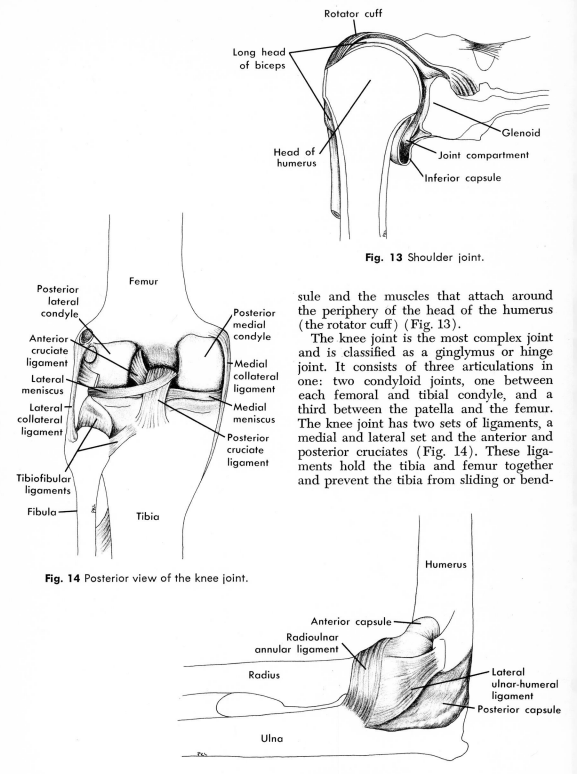

Fig. 13 Shoulder joint.

Fig. 14 Posterior view of the knee joint.

sule and the muscles that attach around the periphery of the head of the humerus (the rotator cuff) (Fig. 13).

The knee joint is the most complex joint and is classified as a ginglymus or hinge joint. It consists of three articulations in one: two condyloid joints, one between each femoral and tibial condyle, and a third between the patella and the femur. The knee joint has two sets of ligaments, a medial and lateral set and the anterior and posterior cruciates (Fig. 14). These ligaments hold the tibia and femur together and prevent the tibia from sliding or bend-

Fig. 15 Elbow joint.

ing sideward (medial and lateral collaterals) and prevent the femur from sliding backward or forward on the tibia (cruciates) while the knee moves through a range of flexion.

The elbow joint is a ginglymus or hinge joint where motion occurs between the humerus and ulna in flexion and extension and between the radial head and outer condyle of the humerus (capitellum) to provide rotation of the forearm in pronation and supination (Fig. 15). Stability between the ulna and humerus is provided by the ulnar collateral ligament, and the radial head is stabilized to the humerus, as well as to the ulna, by the radial collateral and annular ligaments, whose fibers meld into a single structure.

The wrist joint is a condyloid articulation, which means that it is formed by many parts. The major parts are the distal end of the radius and undersurface of the articular disk and the navicular, lunate, and triangular bones (Fig. 16). These articula-

tions are stabilized by the volar and dorsal radiocarpal ligaments and by the ulnar and radial collateral ligaments.

The ankle joint is a ginglymus or hinge joint. The upper surface of the astragalus fits into an inverted U slot in the lower tibia where the sides of the U form the malleoli. The medial malleolus is part of the tibia, the lateral malleolus is part of the fibula, and both malleoli provide an anchor post for the ligaments that stabilize the ankle. The lateral ligament has three separate branches that prevent the astragalus from displacing forward, backward, or medialward, yet permits motion in dorsiflexion and plantar flexion (Fig. 17).

The spine is a series of articulations (amphiarthrodial discs) between the bodies of vertebrae and a series of diarthrodial joints (facets) between vertebral arches. There are twenty-four vertebral arches: seven cervical, twelve thoracic, five lumbar. The fifth lumbar segment articulates with and rests on the sacrum. The sacrum is wedge-shaped and is supported by the iliac wings of the pelvis through the sacroiliac joints strongly supported by ligaments.

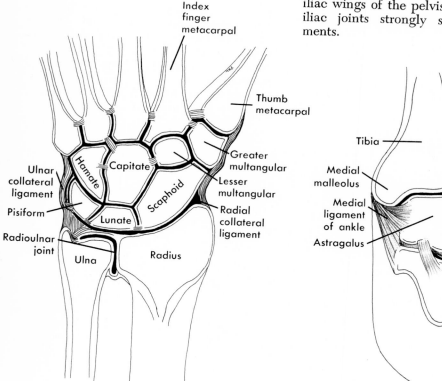

Fig. 16 Wrist joint.

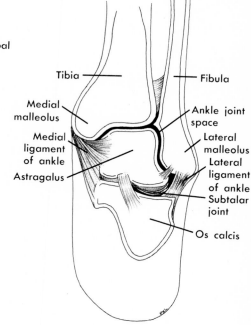

Fig. 17 Ankle joint. Section through midjoint viewed from the rear.

The spine is like a flexible pole rising upward from the pelvis with mild normal curves wherein the lumbar segment has a forward convexity (lordosis), the dorsal segment a backward convexity (kyphosis), and the cervical segment a forward convexity (lordosis). The amount of backward curve is equal to the amount of forward curve so the spine is on balance over the center of gravity, which is just in front of the second sacral segment. Each vertebral segment rests on the segment below, so the entire spinal column can be likened to a series of blocks placed one upon the other with a disk in between (Fig. 18). The stability of each segment is dependent on the intervertebral disk. The disk is composed of a nucleus and an annulus. The nucleus is the center composed of complex mucopolysaccharides that retain water to produce an intradiskal tension or pressure. The nucleus is contained by the annulus, which is composed of fibrocartilaginous tissue arranged much like the elastic wrappings around the center fluid of a golf ball. The annulus is further reinforced by the circumferential longitudinal ligaments that attach to each vertebral body the entire length of the spine. There are also strong ligaments posteriorly between the spinous tips that limit forward flexion between segments and a strong ligament from the pos-

terior arch (lamina) of one segment to the next called ligamentum flavum.

Each vertebral segment has a pair of small joints called facets that articulate with a counterpart facet on the segments above and below. These facets act to guide vertebral column motion and direct it to forward, backward, and lateral bending but block all but a few degrees of rotation.

In the upper cervical spine, the facets come to lie in a more horizontal plane, which permits considerable rotation of the head on the trunk as opposed to the limited rotation in the thoracic and lumbar spine.

The hand is the most versatile member of the body in the matter of providing motion. The major function is grasp; however, grasp must accommodate the many sizes and shapes of objects to be grasped. Fingertip apposition called pinch permits delicate functions such as picking up small objects. Independent function of each digit permits accomplishment of intricate functions such as fingering a musical instrument or a typewriter. The arrangement of the joints of the hand and fingers allows for the versatility of functions when coupled with complex arrangement of muscles available to control the movement of the joints.

The wrist joint (carpal joints) is best described as a compound joint that allows

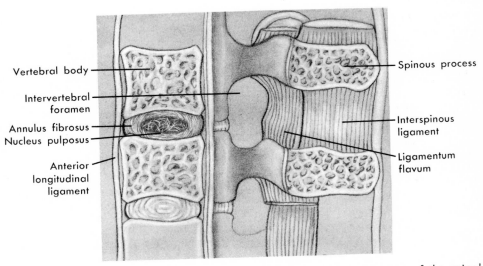

Fig. 18 Median section through two vertebrae illustrating various structures of the spinal column.

radial abduction (Fig. 19), ulnar abduction (Fig. 20), volar (palmar) flexion, and dorsiflexion. The stability is provided by long and short ligaments on the volar and dorsal aspects that essentially connect each of the seven carpal bones to each other and to the radius and to the metacarpals. In any motion, each of the seven bones moves slightly in relation to its neighbor so that the motion is really circumductory (makes a circle similar to a ball-and-socket joint) but is more stable in the process.

The base of the thumb is a saddle joint protected by thickenings in the capsule that serve as ligaments. The short muscles of the thumb (thenar muscle group) aid in the stability of the joint. This joint by its shape allows limited flexion and extension, limited abduction and adduction, and some rotation to allow the tip of the thumb to touch the tip of the little finger (this action is referred to as opponens) (Fig. 55).

The metacarpal phalangeal joints (commonly called knuckles) are condyloid joints. Each joint has a volar and two col-

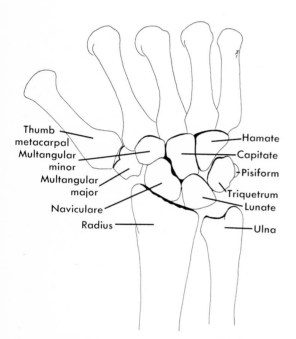

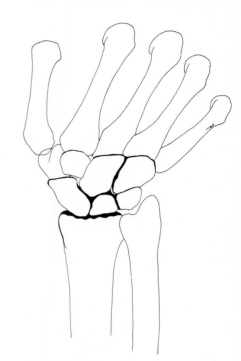

Fig. 19 Hand in radial deviation. Note shift of each carpal bone in relation to ulnar deviation.

Fig. 20 Hand in ulnar deviation. Motion takes place through the carpal joints.

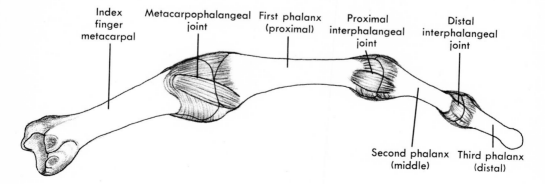

Fig. 21 Arrangement of bones in any finger except thumb.

lateral ligaments that stabilize the joint and permit only flexion from the normal extended position. In the extended position, some abduction and adduction are possible; however, these side-to-side motions are prevented by the collateral ligament that tightens as the joint is flexed.

The interphalangeal joints, two in each finger and one in the thumb, are hinge joints with ligaments similar to those of the metacarpal phalangeal joints except no lateral motion is permitted at any time (Fig. 21).

Structure of movable joints

All movable joints are structured to provide cartilaginous articulating surfaces, enclosed by a joint capsule and a synovial lining to provide joint fluid.

The joint cartilage (hyaline cartilage) covers that portion of each bone end that glides, rotates, or moves in angular motion while in contact with its counterpart. The thickness of the cartilage cap varies with age, being thicker in the young. The deeper layer of cartilage cells proliferates to keep pace with the death of the cells near the frictional surface of the joint cartilage (Fig. 12). However, in disease of the cartilage, as in degenerative arthritis, the cartilage loses its capacity to regenerate and the joint space becomes narrowed (Fig. 376). Hyaline cartilage cannot regenerate once the deeper cells have been destroyed, but repair can occur in the form of fibrocartilage, which does not have the ability to absorb the stress forces compared with hyaline cartilage.

Each joint has a capsule which is a fibroelastic tissue that envelops or encloses the joint (Fig. 13). The capsule may assist the ligaments to stabilize the joint. The intra-articular surface of the capsule is lined by synovium, a membrane that contains secretory and scavenger cells. The synovium is essential to provide nutrients that sustain the superficial layers of cartilage cells and to produce mucin, which is a protein compound that lubricates the joint cartilage. With proper lubrication, the cartilaginous joint surfaces are many times more slippery than ice, which nearly eliminates the friction factor of one joint surface rubbing on the other. The joint fluid covers the cartilaginous joint surfaces by means of a thin film, and movement of the joint acts as a pump to circulate the thin film of fluid. Joint fluid exchange is prevented by immobilization, thus preventing proper lubrication and also interfering with joint cartilage nutrition.

The synovium has another function—that of protecting the joint against invaders such as infection, disease, or injury. The cells of the synovium can produce antibodies, while other cells can phagocytize debris. In either case, the synovium simultaneously pours out excessive joint fluid that distends the capsule and is known as joint effusion.

A sample of the fluid taken by aspiration can yield important diagnostic information. In infection, the fluid will be turbid and carry a very high white blood cell count (up to 250,000 cells/mm). The sugar level will be low compared with blood sugar levels. The fluid contains organisms that can be identified by culture. In rheumatoid arthritis, there will be a similar high cell count but a normal sugar level and no organisms on culture. In effusion that follows injury, the aspiration may indicate hemorrhage into the joint from damaged intra-articular structures. Distention of the capsule from effusion can be painful, and relief can be obtained by placing the joint in the position that affords the most relaxation of the capsule. Most patients will already have found the most comfortable position, which usually is a mild flexion of the joint involved.

The synovium is richly endowed with thin-walled blood vessels and acts as a control membrane to permit nutrients to pass from the bloodstream into the joint fluid. In addition to the essential proteins and glucose, it permits the passage of antibiotics and other drugs into the joint fluid at nearly the same concentration as in the bloodstream.

Whenever the synovium reacts to disease or infection, it has the capacity to hypertrophy (increase in number and length of surface villi), which gives it much more surface area in contact with increased blood flow (hyperemia); this inflammatory response is known as synovitis and usually is accompanied by an increase in joint fluid (effusion).

3 Biomechanics for nursing

The application of mechanical principles to the living human body is referred to as biomechanics. The subject of mechanics deals with forces acting on bodies and the the result of these forces in terms of equilibrium and movement. The human body at rest represents equilibrium, whereas the body at work represents movement. In both instances there are forces acting from within (internal) and forces acting from without (external). An understanding of the forces and how the human body translates them into rest or work is essential in orthopedics, since an improper body response may be responsible for postural defects, painful strains, limps, and other impairments of the musculoskeletal system.

In biomechanics, equilibrium and motion are so closely interrelated that the principles of each will be pointed out as the occasion demands. Mechanics applied to the human body is divided into two main parts: (1) static, which is concerned with the body in balance or erect posture, and (2) dynamic, which is concerned with the body in motion.

STATIC BODY MECHANICS
Erect posture

Standing posture is the ability of the body to remain erect and to maintain this attitude by resisting outside forces with the least amount of energy. The anatomic variations from one individual to another are factors that account for the great differences in postural attitudes that can be observed in any queue at a box office. Postures may be described as erect, good, slouchy, saggy, or tired (Fig. 22), which raises the question: Is there a normal or proper posture?

Statistically, a normal posture would be the posture assumed by the majority of a healthy population. Any investigation to measure what is normal is difficult, because each person's posture may vary from day to day and under various conditions, such as heat, cold, sadness, and joy; thus, normal can never be a fixed value.

Physiologically, posture is known to influence blood pressure, muscle effort, res-

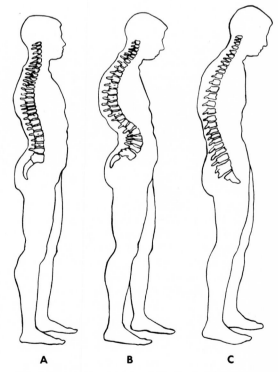

Fig. 22 A, Curves of the spine in good posture. **B,** Curves of the spine in the slump posture. **C,** Obliteration of the spinal curves as in early spondylitis.

piratory efficiency, and energy require-ments. The rigid military posture may require 20% more energy than the at-ease posture. An easy standing position requires relatively little more energy than recum-bency; hence we can say that rigid posture is not ideal.

In order to stand erect, the body of man must resist gravity. We learn in physics that the body has a center of gravity; i.e., a point within the body around which the mass of the body is equally distributed. If the body were supported at this point, it would be in equilibrium. A stable equilib-rium will occur in the erect posture when a vertical line passes through the center

of gravity (situated in front of the second sacral vertebra) and through the base of support (Fig. 23, A). This means an equal amount of body weight is distributed to each side of the line of gravity. If the body leans forward, an unstable equilibrium oc-curs, since the perpendicular line of grav-ity through the body's center of gravity no longer passes through the base of support but is now in front of it. To prevent the body from falling, a muscle force must pull the body back to the stable position over its base of support. If the body were simi-lar to a brick leaning forward on edge, it would continue to fall forward until it came to rest on the flat side that provides a broad base of support with the center of gravity at the lowest point. A broad base of support and the lowest center of gravity provide a stable equilibrium (Fig. 24).

Obviously the human body can compen-sate for an unstable equilibrium, but it will require energy in the form of muscle effort to do so. This capability is balance, which allows the body to resist all outside forces that disturb a neutral equilibrium.

Ideal posture is observed only in the trained individual. The most commonly ob-served posture is by no means ideal. The variations in body build and particularly the inherent inborn length of ligaments ac-count for the marked variations of posture among human beings.

Persons with relaxed ligaments stand with hyperextended knees, hyperextended hips, and very flexible, exaggerated curves of the spine; hence, the individual parts

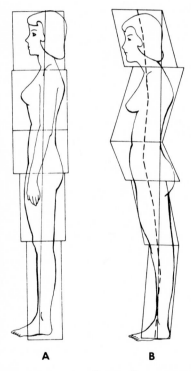

A   **B**

Fig. 23 A, In good standing posture, the weight-bearing line (line of gravity) passes just anterior to the ear, through the shoulder joint, just posterior to the hip joint, and slightly be-hind the patella, striking the floor just anterior to the external malleolus. **B,** Poor standing pos-ture illustrating malalignment of the body seg-ments and a distorted weight-bearing line. Note forward position of the head, round shoulders, increased lordosis, and protruding abdomen. (From Teaching and evaluating posture, Audio-visual Center, The University of Iowa, Iowa City, Iowa; courtesy M. Joan Popp.)

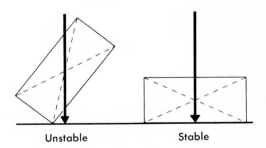

Unstable   Stable

Fig. 24 The arrow represents the downward force of gravity, which comes to rest outside of the narrow base of support. The brick has more weight to the right side of the base and there-fore will fall to the right. The brick will fall until the center of gravity rests over a broad base as depicted in the stable position.

of the body extend farther forward and backward from the line of gravity than do those in individuals with tighter ligaments. (It must be pointed out, however, that as long as there is an equal distribution of weight of the extended parts on each side of the line of gravity, these individuals are as much on line of gravity as others and remain so with no more muscular effort than others.) The posture of these persons necessarily appears slouched although it is efficient. Unfortunately, however, the anterior longitudinal ligaments of the lumbar spine are under more continuous shear strain, which renders the individuals more subject to low back strain. For such persons to strive toward ideal posture would demand constant training and constant muscle energy for which very few people are suited or motivated. To attain the ideal posture would require muscle control in order to stand with knee in neutral extension and trunk control to reduce each vertebral segment toward neutral (reduce the amount of curve). Thus, a more cosmetically accepted posture would be achieved at the expense of constant muscle coordination and energy; the only physiologic gain would be relief of strain on spinal ligaments.

There are a few tricks that are easily learned to improve posture, and these can be accomplished with a minimal expenditure of energy. Head up, chin in, backward pelvic tilt, and standing tall practiced many times for a few seconds at a time will go far toward improving posture. It will eliminate the slouch that accompanies fatigue and diminish ligament strain. It can become a good habit to replace a bad one. For the student nurse, practicing and establishing good posture habits when performing nursing functions should be an essential part of her clinical experience. Good posture not only makes for a more pleasing appearance in contrast to poor posture, which denotes discouragement and fatigue, but also provides for correct functioning of the weight-bearing joints. In addition, since health teaching is an important aspect of nursing today, nurses who understand the necessity for good posture and practice it themselves will be able to demonstrate its importance more effectively by example.

Posture evaluation—nursing assessment skills

As assessment of the musculoskeletal system is made, it must be remembered that the patient and family histories are important aspects of the evaluation. The presence of congenital anomalies, evidence of trauma, complaints of joint pain and deformity, limited motion, muscle weakness, and tremors are of particular significance. Since two of the functions of the musculoskeletal system are support and locomotion, assessment must include observation and evaluation of the individual's posture and ability to ambulate. The ability to stand and to walk with a normal gait and to use coordinated movements necessitates an intact neuromuscular system, as well as a normal skeleton and normal functioning joints.

As the back is examined, the skin should be inspected, noting the presence of scars and abnormal pigmentation. The spinous processes, paravertebral muscles (located on each side of the midline), and paraspinous areas (facet region) should be firmly palpated to elicit the presence of pain and/or muscle spasm.

To evaluate the standing posture, the observer should note the lateral spinal profile and check for the normal anterior and posterior curves of the vertebral column. In the adult, four curves are normally present: cervical, thoracic, lumbar, and sacral. When the trunk is in an erect position, these curves balance the distribution of the body's weight. The extent of the curves is approximately equal both anterior and posterior to the weight-bearing line (Fig. 23, A). Exaggerations of these curves result in poor posture. If the head is carried too far forward of the vertebral support, stress is placed on the vertebrae and there is an increase in the thoracic curve, producing round shoulders. If this deformity is severe, it is referred to as a *kyphosis,* meaning an abnormally increased convexity in the curvature of the thoracic spine. Exaggeration of the lumbar curve causes the pelvis to tilt forward, and the result is a swayback or a *lordosis* deformity, meaning an abnormally increased concavity in the lumbar region.

Posteriorly, the spinal column should be checked for *scoliosis.* Scoliosis means there is lateral bending of the vertebral column;

when this occurs, there is also rotation of the vertebral bodies. This deformity can occur anywhere along the spinal column. As the examiner observes the torso posteriorly, symmetry of the shoulders and scapular levels should be noted. Position of the arms as they hang freely at the sides of the body should be compared. If scoliosis is suspected, ask the individual to bend forward. In this position, the deformity is accentuated, and a mild curve becomes more noticeable. Any asymmetry in the flank areas and the presence of a prominent or higher hip on one side should be noted (see Chapter 13).

Further evaluation of the back includes careful notation of restricted motion or painful motion of the vertebral column. The presence of discrepancies or asymmetry between right and left movements of the spinal column should be evaluated carefully. Accurate measurement of spinal motion is difficult to obtain and varies greatly among individuals. As motion of the cervical spine is observed, the examiner may ask the patient to move the chin toward the chest (flexion), to move the head backward (extension), to turn the head to the right and to the left (rotation), and, for lateral bending, to move the head so that the ear approaches the corresponding shoulder. Range of motion of the trunk is observed in similar fashion by asking the patient to bend forward (flexion), reaching the fingertips toward the floor. Normally as the individual bends forward, the lumbar curve is reversed, and symmetry of the rib cage can be evaluated. Bending backward provides for extension of the trunk. Asking the patient to turn to the right and to the left will permit assessment of rotation (approximately 45° is normal). Lateral bending of the spine is observed by asking the patient to bend to the right and then to the left.

As the examiner continues to evaluate the standing posture, the size and shape of the knees should be observed and compared. Enlargement or deformity (knockknee; bowlegs) should be noted, along with any complaints of discomfort or limitation of activity encountered by the patient. Inability to extend the knee fully (knee flexion contracture) may be apparent as range of motion is checked. In standing and

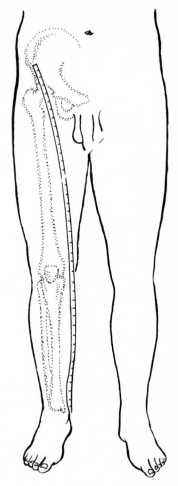

Fig. 25 To determine true shortening of the lower extremity, measure from the anterosuperior iliac spine to the lowest point of the medial malleolus and compare with the measurements of the normal limb. The hip, knee, and ankle must be held in a neutral position.

walking positions, the toes and kneecaps normally point forward.

When a discrepancy in leg length is suspected, accurate measurements of the limbs should be taken. With the hips, knees, and ankles in a neutral postion, measure from the anterosuperior iliac spine to the internal malleolus of each limb (Fig. 25). A leg length difference of one-fourth inch or less is considered to be within normal limits. If muscle atrophy is suspected, circumferential measurements of the thigh or calf areas may be taken and compared (Fig. 26). Accurate recordings of the findings

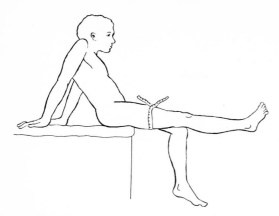

Fig. 26 Atrophy of the thigh muscles may be determined by measuring the circumference of the involved limb and comparing it with the measurement of the normal limb. For subsequent comparisons, measurements must be made at the same location, and the limb should be maintained in the same position.

should include the precise spot measured. This will enable future comparisons.

A persistent limp or complaints of pain in the knee or hip region of the young child, the preadolescent, or adolescent should not go unheeded. Inspection of the limb includes noting the presence of muscle spasm, evaluating hip motion, noting any limitation of activity, and checking for atrophy of the thigh muscles.

When examining an infant or small child, asymmetry in the number and depth of the gluteal and thigh folds should be noted. Discrepancies in joint motion will be detected as the range of motion is checked. Normally, when an infant's hips are flexed to 90° and abducted, the thighs will usually touch the table top. Limitation in hip abduction is indicative of a subluxated or dislocated hip. To compare leg lengths, hold the infant's feet together, flex the hips and knees, and observe for differences in knee levels. The presence of broad buttocks, a wide perineum, and prominent trochanters should be noted as the infant is examined. In the small infant, Ortolani's sign is significant when checking for subluxation of the hip. In the child old enough to stand and walk, observation for Trendelenburg's sign is important when examining hip function (see Chapter 12).

Examination of the child's foot includes checking for deformities: varus, valgus,

calcaneus, and equinus positions (Figs. 243 and 245). However, it should be remembered that the newborn infant normally holds the foot in a varus position, but that when range of motion is done all the other positions may be attained easily. Examination also includes noting the position of the forefoot. Is there adduction (metatarsus adductus; Fig. 87), or does the child walk pigeon-toed (in-toeing)? In infants and most young children, the presence of a fat pad beneath the longitudinal arch (medial aspect) makes the foot appear flat. In some older individuals, the flatfoot position (pes planus) is normal and does not cause discomfort. If symptoms are present, an arch support and foot exercises may be advisable. Likewise, a high arch (pes cavus) may be normal in some individuals, whereas in others it may indicate a neurologic problem. Checking a person's shoes can give the examiner clues as to foot disorders. With a normal walking pattern, there will be some wearing down of the lateral aspect of the heel and sole. Wearing down of the medial aspect indicates a flatfoot position, with the heel tilted to a valgus position.

In the older person, pain and discomfort of the feet are of prime concern. Fallen arches, corns, calluses, and joint deformities such as hammer toes or hallux valgus can be quite painful and make it impossible for the individual to be comfortable in ordinary shoes. Walking is one of the best forms of exercise for elderly persons. However, if weight bearing causes pain, their activities, including walking, will be markedly curtailed. Edema of the feet and ankles and/or the presence of skin abrasions that heal slowly may indicate circulatory problems. All of these affections, plus the fact that many elderly individuals are unable to bathe their feet and to care for the toenails properly, contribute to the foot discomfort of this age group (see also Chapter 17).

Recumbent posture

So far the discussion has related to man's ability to stand erect, which we think of as posture. The strict definition of posture, however, includes other positional attitudes. Lying down is referred to as recumbent posture; lying face down is a prone pos-

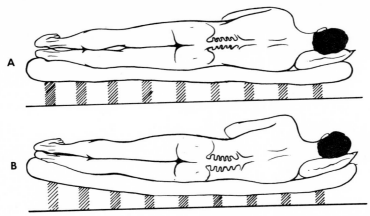

Fig. 27 A, Ideal mattress that allows hips and shoulder sufficient give to maintain a straight spine and an evenly distributed support throughout the body length. **B,** Sagging mattress and spring. This position puts a tension strain on the spinal ligaments at the convexity of the curve and a compression strain at the concavity.

ture, and lying face up is a supine posture. Posture in the sense of description is synonymous with position, the word most commonly used. Gravity continues to exert its force on the body in whatever position it assumes. The effect of that force, however, is altered since the direction of the pull is no longer in the longitudinal axis of the body toward the center of the earth and the base of support is no longer the feet. The body in the supine position supported by a firm bed is pushed against the bed by the force of gravity acting at right angles or downward on each individual segment. Each segment is supported so that there is no energy requirement for balance; therefore, the body is at rest with a zero energy requirement to resist gravity.

This concept is important to the nurse who is responsible for positioning the patient's body in bed. Certain qualifications must be appreciated although the principle remains the same; viz., that wherever a force acts in one direction, there must be an equal force in the opposite direction if the body is to remain at rest.

From a practical view, each body segment has its own shape and weight. A straight hard surface supporting the supine body cannot match the normal curves of the body. The consequence is that the body parts that normally protrude posteriorly must share the bulk of body weight at the mid-dorsal spine, occiput, sacrum, calves

of the legs, and heels. Because these contact points form bridges, the segments of body in between have no base of support and, therefore, sag until the base is reached. The result of this uneven weight distribution clearly places an excessive load at the contact points and thus demands frequent change in body alignment.

An excellent example is a person who has a lordotic contracture of the lumbar spine. Lying supine on the floor would become uncomfortable as the arched back flattens from the forces of gravity but never reaches the base of support. The posterior ligaments bear the strain. A supple individual, on the other hand, may be quite comfortable, since the lumbar spine flattens easily to reach the floor and find support.

The ideal flexibility in the base of support (the mattress) would allow the heaviest and more rigid body segments to sink down just enough to allow the remaining segments to accept support from the mattress and maintain essentially the same body alignment as in standing. Since wide variations exist in the rigidity and weight of body segments in people, a trial-and-error test of spring mattress combinations would be the only way to meet the criteria of need in choosing the proper support (Fig. 27).

In a side-lying position, the body profile is variable; the shoulder segment is broader

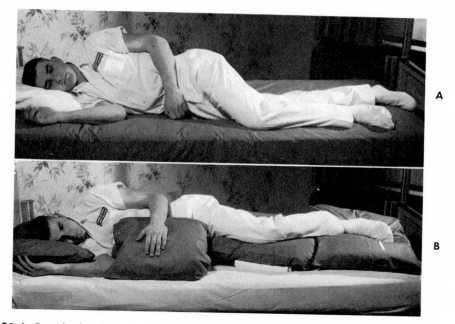

Fig. 28 A, Poor body alignment in the side-lying position. **B,** Good body alignment in the side-lying position. With some patients, to prevent edema of the hand, it will be necessary to maintain the hand even with or higher than the elbow.

and heavier than the pelvis in males, and the reverse is true in females. The head requires pillow support of shoulder width to maintain a straight cervical spine. In an extended position, the lower limbs lying one on the other have a very unstable equilibrium and, therefore, with relaxation tend to rotate unless flexed at the hips and knees. Even in this position the contact points at the knee and ankle provide very small surface areas of support and cannot tolerate the pressure except for short periods. A better base of support is a pillow between the knees (Fig. 28).

Whether the body is in a supine or side-lying position, there is no consistent way to relieve localized pressure points in the recumbent posture. Since relief is obtained only by the frequent shifts of position that normally occur regularly in sleep, the nurse must deliberately and actively provide for frequent changes of position in elderly, weak, and immobilized persons. One of the greatest responsibilities of the nurse is the recognition of the necessity of and the techniques for the implementation of bed positioning and frequent shifting of body positions for those confined to bed.

Body alignment for bed patient

Prolonged poor bed posture can contribute to the development of joint contractures. A sagging mattress encourages the development of hip flexion contractures (Fig. 29). Improperly placed pillows beneath the head and shoulders tend to cause round shoulders. Knees continuously supported with pillows will cause an adaptive shortening of the hamstring tendons and a knee flexion contracture. To help prevent contractures, the mattress supporting the body weight must be firm enough to maintain good body alignment. Increased firmness may be obtained by placing a bedboard beneath the standard innerspring or felt mattress. To permit elevation of the backrest, a hinged board is necessary.

The footboard may or may not be considered a part of the bed, but it is essential for the patient with muscle weakness if a functional position of the feet is to be maintained. It should be several inches higher than the patient's toes, supporting the foot at a right angle to the tibia, maintaining the toes in extension, and holding the bed covers off the feet. If the toes of a paralyzed extremity are permitted to curl

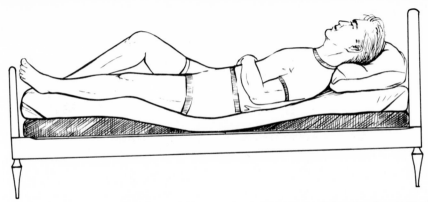

Fig. 29 Sagging mattress contributes to poor body alignment and the development of hip flexion contractures.

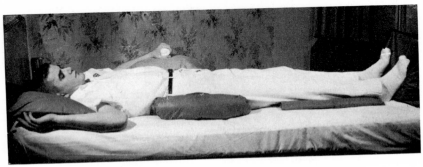

Fig. 30 Good body alignment in the supine position.

over the top edge of a footboard, a toe-drop will develop. When the patient is in the supine position, there should be space for the patient's heels between the end of the mattress and the footboard to protect the heels from pressure. An adjustable foot-board may be shifted to provide support when the patient is moved up in bed and placed in a sitting position.

For a bedfast patient, the addition of a trapeze to the bed is desirable, since it enables him to shift his position and to assist with his care without the leverage of elbow lift from the bed. However, in some instances it is thought that rehabilitees will become more independent if they learn to function without this aid. The bed equipped with an electric control that enables the patient to modify his position is also helpful. In addition to maintaining good body alignment, frequent and regular changes of position are essential to relieve localized pressure points as previously mentioned.

When studying the accompanying illustrations of body positions (Figs. 30 to 36), it should be remembered that an alignment of the body segments that provides good posture for the person in a vertical position will also provide good posture for one who is bedfast or in the horizontal position.

Supine position. A good back-lying position is illustrated in Fig. 30. The footboard holds the covers off the toes and maintains the feet in a functional position, midway between dorsiflexion and plantar flexion. The folded bath blanket placed under the calf of the leg lessens the pressure on the heel. It also provides for a relaxed position of the knee joint and avoids pressure on the popliteal space. A bilateral trochanter roll may be made by folding one or two bath blankets lengthwise in thirds. The folded blankets are placed crosswise on the bed beneath the patient's buttocks. The outer ends are rolled (under) firmly against the corresponding

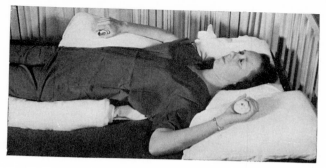

Fig. 31 Positions of rest for the arms. The right arm illustrates a position of abduction with internal rotation. The left arm illustrates a position of abduction with external rotation. Note the position of the wrist and fingers.

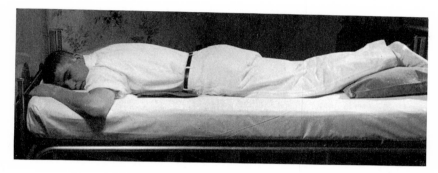

Fig. 32 Good body alignment in the prone position.

hip and thigh. The roll supports and maintains the limb in a neutral position, preventing external rotation. A small pillow or pad placed under the lower portion of the back gives support to the normal lumbar curve. This nursing measure will provide considerable comfort for the patient with lordosis who must remain on his back for an indefinite period of time.

The patient with paralysis or weakness of the upper extremity muscles needs frequent and careful positioning of the arm and hand. The involved arm may be placed on the bed with the elbow and wrist in extension and the forearm pronated or supinated. At other times, the arm should be abducted with the elbow flexed and the forearm supported on a pillow with the hand maintained in a functional position. Another position for the arm is that of abduction with external rotation (Fig. 31).

Prone position. When a patient is turned onto his abdomen with no support beneath the ankles, the feet are forced to remain in an equinus position (plantar flexion). To prevent plantar flexion, a pillow may be used to support the ankles (Fig. 32), or the patient may be positioned so that his feet extend over the end of the mattress. Use of a head pillow in the face-lying position may cause hyperextension of the cervical spine. Some individuals in the prone position have better body alignment and are more comfortable with a thin pillow placed beneath the abdomen. Other patients, however, can be made comfortable without this pillow and still maintain good body alignment. The abducted and externally rotated (spread-eagle) position of the arms is restful for many patients (Fig. 32).

Side-lying position. When a patient is turned on his side, the entire length of the uppermost limb should be supported with pillows to prevent an adducted position. Maintaining the hip and knee in the same plane lessens strain on the hip joint and is of particular importance for the

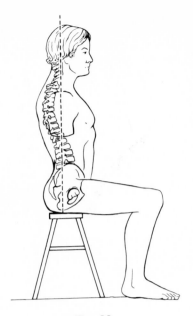

Fig. 33

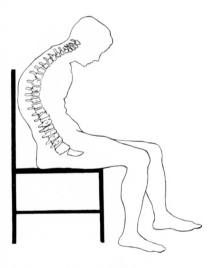

Fig. 34

vide different positions for the joints of the uppermost arm.

Sitting posture

In the usual sitting position, the ischial tuberosities supplant the feet as the base of support for the trunk and head. The head, trunk, and upper extremities constitute 80% of the weight of the total body. A new segmental center of gravity for the trunk, upper extremities, and head has been said to be just in front of the eleventh dorsal vertebra. The perpendicular line passing through the new center of gravity must also pass through the very narrow base of support, the ischial tuberosities (Fig. 33). This

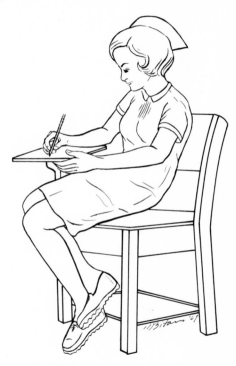

Fig. 35 Poor sitting posture. In this position, there is more strain on the posterior longitudinal ligaments and the interspinous ligaments of the spine than elsewhere. In addition, there is an abnormal amount of pressure placed on the anterior portion of the intervertebral disc. If sustained for any length of time, this compression may be a factor in initiating the degeneration of a disc, and it certainly can perpetuate it. The depth of the seat on many upholstered chairs does not provide for good sitting posture but tends to encourage the individual to sit with most of the weight on the lower back region.

patient who has had hip or back surgery. Also it is desirable that the uppermost limb be positioned to avoid pressure on the underneath limb. When the patient is placed in the side-lying position, the underneath arm and shoulder must be made comfortable, and pillows may be used to support the uppermost arm and back as needed (Fig. 28, B). Variations of this position may be utilized to change pressure points on the hip and shoulder areas and to procan be considered as unstable equilibrium or at least a narrow base equilibrium. If the upper thighs are added to the sitting base, the base obviously becomes more stable. Without the upper thighs, a back rest on the seat provides stability if it is inclined backward just enough to move the perpendicular back of the tuberosities.

It is common for an individual to slide forward in a chair to assure the perpendicular of gravity to be back of the tuberosities (Figs. 34 and 35). Such a position places the entire spine in a convex curve pointing backward, and this position, if sustained, places excessive strain on the posterior ligaments.

The ideal sitting posture can be achieved in a chair that allows the upper thighs to

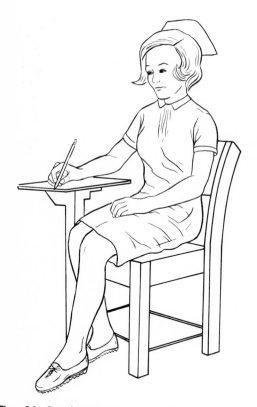

Fig. 36 Good sitting posture. To provide for good sitting posture, the height and depth of the chair seat should permit the person to sit with the feet resting flat on the floor, the knees and hips flexed at right angles, and the back supported by the chair back. When sitting, the body weight should rest on the ischial tuberosites and proximal portion of the thighs.

add to the sitting base (Fig. 36) while the ischial tuberosities provide the major base, the lumbar spine is in mild flexion, and the entire spine is supported with the slightest backward inclination from the perpendicular. This posture is impossible in soft, deep, upholstered chairs, modern dish-shaped chairs, or bleachers without back-rests. Many automobile seats are either too soft and deep or have too much backward inclination of the backrest and improper seat length for thigh rest to permit a stable equilibrium in sitting. Adjustments can be made with pillow buildups or electrically powered adjusters.

DYNAMIC BODY MECHANICS

Kinesiology, the science of human motion, is studied in many fields such as anatomy, physics, mathematics, orthopedics, and engineering. A number of textbooks are geared to the specific needs of each discipline and include those for occupational and physical therapy. To be of practical value for nurses, this discussion is intended only to provide a new viewpoint for nurses as they deal day to day with mechanical problems in patient care. It is hoped that some insight into biomechanics as it relates to gait, traction, and the performance of mechanical tasks may aid the nurse to understand the energy costs and ways to avoid musculoskeletal strains.

Kinematics is concerned with measurement and recording of body motions and combinations of several joints to produce certain acts such as throwing a baseball. Such a series of motions constitutes a kinematic chain.

Kinetics deals with forces that produce motions and the effect of these motions on body equilibrium. The laws of forces and the classes of levers must be identified as they apply to produce bodily motions.

Laws of force

The musculoskeletal system is designed to accomplish two main objectives: (1) overcome or resist the forces of gravity and (2) perform work. The anatomic structures of the body are arranged to achieve both with a conservation of energy—in other words, the least amount of energy needed to accomplish the job.

The same laws of force, known as Newton's laws, and the same classes of levers that apply to simple machines apply to the human body as it overcomes gravity and produces work.

Newton's laws

Law I

A body will remain at rest or in motion in a straight line until acted upon by a force.

Example: Once a heavy object, such as a bed, is put into motion, it is much easier to keep it moving than to start and stop it continually.

Law II

A force acting on a body causes the body to accelerate in the direction of the force.

Example: Pushing a heavy patient in a wheel-chair will require more force for a comparable acceleration than pushing a lighter patient.

Law III

For every force there is an equal and opposite reaction force.

Example: A patient in bed places a force (body weight) against the mattress, and the mattress produces an equal push against the patient. Pressure sores occur where heavy body parts press firmly against a mattress and receive an equal force in return. A person who is standing places a force (body weight) downward through the base (foot) against the floor, and the floor pushes an equal amount upward against the foot.

A knowledge of these laws of force and motion has application to every physical effort the nurse makes in the course of her work and also applies to the patient provided with nursing care. The alert nurse will think in terms of body mechanics as each act of nursing is performed in order to protect against strains that are avoidable if the proper mechanical advantage is applied to the task.

Body levers

A lever is a machine, a device for transmitting energy derived from muscle contraction to move body segments which, in turn, transmit energy to external objects. All levers have a fulcrum, an effort arm, and a resistance arm. Depending upon the relative location of the fulcrum to the effort and resistance, levers are designated as Class I, II, or III.

Class I

Class I lever is a seesaw where the weight R can be balanced by an equal force E across fulcrum F. If R is heavier than E, the seesaw is unbalanced and the lever will tilt downward. If the fulcrum is moved half the distance toward R, the lever arm for E is lengthened and E will balance R with half the effort (Fig. 37, A).

Example: A man using a shovel (Fig. 37, B).

Class II

In Class II lever, the fulcrum is at one end, and the energy E is applied at the opposite end to lift a weight R somewhere between (Fig. 38, A). The advantage of this lever is obvious if the mathematics is understood. The energy in pounds times the lever arm distance to the fulcrum will lift a weight R times the lever arm distance from the fulcrum (formula at top of first column on opposite page).

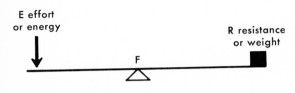

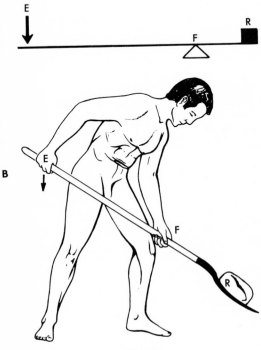

Fig. 37

18 lb (R) × 1 ft (lever arm) = lb E × 3 ft (lever arm)

From this formula, x equals 6 lb. It will take 6 lb of energy to lift 18 lb of weight if the energy is applied at the lever arm three times as far from the fulcrum as the weight.

Example: A man pushing a wheelbarrow (Fig. 38, B).

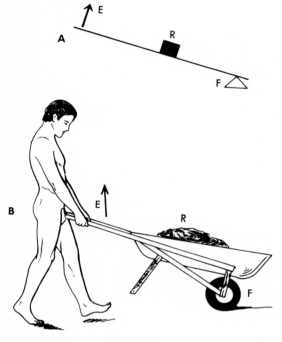

Fig. 38

Class III

In Class III lever the energy is applied to the lever somewhere between the fulcrum and the weight or resistance (Fig. 39, A). The energy requirement is greater than the resistance to be lifted; however, the resistance of weight can be lifted a greater distance more rapidly. The majority of single muscle levers in the body are Class III.

Example: In Fig. 39, B, the fulcrum is the elbow joint, the lever the forearm, and the hand with its contents the resistance. The energy is supplied by the biceps muscle inserted into the radius. Since the insertion is 2 inches forward of the fulcrum and the resistance is at least 10 inches forward of the fulcrum, it means that the biceps must pull upward with a force of 25 lb to hold a weight of 5 lb in the hand.

The illustration serves to point out another important fact in body mechanics—vig., the position of the fulcrum. The fulcrum can be moved to any position required to do a lifting job and must be held or stabilized in that position. Movement of the shoulder can place the elbow fulcrum and stabilize it in whatever position is required. The shoulder muscles are acting throughout the effort in exactly the same fashion as the biceps. The shoulder holds the elbow lever that holds the weight (Fig. 39, C).

The more forward the hand is held from the body, the harder the shoulder muscles must work to stabilize the position of the elbow. When the elbow is extended, the biceps muscle continues to hold the 5 lb in the hand; however, the lever arm now is lenghtened the distance from the hand to the shoulder; there-

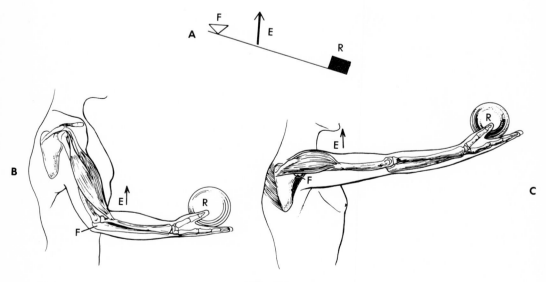

Fig. 39

fore, the shoulder muscles become the energy for a new lever system. The length of the lever from hand to shoulder is now 20 inches so the shoulder muscles must use 25 lb of force additional to the 25 lb of force of the biceps at the elbow to sustain the 5-lb weight in the hand.

The foregoing concept is important for nurses to understand since some positions for lifting require less energy than others for the same job. To better understand this concept requires a knowledge of torque stresses.

Torque stresses

When a force acting on the body tends to rotate that body, the force is called a couple, and the moment of that couple is the torque. The direction of torque is either clockwise or counterclockwise. The moment is the distance from the center of rotation (fulcrum) to the resistance (weight). For a body to be in equilibrium and not rotate, there must be a force in the opposite direction equal to the resistance. The fulcrum in this situation is the axis of motion or center of rotation (Fig. 40).

The principle of torque explains why there are some positions in work that are better than others because they require less energy and produce less strain on soft tis-

sues. An example is lifting (Fig. 41). R is the weight that tends to rotate the body forward (clockwise) at the center of rotation (hip) with a force equal to the weight being lifted times the distance from the weight to the hip. To produce equilibrium and prevent the body from falling forward, the posterior muscles of the back must produce an equal force to resist the clockwise fall. The counterclockwise torque or distance from the center of rotation (hip) to the origin of the back muscles is very short compared to the clockwise torque. Therefore, the muscles must generate a force of 30 lb for the individual to hold a weight of 5 lb.

A more efficient position for weight holding or lifting can be seen in the example of proper lifting position (Fig. 42, *B*). In this position, the counterclockwise torque (distance from weight to hip) is reduced to one-half so that the force of the back muscles will require only 11 lb of force to hold or lift 5 lb in the hand.

The case of a man lifting a 5-lb ball is an excellent example of a Class III lever because it indicates the internal muscle

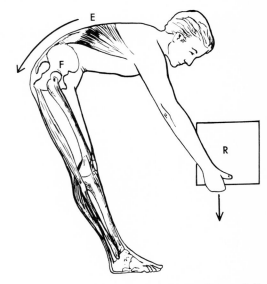

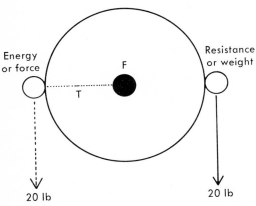

Fig. 40 The diagram appears as a wheel with the axis of rotation at **F** (fulcrum). If a force (weight) pulls the wheel clockwise, the wheel will rotate clockwise at the axis of motion **F**. The wheel will not rotate if an equal force (energy) pushes it counterclockwise. If the wheel does not rotate, it is said to be in equilibrium. **T** (moment) is the distance from fulcrum to weight (resistance).

Fig. 41 This illustrates the torque force of **R**, which must be equaled by **E** where the fulcrum **F** is an unequal distance from **R** and **E**. The moment of **R** is six times the moment of **E** (the distance from **R** to **F** compared to the distance from **E** to **F**). Therefore, the force (torque) generated by the back muscles must be six times the force (weight) of object **R**.

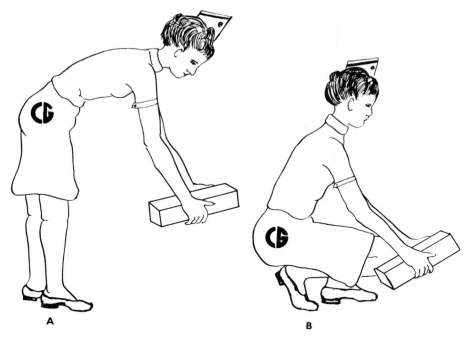

Fig. 42

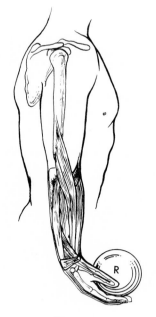

Fig. 43

forces at equilibrium with the weight. This is only a part of what actually happens since the arm is one segment of the total body. The 5-lb weight away from the line of gravity of the body has upset the pos-

tural (torque) equilibrium by adding weight to the front of the body's center of gravity. The body will fall forward unless a new force acting posteriorly on the body neutralizes the 5-lb weight. The center of gravity acts as a fulcrum or axis.

The rotary equilibrium of the body at the center of gravity axis is unstable, since the 5-lb weight as an external force has added a clockwise torque. To restore equilibrium, an equal counterclockwise force must be added. Ordinarily, the contractile force of extensor muscles of the back and pelvis will be sufficient to restore equilibrium.

If the weight is carried at the side as illustrated in Fig. 43, there is little or no torque and no need for a lever system. The only energy requirement will be a 5-lb finger grip to hold the weight. If the weight then must be placed at a higher level, such as a shelf, the energy requirement for the Class III elbow lever (Fig. 39, *B*) will suffice. If the shelf is at a higher level, much more energy is necessary for the extended lever, and body torque is increased (Fig. 39, *C*). It is obvious that the closer the weight is to the line of gravity of the body, the less the energy force required to do the work. The nurse can apply this principle to lifting in general. However, there are exceptions, such as when the object to be lifted cannot be brought close to the nurse's center of gravity, as in the case of a patient in bed. Here, a knowledge of lever systems can be helpful.

With a hand placed under the patient while the elbow of the same extremity rests on the bed, the fulcrum of the lifting lever has a stable base. (This is sometimes referred to as the elbow lift.) The only force required in this position will be the pull of the biceps (energy) acting on a Class III lever to lift weight. The shorter lever arm will require less energy than lifting from the shoulder, and there will be no torque of the center of gravity of the body.

In the examples of proper lifting and proper holding, there is not only conservation of muscle energy, but also much less strain on the other tissues.

Strains are the deformations of materials under loads; e.g., the stretch of a rubber band or the bend of a wire. There are three types of strain: compression, tension, and shear.

Loads are forces or weights applied externally to a structure. Whenever a structure is loaded by a force, it must resist that force and the resistance becomes another force within the structure. The forces within a structure are called stresses and are intermolecular forces to resist certain loads; these are referred to as compression stress, tension stress, and shear stress. Stress forces within a structure such as bone, intervertebral disk, or ligament are not to be confused with strain.

Strain, to repeat, is another property of materials which allows the material to respond to loads by changing shape. This is called deformation. The material elongates under tension (stretching) loads and shortens under compression loads; each material has a limit to which it can alter its shape without breaking. Solid materials have another property, which is the ability to return to an original shape after the load is removed. This is called elasticity, and whereas the deformation of tension on a rubber band is easily visible as stretch, the same deformation occurs in ligaments or even bone but is too small to be visible.

This is true also in compression and shear strains. As in the case of a bone or ligament, each material has for its shape and size a certain measurable strain called Young's modulus of elasticity. When this is exceeded, the bone or ligament no longer returns to its original shape but rather it ruptures or breaks.

Bones and ligaments are living tissues that are capable of change in response to the load demands placed on them. The modulus of elasticity can change as the tissues grow stronger or weaker. For this reason, excessive loading should be avoided if the bones or ligaments are unaccustomed to sudden excessive loading since the modulus of elasticity may be exceeded and the tissue will remain deformed. Conditioning programs can stimulate the living tissues to grow stronger to meet the demands of loads placed on them. This is just as important a part of conditioning as the development of strength in muscles by exercise. Good body mechanics will avoid excessive loading, whereas poor mechanics will produce excessive loading, and if the modulus of elasticity of the loaded tissues is exceeded, the tissues, particularly ligaments, will be strained and actually become painful. This type of strain can be avoided by the application of proper body mechanics to each task.

One of the most common areas of the body to be strained is the low back. This is understandable because great forces of torque are transferred to the disk and ligaments of this area in stooping and lifting. Application of good body mechanics will lessen the torque loading on the low back throughout the working day. Good body mechanics applied to specific jobs will help the nurse to develop good habits for herself and teach good habits to patients.

The nurse must remember that the laws which govern balance in the standing position also apply when the body is in motion and that maintaining correct alignment of the body segments (weight-bearing line) in relation to the base of support is important in preventing strain of supporting muscles and ligaments. Balance and motion of the human body are produced and controlled by the contraction of muscles attached to the skeletal system. Contraction of a muscle supplies the force necessary to overcome gravity and to provide for motion and work. When the nurse carries a heavy tray, the biceps muscle inserted in the radius contracts and supplies the effort needed to support the resistance offered by the tray. Carrying the tray close to the body enables the nurse to maintain correct alignment of the body segments and requires less muscle effort than holding the tray farther from the body.

If a nurse working at the bedside bends forward by flexing the hips and spinal column (with knees extended), the work placed on the spinal ligaments and low back muscles is very great. Lifting or working in such a position (Fig. 44) may result in backache due to strain of the low back muscles and spinal ligaments and also may be a factor in causing rupture of a disc. In this position there is increased pressure placed on the anterior aspects of the vertebral bodies and on the intervening nucleus pulposus. However, if the nurse, when positioning a bed patient, flexes the hips and knees, faces the work, and assumes the foot-forward position, correct alignment of the shoulders and pelvis in relation to the line of gravity and base of support will be maintained. In this position (Fig. 45) she is able to use the strong muscles of the thighs and arms for moving the patient. Stabilization of the pelvis is accomplished by tightening the abdominal and gluteal muscles. In some instances, moving the bed patient may be accomplished with less effort by using a lifting sheet. The amount of friction between the patient's body and the bed surface is lessened. If the nurse wishes to move the mattress or the patient up in bed, the head of the bed is lowered, unless the patient's condition contraindicates the change of position. Sliding an object on a level surface requires less effort than moving it on an inclined plane. The nurse soon learns, when caring for the helpless individual, that the patient's position can be changed with less exertion by turning or sliding his body than by lifting him and that it is easier and safer for both the patient and the nurse to slide or turn the patient toward rather than away from the nurse.

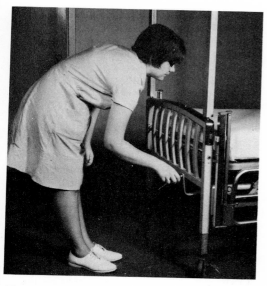

Fig. 44 When the kind of bed shown here is used, nursing personnel raise and lower the headrest many times a day and, in addition, frequently raise and lower the bed. When these activities are done with the body in the position illustrated (feet parallel and knees in extension), strain is placed on the muscles and ligaments of the lumbosacral area.

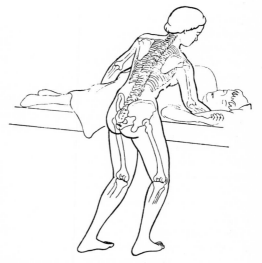

Fig. 45 When working at the bedside, the nurse should assume the foot-forward position, face the work, flex the knees and hips slightly, and maintain the shoulders in the same plane as the pelvis. In this position the small muscles of the back are protected and the large muscles of the thigh are used. (Courtesy National Advisory Service for Orthopedics and Poliomyelitis, and Alfred Feinberg, artist, College of Physicians and Surgeons, Columbia University, New York, N. Y.)

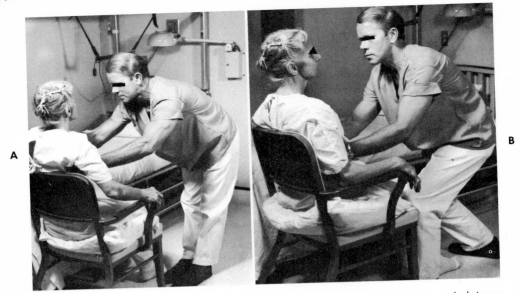

Fig. 46 A, The nurse illustrates the use of poor body mechanics preparatory to helping a patient assume the standing position. **B,** The nurse demonstrates correct body mechanics and in this position is able to lift and support the unsteady patient without strain to his own back muscles.

Nursing procedures and correct body mechanics can be practiced concurrently (Fig. 46). Once the student has learned to carry out procedures while using correct body mechanics, it becomes a conditioned skill likely to be carried into similar situations on the patient unit. The carryover to the patient will not be automatic. The situation facing the beginning student is very complex, and there are many things to remember in the early days in the clinical area. Guided instruction will be needed. The material on body mechanics cannot be given in one gigantic dose; it must be offered in suitable small doses and repeated often. That is why it is so important for all teaching personnel and nurse clinicians who come in contact with the student to be well grounded in the subject and convinced of its importance.

The following reminders will help the nurse who is working at the bedside to use the body's many lever systems in an efficient manner, thus minimizing fatigue and the possibility of strained ligaments:

1 Carry or lift heavy burdens close to the body. Since the object carried becomes a part of the body's weight, there occurs less displacement of the body's center of gravity (Fig. 39).

2 To attain a lower work level, flex the knees and keep the back straight (Fig. 42, B). If the shoulder and pelvic girdles are maintained in the same plane, the body's center of gravity is kept over the the base of support. Rounding the back and reaching forward or downward to lift with the arms displaces the weight of the trunk forward (Fig. 41). To maintain body balance in this position, excessive strain is placed on the hip and back extensors, and, in addition, the strain of any lifting is placed on the small back muscles rather than on the stronger, more massive muscles of the thighs and buttocks.

3 Increase the body's base of support toward the object to be lifted or moved. A broader base of support increases stability.

4 When lifting, face the work situation and avoid rotary movements of the spine.

5 Stand close to the object being moved or lifted. This helps to maintain the body's center of gravity over the base of support and increases stability.

6 More efficient use of muscle force occurs when the object is turned or

moved toward the worker's body. To move an object toward oneself, the flexors of the elbows supply the force. These muscles are stronger than the elbow extensors, which are used when pushing or turning an object away from oneself. It should also be remembered that this is a safer procedure since the nurse has greater control over the patient's body when the turning is done toward herself.

7 When possible, move a patient by sliding or turning, as opposed to lifting. If an object is lifted, additional effort must be used to overcome the force of gravity.

8 Move a patient on a level surface as as opposed to an inclined plane. Lower the headrest (unless contraindicated) when sliding a patient toward the head of the bed.

9 Utilize smooth continuous movements as opposed to jerky start-and-stop movements. Less effort is needed to keep an object moving than to start its movement.

10 Use of a lifting or turning sheet decreases the amount of contact surface and, by so doing, lessens the friction between the patient and the supporting surface. When using a lifting sheet, it is helpful (when possible) to have the patient flex his knees and hips and to raise his head off the mattress.

11 When feasible, support a patient's body or extremity by utilizing the elbow lift.

12 When strenuous activity is required, prepare for it by setting the pelvis; i.e., retract the abdominal muscles and contract the gluteal muscles. Sometimes this is referred to as pelvis tilt. "Up in front, down in back" and "pull and pinch" are instructions sometimes used to convey this concept to the student.

13 Never lift an excessive load in an attempt to keep from asking for help.

Joint motion—nursing assessment skills

Examination of the musculoskeletal system involves testing for function as well as structure. Thus, observation of the patient's ability to move about, to sit, and to stand will provide the observer with valuable information. The presence of joint stiffness and deformity, lack of muscle coordination, signs of muscle weakness, and evidence of pain or discomfort may be apparent when an activity such as walking is observed.

As each joint is examined, the alignment, range of motion, contour, and size are noted and compared with the opposite side. Surrounding muscles are observed for atrophy, and the general skin condition is checked. The presence of tenderness, increased amounts of fluid, swelling, a thickened synovial membrane, and increased warmth of the overlying skin may be detected by gentle palpation about the joint area. When swelling (effusion) of a joint is present, or there is thickening of the synovial membrane, the normal hollow areas about the joint may be absent depending on the degree of swelling. Normally one is not able to palpate the synovial membrane, which lines the joint capsule. However, a thickened synovial membrane feels "doughy" or "boggy." The presence of an inflamed and enlarged bursa should not be confused with joint swelling. Usually the bursa swelling is smaller. Sometimes a grating sensation, caused by a roughening of the joint cartilage, may be heard or felt as the joint is moved. This is known as crepitus. Cupping the hand over the joint area as motion is checked enables the examiner to detect the presence of crepitation.

To record range-of-motion findings, a vocabulary to describe position and motion is necessary, and for this reason the following explanation of various terms has been included.

abduction means moving or withdrawing of a limb away from the medial line of the body, hand, or foot.

adduction means moving or drawing of a limb toward the medial line of the body, hand, or foot.

circumduction involves circular movements of a limb or part of the body around a stationary disk; this motion is a group of motions that include flexion, abduction, extension, and adduction.

eversion as applied to the foot means turning the sole of the foot outward.

extension means to straighten; with this motion the joint angle is increased, and the adjoining

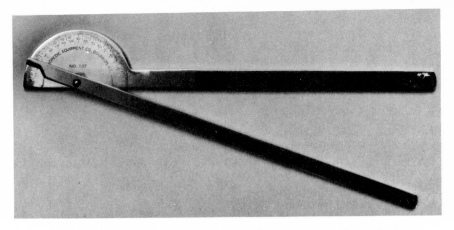

Fig. 47 Goniometer—instrument used for measuring joint motion.

segments of a limb or part of the body are moved toward a straight position.

external rotation involves turning of the limb away from the midline of the body.

flexion means to bend; with flexion of a joint, the joint angle is decreased and the adjoining segments of the limb or body parts come closer together.

dorsiflexion of the ankle means the top surface of the foot approaches the anterior surface of the lower leg.

dorsiflexion of the wrist means the hand is moved so that the back of the hand approaches the posterior aspect of the forearm.

palmar flexion of the wrist means the hand is moved so that the palm of the hand approaches the anterior aspect of the forearm.

plantar flexion is used to describe extension of the ankle; the foot is bent down into the toe-walking position.

hyperextension means excessive extension of a limb or part of the body, beyond the normal arc of motion; an example is recurvatum deformity of the knee joint (Fig. 75).

internal rotation involves turning of the limb toward the midline of the body.

inversion as applied to the foot means turning the sole of the foot inward.

opposition is a term used to describe the movement involved in placing the palmar surface of the thumb against the fingers.

pronation as applied to the forearm means turning the palm downward with the thumb toward the body.

rotation is the process of turning around a central axis.

supination as applied to the forearm means turning the palm forward or upward with the thumb away from the body.

The motion that is normally present for any given joint is known as the range of motion. Joint motion is measured in degrees of a circle by means of a goniometer

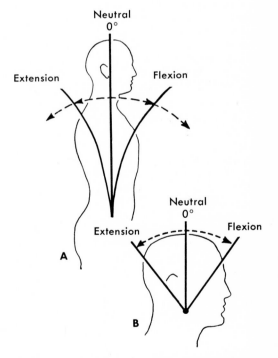

Fig. 48 A, Flexion and extension of the thoracic and lumbar segments of the spine. Lateral bend or flexion (not illustrated) consists of moving the trunk laterally from the neutral position. **B,** Flexion and extension of the cervical segment of the spine. Lateral bend or flexion (not illustrated) consists of moving the head from the neutral position laterally. The ear approximates the corresponding shoulder.

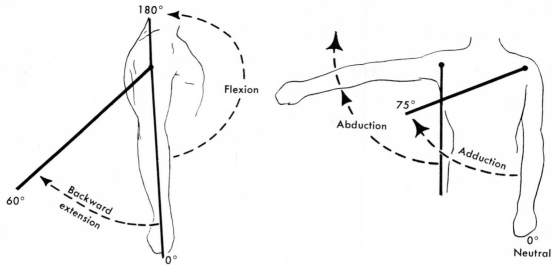

Fig. 49 Flexion and extension of the arm. With the arm in a neutral position, flexion to approximately 180° is accomplished by moving the arm forward and upward. Flexion to 180° includes scapular motion. Extension consists of moving the arm down and backward to the side of the body. Approximately 60° of backward extension is possible—from the neutral starting position.

Fig. 50 Abduction and adduction of the shoulder. With the arm in a neutral position, abduction to approximately 180° may be accomplished by moving the arm outward and upward from the side of the body. Abduction to 180° includes scapulothoracic motion as well as glenohumeral motion. Adduction consists of returning the arm toward the midline of the body. This motion may be continued in an upward direction beyond the midline of the body to approximately 75°.

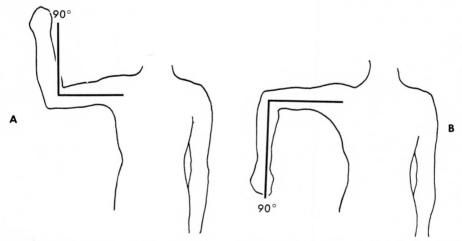

Fig. 51 Rotations at the shoulder joint are measured in two positions: (1) with the elbow at the side and flexed 90° from the anatomic position and (2) with the arm abducted 90° and the elbow flexed. The diagrams indicate the second method—the more common measurement. **A,** External rotation of the shoulder to approximately 90°. This is accomplished by raising the forearm and hand from the neutral position. **B,** Internal rotation of the shoulder to approximately 90°. The forearm and hand are lowered from the neutral position.

(Fig. 47). The "neutral zero method" (approved by The American Academy of Orthopaedic Surgeons) provides that the motion be measured from a defined starting point known as the neutral zero position. The neutral zero position for each joint is the position of that joint in the anatomic position. When the term *anatomic position* is used, it refers to the body in the standing position with the palms of the hands facing forward and the toes and kneecaps pointing forward. Thus, the neutral zero position for several of the body joints is that of extension. The following example will serve to illustrate this method of measuring and recording joint motion. The elbow joint in extension is at 0° (neutral zero method). As the forearm and hand are moved toward the shoulder, degrees of motion may be estimated or measured with the goniometer. Normal range of motion for the elbow is 0-150° (approximately). If an individual is unable to extend the elbow beyond a right angle, this would be referred to as a flexion deformity of 90° with further flexion to 150°. The range of motion for this elbow would be 90-150°. The student interested in obtaining detailed information pertaining to joint range of motion and the measuring and recording of joint motion should consult the American Orthopaedic Association's *Manual of orthopaedic surgery*.[17]

Knowledge of the range of joint motion enables the nurse to detect early limitations of motion. When limitations are anticipated or are recognized early, preventive measures against further restrictions can be instituted.

Figs. 48 to 62 will help the nurse gain an understanding of normal ranges of joint motion. Such knowledge is considered fundamental to the application of nursing care that will minimize or prevent any limitations from disuse. However, all degrees of motion illustrated must be interpreted as the approximate degrees of motion possible and not as a standard or an average. Since ranges of joint motion vary widely among individuals, the patient's normal extremity may better serve as a standard or a guide pertaining to his range of motion.

The presence of joint stiffness or limitation of motion in the upper extremity may

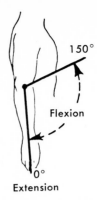

Fig. 52 Flexion and extension of the elbow.

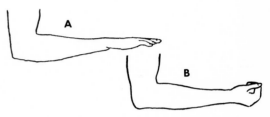

Fig. 53 Pronation and supination of the forearm. In the neutral position, the forearm is supported so that the thumb and index finger are uppermost, weight of the forearm rests on the little finger or ulnar side, and the elbow is flexed 90°—not illustrated. **A**, Pronation is accomplished by turning the forearm 80° to 90° so that the palm side of the hand is facing downward. **B**, Supination consists of turning the forearm from the neutral position, 80° to 90°, so that the palm side of the hand is facing upward.

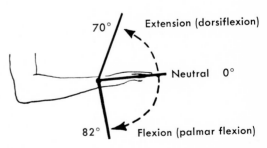

Fig. 54 Wrist flexion and extension. Ulnar deviation and radial deviation are not illustrated. Ulnar deviation consists of moving the hand from the neutral position toward the ulnar or little finger side of the hand. With radial deviation, the hand is moved toward the radial or thumb side of the hand (see Fig. 68, **D** and **E**).

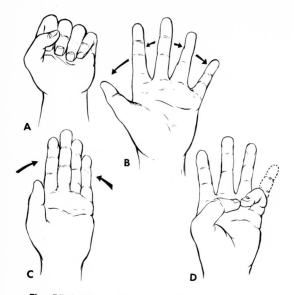

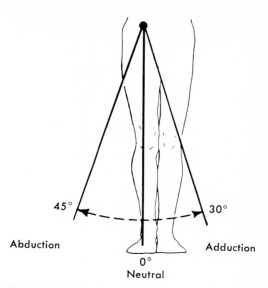

Fig. 55 A, Finger flexion. **B,** Finger extension and abduction. **C,** Finger extension and adduction. **D,** Thumb opposition—thumb is moved in a circling motion (outward and around) to the little finger.

Fig. 57 Abduction and adduction of the hip. With the limb in a neutral position, abduction of the hip to approximately 45° is accomplished by moving the limb outward from the body's midline. Adduction to approximately 30° is accomplished by moving the limb toward and across the body's midline.

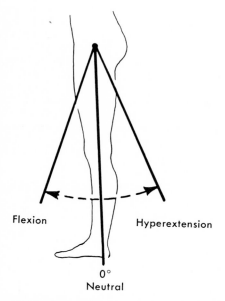

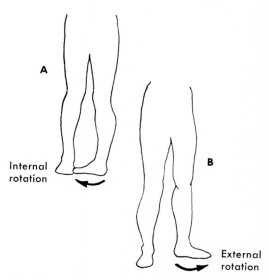

Fig. 56 Flexion and extension of the hip. With the limb initially in a neutral position, flexion is accomplished by bringing the limb forward. To measure the true extent of hip flexion, the knee must be simultaneously flexed to relax the hamstring restraint. Extension consists of lowering the limb to the neutral position. Further extension (hyperextension) may be produced by moving the limb backward.

Fig. 58 Internal and external rotation of the hip. (In the neutral position, the limb is in a position of extension with the kneecap and foot pointing forward—not illustrated.) **A,** Internal rotation is accomplished by turning the limb toward the midline of the body. **B,** External rotation is accomplished by turning the limb away from the midline.

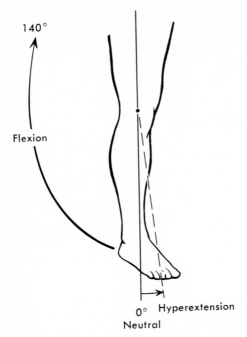

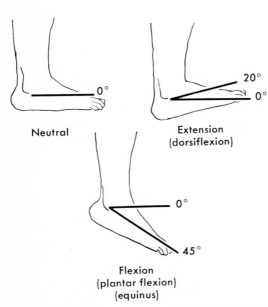

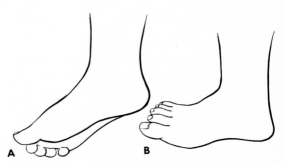

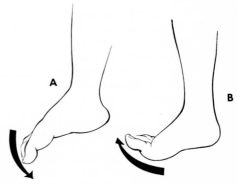

50

be noted by simply asking the patient to do the following:

1 Spread and close the extended fingers; this provides for extension of the phalangeal joints and for abduction and adduction of the metacarpal phalangeal joints.
2 Make a fist, with the thumb crossing the fingers; this provides for flexion of the phalangeal joints.
3 Reach the arms forward; this provides for flexion of the shoulder joints and extension of the elbow joints.
4 Turn the palms up and down; this provides for supination and pronation of the forearms.
5 Raise the arms over the head and place the hands behind the head; this provides for flexion of the elbow joints and abduction and external rotation of the shoulder joints.

Fig. 59 Flexion and extension of the knee. With the knee in the neutral position, flexion to approximately 140° is accomplished by bending the knee. Extension to the neutral position is the motion opposite to flexion. A small amount of motion beyond the neutral position is possible. This is an unnatural position known as hyperextension.

Fig. 61 A, Inversion—sole of the foot turned toward medial aspect of the body. **B,** Eversion—sole of the foot turned toward lateral aspect of the body.

Fig. 60 Dorsiflexion and plantar flexion of the ankle.

Fig. 62 A, Flexion of the toes. **B,** Hyperextension of the toes.

Normally, movements of the body parts will maintain joint motion and prevent tightness of soft tissue. When motion is present, connective tissue is reorganized and replaced in proper alignment. This permits stretching and shortening of the muscle fibers and is essential to good range of motion. When disuse of a muscle occurs, the areolar connective tissue becomes dense and fibrous, and this tends to limit motion or make it difficult. The avoidance of a shortened or stretched position of a muscle for long periods of time is necessary to prevent fibrosis of the tissue and limited motion of the involved joint. With immobilization, degenerative changes also occur in the joint. The intracapsular fatty connective tissue grows excessively and forms adhesions with the nonweight-bearing surfaces of the ligaments and bones. Narrowing of the joint space occurs, and the joint cartilage becomes thin. Restriction of motion accompanies these changes. Self-care activities, passive or active exercises, and frequent change of body positions are preventive measures.

There is no active contraction of the muscle fibers with passive motion exercise. The extremity is moved through a range of motion by the therapist or nurse. This type of exercise is prescribed in the presence of paralysis or marked weakness of muscles. Passive exercise does not maintain or develop muscle strength but helps to prevent adaptive shortening or stretching of involved muscles and the tightening of the joint capsule and ligaments.

With active motion exercise, there is contraction of muscle fibers and movement of extremities. This type of exercise, in addition to maintaining range of motion, helps to maintain or increase muscle strength and function. Active assistive exercise may be utilized when the muscle contraction is too weak to produce motion of an extremity without assistance. Varying degrees of assistance may be provided by the therapist or by some mechanical device. In some instances, relieving the pull of gravity is sufficient to make motion possible. To increase muscle strength, resistive exercise may be prescribed. As the patient moves an extremity through a range of motion, resistance to the motion is provided.

Isotonic exercise is an exercise in which the length of the entire muscle changes. It may become shorter or longer and in so doing causes movement of the part of the body to which it is attached. Concentric contraction means a shortening of the muscle, and eccentric contraction means a lengthening. When an isometric exercise is performed, the length of the total muscle does not change and there is no movement of body parts. This type of exercise may be used to maintain the strength of a particular group of muscles when movement of the involved joint is undesirable. The quadriceps setting exercise is an example of isometric (static) exercise. With the knee in extension, maximum tensing of the muscle can be produced without movement of the knee joint (Fig. 415). This may be an important exercise for a patient in traction or for one wearing a cast. Isometric or muscle-setting exercise of the abdominal, gluteal, and quadriceps muscles may be very beneficial to the patient confined to bedrest. These exercises help to strengthen the antigravity or postural muscles of the body.

Many self-care activities provide for some degree of active exercise and range of motion. The patient who brushes his own hair or ties the neck strings of his hospital gown abducts and externally rotates his arms. Active use of the uninvolved extremities and joints is not considered corrective therapy but is aimed at preventing disuse problems related to the musculoskeletal system. However, when planning range-of-motion exercises and self-care activities, care and judgment must be used to make certain that the activity utilized is in keeping with the patient's general physical condition. With some patients, the nurse needs specific orders for an exercise program, and she also must be aware that any exercise regime for the involved extremity or joint is prescribed by the physician.

Passive range-of-motion exercise may be a part of the bath procedure for the patient with paralyzed extremities. When bathing the axillary region, the nurse moves the arm away (abduction) from the patient's side. Bending and straightening the elbow provides for flexion and extension. The movements of the wrist, plus closing and opening the hand for finger flexion

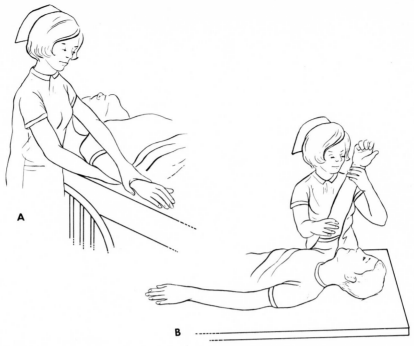

Fig. 63 Flexion and extension of the shoulder joint. **A,** With the patient in the supine position and his arm lying at his side (thumb side uppermost), support the elbow and hand as illustrated. **B,** Lift the arm straight up and toward the head of the bed (flexion). Return the arm to the patient's side (extension). Do not abduct the shoulder. Note that the patient's elbow may need to be flexed as his hand nears the head of the bed.

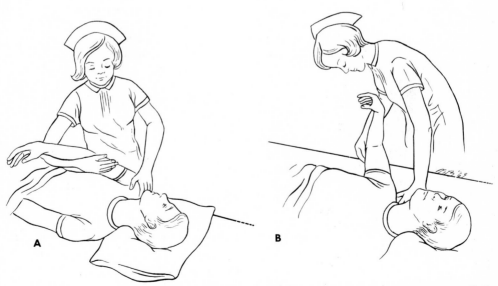

Fig. 64 Abduction of the shoulder joint. **A,** With the patient in the supine position, "cradle" his arm as illustrated. Use your other hand to hold his shoulder in a fixed position. **B,** Move the patient's arm away from his side (maintain the arm at bed level).

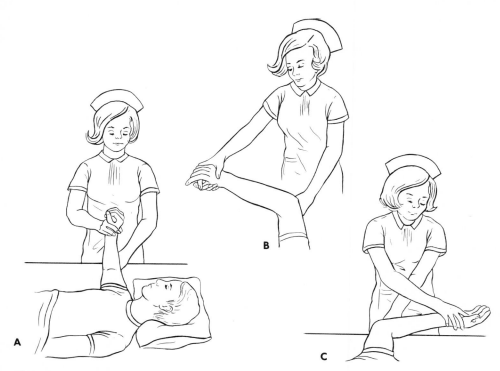

Fig. 65 Internal and external rotation of the shoulder joint. **A,** With the patient in the supine position, the upper arm supported on the bed in a position of abduction (90°) and the elbow flexed (90°), grasp his hand, supporting his thumb with your fingers. Your thumb is on the dorsal aspect of his hand. **B,** Move the forearm toward the bed, palm downward (internal or medial rotation). **C,** Return the forearm to the starting position and move it backward toward the bed with the palm upward (external or lateral rotation).

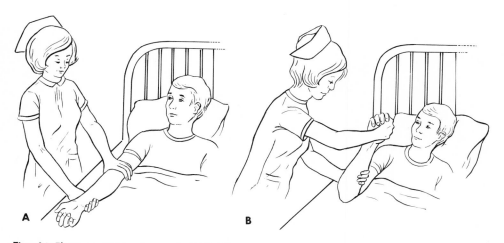

Fig. 66 Flexion of the elbow. **A,** With the patient in the supine position, his arm resting at his side, palm side uppermost, support his hand and wrist as illustrated. **B,** Flex his elbow, moving the hand toward his shoulder. Straighten the elbow by returning his hand to the bed (extension).

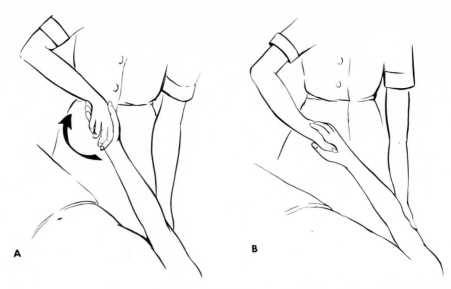

Fig. 67 Supination and pronation of the forearm. **A,** With the patient in the supine position, and supporting his hand in a hand-shaking position and his bent elbow with your other hand, turn the palm of his hand upward (supination). **B,** Turn the palm of his hand downward (pronation).

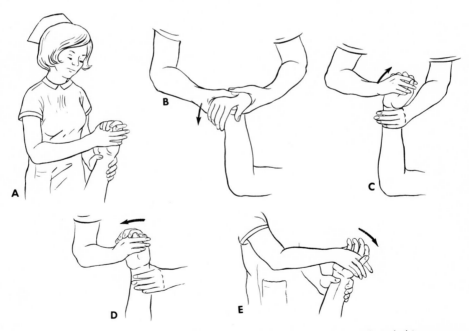

Fig. 68 Wrist motion. **A,** With the patient in the supine position and with his upper arm resting on the bed and his elbow flexed, support his forearm with one hand, and with your other hand grasp his hand, supporting his thumb with your fingers. **B,** Flex his wrist by moving the palm of his hand toward his forearm. **C,** Move his hand backward, with palm turned upward (dorsiflexion or extension). **D,** Supporting his wrist in the neutral position, move his hand toward the "little finger" side (ulnar flexion). **E,** Move his hand toward the "thumb side" of his hand (radial flexion).

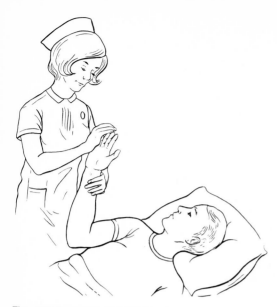

Fig. 69 Finger flexion. With the patient's elbow flexed and resting on the bed, support his extended wrist with one hand. Place your other hand and fingers (palm side) over the dorsum of his hand and fingers. Flex his fingers to make a fist. Fingers are then straightened. Thumb opposition (not illustrated)—with the elbow resting on the bed and the fingers held in extension, move the thumb in a circling motion (outward and around) toward the little finger.

and extension, can be accomplished nicely as the extremity is bathed and dried. Raising and lowering the leg and bending the knee provide for flexion and extension of the hip and knee joints. Moving the leg toward the edge of the bed helps maintain the motion of abduction, and rolling the limb in provides for internal rotation. Simple dorsiflexion of the foot during the bath procedure will help prevent tightening of the heel cord (Achilles tendon). These joint motions performed by a nurse who knows how to support and move a paralyzed extremity can be most helpful in preventing joint contractures.

When performing passive range of motion, care must be taken that all movements are done slowly and smoothly. The patient should be relaxed and in a comfortable position. Movements should be pain-free, and the existing range of motion should not be exceeded unless the attending physician has prescribed passive exercise to provide for stretching of tight muscles. The person performing passive exercises supports the patient's extremity by cradling it in his arm (Fig. 64) or by cupping his hands beneath the joints (Fig. 65). Grasping of muscle bellies is uncomfortable to the patient and should be

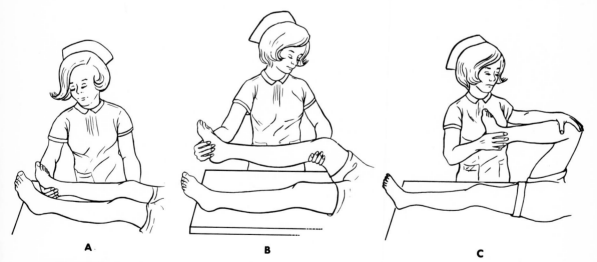

A   **B**   **C**

Fig. 70 Flexion and extension of the hip and knee. **A,** With the patient in the supine position, place one hand beneath his knee and use the other to support his heel. **B,** Flex the knee and hip as the limb is lifted off the bed. Maintain the limb in a neutral position (without external rotation or abduction). **C,** As you move and guide the knee toward the patient's chest, move your hand from beneath the knee to the patella region. As you slowly return the limb to the bed, support the knee again with your hand as shown in **B.**

avoided. Figs. 63 to 74 will be helpful to the nurse who is responsible for providing passive range-of-motion exercise for a paralyzed or otherwise inactive patient.

Joint deformities

In addition to the terminology used to describe joint movements, an understanding of the following terms used to describe joint deformities will be helpful.

calcaneal indicates a deformity in which only the heel touches the ground.
coxa refers to the hip joint.
  coxa plana indicates a flattening of the epiphysis of the head of the femur.
  coxa valga describes an increase in the joint angle (Fig. 75).

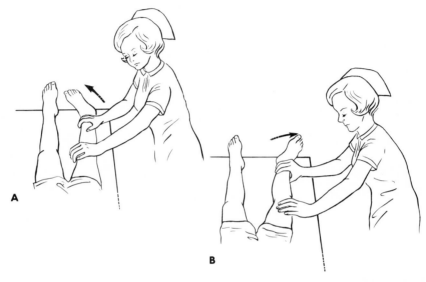

Fig. 71 Internal and external rotation of the hip joint. **A,** With the patient in the supine position, place one hand above his ankle and the other above his knee. Gently roll the thigh and lower leg toward the midline and then return to the neutral position. **B,** Roll the entire leg outward, away from the midline.

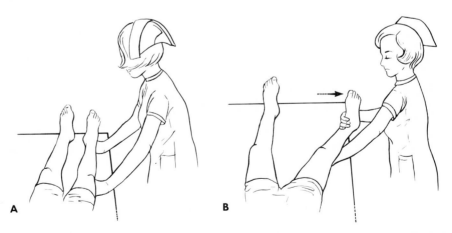

Fig. 72 Abduction and adduction of the hip joint. **A,** With the patient in the supine position, place one hand beneath his ankle and heel, and the other hand beneath his knee. **B,** Move the limb slowly and gently toward the edge of the bed, keeping it at bed level and in a neutral position (no external rotation). Then move it back toward the midline of the body as shown in **A.**

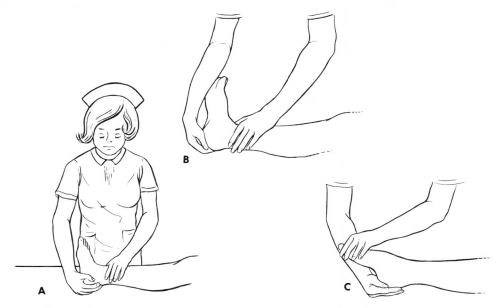

Fig. 73 Dorsiflexion and plantar flexion of the foot. **A,** With patient in the supine position, grasp his heel with one hand, permitting the sole of his foot to rest against your forearm. Support the limb just above the ankle with the other hand. **B,** Use the forearm to dorsiflex the foot. **C,** Move the hand on the ankle to his forefoot and place the foot in a plantar-flexed position.

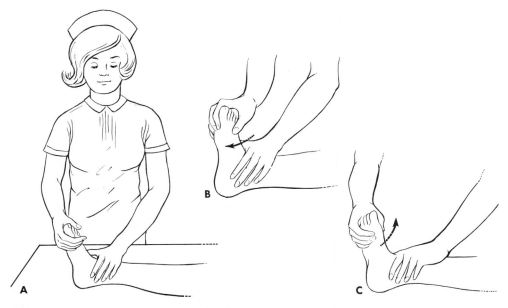

Fig. 74 Inversion and eversion of the foot. **A,** With the patient in the supine position, grasp his forefoot with one hand (fingers on the plantar surface of the foot). With the other hand, hold the limb at the ankle region. **B,** Move the foot toward the "little" toe side of the foot (eversion). **C,** Move the foot toward the midline of the body (inversion).

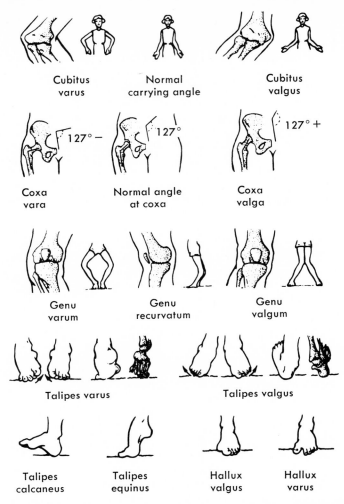

Cubitus varus   Normal carrying angle   Cubitus valgus

Coxa vara   Normal angle at coxa   Coxa valga

Genu varum   Genu recurvatum   Genu valgum

Talipes varus   Talipes valgus

Talipes calcaneus   Talipes equinus   Hallux valgus   Hallux varus

Fig. 75 Common orthopedic deformities. (Adapted from American Orthopaedic Association: Manual of orthopaedic surgery, Chicago, 1970.)

coxa vara indicates a decrease in the joint angle.

cubitus means elbow; when combined with the adjectives varus or valgus, it describes a deformity of the elbow (Fig. 75).

equinus is a deformity in which the individual walks on the toes or anterior part of the foot; the foot is in a fixed plantar flexion position.

genu refers to the knee joint; when combined with the terms varum or valgum, it describes a deformity of the knee joint.

hallux refers to the great toe; when combined with the word valgus, it describes a position wherein the big toe inclines excessively toward the outer toes.

pes cavus deformity designates an exaggeration of the plantar arch (longitudinal arch) of the foot.

planus designates a "flatfoot" position; the longitudinal arch is absent.

recurvatum means a backward bending or curvature; an example is genu recurvatum—hyperextension of the knee.

talipes (*talus* plus *pes* means ankle-foot) refers to a deformity of the foot; when combined with the words calcaneus, equino-, varus, or valgus, it describes a specific deformity of the foot.

valgus deformity means that the part of the body distal to the joint is directed away from the midline.

varus describes a change from normal alignment wherein that part of the body distal to the joint is directed toward the midline of the body.

Muscle evaluation—nursing assessment skills

Assessment of the muscles involves observation, palpation, and measurement for size and possible atrophy. *Atrophy* means loss of muscle mass and is found secondary to disuse or paralysis. The reasons for disuse of a muscle or group of muscles are numerous and include such causes as loss of nerve supply due to injury or disease, the presence of pain in an extremity, or immobilization produced by a cast or other apparatus. When a muscle is not used in a normal fashion, muscle wasting occurs. Symmetry of the right and left extremities is checked, and for accurate comparison the circumference of the thighs, calves, and upper arms may be measured (Fig. 26). Posture and muscle contours are checked for symmetry. Wasting of the small muscles of the hand may become apparent as the hands are compared. In addition, abnormalities of muscle tone are evaluated as the extremity is moved passively. Diminished muscle tone can be expected with general disability, inactivity, emaciation, and malnutrition. Any evidence of muscle spasticity, rigidity, or flaccidity also is noted.

With *flaccid* paralysis the muscles are small, flabby, atrophic, and weak. When a paralyzed muscle is opposed by a normal muscle, deformity of the involved joint may be present. A weak or paralyzed dorsiflexor of the foot opposed by a healthy gastrocnemius muscle will result in an equinus (drop-foot) deformity. Gravity and the unopposed gastrocnemius muscle maintain the foot in a position of plantar flexion.

With *spastic* paralysis, the muscle is tight and tense and movements will be uncoordinated. This type of paralysis is seen with upper motor neuron lesions.

Hypertrophy or overdevelopment of muscles may be observed in the person who does heavy labor or actively engages in sports. A vigorous exercise program is prescribed for the paraplegic individual to help him overdevelop the muscles of his upper extremities to do transfer activities as substitutes for lack of function in the legs.

When *pseudohypertrophy* (false) of muscles is present (dystrophies), the muscle appears large but has little strength due to replacement of muscle fibers with fatty tissue.

Strength of the various muscles is tested as joint movements are done. Corresponding muscles on each side of the body are compared. The examiner may test and compare the strength of the finger muscles by asking the patient to use full strength in a handclasp. The strength of the biceps (elbow flexor) and the triceps (elbow extensor) may be evaluated and the right and left arms compared by asking the patient to flex the elbow partially and to maintain that position as the examiner grasps the hand or wrist and pulls or pushes in an attempt to increase flexion or extension of the elbow. Strength of the quadriceps muscle may be checked by asking the patient (in the supine position) to elevate his leg to 45° keeping the knee in extension, and to hold this position for fifteen to twenty seconds (Fig. 416). Inability to prevent "wobbling" or "drifting" is a sign of muscle weakness. Inability to walk on the toes or the heels may indicate weakness of the muscles in the lower extremities.

It is important that evaluation of muscle strength be recorded in terms of general use. This makes it possible to compare and determine increases or decreases in strength at a later date.

Mechanics of human gait—nursing assessment skills

Gait is man's self-powered means of travel from one place to another, to reach a position to see, to hear, or to perform a task. There is no means of transportation as versatile as man's bipedal locomotion to adapt to diverse terrain and simultaneously protect the brain and vital organs against sudden impacts of heel strike.

Normal gait is accomplished by a series of intricate and coordinated muscle and joint actions of the legs and trunk. The coordinated actions require energy (or force) and direction to carry the body forward in a smooth gliding fashion. A normal person tends to walk at a fairly well-defined velocity of 2.5 mi/hr, at a cadence of 90-110 steps/min, and an average step length of 30-40 in. Energy consumption at this velocity seems to be optimal. Whenever a person lacks the required range of motion in the joints or muscle strength and central nervous system balance and coordination, he will limp or have to exaggerate other actions to compensate for the deficiencies.

Children up to 3 or 4 years of age whose early walking patterns are evolving from the stage of support to no support have less uniform gait patterns than older children and adults. From step to step they show variability in speed, stride length, cadence, and knee and ankle motion patterns. A limp in a young child must be consistent before it can be qualified as a gait abnormality. Not infrequently a show-off tendency, mimicry, or a bid for attention will be responsible for gait pecularities in young children, so that again a consistent presence and a consistent pattern should be observed before a pathologic cause is ascribed to the abnormality.

To recognize and appreciate abnormal gaits, it is necessary to have some understanding of what constitutes a normal walking pattern. With a normal walking pat-

tern, forward progression of the body is accomplished with a minimal amount of energy and time, and, in addition, a smooth, nonjarring ride is provided for the body's vital organs.

In the normal standing position, the body's center of gravity is centrally located and the body's weight is supported by both lower extremities. As a step is taken, one support is removed. To prevent falling, the individual must counteract the pull of gravity by shifting his body weight over the supporting hip and extremity, or by applying a force in the opposite direction that is equal to the pull of gravity. Con-

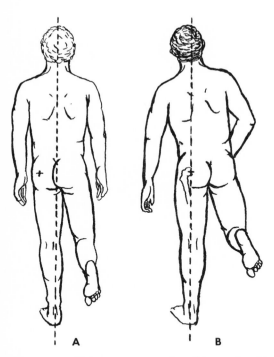

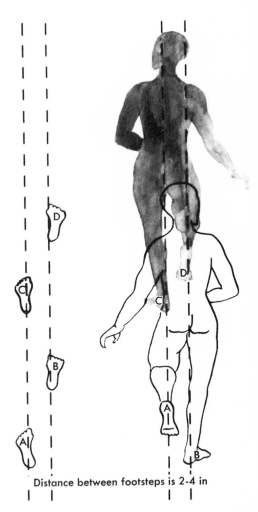

Distance between footsteps is 2-4 in

Fig. 76 A, Illustrates a normal walking gait with a small amount of side-to-side movement of the torso. **B,** Illustrates an abnormal amount of swaying from side to side. This sideward shift of the body enables the individual to maintain his balance (center of gravity is shifted over the weight-bearing limb) and is necessary when the abductor muscle of the hip is not functioning in a normal manner.

Fig. 77 The body shifts gently from side to side to assure that the center of gravity is supported on a single leg alternately.

traction of the gluteus medius (hip abductor) supplies this massive holding force and enables the individual to maintain his balance and to move forward without an abnormal side-to-side movement of the torso with each step (Fig. 76).

In a normal walking pattern, the individual walks with his feet two to four inches apart and shifts his body laterally about one inch (Fig. 77). If the abductor muscle of the hip is not capable of functioning, the person will walk with a marked lateral shift of the torso toward the weight-bearing limb (Fig. 76). The lateral shift is necessary to maintain balance. This gait is referred to as an "abductor lurch" or a "Trendelenburg gait" and may be observed in the individual with paralysis of the abductor muscle or with a mechanical insufficiency of the hip joint due to injury or disease. It is evident to the observer that walking with this type of gait not only is time-consuming, but also requires more energy and consequently is more fatiguing.

Observing the normal walking pattern in the lateral plane reveals the individual bearing weight on the forward limb while his center of gravity is behind the forward weight-bearing limb (Fig. 78, A). Falling

backward is resisted by contraction of the hip flexors (iliopsoas). As the forward motion of the body continues (Fig. 78, B), the body's center of gravity is balanced over the hip joint, and with continued forward movement of the body and movement of the opposite limb forward, the center of gravity shifts to a position anterior to the weight-bearing limb (Fig. 78, C). In this position the gluteus maximus (hip extensors) contracts and resists the body falling forward. Thus with each step forward, there is alternate use of the hip flexors and extensors and alternate use of the right and left hip abductors. The actions of these muscles enable the individual to maintain the upright position, even though his center of gravity is not directly over the limb supporting his weight. The contraction of each of these muscles during various stages of each step impacts a force roughly equivalent to balancing the weight of the torso. Consequently, during various phases of walking, a load equal to three body weights is placed on the hip joint (gravity, abductor balance, and flexor-extensor balance.)[17]

As one of the limbs is moved forward to take a step, there must be some means of

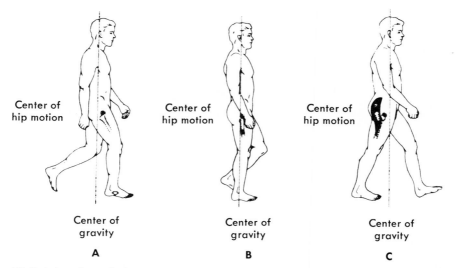

Center of hip motion   Center of hip motion   Center of hip motion

Center of gravity   Center of gravity   Center of gravity

A   B   C

Fig. 78 Gait in a lateral plane. **A,** As weight is taken on the forward limb, the individual's center of gravity (indicated by the vertical line) is behind the weight-bearing foot. **B,** As forward movement progresses, the individual's center of gravity is directly over the hip joint and the weight-bearing foot. **C,** With continued forward movement, the body's center of gravity moves in front of the weight-bearing foot. (From American Orthopaedic Association: Manual of orthopaedic surgery, Chicago, 1972.)

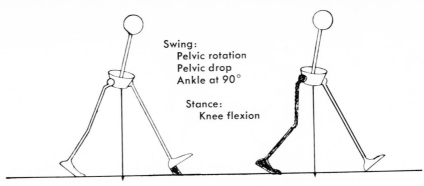

Fig. 79 Adjustment of limb length. To reach the desired point of ground contact without dropping abruptly, the reaching limb is lengthened relatively by pelvic rotation and pelvic drop and by holding the ankle at a right angle. The demand is lessened by slight flexion of the stance limb. (Reprinted from Perry, J.: The mechanics of walking, Phys Ther **47:**778-801, Sep 1967, by permission of the American Physical Therapy Association.)

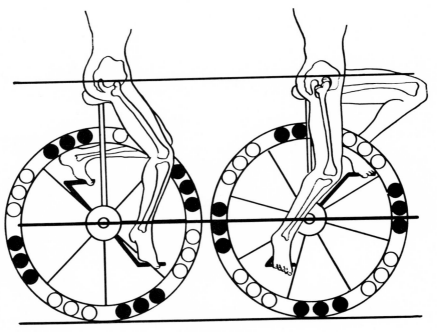

Fig. 80

enabling the forward limb to reach the floor, since the diagonal distance is greater than the vertical distance (Fig. 79). As the reaching limb is moved forward to take a step, the pelvis rotates forward and drops on that side. Also, the foot of the progressing limb is held at a right angle, allowing for heel strike, which provides additional length. In addition, some flexion of the weight-bearing knee lessens the vertical distance. These changes allow for adjustment of limb length and provide for a minimal up-and-down shift of the body's center of gravity, as forward progression is accomplished. If fused joints, paralyzed muscles, or joint contractures prevent this adjustment, the walking gait is altered considerably. More energy is consumed as the

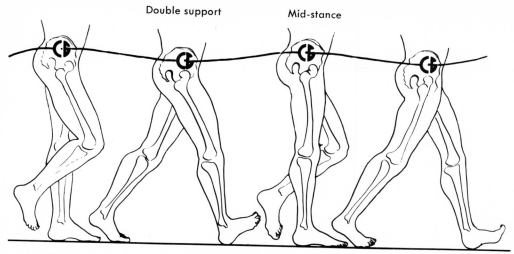

Double support   Mid-stance

Fig. 81 The heavy line follows the pathway of the body's center of gravity. The low point is at the moment of double support; the high point at mid-stance. The small rise and fall throughout the cycle of walking conserve energy.

body travels up and down as well as forward, and the forward movement is less smooth.

If the human body operated or moved like a wheel, the hub of the wheel (its center of gravity) would not oscillate up and down on smooth ground but would follow a straight line (Fig. 80). The center of gravity of the human body in walking follows a pathway that shifts up and down as well as from side to side in a smooth undulating fashion (Figs. 77 and 81). These shifts of body weight are kept to a minimum, since energy is required for each shift of lowering and raising the body weight in each cycle of gait. The shift, although minimal, is necessary in order to meet two requirement of bipedal gait:

1 One leg must support the body weight while the other leg swings (Fig. 77) forward to take a step (single leg stance).

2 The swinging leg cannot reach the ground unless the pelvis on the swing side is lowered and rotated forward to make heel contact with the ground (Fig. 79).

The pelvic dip and rotation are insufficient to allow the forward-swinging leg to contact the ground unless the knee of the weight-bearing limb is flexed simultaneous-

ly. The knee flexion lowers the center of gravity.

The two phases of a normal walking gait—*stance* and *swing*—occur simultaneously. One limb is in the stance phase while the other is in the swing phase. The swing phase begins as the weight is shifted off the leg (Fig. 81, left leg). The hip and knee are flexed. The limb is swung forward, and the knee is extended as the heel strikes the floor. The stance phase (Fig. 81, right leg) begins as the heel strikes the floor and ends after the foot is placed in a plantar-flexed position and the body weight has been shifted over to the opposite extended leg. As the heel strikes the floor, the ankle is at a right angle, the knee is fully extended, and the hip is flexed about 30°. Following heel strike, there is plantar flexion of the foot, decreased flexion of the hip, and, with toe-off, increased knee flexion. As the weight-bearing leg with the bent knee prepares to push the body forward at toe-off, the knee goes into extension at the same time that the foot pushes off from a position of equinus. The knee extension plus ankle extension in effect lengthen the trailing leg to prevent a rapid fall of the center of gravity. The center of gravity is at the low point when both feet are on the ground (double support) (Fig. 82) and at the high point at mid-

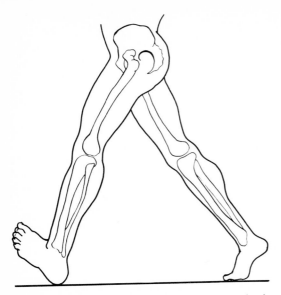

Fig. 82 When the leading foot receives body weight (heel strike) and the trailing foot pushes the body forward (push-off), double support takes only a fraction of the walking cycle time. This is the low point for the center of gravity of the body. The forward progression would be a sudden surge from the push-off energy unless the surge is modified by the heel strike, which receives the momentum and slows it to a steady progression by lowering the foot to the floor gradually.

stance. The walking base controls the horizontal side-to-side shift.

The muscle effort of push-off, which comes mainly from the gastrocnemius, is the force that accelerates the body forward. In order that each push does not constitute a forward surge, other muscles decelerate the body to keep the momentum smooth and uniform. The greatest acceleration of the forward progression of the body occurs as the heel of the reaching foot strikes the floor. The anterior tibial muscle is holding the foot in dorsiflexion at heel strike. The muscle lowers the foot slowly into a flatfoot position, and this serves to lessen the impact to the body at heel strike as well as to decelerate the forward momentum of the body.

In summary, the functional tasks of walking are forward progression, single-leg balance, and limb-length adjustment. When these are accomplished by proper body mechanics, normal walking becomes a

smooth, minimal rise and fall of the center of gravity and a fairly uniform forward acceleration with an optimal expenditure of energy.

A limp occurs whenever any individual component of joint motion or muscle force is abnormal. If the abnormality is known, it is possible to predict the type of limp to be expected. This approach may serve to focus the viewpoint of the observer on that portion of gait which is abnormal.

Classes of limp

The commonplace limps encountered may be more meaningfully reviewed if illustrated by specific abnormalities such as those related to hip pathology, knee problems, muscle diseases, etc.

Hip limps. The hip joint is the major weight-bearing joint in the body and must function properly to produce a normal gait. Body weight is balanced over a single ball-and-socket joint in stance phase. The hip joint is the fulcrum over which muscle force must provide balance. If the pelvis is to remain level when body weight is balanced on one hip, the mechanical arrangement resembles a seesaw (Fig. 83). The force of the abductor muscle on the outer end of the lever must equal the weight of the body at the inner end of the seesaw. The Trendelenburg test is negative if the pelvis remains level during the single-leg stance. The test is positive if the pelvis drops on the nonweight-bearing side (Fig. 84). A positive test indicates an abnormality in the abductor mechanism and will show an associated limp. In normal gait the pelvis must be tilted and rotated during the stance phase, as previously described. Also, the pelvis must be shifted laterally to receive body weight and keep the center of gravity over the base of support.

Limp in congenital dislocation of hip. In congenital dislocation of the hip, the pelvic fulcrum at the hip joint is lacking, which affects single-leg balance. As the body center of gravity shifts laterally to provide single-leg balance, the hip abductor cannot regulate pelvic tilt, which becomes excessive. Thus, the body falls sideways away from the dislocated side unless it can compensate by bending the spine toward the dislocated side. This can be observed in gait as a body lurch to the dislocated

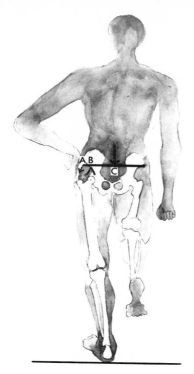

Fig. 83 The abductor mechanism of the hip allows single-leg stance to support the entire body weight. The pelvis is balanced on fulcrum **B,** the hip joint. The body weight at **C** must be balanced by an equal force at **A,** the abductor muscle. Ability to balance body weight and maintain a level pelvis in single-leg stance is known as a negative Trendelenburg test. If the abductor mechanism fails and the pelvis drops on the nonsupport side, the Trendelenburg test is positive.

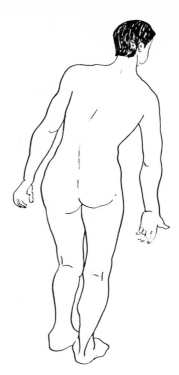

Fig. 84

side each time body weight is transferred to the dislocated limb. This has been called an abductor lurch or Trendelenburg gait (Fig. 84). It is indistinguishable from the gait caused by a paralyzed abductor muscle as often seen in a poliomyelitis victim. In bilateral dislocations the gait has been described as waddling.

Paralysis of the hip abductors. Paralysis of the hip abductors results in a limp similar to that seen in congenital dislocation of the hip. However, the lurch is likely to be of greater magnitude since the loss of all control of one end of the lever requires a greater compensatory shift of the body.

Stiff-hip gait. The word limp is deliberately not used here since an individual with

a hip that is stiff in a position of slight adduction, mild external rotation, and 30° of flexion will show very little abnormality in gait. If the hip is stiff in a position of 50° flexion, the gait will be altered in two components:

1 The pelvis cannot rotate forward or tilt downward when the stiff hip is in stance phase; thus the length of stride of the opposite limb is diminished.
2 At push-off, the hip cannot be extended; therefore, to compensate the lack of hip extension, the lumbar spine extends to allow an upright posture for the trunk (Fig. 85).

Limp in slipped capital femoral epiphysis. In slipped capital femoral epiphysis, the range of motion in the hip joint is altered, resulting in a limp. The hip lacks internal rotation. Therefore, pelvic rotation to extend the length of stride for the opposite limb will be lessened; however, the pathway of the center of gravity remains quite normal. As the gait is observed, two deviants are likely: (1) the involved limb will be externally rotated throughout the walk-

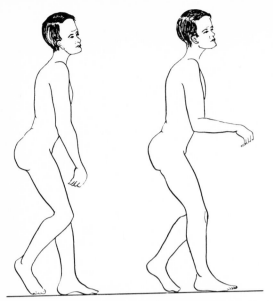

Fig. 85 Note that in bilateral stiff hips the angle of flexion remains constant and there is no swing phase of gait. The entire propulsion and limb-length adjustment occur at the knee and ankle.

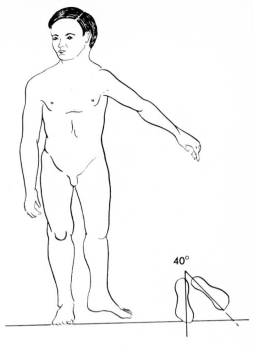

Fig. 86

ing cycle, and (2) the step length will be slightly shortened on the opposite side (Fig. 86). An antalgic component may be present if the hip is also painful.

Knee limps. In the consideration of knee limps, it should be kept in mind that both flexion and extension are needed in the knee to provide the center of gravity a smooth ride, to clear the floor for the swing-through limb, and to extend the leg to reach the floor at heel strike.

Knee flexion–deformity limp. Fixed flexion of 40° at the knee shortens the length of the limb; therefore, as the limb reaches forward for heel strike, the opposite knee must bend to lower the center of gravity more than usual. This has three observable effects on gait:

1 The rise and fall of the center of gravity will be more abrupt and greater from the mid-stance of the good limb to mid-stance of the flexed limb.
2 There will be a shorter step on the flexed limb.
3 Often, the flexed limb will walk on tiptoe to gain length.

If the deformity at the knee is 20°, the

compensatory mechanisms will allow a gait that seems almost normal to the casual observer.

Stiff-knee gait. If the leg length is normal and the knee is stiff in the extended position, there are two main problems:

1 Heel strike will be quite normal, but the knee flexion that occurs immediately after will be absent; this means that the center of gravity, starting low at heel strike, will rise to the normal height of mid-stance but in a more abrupt rather than gradual curve.
2 In the swing phase of the limb with the stiff knee, the foot will have difficulty clearing the ground; thus, in order to assure clearance, the limb will circumduct (swing out in an abduction circle) as the foot swings over the ground.

To the observer, the stiff knee gait in the stance phase can best be described as vaulting when the body is carried forward over the stiff-kneed limb, and in the swing phase there is a sweep of the leg laterally to replace the absence of flexion at the knee.

Other common limps. Other common

limps include short-leg limp, in-toeing, and antalgic and slap-foot (drop-foot) gaits.

Short-leg limp. A short leg will affect the limb-length adjustment and require the center of gravity to be lowered more than usual for the short limb to reach the floor

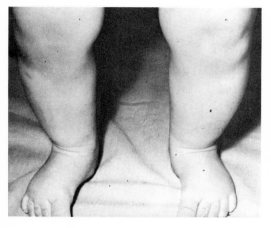

Fig. 87 Bilateral metatarsus adductus.

at heel strike. This can best be observed by watching the entire body drop more at heel strike on the short leg than at heel strike of the normal leg.

In-toeing. The most common gait problem in children under 5 years of age is that of in-toeing (pigeon toe). Whereas recognition of in-toeing is simple, the cause is not so clearly discernible. Three primary defects produce in-toeing, and the gait appears the same in each. To differentiate the primary defect, whether it be hip, knee, or foot, the observer must have knowledge of normal leg alignment. Normally in two-legged standing, the feet are separated 2-4 in, slightly toed out, the tibias are parallel to each other and perpendicular to the ground, the femurs angle outward from the knee the distance required to place the femoral heads into the acetabular sockets, and the kneecaps point straight ahead. The normal alignment just described will show three variants to account for in-toeing:

1 Metatarsus adductus, in which the feet appear toed-in because of the adducted

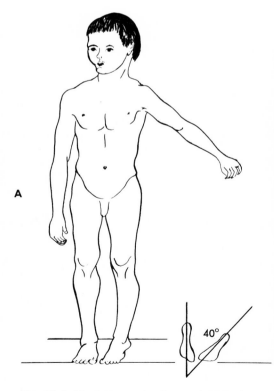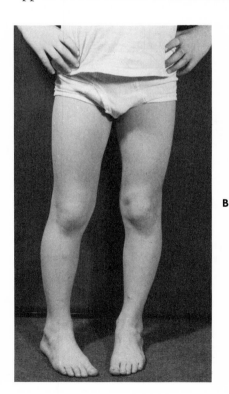

Fig. 88 A, The knees point forward properly, yet the left foot is toed-in because of internal torsion of the tibia. **B,** Internal torsion of the right tibia.

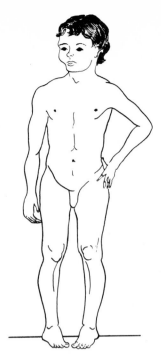

Fig. 89 Kneecaps point inward as do the feet, which indicates that the entire extremity is rotated inward at the hip joint. The usual cause is excessive anteversion of the femoral neck, which is normally 12° at growth completion. The anteversion in this in-toeing could well be 35°.

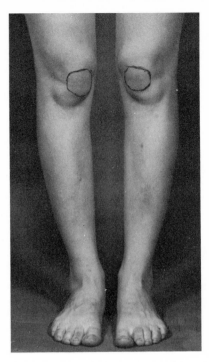

Fig. 90 Actual case of a 17-year-old girl with anteversion of 35° by roentgenographic measurement. Note the knees pointed inward and the feet straight ahead. Frequently the tibias show a compensatory external torsion.

position of the forefoot, which appears exaggerated in walking (Fig. 87).

2 Internal torsion of the tibia, in which the entire foot appears toed-in while the kneecap points straight ahead (Fig. 88).

3 Anteversion of the neck of the femur, in which the foot and kneecap are in proper alignment but both appear to be rotated internally; the internal rotation of the entire limb is an accommodation at the hip to rotate the trochanter forward for better mechanics of the abductor mechanism—a compensation to relieve the posterior position of the trochanter caused by anteversion (Figs. 89 and 90).

Antalgic gait. The word antalgic means relieving pain and often is used to refer to a limp. The term does not describe the limp, nor does it imply a specific mechanical component of gait; it is the same

as saying the limp relieves pain. Although the condition may appear in a variety of forms, there is one common denominator of all antalgic limps—viz., that the less time weight rests on the painful joint, the less pain; hence, the average antalgic limp is a "quick-step" gait, which is obvious to the observer. Other abnormalities of gait may be associated in the same individual; however, the associated limps are usually explainable by known associated deformities, limited motions, or muscle deficiencies. An antalgic limp relieves pain in any joint (the hip, knee, or ankle) or even pain caused by a nail in the shoe.

Slap-foot (drop-foot) gait. In the beginning of the stance phase of gait, at the time of heel strike, the limb is suddenly loaded by body weight that has just been propelled forward by the push-off limb. At the next instant, the dorsiflexed foot would be forced rapidly to the ground with a slap sound unless the foot were lowered more gradually. The gradual lowering is

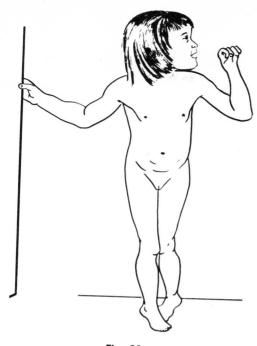

Fig. 91

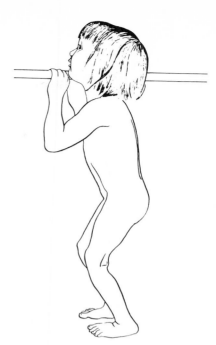

Fig. 92

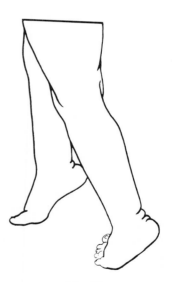

Fig. 93

accomplished by the anterior tibial and toe extensor muscles whose forces hold the foot dorsiflexed. A weakness of these muscles, as in peroneal palsy, allows the foot to slap to the ground. Likewise, if these muscles are absent, the foot is never dorsiflexed; instead of heel strike, the entire foot slaps flatly to the ground. In this instance, the observer will note two things: (1) the knee is raised higher in the swing phase to keep the dropped foot from scraping the ground and (2) there will be an audible slap as the foot strikes the ground.

Miscellaneous limps. Cerebral palsy, poliomyelitis, and neuromuscular defects are responsible for an array of limps and gait abnormalities that defy accurate description. Often the compensatory mechanisms alter the anticipated limp in the case of known muscle deficits. Inability of reciprocal muscle relaxation may restrict a joint movement in an otherwise normal joint. Cerebral imbalance from brain damage may produce a drunken gait. Lack of proprioceptive positional feedback will exaggerate the movements of an otherwise normal gait. Some individuals may be unable to walk in darkness since eyesight gives the only positional feedback.

Extensive spasticity is most commonly displayed by the scissor gait in which the extended legs become crossed from persistent overwhelming adductor muscle spasm. A jerky, slow deliberate effort manages to swing one leg past the other in each step (Fig. 91).

If the knees are simultaneously held in flexion by quadriceps and hamstrings in unrelenting spasticity, neither of which will relax to allow alternating motion, each leg will suddenly spring forward as though released from a spring trap at each step. The body center of gravity, usually riding with smooth even undulations, is now moved by a series of jerks (Fig. 92).

Add permanent spastic equinus to the flexed knees and scissored legs, and the commonly described jump gait is produced (Fig. 93). Take away the gastrocnemius, as in myelomeningocele, and the individual displays a calcaneal gait.

4 Nursing care problems associated with inactivity and immobilization

Muscle atrophy and joint contracture

Inactivity or prolonged bed rest can contribute to a number of complications by interfering with the physiologic processes of the body. Prolonged inactivity results in atrophy of muscle tissue, decreased endurance, and increased fatigability. Consequently, the individual is less active, and further muscle atrophy occurs. Muscle atrophy caused by disuse may be readily observed after removal of a plaster cast that has been worn for several weeks. The circumference of the involved leg is less than that of the normal limb, and the muscles appear flabby. Extended bed rest will cause similar atrophy. The antigravity muscles of the lower limb (glutei, quadriceps femoris, and gastrocnemius) are the muscles most affected.

From the study of physiology the student will remember that, in order to move joints, muscles must contract or relax. For maintaining the upright posture, however, they must have a constant slight contraction. This constant slight contraction is called muscle tonus or tone. A higher degree of muscle tonus is required to maintain the body in a standing position than is required for lying in bed. After a day of bed rest, one often feels a weakness out of all proportion to the minor illness he has experienced. From this common observation the student can easily understand that muscle tone may be greatly depleted when bed rest is continued over a considerable period of time. Muscles with diminished tone may become permanently stretched from being held in a lengthened position, or they can become contracted from being held in a shortened position, thus producing so-called myostatic contractures. In terms of the patient's well-being, these problems may mean a longer convalescence, discomfort on assuming the upright position, and possibly a persistent joint deformity. Even two weeks of bed rest in faulty positions may be sufficient to bring about contractures of important muscle groups.

If joint mobility is impaired by beginning contractures, more muscle energy is required to produce motion. This situation may be encountered when ambulation is attempted by the patient who has developed a hip-flexion contracture. Inability to fully extend the hip joint in the standing position interferes with easy balance of the body weight; therefore, increased muscle activity and strength are necessary to maintain the upright position and to ambulate.

The nurse also realizes that after a period of bed rest, even though there are no contractures, the patient will tire more quickly and his endurance for sitting in a chair or for walking will be markedly decreased. Walking short distances or sitting in a chair for short periods several times daily is more beneficial than extended periods of activity, which result in physical exhaustion.

A patient who is gravely ill sometimes receives less attention to body mechanics than do others on the unit. It is said, and with some reason, that the problem of keeping such a patient alive takes all the nurse's strength and energy and that effort should not be dissipated on minor details, but it is a mistake to forget that the desperately ill patient may recover. Indeed, one of the primary purposes of nursing is to help the patient get well if it is at all possible. No nurse wants a patient to recover from his original illness only to find that he has another handicap as a result of his confinement to bed. Our concern for the horizontal man must not allow us to forget the vertical one.

Many deformities develop in patients with debilitating illnesses because they lie in bed in positions of adduction and flexion. The student should understand that use of flexion is one of the ways the patient learns to relieve discomfort in his back, hips, and knees. Sometimes he assumes these positions to keep warm when he has insufficient circulation or covers. Proper nursing care should overcome at least some of these discomforts. Sometimes making the patient comfortable may be as simple as giving support to the lower portion of the back, a little gentle massage perhaps, or an extra blanket.

Change of position is also important. Any position, however adequate it may be as far as posture is concerned, will need frequent alteration. Human beings are not static, nor were they ever intended to be; movement is the very sine qua non of life itself. Sometimes these necessary alterations—from one type of good bed posture to another one equally good—will require all the nurse's ingenuity.

In all of these considerations, as in all treatment, the irreducible and stubborn fact remains that patients are human beings; they do not stay where they are put. They have their likes and dislikes about these things. The nurse may know that positions of good alignment usually produce more lasting comfort for the patient; nevertheless, if the patient has been in poor alignment so long that he has become accustomed to it, a little teaching and persuasion may be necessary. The student must understand that deformity cannot be corrected in a day and that zealousness should be tempered with patience and understanding. The patient's confidence and courage cannot be sacrificed in the attempt to overcome the results of neglect. Over-determination, nagging, or sharpness demonstrates a fractional approach to the patient's total problem.

Drop-foot deformity

Of particular significance in nursing is the fact that the tendon of the muscles of the calf tends to shorten if the foot is allowed to rest in an unsupported position, whereas the muscles in the anterior portion of the leg become stretched. Even a mild degree of this muscle imbalance can cause many weeks of painful discomfort. In the standing position, an individual with drop-foot deformity (equinus position) is unable to place his heel on the floor, and walking becomes difficult and tiring. With severe deformity, the patient is unable to wear shoes and must resort to a soft knit slipper. The cosmetic value of maintaining the foot in a functional position should not be overlooked.

Conscientious nursing care can do much to eliminate this unnecessary sequela of illness. Adequate support that maintains the feet (including the toes) in a functional position should be furnished during confinement to bed and exercises to maintain muscle strength and to prevent joint contractures should be utilized.

The patient should wear shoes rather than nonsupporting bedroom slippers when weight bearing is started after a period of bed rest. As previously stated, inactivity produces generalized weakening of the muscles and attritional thinning of the ligaments. With weight bearing, these ligaments and muscles, which support the arches of the feet, need the support of a well-fitted shoe. Arch strain caused by disuse atrophy of ligaments can be quite painful and disturbing to the patient.

Knee-flexion contractures

Another set of muscles that tends to contract quickly is the hamstring group of the posterior aspect of the thigh, whose tendons pass under the knee. Flexion of the knees continuously supported by pillows may bring about contractures in this group in a surprisingly short time. The nursing measures to counteract this are quite simple and obvious: pillows under the knees must be used with caution and with constant awareness that the position of the knees must be altered from flexion to extension at frequent periods.

Preventing flexion contracture of the knee is of special significance for the arthritic patient, since painful joints are more comfortable in the flexed position. The ability to fully extend the knee joint is also important for the below-the-knee amputee. A slight flexion contracture makes the fitting of a prosthesis difficult, if not impossible. To prevent flexion contracture of the knee, a posterior splint or traction that holds the joint in extension may be prescribed. With some patients, instruction in active exercise is needed. This includes quadriceps setting and straight leg raising (Figs. 415 and 416), as well as flexion and extension of the knee joint. Long periods of sitting with the knees flexed should be avoided. When flexion contracture is present at the knee joint, increased muscle strength is needed for walking, and consequently the act of walking is very tiring, frequently resulting in discouragement and decreased activity.

Hip deformities (flexion; adduction; external rotation)

Consider the problem of the patient with an acute condition of the abdomen that requires prolonged semisitting in a Gatch bed. Such a patient may develop flexion contractures of the hips and knees as well as drop foot. If he sits in a slumping position on the lumbar spine with his chest caved in and his shoulders sagging forward, pulled down by the weight of his arms, pain and muscle spasms are likely to occur in the muscles of the back, particularly those between the scapulae. The patient confined to bed is most likely to lose tone in the abdominal, gluteal, quadriceps, and tibial muscles and in those of the interscapular group—all muscles that will be of great importance when he becomes ambulatory again.

Even though the patient's condition is such that he must be kept in the sitting position, certain measures can be used that will afford him greater comfort and also minimize the after-effects of his illness. The nurse who understands the principles of

sitting posture will know that the weight of the body should be borne on the ischia and the thighs and therefore will make certain that the hips are back as far as possible in the angle of the bed in order to prevent the patient from slumping down and sitting on his sacrum or lumbar spine. Although flexion of the knees is necessary to relax the spinal extensor muscles, the knees must be extended fully several times during the day. The back should be supported in its entirety, and pillows must not be allowed to bunch up under the shoulders and head, thereby forcing the spine out of its normal curves. Recognizing the dangers of prolonged outward rotation at the hips, which so often accompanies such bed posture, the nurse can improvise a simple piece of equipment for overcoming this tendency— e.g., a sandbag, a pillow, or a trochanter roll. The customary type of footboard or a folded pillow (placed between the soles of the feet and the bed) may be used to maintain the patient's feet in a neutral position. Pillows placed under the forearms will eliminate the pull on the shoulders. When it is finally permissible for the patient to lie flat in bed for certain periods during the day, the nurse will be alert to the necessity of restoring full extension to the hips and knees to overcome the results of long-continued flexion to those joints. Turning the patient to the prone position for short periods of time is also helpful in preventing the development of a hip-flexion contracture. A firm support beneath the hips is important. A sagging mattress can be the cause of insidious deformity, even though the nurse is careful to arrange the patient in positions of good body mechanics and is conscientious about teaching him his role in his own recovery. A depression in the mattress at the hip level may bring about contracture of the hip flexor muscles that may make the upright position of full extension at the hips almost impossible.

The development of a sacral decubitus always presents a grave situation, particularly in a thin, elderly patient or in one in whom dehydration and pyrexia persist over a long period. The potential danger to pressure areas is always in the mind of the nurse caring for such a patient. This is one preventive measure about which no nurse is uninformed today. Sometimes, however, the problems involved in preventing a breakdown of the skin in the threatened area are so manifold that the nurse may forget the rest of the patient's problem entirely. Perhaps he is turned on his side and allowed to lie a great portion of the time with his legs adducted and his hips and knees flexed. The danger of decubitus may be overcome, but unless pillows are placed between the thighs for alignment of the extremities, by the time the patient is ready to sit up and walk he has a dislocation of the hip that lay adducted and unsupported for so long. A crippling condition results, that will require many months, or even years, to remedy. This outcome is no hypothetical possibility; it has happened often enough to make it essential that students be taught the important part they play in the prevention of such disasters. They should be well aware of the response of the musculoskeletal system to disease, to fever, and to disuse. The necessity for good body alignment in bed will become more reasonable and immediate as these matters are more fully understood.

Deformities of upper extremity

Another group of muscles that develops contractures because of faulty or unphysiologic positions in bed are the muscles at the axillary level, particularly the pectoral group. The value of providing for active range of motion of the shoulder joint following mastectomy is well known. It also should be remembered that the individual wearing a sling to support the forearm needs range-of-motion exercise for the shoulder joint to prevent tight pectoral muscles and an adduction contracture. Patients lying in bed tend to be very limited as far as activity of the upper arms and shoulders is concerned. Many ambulatory patients, are also somewhat restricted in this respect. The muscles that bring the arms away from the side and those that rotate them outward are used so infrequently that they undergo considerable atrophy. The patient with a debilitating illness is likely to lie in bed with the arms held closely to the sides of the body, elbows flexed at right angles, and wrists crossed and dropped. There is usually no reason why he must lie this way; he does it out of apathy or lack of knowledge that it may be harmful to him. Skillful nurses will find reasons for making the patient use his arms in positions of abduction and outward rotation. They will have him reach upward toward the head of the bed, comb his hair, or fasten his gown at the back of the neck. At other times they will arrange for him to lie with his arms in a position opposite to the one he tends to assume constantly; i.e., they will see that the upper arms are abducted, the elbows extended, and the hands turned palm upward. By doing this, the nurse may be able to prevent the troublesome bursitis and synovitis that sometimes follow long-continued restriction of motion in the shoulder and certainly will be able to prevent the tightness in the axilla that so frequently follows long illness. If, however, the patient has been in a restricted position for a long time at home, such activity must be resumed gradually and cautiously.

With paralysis of the upper extremity, positioning and change of position of the forearm, wrist, and fingers are vital to prevent fixed deformity. The wrist and fingers of the paralyzed hand may be maintained in a functional position by means of a hand roll or a posterior splint. Functional position implies a position of use: the wrist is in extension, the fingers are semiflexed, and the thumb opposes the fingers. Change of position and passive exercise will prevent tightening of the joint structure.

• • •

The foregoing are only some of the mishaps of poor bed posture. There are others that may cause the patient discomfort, if not actual disability, after a period of bed rest. As students go through the clinical services, they will become increasingly aware of situations in which knowledge of elementary body mechanics is of importance. In the obstetric nursery an infant may be noted whose head seems habitually to rest a little to one side with the chin pointed in the opposite direction. The baby may normally lie that way part of the time, but is he lying that way all of the time? And does he resist having his head turned the other way? Again, a patient receiving oxygen may be observed to have two or three pillows under his head but no support whatever to the back or shoulders, with the result that the chest is concave and sunken. The student knows, of course, that the oxygen is being given to support a failing respiratory system. The incongruity of this in the face of such a sunken and depleted chest capacity should be apparent at once.

Charcot, the great French neurologist, once said that it was the mind that was truly alive and saw things but that it would hardly see anything without instruction. This wise observation might well serve as a professional axiom for all teachers of student nurses. The difference between a trained observer and an untrained observer is never more important than it is in these instances. Unaided observation has little value for the young student.

. . .

Prevention of crippling, of course, includes far more than attention to bed posture. Disease and accidents are the causes of a large percentage of crippling conditions today. The nurse's function in the prevention and control of disease will be emphasized in all phases of professional education, but her role in accident prevention may not be so apparent unless it is given considerable thought and analysis both in the classroom and at the bedside.

Accidents in the home cause a high percentage of fatalities each year. Besides the fatalities, the innumerable disabilities (temporary and permanent) and the resulting economic losses they engender must be considered. When the situations in the home and hospital that are most likely to result in accidents are brought to the student's attention, her horizon for observation is enlarged immeasurably. A clear comprehension of what constitutes individual responsibility for community health and betterment is not the least of the lessons the nurse must learn.

Hypostatic pneumonia

Prolonged bed rest with infrequent change of position is a contributing factor in the development of hypostatic pneumonia. The patient's position in bed, presence of a tight bandage around the chest or abdomen, abdominal distention, severe pain, administration of sedatives or anes-

thetics (which depress the respiratory center in the medulla), and decreased innervation of the respiratory muscles are factors that can contribute to lung congestion and decreased rib cage expansion. Also, with inactivity, basal metabolism is lowered. This results in a decreased amount of carbon dioxide being produced, and thus the need for oxygen is lowered. Consequently, the respiratory center does not stimulate breathing and respirations are slower and more shallow. The horizontal position tends to permit secretions to pool, and ciliary action is inhibited. The resulting stasis of the bronchial secretions provides an ideal media for the growth of pathogenic organisms, and if dehydration occurs, the secretions are more tenacious and difficult to expectorate. When lung congestion or pneumonia is present, the patient becomes lethargic, rales may be heard, dyspnea is present, respirations are rapid and noisy, chills and fever with diaphoresis may occur, blood-tinged sputum may be expectorated, and blood studies reveal leukocytosis. To help prevent a patient from developing lung congestion, nursing care must include changing his position at specified times, encouraging activity, and helping him to cough and breathe deeply at frequent intervals. With some patients, use of the intermittent positive pressure breathing machine is indicated to accomplish deep breathing and to stimulate coughing. Also, the use of suction may be necessary to help remove secretions from the respiratory tract.

Pressure necrosis (decubitus ulcers; pressure sores)

Prolonged pressure from the body weight on vulnerable areas such as the sacrum, heels, malleoli, or even the greater trochanters frequently results in breakdown of the skin and the underlying tissues. Continuous pressure from the body weight compresses the capillaries and venules and causes a decrease in the blood supply (ischemia) to the involved tissues. When circulatory exchange is inadequate, anoxemia of the tissue and the accumulation of catabolic waste products cause cell death. An ischemic area of skin appears white but immediately becomes red (hyperemia) when body pressure is relieved. If the redness of such an area does not disappear within a relatively short time (approximately one hour) following relief of the pressure, tissue damage has very likely occurred.

To prevent tissue necrosis, nursing care should be directed at relieving pressure and providing good skin care. To relieve pressure, a turning schedule that includes the prone, side-lying, and supine positions, as well as variations of these positions, should be established. In addition, the use of synthetic lamb's wool or other such device beneath the involved area will provide for the distribution of the body weight over a larger area. Additional preventive and therapeutic measures for the patient in traction are discussed in Chapter 7. Along with relief of pressure, nursing care should provide for such things as cleanliness, adequate protein and liquid intake, the prevention of breaks in the skin, and the maintenance of normal skin oils. Gentle massages of normal tissue increases the circulation and is beneficial. However, vigorous massage of a reddened area may cause further injury to damaged tissue. Other health factors such as circulatory problems, nutritional status, sensory deficits, and age will greatly influence the condition of the skin and the speed with which pressure necrosis can occur.

Disuse osteoporosis

Bone formation and bone resorption are normal and continuous processes that go on throughout life. The osteoblasts (bone-building cells) lay down bone matrix, and resorption of bone is the function of the osteoclasts (bone-destroying cells). Osteoporosis (loss of calcium) occurs when the balance between the osteoblasts and osteoclasts is disturbed; the destruction of bone occurs at a faster rate than the bone-building process. The mechanism of normal bone formation and resorption is not understood; consequently, the cause of osteoporosis is not known. It is known, however, that inactivity and the absence of weight-bearing stress on the lower extremities will result in a loss of calcium from the skeletal system. This loss increases rapidly and reaches a peak in approximately five weeks and will continue as long as the individual is inactive and not weight bearing. The calcium is excreted primarily by the kid-

neys through the urine. Possible complications include the formation of renal stones and ensuing urinary tract problems (see following discussion) and the development of fragile bones that fracture with little or no trauma. To slow down and prevent the calcium loss, bracing and the early use of the tilt table with weight-bearing stress are recommended and used as soon as the patient's general condition permits.

Renal calculi

When disuse osteoporosis occurs, the increased excretion of calcium salts by the kidneys may lead to the formation of stones. Other factors that favor precipitation of calcium and stone formation are stasis of urine, decreased urinary output, urinary tract infection, and an alkaline urine. With decreased muscle activity, urine becomes more alkaline, and it is known that an alkaline urine favors precipitation of calcium salts. The presence of infection in the urinary tract favors stone formation by reducing the acidity of the urine and by increasing the amount of cellular debris that acts as nuclei for stone formation. Such symptoms as hematuria, severe coliclike pain, nausea and vomiting, and backache may indicate renal calculi. This is a very painful and distressing complication that can accompany continued bed rest. Preventive measures should include increased fluid intake to help prevent urinary stasis and to decrease the concentration of calcium in the urine. In addition, frequent change of position is essential and should include sitting and standing whenever possible. In the supine position, the hilus of the kidney is uppermost, and thus gravity does not assist in the drainage of urine from the kidney. Also, providing for muscle activity and, as previously stated, for weight-bearing stress will lessen the amount of calcium lost from the skeletal system and consequently the amount of calcium to be excreted by the kidney.

Bowel and bladder problems

It is not uncommon for a patient confined to bed and the supine position to have difficulty in voiding. Lack of privacy and attempting to use a bedpan or urinal in an unnatural position may make it difficult for the individual to consciously relax the perineal muscles, including the external sphincter.

The nurse needs to recognize that the patient who asks for the urinal or bedpan often but voids only small amounts and the older patient who is frequently incontinent may be having bladder distention with overflow incontinence. If this condition is permitted to continue, serious urinary tract complications may follow.

In many cases, constipation and fecal impactions become a problem for the immobilized or bedridden patient. Defecation depends upon both smooth and skeletal muscle action plus a complex visceral reflex pattern. Lack of adequate privacy and the use of an uncomfortable position tend to encourage poor habits in the bedfast patient. Neither the supine position nor a sitting position with the knees extended promotes the normal reflexes and pelvic muscle action desirable for defecation. Fecal material remaining in the lower bowel and rectum becomes increasingly hard and dry due to absorption of water by the gut. The patient with a fecal impaction may repeatedly ask for the bedpan and will frequently pass a small amount of liquid stool; the older patient, because of relaxation of the anal sphincters, may have continuous or repeated incontinence of liquid fecal material.

Generalized weakness, loss of muscle strength, lack of activity, and changes in dietary habits and the daily routines also contribute to bowel problems for the bed patient. To remedy or prevent these problems, it is helpful to know the patient's toilet and dietary habits. If these can be continued in the hospital situation, bowel problems may be avoided. Provision for a high-residue diet, adequate liquid intake, and the use of the bedside commode as soon as permissible are helpful nursing measures. Frequently, a stool softener may be desirable.

Thrombosis and pulmonary embolism

See discussion on pp. 87 and 88.

Postural hypotension

Patients who have been confined to bed may experience dizziness (vertigo) upon assuming the vertical position. In some instances, fainting will occur. This is known as postural hypotension and is caused by a pooling of the blood in the muscles and abdominal viscera. Following a period of bed rest, the ability of the peripheral vessels to constrict when the individual assumes the upright position is diminished. The reason this occurs is not completely understood. However, when it does take place, it results in a diminished circulatory blood volume with a corresponding drop in blood pressure. When ambulatory activities are prescribed after a period of extended bed rest, the nurse will realize that rolling the head of the bed up for short periods or permitting the patient to sit on the side of the bed can be helpful in preventing dizziness and fainting. In many instances, placing the individual on a tilt table (Fig. 445) and gradually permitting him to assume a vertical position is necessary. The application of elastic bandages or stockings to the lower extremities is helpful not only in preventing pooling of blood but also in preventing edema of the dependent extremities.

Chronic illness

It has been said that ward aides and practical nurses give more satisfactory care to chronically ill patients than do professional nurses. If this is true, teaching methods should be examined rather carefully to determine how students might be better prepared for this type of nursing. Every orthopedic nurse encounters again and again the problem of the patient who has been ill a long time—the patient exhausted in courage, short in patience, and unreasonable, fearful, and demanding.

Many of these problems will be apparent to the nurse as she works with the arthritic patient and the elderly individual. Nurses working with the chronically ill patients are urged to read again Florence Nightingale's *Notes on nursing,* especially those passages having to do with the patient who has been confined to a bed or chair for a long time. No one has ever written of this matter with greater feeling and common sense than Florence Nightingale.

There are certain recurring problems regarding chronically ill patients that the nurse should bear in mind whether the patients are young or old. The very act of entering a hospital, for instance, may be a source of profound apprehension and fear to the patient. Perhaps he has had prolonged care in the home, care that he himself directed, wisely or unwisely. Every innovation that hospital nurses make is viewed with disfavor and suspicion, often because of the threat it offers to his comfort, but often, too, because he has come to take a negative attitude regarding any suggestion of change in his care. The student should realize that many of the characteristic reactions of such patients come from a single source—fear. Nurses must recognize that they may be the cause of this reaction and accept the challenge to eliminate it. All experienced orthopedic nursing personnel have seen patients forcibly removed from the health care setting by what we justly think of as unreasonable and short-sighted relatives after a day or two of preliminary treatment. Perhaps a large number of these withdrawals are unavoidable. But let us look to ourselves and to the initial treatment we give to cherished children or sheltered individuals.

The problem is resolved by use of the golden rule. It is just that simple, commonplace, and undramatic. It means that the nurse must understand that the habitual response to these situations must be the response to a patient who is also a unique individual, a worthwhile human being.

If one quality could be singled out as basic to every nursing skill, that quality must be **gentleness.** Too often this indispensable component of patient care is taken for granted. It is presupposed that providers of health care, as decent human beings, will treat their patients with gentleness. Certainly no nurse worthy of the name would consciously mistreat another person. However, one cannot safely assume that gentleness is a major objective that will be integrated automatically into all patient care activities. Gentleness may be inherent in some person's behavior; yet for most it

is a skill and an attitude that must be developed and practiced. Its importance cannot be overemphasized, particularly for patients whose very identity may be threatened by the automated, impersonalized processing characteristic of many health care institutions today. Gentleness, kindness, understanding—these are often only words, not actions essential to the nurse's skills and the patient's well-being.

Gentleness in using one's voice and hands needs to be a conscious habit because it is good treatment. This thoughtful, objective gentleness is based not on compassion alone but on the knowledge that sickness is an unremitting source of human fear. It recognizes that the emotional components of the patient's illness are as important as other common symptoms observed and recorded.

Habitual gentleness is based on understanding, experience, and empathy and reflects intelligence as well as emotion. It seems that nursing often loses sight of this. Whether the patient suffers from an acutely inflamed joint, fear of an oncoming treatment, or apprehension about a suspected malignancy, gentleness is a primary requisite in effective treatment. It cannot be taken for granted that nurses understand and apply gentleness simply because they have elected nursing as their profession.

Biographers of Sir Robert Jones, the famous British orthopedist, have written often and with deep appreciation of the cordial spirit with which he received and handled his patients. They describe his methods of supporting a limb during examination—gently and with great skill in avoiding movement that would cause pain. Part of this skill, the cordial spirit, certainly was from the heart, but much of the rest of it must have been painstakingly learned. Both characteristics are greatly needed by nurses, particularly those working with orthopedic patients.

5 Emergency nursing on the orthopedic patient unit

DOLORES J. WHITEHEAD, R.N., M.S.

Emergency nursing is the care and management given to the patient with critical and urgent needs. The primary objective of this care is to preserve life and prevent further complications.

In the absence of a physician or while awaiting his arrival, the nurse on the orthopedic unit may have to take responsibility for initiating appropriate action as adverse signs and symptoms present themselves. Often there will be hospital policies to guide her that have been established with the physicians. But when the physician is not immediately available, the nurse is the skilled professional whose judgment and action are needed to diagnose and treat life-threatening conditions.

The nurse must, however, operate within the constraints of good practice. She should be familiar with the standard emergency procedures and be able to act quickly and knowledgeably. She must systematically evaluate the status of the patient and act to maintain life and function until the physician arrives. Continuity of care from the onset of signs and symptoms of serious difficulty until the condition of the patient is stabilized is essential.

Commonly accepted emergency measures for the life-threatening situations that arise in orthopedic units are presented in this chapter. Priorities for the initiation of treatment are determined by the comparative threat to the patient's life. Those conditions that interfere with vital physiologic function take precedence: obstructed airway, cardiac arrest, hemorrhage.

Basic emergency management

The following steps should be taken in the management of an emergency:

1 Establish and maintain an effective airway. Use resuscitation when necessary.
2 Evaluate and restore cardiac output.
3 Stop the bleeding.
4 Prevent and treat shock.
5 Start a timed record of the patient's vital signs. Monitor blood pressure, pulse, and respirations at intervals of five to fifteen minutes. Record fluid intake and output, medications, and procedures.
6 Carry out an ongoing assessment of the patient's condition. (The clinical course of the seriously ill person is seldom static.)
7 Assure patient comfort insofar as is possible by proper positioning and by control of pain. Explain treatments or procedures in an effort to relieve anxiety.

Psychologic support of patient

As indicated in the last step in the foregoing list, it is important to relieve patient anxiety. The patient who develops a sudden complication or is the victim of accidental injury and requires emergency action is often overwhelmed by anxiety since he has not had time to mobilize his resources to adapt to the crisis. In pain, and feeling very much alone, he may experience real and terrifying fear—of death, mutilation, isolation, loss of control (physical and mental), or other assaults on his personal identity.

Those caring for the patient should be prepared to act confidently and completely. They must know what to expect and what to do. Any indication that the professional staff members in charge are unsure of themselves may be perceived by the patient, who will react with a greater fear. At the same time, knowing how to handle acute illness skillfully will do much to alleviate the nurse's own anxiety and will likely increase the patient's confidence. Explanations should be given on a level that the patient can understand and grasp, for this will assist him to cope with the psychologic and physical stress in a more positive manner.

The effort spent on providing the patient a sympathetic, clear explanation of procedures within his ability and wish to understand carries, as well as the value of human comfort, the reward to the nursing staff, of a more cooperative patient. How much and what to say will vary with each patient and each emergency—a difficult task but one that must not be ignored in the all-out effort to meet the physiologic demands of the moment. In an emergency situation, an ongoing contact between the patient and the nurse or physician helps to reduce panic; reassuring words aid in dispelling fear.

Time should likewise be found to inform the family or friends of the situation and of the action being taken; again, this should be done in a calm, matter-of-fact, reassuring manner.

Emergency cart

An emergency cart stocked with equipment, supplies, and drugs commonly used in medical emergencies (Fig. 94) should be available in each nursing unit. A list of the drugs, including emergency drug doses for the adult patient, or, on the pediatric unit, for the infant and child, should be attached to the cart. The nurse must be knowledgeable of the contents of the cart as well as skilled in the use of the equipment. A review of the emergency procedures and of the equipment, supplies, and drugs on the cart might well be made part of regular in-service training. Typically, the cart is stocked with the items listed.

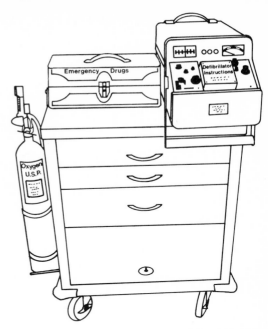

Fig. 94 The well-equipped emergency cart is a time-saving device in a medical emergency. Equipment and supplies and drugs commonly used in medical emergencies can be taken to the bedside without delay.

Equipment and supplies

Air mask/bag unit (Ambu)
Alcohol swabs
Blood gas kit
Blood specimen tubes
Bulb syringe
Cardiac needles (3½ in)
CVP manometer and 24-in intracatheter
Endotracheal tubes (various sizes)
Hemostats
IV equipment
  Needles
  Cannulas
  Administration sets
  Stopcocks
  Fluids—lactated Ringer's, normal saline, dextrose 5%
Laryngoscope handle with blades
Nasogastric tube and lubricant
Nasopharyngeal airways
Oral airways (infant, child, and adult sizes)
Oxygen supply, flowmeter, connecting tubing
Sterile 4 × 4 sponges
Sterile gloves
Suction catheters (various sizes)
Suture scissors
Syringes (various sizes)
Tape

Tourniquet
Venesection set

Drugs

Aminophylline
Atropine sulfate
Calcium chloride
Dextrose 50%, 50 ml
Diazepam (Valium)
Digoxin (Lanoxin)
Phenytoin sodium (Dilantin)
Diphenhydramine HCl (Benadryl)
Dopamine (Intropin)
Epinephrine (Adrenalin)
Furosemide (Lasix)
Glucagon HCl
Hydrocortisone (injection)
Isoproterenol HCl (Isuprel HCl)
Levarterenol bitartrate (Levophed)
Lidocaine HCl (Xylocaine HCl)
Metaraminol bitartrate (Aramine bitartrate)
Naloxone HCl (Narcan)
Procaine amide (Pronestyl)
Propranolol HCl (Inderal)
Protamine sulfate (injection)
Sodium bicarbonate

Respiratory insufficiency and airway obstruction

The first requisite in the management of an emergency condition is the establishment of an open airway. An obstructed airway or interference with adequate pulmonary ventilation constitutes an immediate threat to life. If the airway is obstructed, the ensuing hypoxia will produce brain damage or death within three to six minutes.

The anesthetized patient, the patient with paralysis, the patient with poor pulmonary exchange due to severe thoracic deformity, the patient with laryngeal edema, and the patient with excessive pulmonary secretions require intensive airway surveillance.

The signs of airway obstruction are ominous; they will vary according to the cause and the rapidity of onset. There are dyspnea and inspiratory or expiratory stridor (harsh high-pitched sound). The obvious difficulty in breathing causes characteristic retraction noticeable in the supraclavicular and intercostal spaces. In children, the sternum and epigastrium may be drawn in. Cyanosis is often present. Severe obstruction may result in an ashen-gray appearance.

In the early stages of obstruction, the lack of oxygen in the blood and the retention of carbon dioxide are evidenced by restlessness, disorientation, headache, and uncooperativeness. If untreated, the condition progresses to cerebral depression causing lassitude, decreasing respiratory effort, unresponsiveness, and, finally, coma and death.

Initially, the pulse is usually rapid and hypertension is present. Continued obstruction is indicated by a weak, thready pulse, hypotension, and evidence of circulatory collapse.

Astute assessment of the respiratory distress signs and symptoms in conjunction with the patient's general condition may indicate the most effective emergency measures to be used. In assessing respirations, (1) look for breathing movements, (2) listen for airflow at the nose and mouth, and (3) place the palm of the hand over the patient's nose and mouth to feel for air exchange. If there is complete obstruction, there will be no detectable movement of air. If there is partial obstruction, there will be noisy breathing. A nosiy breathing condition should be treated promptly to avoid further complications.

One of the common postoperative complications is pulmonary atelectasis (collapse of portions of the lung). It usually occurs within the first forty-eight hours following surgery. Obstruction of the bronchial tree is caused by retained bronchial secretions. Factors that contribute to atelectasis are ineffective coughing, pain, and analgesics, all of which may lead to shallow respirations and inadequate ventilation. Atelectasis is characterized by fever, increased respiratory and pulse rates, and cyanosis (when large portions of the lung are affected). Effective coughing and deep-breathing exercises are essential to clear the bronchial tree of these secretions. Intermittent positive-pressure breathing (IPPB) treatments also may be helpful. The patient should be turned frequently to promote full ventilation of the lungs.

The unconscious patient may not require artificial ventilation but merely proper positioning of the head to allow adequate breathing through an open airway. For example, the patient who has suffered a stroke should be placed on his side (Fig. 95) or in a semiprone position with the

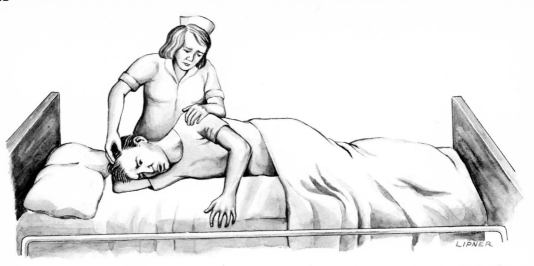

Fig. 95 The patient should be placed on his side or in a semiprone position with the mouth lowered to prevent the tongue from slipping back and to facilitate drainage of secretions.

mouth lowered to prevent the tongue from slipping back and to facilitate drainage of secretions. This may allow adequate respiration.

When the major signs of airway obstruction occur, the immediate action is to clear the blood, vomitus, mucus, or any foreign material. This can be done quickly by sweeping a finger deep in the patient's mouth. A suction machine may be used if it is immediately available.

The patient is positioned on his back. The lower jaw is manipulated and moved so as to prevent the tongue from resting on the back of the pharynx. Placing the fingers behind the angles of the jaws and pushing the mandible upward manually opens the air passages for maximum ventilation (Fig. 96). The fastest and best method of opening the airway for resuscitation is maximum extension of the head. Lift the neck with one hand and tilt the head back with the other. This allows an immediate assessment of the patient's condition. If the head-tilt position opens the airway and the patient starts to breathe spontaneously, maintain the poistion and go no further. If tilting the head back does not open the airway, force two or three deep breaths quickly into the patient's lungs through the mouth (see discussion on cardiopulmonary resuscitation, p. 83). This ventilation measure may be enough to clear

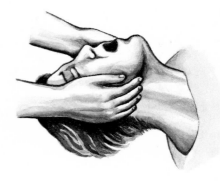

Fig. 96 The airway may be improved by placing the fingers behind the angles of the jaws and pushing the mandible upward manually.

the air passages and start spontaneous respiration.

Mechanical devices, the nasopharyngeal or the oropharyngeal airway, may be inserted to ensure ample air passage to the pharynx but will not relieve lower obstruction. The use of a bag and mask may provide a satisfactory temporary means of artificial respiration.

Endotracheal intubation is often the most rapid method of establishing an airway in patients with acute respiratory insufficiency who cannot be treated satisfactorily with the nasopharyngeal or oropharyngeal airway. Intubation may be accomplished by exposure of the larynx with a laryngoscope and insertion of an endotracheal tube (or a catheter) into the trachea. It is important to position the patient properly with the neck flexed and the head extended to bring the mouth, larynx, and trachea in alignment. An air mask/bag unit (Ambu) attached to the endotracheal tube is used to artificially ventilate the patient in the absence of spontaneous respiration.

Because endotracheal intubation is complicated, the nurse who is expected to carry out this procedure must have received appropriate training and supervised practice. Usually intubation is done by the physician.

If attempts at maintaining sufficient airway fail and there is a respiratory arrest, resuscitation must be initiated at once.

Cardiac complications

The cardiovascular-pulmonary system is a closed system whose functions are interrelated and interdependent. When normal cardiovascular and pulmonary functions are endangered, cardiovascular dysfunction or a cardiac emergency will occur. Collapse of the cardiovascular system will result in inadequate oxygenation and nourishment of the body tissues. If a cardiac arrest occurs, it is essential to preserve cardiac output in order to provide an oxygenated blood supply to the vital centers (see discussion on cardiopulmonary resuscitation that follows).

Reduced cardiac output may be due to hypovolemia (insufficient blood volume) arising from trauma or hemorrhage following surgery. Impaired cardiac output also may be due to cardiac dysrhythmias arising from organic heart disease or insufficiency of blood in the myocardium (myocardial ischemia) arising from respiratory insufficiency or airway obstruction.

The symptoms of decreasing cardiac output or impaired cardiac status are persistent chest pain, shortness of breath, significant decrease in blood pressure, changes in heart rate or rhythm (tachycardia, bradycardia, irregular rhythm), decreasing urinary output (less than 25-30 ml/hr), decreasing level of mentation, lethargy, dizziness, and diaphoresis.

The two most common symptoms that alert the nurse to a potential problem are cardiac dysrhythmias and severe and persistent chest pain. The physician should be summoned when these symptoms are noted. He will need to know the character of the chest pain—location, severity, onset, duration, association with respiratory or position changes. And on that basis he may advise the nurse by phone on the procedures to follow.

The patient who complains of severe chest pain or other symptoms should be connected to a monitor in order to detect abnormal rhythms. A defibrillator should be made available in anticipation that its use might become necessary. As in all emergencies, vital signs should be monitored frequently. Medication may be ordered to relieve the chest pain. An intravenous infusion should be started with a stopcock attached to the tubing for the administration of any medications ordered, such as sodium bicarbonate, epinephrine, or calcium chloride. These drugs should be part of the medication box on the emergency cart brought to the bedside. The patient may be ordered transferred to a special care unit. If cardiac or respiratory arrest occurs, cardiopulmonary resuscitation must be initiated at once.

Cardiopulmonary resuscitation

The indications for cardiopulmonary resuscitation (CPR) are cardiac arrest and respiratory arrest. The purpose of the procedure is to promptly establish effective circulation and ventilation until the patient recovers the ability to breathe on his own or until advanced life support is available. The steps to follow vary slightly when one or two persons are at the bedside.

Procedure with one person

1 Check the responsiveness of the patient by verbal and tactile stimulation (call his name; shake him). Note the time of the cardiac arrest. A lack of effective circulation to the central nervous system for more than three to six minutes may result in irreversible changes.
2 Open the airway. Remove the pillow so as to be able to hyperextend the head effectively. This tilting back of the head tends to lift the tongue off the back of the pharynx and opens

the airway. In an infant, the tilt position should not be exaggerated, because with an infant's very pliant neck, hyperextension of the head may actually obstruct the air passages.

3 Check for breathing. Place your ear over the patient's nose and mouth while looking toward his chest. In this position you can feel and listen for breathing and at the same time observe the chest to see if it is rising.

4 If no breathing is noted, prepare to ventilate the patient. Keep the head tilted back, pinch the nostrils, and get a good seal around the mouth with your own mouth.

5 Ventilate four times. (For infants, blow only puffs from the cheeks.) Take deep breaths and blow quickly and forceably into the patient's mouth. The chest should be seen to rise. Absence of chest expanison is a sign of airway obstruction.

6 Check for carotid pulse.

7 Call for help. Use the bedside call system; if necessary, send another patient or a visitor.

8 Start external cardiac massage. Find the correct sternal position: pressure will be applied on the middle third of the sternum. Place one hand on top of the other.

 a *For adults*, compress the sternum fifteen times at a rate of 80 compressions/min and a depth of 1½-2 in.

 b *For children*, compress in the middle of the sternum, using the heel of one hand only, a rate of 100 times/min and a depth of ¾-1½ in.

 c *For infants*, use only the index and middle fingers and compress the sternum only ½-¾ in. In small infants, one hand can be used to support the back while external massage, at a rate of 100 times/min, is given with the other.

To allow for the chest expansion part of the cycle, do not remove the hands or fingers from the sternum but simply release the pressure from the chest. The compression cycle must be regular and smooth.

9 After fifteen cycles of cardiac massage, change your position to the head for ventilation. Quickly lift the neck, tilt the head, pinch the nose, cup the patient's lips, and secure a good seal. Ventilate two times.

10 Return to cardiac massage. Position the hands correctly on the exact sternum location and compress fifteen times as before.

11 Repeat until help arrives or the patient shows signs of effectiveness of the procedure: good pulse, return of respiration, good color, purposeful movement.

12 During the procedure, check the pupils occasionally to see if they are dilated or reacting. Constriction of the pupils is a sign that CPR is being effective.

Procedure with two persons

The first person to reach the patient begins the resuscitation measures as just outlined. The second person calls the physician, obtains advanced life support equipment (heart monitor, defibrillator, emergency cart), brings it to the bedside, and proceeds to assist the first person with the resuscitation. One person can then act as the compressor, while the other is the ventilator and takes a position at the head.

1 At a sternal compression rate of 60 compressions/min, there will be five compressions to each breath. The ventilator must get her breath in quickly and forcefully while the compressor has the pressure on the chest released. The person compressing must not pause to let the ventilator get her breath in. The ryhthm is to continue smoothly.

2 The ventilator should check every two minutes for signs of effectiveness between ventilations. Palpate for carotid pulse and look at the size of the pupils. The presence of a palpable pulse and constriction of the pupils are evidence of effective circulation of oxygenated blood.

3 When medical assistance arrives, the nurse attaches the patient to the monitor, prepares medication for administration, and assists with establishing IV site and with endotracheal intubation.

As the physician requests, the following may need to be prepared: a bottle of intravenous solution with three-way stopcock attached to the tubing; IV sodium bicarbonate to be given every five to ten minutes to offset the marked metabolic acidosis that occurs at the time of cardiopulmonary arrest; epinephrine attached to a cardiac needle; suction equipment, oxygen equipment, and the defibrillator.

Control of hemorrhage

The commonest cause of shock on a surgical unit is reduction in the circulating blood volume—hypovolemic shock.

Hemorrhage may occur within the first few hours after surgery, or it may occur some time later due to slipping of a ligature or for some other reason. During the immediate postoperative period, observations must be made of the blood pressure, pulse rate, wound, and drain sites. Because rising pulse rate and a slowly falling blood pressure may indicate persistent bleeding, the physician should be promptly notified. Early detection with prompt treatment may prevent the condition from becoming an emergency.

The most effective method of controlling external bleeding is direct pressure on the wound. When the bleeding is relatively mild, pressure applied to the wound with a bulky sterile dressing (or reinforcement of the existing dressing) will usually control bleeding. A sandbag or a firm trochanter roll may be used, if ordered, to apply pressure to oozing wound sites following hip surgery. If bleeding is profuse, firm manual pressure applied to the wound with a bulky dressing or direct pressure to the artery involved will usually control bleeding. Elevate the affected extremity.

The patient who has an amputation should be carefully observed for signs of hemorrhage. As a precaution, the surgeon may request that a tourniquet be kept at the bedside. If severe bleeding occurs, the tourniquet should be applied to the stump and pulled sufficiently tight to stop the bleeding. The tourniquet is used only when other measures—elevation and pressure—have failed to stop the bleeding.

Internal bleeding may occur as a result of fracture or other trauma or for some other reason (e.g., peptic ulcer).

The patient with a closed fracture may have marked swelling and tenderness about the fracture site—an indication of some bleeding into the surrounding tissues. A closed fracture of the femur may cause loss of one to three pints of blood into the surrounding tissue. In a pelvic fracture where major blood vessels are severed by jagged bone fragments, there may be a severe blood loss in the pelvic cavity and tissues around the pelvis.

Internal hemorrhage may or may not have outward indicators. The patient may cough up bright red blood, or he may vomit blood that has the appearance of coffee grounds. Stools may contain bright red blood, which may indicate bleeding from the lower bowel, or they may have a tarry appearance, which is an indication of bleeding in the small intestine or upper region of the colon.

The physician should be notified when any unexpected signs of bleeding occur.

Hypovolemic shock

Shock is an abnormal state in which there is failure of the cardiovascular system to provide adequate blood flow to sustain normal cell activity; i.e., there is inadequate tissue perfusion. Signs of shock do not usually appear until 10% or more of the blood volume is lost.

Hypovolemic shock is seen where there is significant loss in circulating blood volume. It is characterized clinically by cool skin, pallor, a rapid, weak pulse, rapid respiration, and lowered blood pressure. The physician should be alerted at the first signs of shock—an increasing pulse rate and cool skin. If blood loss is the primary factor and the source of bleeding can be controlled, the condition should be amenable to adequate blood replacement. The patient will show signs of apprehension.

The patient who is bleeding will require constant observation, including measurement of vital signs every five to fifteen minutes. Urine output should be measured, since it is one of the most valuable indices in determining the adequacy of tissue perfusion. An output below 30 ml/hr is suggestive of inadequate fluid replacement (or cardiac failure).

Since fluid and blood replacement is determined by the amount and type lost, an accurate measurement or estimate of blood loss is essential in order for the physician to plan proper therapy. If blood loss is extensive, blood and fluid replacement will be needed. An intravenous infusion should be started using 5% dextrose or lactated Ringer's solution until other fluids are ordered. Blood samples for typing and cross-matching, blood count, and blood chemistries should be sent immediately.

The physician should be notified when any unexpected signs of bleeding occur. As usual, the patient should be carefully monitored, including frequent measurement of vital signs, so that his condition can be precisely evaluated by the physician. Laboratory results will help the physician determine fluid and blood replacement.

It is essential that an adequate airway be maintained. If breathing difficulty is noted, oxygen should be administered by face mask or nasal catheter. (Use resuscitation procedures if necessary.) Blood gases may be ordered to measure arterial oxygen levels.

The physician may wish to insert a central venous pressure (CVP) catheter into the superior vena cava. Measurement of the central venous pressure reflects the pressure of the right atrium and aids in determining the heart's ability to tolerate the circulating blood volume. When the blood volume is reduced, as in hypovolemic shock, the CVP is lower than normal (5-10 cm of water); and conversely, when the circulatory system is overloaded, as by excessive infusion of blood and fluids, the CVP is higher than normal.

Because body temperature tends to be reduced by the shock condition, it should be maintained by application of a light blanket. However, the patient should not be overheated.

If there are signs of gastrointestinal bleeding, a nasogastric tube connected to suction may be ordered. The nurse is responsible for observing the drainage and maintaining the suction. Other drugs and procedures may be ordered depending upon the patient's condition.

Bleeding as complication of anticoagulant therapy

When anticoagulant therapy is given to patients with pulmonary embolism or thrombophlebitis, the major complication nurses will encounter is bleeding. Minor bleeding, often manifested by easy bruising, usually requires only that the level of anticoagulation be reduced. Severe hemorrhage is more likely to occur in patients with hypertension or in those with a history of peptic ulcer. Members of the nursing staff should be aware that patients taking corticosteroids may have a history of peptic ulcer.

As a complication of anticoagulant therapy, there may be bleeding into the skin, central nervous system, gastrointestinal tract, or genitourinary tract. If a severe bleeding problem develops, rapid reversal of anticoagulation with appropriate antidotes and replacement of blood loss are mandatory. Vitamin K is the most effective antidote for oral anticoagulants. Vitamin K can be given orally or slowly intravenously. The antidote for heparin, protamine sulfate, which may be given via slow intravenous injection, will usually return the clotting time to normal within five minutes.

When a severe bleeding problem develops, the nurse must make frequent observations, including determination of the vital signs, and make preparations for the patient to receive blood replacement. This continued close monitoring is essential until bleeding is controlled and the patient's condition is stabilized.

Hemophilia—measures for control of bleeding

Hemophilia is an inherited, congenital blood disorder characterized by a deficiency in blood-clotting factors. The most common factors involved are Factors VIII, IX, and XI. Factor VIII deficiency is the most common. It appears in males but is transmitted by females.

The severity of the bleeding tendency is well correlated with the plasma concentration of the factor in question. Spontaneous hemorrhage is rare, but serious hemorrhage may follow trauma or surgery.

Common clinical manifestations include bleeding into joints (elbows, knees, ankles), causing pain, swelling, and limitation of movement, bleeding from the mucous membranes of the nose and mouth, bleeding into soft tissue, bleeding from wounds, or bleeding from the urinary tract (spontaneous hematuria). Intracranial hemorrhage is rare. The nurse must be alert to these adverse signs and report them promptly to the physician.

The following emergency supportive measures are instituted to prevent further bleeding:

1 Handle the patient carefully.
2 Immobilize and elevate the affected part. Splints may be useful in patients who have suffered joint or muscle hemorrhage to prevent motion and further bleeding and to provide comfort.
3 Apply local pressure as an aid in controlling epistaxis. Packing of the nose may be necessary.
4 Apply ice packs.
5 Medications given as prescribed (sedatives or narcotics to alleviate pain) should be administered orally if possible. Intramuscular medications should be given slowly, followed by gentle pressure to the area for five minutes. Injection sites should be rotated.
6 Control bleeding from wounds by applying pressure.

The basis of treatment for hemophilia is replacement of the deficient clotting factor. Therefore, the nurse should prepare to administer blood, plasma, or factor concentrates as directed by the physician.

Pulmonary embolism

Pulmonary embolism is an obstruction to the pulmonary vascular bed. It is most typically caused by a dislodged thrombus (blood clot) but can be caused by any foreign substance, such as fat, air, or cells released from a tumor.

The true incidence of the disease is unknown, but autopsy studies indicate that it is much more common than is suspected clinically. The incidence is difficult to determine because the clinical picture varies from that of vague, easily missed symptoms to those that result in shock, cardiac arrest, and death.

Pulmonary emboli most commonly originate as thrombi within the deep veins of the leg. The clots become dislodged and travel through the vena cava and the right side of the heart and become lodged in the pulmonary artery or one of its branches. Other sources include the veins of the pelvis and the right atrium of the heart.

Three conditions favor the development of thrombus formation: (1) prolonged immobilization with peripheral venous stasis, phlebothrombosis, and thrombophlebitis, (2) damage in the vessel wall secondary to trauma or inflammation, as in phlebitis, arthritis, or fracture of the hip or of the pelvis, and (3) changes in the composition of the blood predisposing to coagulation—dehydration, fever, myocardial infarction.

Certain patients are predisposed to peripheral vein thrombosis: elderly surgical patients (particularly those with a hip fracture), patients with traumatic fracture of the pelvis, obese patients, patients with a malignancy, patients with previous emboli, and patients with congestive heart failure. Thus, prevention of peripheral thrombosis formation will do much to obviate the problem of pulmonary embolism.

The nurse can aid in prevention of the problem by assisting the patient to develop a routine so that he remembers to do his exercises and is alerted to avoid those situations that are more likely to cause thrombus formation. The high-risk patients should be taught to exercise their legs and feet (dorsiflexion and plantar flexion exercises) so as to speed up blood flow and prevent venous stasis. Antiembolism elastic stockings are frequently prescribed, for the compression on the legs aids in increasing the venous velocity. The nurse should routinely check the calf for signs of tenderness and edema and for a positive Homans' sign (pain in the calf generated by dorsiflexion of the foot). A liberal fluid intake should be encouraged. Deep-breathing exercises should be done routinely. The patient should not be permitted to dangle his legs in a dependent position for long periods of time. Ambulation is encouraged as soon as his condition permits. The nurse should explain the reasons for ambulation and assist the patient as needed.

The symptoms of pulmonary embolism vary greatly. A so-called typical clinical picture includes dyspnea, tachypnea, tachycardia, and apprehension. Cough with pleuritic chest pain, hemoptysis, and fever also may be present. A lung scan may be done as an aid in establishing diagnosis. Massive pulmonary emboli produce shock, cyanosis, restlessness, extreme dyspnea, and chest pain. Death may occur in a few minutes or a few days.

Treatment, of course, will depend upon the severity of the attack and the degree of cardiovascular involvement accompanying the pulmonary artery obstruction. In those instances in which shock occurs, the treatment is directed toward support of vital functions.

When cardiopulmonary function is not seriously compromised and life is not immediately threatened, treatment consists of the following measures:

1 Bedrest to prevent further embolization.
2 Gentle handling (e.g., if an x-ray film of the chest is ordered, the patient should be moved in a gentle manner).
3 Administration of oxygen by mask or nasal catheter.
4 Administration of heparin intravenously by continuous infusion or by intermittent injections; if administered by continuous infusion, frequent observations of the IV solution should be made to assure that the infusion is running at the prescribed rate, and the injection site should be observed for evidence of infiltration of the fluid into the surrounding tissues.

Continuous close observation is necessary until the patient's condition is stabilized. Frequent, regular assessment should be done following the acute episode.

Fat embolism

Fat embolism occasionally occurs in patients who have multiple severe injuries or massive trauma to long bones. Signs and symptoms are seemingly related to the appearance in the bloodstream of many fat droplets released from the bone marrow that act as emobli.

The most prominent and most serious symptoms are those derived from involvement of the lungs and brain. A steady rise in the pulse rate, respiratory rate, and temperature without apparent cause occurring within the first day or so following injury may be the clue to the diagnosis. Cyanosis may be present. Petechiae frequently appear early on the skin of the anterior aspect of the chest. The patient may be mildly agitated, apprehensive, or confused. As the condition progresses, the symptoms become more pronounced, and the patient may convulse and lapse into a coma. As soon as the first signs are noted, the physician should be notified, for therapy must be instituted promptly if the patient's life is to be saved.

X-ray films of the chest may be requested. Blood, fluid, and electrolyte replacement will be needed. A major factor in the treatment of this condition is the provision of adequate oxygenation at the tissue level, specifically to the brain and heart. The determination of arterial blood gases is necessary to evaluate the results of treatment. Oxygen may be supplied through a nasal catheter or mask, or, if pulmonary damage is more extensive, positive-pressure oxygen by means of a tracheotomy and a respirator may be needed. Heparin and steroids are sometimes ordered. Vital signs should be determined at least every hour, or more often, until stable. Mental status should be carefully evaluated and measures taken to prevent the confused patient from injuring himself. Blood gas determinations may be repeated, since they serve as a guide in determining the continued need for oxygen therapy.

Complication of diabetes mellitus—hypoglycemia

The nurse on the orthopedic unit frequently encounters a patient with a history of diabetes mellitus. Usually the diabetic status is stabilized, his diet is controlled, and his insulin or oral hypoglycemic medication is regulated. However, the patient, particularly the young diabetic or the severe diabetic, is subject to hypoglycemia (insulin shock or insulin reaction) if his blood glucose level drops abnormally low.

Hypoglycemia may be caused by too large a dose of insulin, failure to ingest an adequate amount of food after taking medication, unusual exercise, vomiting, diarrhea, or unusual stress imposed by surgery or trauma. Also, hypoglycemia may develop without warning. The postoperative patient should be closely observed to see that he eats properly; if calorie or fluid intake is inadequate, intravenous glucose replacement may be needed.

The signs and symptoms of hypoglycemia are extremely variable, but each person tends to follow a reproducible pattern.

The nurse should become familiar with each patient's pattern. The most common complaints of insulin shock are a trembly feeling inside, a gnawing sensation in the stomach, weakness, profuse sweating, rapid pulse, pallor, and tremor of the hand. Other symptoms are disorientation, aphasia, coma, and convulsion. Death can result from prolonged hypoglycemia.

The diagnosis of hypoglycemia can be confirmed only by the demonstration of a markedly decreased blood glucose level—usually 60 mg or less. When the condition is suspected, blood should be drawn and sent immediately for a blood sugar determination. Urinalysis is undependable in this regard since urine specimens obtained at the onset of a hypoglycemia episode may or may not contain glucose. Urine that has been in the bladder over a period of several hours may still contain a considerable amount of glucose.

The diagnosis must be established promptly. The administration of sugar is the treatment for insulin shock. A glass of orange juice or anything sweet usually will relieve the symptoms in a few minutes. If the patient cannot swallow, 20-40 ml of 50% glucose may be given intravenously. Once the hypoglycemia and symptoms are controlled, the physician usually will request that the blood sugar levels be determined at periodic intervals thereafter.

Acute adrenal insufficiency

The hormones derived from the adrenal cortex are of importance in orthopedic surgery because of their use as potent anti-inflammatory agents in the treatment of rheumatic and arthritic disorders. Since many patients undergoing orthopedic surgery have some type of rheumatic complaint, it is quite common to find that they are taking, and may have been taking for some time, one of the adrenocorticosteroids. Three of the important adrenocorticosteroids are cortisone, hydrocortisone, and prednisone.

Cortisone and hydrocortisone have a rather strong effect on electrolyte balances. They tend to promote the retention of sodium and the loss of potassium. When these drugs have been used on a long-term basis, the physician will periodically order blood studies to determine the serum levels of sodium and potassium. If these electrolyte values are abnormal, it is necessary that corrective therapy be instituted.

The long-term administration of steroids produces atrophy of the adrenal glands, thus diminishing the body's adaptive reactions to stress. Therefore, during periods of stress, such as surgery or trauma, the dosage of cortisone must be increased because the body is unable to produce the additional amount of steroid hormone demanded by these circumstances. Acute adrenal insufficiency may develop if the replacement dosage of the hormone is inadequate to meet body needs.

The earliest symptoms of adrenal insufficiency are lassitude and easy fatigability, followed by anorexia, thirst, cramping, abdominal pain, and fever. If the condition remains untreated, the patient may develop hypotension and shock.

Emergency treatment of this condition consists of the rapid correction of the insufficient steroid blood level by the intravenous injection of hydrocortisone. An intravenous infusion should be started so that additional fluids or drugs may be given if needed. Blood studies, including a complete blood count, potassium, sodium, chloride, blood urea nitrogen, glucose, and plasma cortisol level, may be requested. A blood culture may be ordered. Careful monitoring of vital signs must continue until the patient's condition is stabilized. Decreasing blood pressure or failure of pressure to rise after therapy should be promptly reported to the physician.

Since the patient in acute adrenal crisis is unable to adapt to any increase in stress, it is important to avoid making unnecessary demands upon him. Attention should be given to correct body positioning and other general comfort measures.

Cerebrovascular accident—stroke

A stroke occurs when the blood supply to part of the brain is cut off, impairing the function of the cells in that particular part of the brain. The part of the body controlled by the affected cells also is impaired. The effects range from slight to severe and may be temporary or permanent.

The most common cause of stroke is a blockage of the cerebral artery by a clot that forms within the artery. The condition is called cerebral thrombosis. A clot is more likely to develop in arteries damaged by arteriosclerosis, but blockage of the cerebral artery also may be caused by an embolus carried to the brain via the bloodstream from a distant part of the body.

Another cause of stroke is cerebral hemorrhage, which can occur in the distribution of any artery but most commonly occurs deep within one hemisphere or in the vital areas of the brainstem. It is more likely to occur in a patient who suffers from a combination of arteriosclerosis and hypertension. A stroke may be the result of both thrombosis and hemorrhage occurring at the same time.

The onset of a stroke is generally quite sudden. The state of consciousness may vary from alert to comatose. The pupils of the eyes may be unequal in size, and there may be a brisk, sluggish, or absent response to bright light. There may be facial drooping. Respirations may be abnormal—the slow, snoring type, where the cheeks puff out with each exhalation or the Cheyne-Stokes types of respiration—or there may be a deep, forceful regular breathing pattern. Usually there is weakness or paralysis in only one side of the body. Frequently, this weakness will be noted in the arm. Disturbance of speech and comprehension may be present. The physician should, of course, be promptly notified when such signs or symptoms are detected.

The nurse should be alert to and carry out those measures aimed at the prevention of complications. Because the patient may develop difficulty in breathing, maintenance of the airway through proper positioning and adequate suctioning is vital. The patient should be placed in a side-lying position to prevent aspiration of secretions and obstruction of the airway. Oral or tracheal suctioning should be done as needed to clear the airway.

The quantity and consistency of secretions should be noted. Oral fluids should be withheld if the patient has difficulty swallowing. Total fluid intake may be restricted in an effort to control cerebral edema. The vital signs—blood pressure, pulse, respirations—should be observed at least every hour until stable. The rate, rhythm, and quality of respiration should be noted. The temperature should be taken initially and at regular intervals, for the patient may develop a markedly elevated temperature. The size and equality of the pupils and pupillary response to light (flashlight) should be evaluated at regular intervals. The level of responsiveness, as evidenced by movement, response to painful stimuli, verbal requests, orientation to time, person, and place, should be evaluated every hour until a stable reaction is obtained. Bladder function following a stroke is frequently abnormal in the form of incontinence and/or retention. Urine output, therefore, should be accurately recorded. The physician may request that a Foley catheter be placed.

An explanation to the patient of what has happened and what is being done will help combat mental confusion and despair. Also, explanation of the condition and reassurance should be given family members.

Anaphylactic shock (extreme allergic reaction)

Anaphylactic shock is a condition that should be considered a true emergency. Anaphylactic reactions occur when a patient contacts something (allergen) to which he is extremely allergic. These reactions are uncommon but occasionally occur in patients with extreme degrees of sensitization; the patient with a history of allergies is more susceptible to such reactions than are those without such a history.

Drugs and other substances can cause a violent allergic reaction in a sensitized person. Penicillin (ingested or injected) and other drugs, antibiotics, or sera may cause a severe allergic reaction. Other substances such as pollen, dust, foods, and bee and wasp stings also may cause such a reaction. In an effort to prevent anaphylactic reaction, the patient should be questioned about sensitivity to drugs and to other substances. When a drug sensitivity is known, the medication or injection should not be given. Those substances to which the patient is known to be allergic should be noted clearly on the nursing care plan, on the medication card file, and on the front cover of the patient's medical record.

The nurse should be aware that an anaphylactic reaction may occur within a few seconds after exposure to an allergenic substance; thus, prompt recognition and treatment of the problem are vitally important.

The initial signs and symptoms of anaphylactic shock are itching about the face, chest, or site of injection, edema of the face, hands, and other parts of the body, and hives over large areas of the body. More serious symptoms are tightening or pain in the chest, dyspnea, wheezing, cyanosis, rapid and weak pulse, dizziness, faintness, and falling blood pressure. Circulatory failure leading to death may follow in a few minutes.

Epinephrine (Adrenalin) should be given subcutaneously by the nurse for immediate anaphylactic reaction in a dose appropriate to the patient's age and weight. The nurse should initiate other life-support measures as required, including cardiopulmonary resuscitation, establishment of an intravenous site, treatment of shock, and administration of oxygen until the physician arrives. The physician may request that hydrocortisone or antihistamine drugs (Benadryl) be given intravenously if the patient has a prolonged reaction. The slow intravenous administration of aminophylline may be ordered for patients with severe bronchospasm. Other drugs and the intravenous administration of fluids may be ordered if the response is not satisfactory.

Unit I STUDY QUESTIONS

STRUCTURE AND FUNCTION OF BONE AND JOINTS

1 List three types of bone cells and give the function of each.
2 Discuss the functions of bone.
3 List several laboratory tests for mineral metabolism, including normal values.
4 Discuss briefly several types of rickets and the necessary treatment.

BIOMECHANICS FOR NURSING/NURSING CARE PROBLEMS ASSOCIATED WITH INACTIVITY AND IMMOBILIZATION

1 List criteria for evaluating the following:
   a Standing posture
   b Sitting posture
2 Demonstrate use of correct body mechanics when doing the following:
   a Moving a patient to the side of the bed
   b Assisting a patient from the bed to a chair
   c Giving back care to a bed patient
3 Describe or demonstrate the normal range of motion at each of the following joints:
   a Shoulder
   b Elbow
   c Wrist
   d Metacarpophalangeal
   e Hip
   f Knee
   g Ankle
4 Be prepared to demonstrate good posture for the bed patient in the following positions:
   a Supine
   b Prone
   c Side-lying
5 What nursing care would you suggest to prevent the following:
   a Footdrop
   b Knee flexion contracture
   c Hip flexion contracture
6 Bed rest or inactivity may contribute to a number of complications by interfering with the physiologic processes of the body. Discuss nursing interventions that will help to minimize these problems.
7 What is meant by the stance and swing phases of a normal walking gait?
8 Discuss factors that should be included with nursing assessment of the musculoskeletal system.

EMERGENCY NURSING ON THE ORTHOPEDIC PATIENT UNIT

1 Discuss early signs and symptoms of airway obstruction and the necessary nursing interventions.
2 List factors to be considered when assessing respirations.
3 List nursing interventions that will aid in the prevention of pulmonary embolism.
4 List early signs and symptoms of shock.
5 Discuss and demonstrate cardiopulmonary resuscitation:
   a In the adult patient
   b In the infant patient
   c The procedure with one person
   d The procedure with two persons

Unit I REFERENCES

STRUCTURE AND FUNCTION OF BONE AND JOINTS

1 Atkinson, P. J., and Woodhead, C.: The development of osteoporosis, Clin Orthop 90: 217-228, Jan-Feb 1973.
2 Dunn, A. W.: Senile osteoporosis, Geriatrics 22:175-180, Nov 1967.
3 Hass, H. G.: Osteoporosis, Geriatrics 22:100-111, Dec 1967.
4 Hegsted, D. M.: Osteoporosis and fluoride deficiency, Postgrad Med 41:A49-53, Jan 1967.
5 Hohl, J. C., guest editor: Symposium on metabolic bone disease, Orthop Clin North Am 3:501-840, Nov 1972.
6 Jowsey, J.: Osteoporosis; its nature and the role of diet, Postgrad Med 59:75-79, Aug 1976.
7 Jowsey, J., Riggs, B. L., and Kelly, P. J.: New concepts in the treatment of osteoporosis, Postgrad Med 52:62-67, Oct 1972.
8 Lonergan, R. C.: Osteoporosis of the spine, Am J Nurs 61:79-81, Jan 1961.
9 Lutwak, L.: Osteoporosis: a public health problem, Am Assoc Industr Nurses J 14:21-23, Sep 1966.
10 Lyford, B.: Implications of osteoporosis, J Am Phys Ther Assoc 42:106-110, Feb 1962.
11 Moncrieff, M.: Rickets, Nurs Times 73:199-201, 10 Feb 1977.
12 Pinel, C.: Metabolic bone disease in the elderly, Nurs Times 72:1046-1048, 8 Jul 1976.
13 Riggs, B. L.: Diagnosis and treatment of primary osteoporosis, Postgrad Med 44:224-229, Oct 1968.

14 Soika, C. V.: Combatting osteoporosis, Am J Nurs **73**:1193-1197, Jul 1973.

15 Tapia, J., Stearns, G., and Ponseti, I. V.: Vitamin-D resistant rickets; a long-term clinical study of eleven patients, J Bone Joint Surg [Am] **46**:935-958, Jul 1964.

BIOMECHANICS FOR NURSING/NURSING CARE PROBLEMS ASSOCIATED WITH INACTIVITY AND IMMOBILIZATION

16 Alexander, M. M., and Brown, M. S.: Physical examination. Part 16: The musculoskeletal system, Nursing (Jenkintown) **6**:51-56, Apr 1976.

17 American Orthopaedic Association: Manual of orthopaedic surgery, Chicago, 1972.

18 Anderson, T. M.: Human kinetics and good movement, Physiotherapy **57**:169-176, Apr 1971.

19 Bates, B.: A guide to physical examination, Philadelphia, 1974, J. B. Lippincott Co.

20 Brower, P., and Hicks, D.: Maintaining muscle function in patients on bed rest, Am J Nurs **72**:1250-1253, Jul 1972.

21 Browse, N.: Physiology and pathology of bed rest, Springfield, Ill, 1965, Charles C Thomas, Publisher.

22 Cadogan, D.: Handling the handicapped, Physiotherapy **57**:467-470, Oct 1971.

23 Carnevali, D., and Brueckner, S.: Immobilization—reassessment of a concept, Am J Nurs **70**:1502-1507, Jul 1970.

24 Ciuca, R., Bradish, J., and Trombley, S. M.: Range of motion exercises, active and passive: a handbook, Nursing (Jenkintown) **3**: 25-37, Dec 1973.

25 Coles, C., Grendahl, B., Hannan, V., Plass, J., and Ulrich, P.: Rehabilitative nursing techniques. 3. A procedure for passive range of motion and self-assistive exercises, Minneapolis, 1964, Kenny Rehabilitation.

26 Cooper, J. M., and Glassow, R. B.: Kinesiology, ed. 4, St. Louis, 1976, The C. V. Mosby Co.

27 Drapeau, J., and Prave, M.: Getting back into good posture: how to erase your lumbar aches, Nursing (Jenkintown) **5**:63-65, Sep 1975.

28 Farrell, J.: Physical assessment of the extremities, ONA J **3**:80-83, Mar 1976.

29 Fixsen, J. A.: Common postural deformities in children. Nurs Times **68**:1086-1088, 31 Aug 1972.

30 Ford, J. R., and Duckworth, B.: Moving a dependent patient safely, comfortably: part I—positioning, Nursing (Jenkintown) **6**:27-36, Jan 1976.

31 Ford, J. R.: Duckworth, B., and Strong, G. F.: Moving a dependent patient safely, comfortably: part 2—transferring, Nursing (Jenkintown) **6**:58-65, Feb 1976.

32 Foss, G.: Use your head and save your back . . . body mechanics, Nursing (Jenkintown) **3**:25-32, May 1973.

33 Foss, G.: The "how to's" of bed positioning, Nursing (Jenkintown) **2**:14-16, Aug 1972.

34 Frankel, V. H., and Burstein, A. H.: Ortho- paedic biomechanics; the application of engineering to the musculoskeletal system, Philadelphia, 1970, Lea & Febiger.

35 Greenwood, M. W.: An illustrated approach to medical physics, ed. 2, Philadelphia, 1966, F. A. Davis Co.

36 Griffin, W., Anderson, S. J., and Passos, J. Y.: Group exercise for patients with limited motion, Am J Nurs **71**:1742-1743, Sep 1971.

37 Grimes, D. W., and Caley, J.: Ward physiotherapy, ONA J **4**:40-41, Feb 1977.

38 Gruis, M., and Innes, B.: Assessment: essential to prevent pressure sores, Am J Nurs **76**:1762-1764, Nov 1976.

39 Hirschberg, G. G., Lewis, L., and Vaughan, P.: Promoting patient mobility and other ways to prevent secondary disabilities, Nursing (Jenkintown) **7**:42-47, May 1977.

40 Hogberg, A.: Orthopedic nursing. Part 2. Preventing orthopedic complications, RN **38**:34-37, Mar 1975.

41 Jones, E.: Immobilisation syndrome in the elderly, Nurs Times **72**:1009-1011, 1 Jul 1976.

42 Jordan, H. S., and Kavchak, M. A.: Transfer techniques, Nursing (Jenkintown) **3**:19-22, Mar 1973.

43 Kamenetz, H. L.: Exercises for the elderly, Am J Nurs **72**:1401, Aug 1972.

44 Kern, F. C., and Poole, L.: Transfer techniques, Nursing (Jenkintown) **2**:25-28, Jul 1972.

45 Kottke, F. J.: Deterioration of the bedfast patient; causes and effects, Public Health Rep **80**:437-447, May 1965.

46 Krusen, F. H., Kottke, F., and Ellwood, P.: Handbook of physical medicine and rehabilitation, ed. 2, Philadelphia, 1971, W. B. Saunders Co.

47 Lilla, J. A., Friedrichs, R. R., and Vistnes, L. M.: Flotation mattresses for preventing and treating tissue breakdown, Geriatrics **30**:71-75, Sep 1975.

48 Millen, H. M.: Physically fit for nursing, Am J Nurs **70**:520-523, Mar 1970.

49 Müller, E. A.: Influence of training and of inactivity on muscle strength, Arch Phys Med Rehabil **51**:449-462, Aug 1970.

50 Nursing 74: How to negotiate the ups and downs, ins and outs of body alignment, Nursing (Jenkintown) **4**:46-51, Oct 1974.

51 Olson, E. V., Johnson, B. J., Thompson, L. F., McCarthy, J. A., Edmonds, R. E., Schroeder, L. M., and Wade, M.: The hazards of immobility, Am J Nurs **67**:779-797, Apr 1967.

52 Perry, J.: The mechanics of walking, Phys Ther **47**:778-801, Sep 1967.

53 Rantz, M. J., and Courtial, D.: Lifting, moving and transferring patients, St. Louis, 1977, The C. V. Mosby Co.

54 Saunders, J. B. de C. M., Inman, V. T., and Eberhart, H. D.: Major determinants in normal and pathological gait, J Bone Joint Surg [Am] **35**:543-558, Jul 1953.

55 Works, R. F.: Hints on lifting and pulling, Am J Nurs **72**:260-261, Feb 1972.

56 Young, C.: Exercise; how to use it to de-

crease complications in immobilized patients, Nursing (Jenkintown) 5:81-82, Mar 1975.

EMERGENCY NURSING ON THE ORTHOPEDIC PATIENT UNIT

57 The American National Red Cross: Advanced first aid and emergency care, New York, N. Y., 1973, Doubleday & Co., Inc.

58 Blount, M., and Kinney, A. B.: Chronic steroid therapy, Am J Nurs 74:1626-1631, Sep 1974.

59 Brunner, L. S., and Suddarth, D. S.: The Lippincott manual of nursing practice, Philadelphia, 1974, J. B. Lippincott Co.

60 Campbell, E. B.: Nursing problems associated with prolonged recovery following trauma, Nurs Clin North Am 5:551-562, Dec 1970.

61 Clark, N. E.: Pump failure, Nurs Clin North Am 7:529-539, Sep 1972.

62 Cohen, S.: Blood gas and acid base concepts in respiratory care, Am J Nurs 76:973-992, Jun 1976

63 Crenshaw, A. H., editor: Campbell's Operative orthopaedics, ed. 5, St. Louis, 1971, The C. V. Mosby Co.

64 Erikson, R.: Cranial check; a basic neurological assessment, Nursing (Jenkintown) 4:67-72, Aug 1974.

65 Gordon, A. S., chairman: Standards for cardiopulmonary resuscitation (CPR) and emergency cardiac care (ECC), JAMA 227(suppl):837-851, 18 Feb 1974.

66 Grant, H., and Murray, R.: Emergency care, Bowie, Md., 1971, Robert J. Brady Co. (subsidiary of Prentice-Hall, Inc.)

67 Higgins, H.: Your patient's illness is a family affair, RN 39:48-49, Nov 1976.

68 Hogberg, A.: Orthopedic nursing. Part 2. Preventing orthopedic complications, RN 38:34-37, Mar 1975.

69 Houser, D.: What to do first when a patient complains of chest pain, Nursing (Jenkintown) 6:54-56, Nov 1976.

70 Houser, D. M.: Emergency cardiac care, Nurs Clin North Am 8:401-411, Sep 1973.

71 Johnson, C. F., and Convery, F. R.: Preventing emboli after total hip replacement, Am J Nurs 75:804-806, May 1975.

72 Kempe, C. H., Silver, H. K., and O'Brien, D.: Current pediatric diagnosis and treatment,

ed. 3, Los Altos, Calif., 1974, Lange Medical Publications.

73 Kintzell, K. C., editor: Advanced concepts in clinical nursing, Philadelphia, 1971, J. B. Lippincott Co.

74 Krystowski, K., and Nelson, C.: Total hip-replacement arthoplasty: postoperative care of patient, Hosp Topics 71:69-72, Nov 1971.

75 Law, J.: Symposium on current surgical nursing: the fat embolism syndrome, Nurs Clin North Am 8:191-198, Mar 1973.

76 Liechty, R., and Soper, R.: Synopsis of surgery, ed. 3, St. Louis, 1976, The C. V. Mosby Co.

77 Meltzer, L. E., Abdellah, F., and Kitchell, J.: Concepts and practices of intensive care for nurse specialist, Philadelphia, 1969, The Charles Press Publishers, Inc.

78 O'Dell, A. J.: Emergency care in establishing an effective airway, Nurs Clin North Am 8:413-424, Sep 1973.

79 Plum, F., and Posner, J. B.: The diagnosis of stupor and coma, ed. 2, Philadelphia, 1972, F. A. Davis Co.

80 Quesenbury, J. H., and Lembright, P.: Observations and care for patients with head injuries, Nurs Clin North Am 4:237-247, Jun 1969.

81 Ryan, M. A.: Helping the family to cope with a cardiac arrest, Nursing (Jenkintown) 4:80-81, Aug 1974.

82 Shapiro, R. M.: Anticoagulant therapy, Am J Nurs 73:439-443, Mar 1974.

83 Stein, A. M., Mandell, D., and Ferguson, J.: Multiple fractures: look out for those pulmonary complications, Nursing (Jenkintown) 4:26-32, Nov 1974.

84 Steinberg, J., and Hurst, J. W.: Role of nurse in cardiac arrest, Nurs Clin North Am 2:245-254, Jun 1967.

85 Wiley, L.: Shock 2. Different kinds—different problems, Nursing (Jenkintown) 4:19-27, Apr 1974.

86 Wyper, M.: Pulmonary embolism: fighting the silent killer, Nursing (Jenkintown) 5:31-38, Oct 1975.

87 Young, J. F.: Recognition, significance, and recording of the signs of increased intracranial pressure, Nurs Clin North Am 4:223-235, Jun 1969.

6 The patient in a cast

To preserve the efficiency of a cast while maintaining the patient in cleanliness and comfort taxes the ingenuity of the best nurse. This skill is important in orthopedic nursing, and physicians frequently judge the competency of the nursing staff by the care given to patients in casts. No one way of caring for these patients can be arbitrarily defined, and nurses are learning new and better methods daily.

Although it is the nurse's responsibility to safeguard the efficiency of the cast (i.e., its ability to maintain the position for which it was applied over the period of time necessary for the accomplishment of treatment) her first concern must be the patient in the cast. One thing to understand clearly from the outset is that the patient's every complaint must have prompt attention, even though it may seem trifling and the nurse may privately consider the patient to be a chronic complainer. The patient who seldom complains is given solicitous attention when he reports a burning sensation over common points of pressure, such as the heel, the malleoli, or the sacrum. It is the constantly complaining patient who may be overlooked, so that when the cast is finally removed a sloughing sore may be found over an area he had told the nurse about at one time—an orthopedic version of the story about the boy who cried "wolf."

Neurovascular evaluation—nursing assessment skills

Nurses have been warned repeatedly about the dangers of impaired circulation in an extremity just placed in a cast, and it seems that the subject could be passed over with little more than a word. However, inspecting the fingers or toes of an extremity encased in plaster is as important as taking a pulse rate after an operation. It is important to watch for signs of circulatory impairment, as well as for signs of hemorrhage. The rapidity with which such an impairment may progress from bad to worse is difficult for the inexperienced nurse to comprehend. Permanent paralysis may be produced within a twenty-four–hour period.

Neurovascular evaluation of an extremity following application of a cast includes noting the color of the digits and comparing it with that of the digits of the opposite extremity. Cyanotic toes or fingers indicate venous stasis or interference with the return flow of blood, whereas whiteness or pallor is an indication of arterial impairment. Nurses should be familiar with the blanching sign, which is particularly important in caring for patients with casts applied to the leg or arm. The nail of the thumb or great toe is momentarily compressed and the return flow of blood to the nail observed. The compressed area should refill with blood immediately upon the release of pressure; i.e., the nail should turn from white to pink at once.

The skin temperature of the involved digits should be compared with that of the digits of the opposite limb. Cold fingers or toes can indicate poor circulation. However, a newly applied cast, which is still wet, and the application of cold to an extremity may be factors the nurse needs to consider. The toes or fingers should be checked for edema and the patient's complaints of discomfort or pain heeded carefully. The testing of digits for sensation and motion is important. Numbness, a tingling sensation, and the absence of feeling or motion are indications of pressure and/or damage to a peripheral nerve. Pressure on a peripheral nerve can be caused by circulatory impairment and edema or by direct pressure from the cast. An example in the lower extremity is that of peroneal paralysis. Pressure on the lateral aspect of the leg over the head of the fibula compresses the peroneal nerve against the bone. If there is injury to the nerve, weakness or paralysis of the muscles will occur, and dorsiflexion and inversion of the foot will not be possible. If the cast permits, the presence or absence of peripheral pulses should be noted and compared with the normal side. A diminished pulse or failure to feel the pulse warrants notifying the physician at once. Marking the spot where a hard-to-find pulse may be felt is also helpful for other nurses involved with the patient's care. Coldness, pallor, blue-

ness, edema, loss of motion, numbness, pain, and a slow return of blood to a part upon blanching are cardinal symptoms. It is important that all the fingers and toes are visible. Further, the nurse should not be satisfied with twelve or twenty-four hours of close observation. The extremity must be watched during many succeeding days.

It is essential that the neurovascular evaluation be recorded on the patient's chart. The notations should indicate the time frequency and the findings, as well as any action taken by the nurse. Nurses responsible for checking extremities enclosed in plaster should have a working knowledge of the nerves supplying the extremi-

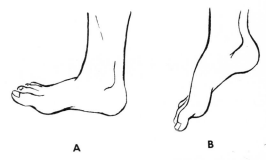

A   B

Fig. 98 Assessing motor function of the nerves of the lower extremity. **A,** Peroneal nerve—observe the patient's ability to dorsiflex his foot. **B,** Tibial nerve—observe the patient's ability to plantar flex his foot.

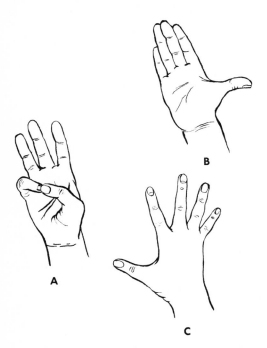

Fig. 97 Assessing motor function of the nerves of the upper extremity. **A,** Median nerve—observe the patient's ability to touch the end of his little finger with his thumb (opposition). **B,** Radial nerve—observe the patient's ability to hyperextend his thumb or wrist. **C,** Ulnar nerve—observe the patient's ability to spread his fingers.

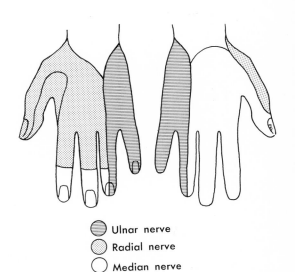

Ulnar nerve
Radial nerve
Median nerve

Fig. 99 Sensory map of hand.

ties as well as methods of checking their sensory and motor function (Figs. 97 to 99).

Compartment syndrome; Volkmann's contracture

Care of the individual with injury of an extremity involves careful assessment for the development of edema and ischemia of the soft tissues. In the extremities, groups of muscles are enclosed within tough fascial envelopes. Blood vessels and nerves enter and leave these compartments through small openings. In addition to the compartments, each muscle is covered by a fibrous sheath known as epimysium. Compartments in the forearm are the extensor, the deep flexor, and the superficial flexor. Those in the lower portion of the leg are the anterior, peroneal, and posterior.

When trauma to a muscle or group of muscles causes edema of the soft tissues, pressure within the compartment increases greatly due to the restricting fascial envelope enclosing the muscles. The increasing intramuscular pressure causes compression of the small openings, through which the blood vessels and nerves enter and leave the compartment. Sufficient pressure build-up can result in nerve damage and decreased blood supply, producing a progressive irreversible necrosis of the involved muscle tissue. The most important symptom is pain—unrelenting pain that continues to increase in severity. Normally following immobilization of an injured extremity, the amount of pain is not expected to increase but should become less of a problem rather than progressively worse. Passive flexion or extension of the fingers or toes, depending on the compartment involved, causes increased pain due to the pressure placed on the ischemic area. As pressure within a compartment increases, some degree of sensory loss also can be expected, and numbness and tingling will develop. When the forearm is involved, areas supplied by the ulnar and median nerves will be affected. In the lower extremity, involvement of the posterior tibial nerve produces paresthesia of the plantar surface of the foot and involvement of the peroneal branch causes paresthesia in the web space between the

first and second toes. Loss of motor function also can be expected to occur as the pressure and ischemic condition progress. Assessing the individual's ability to actively flex and extend the fingers or the toes is important. A decrease or loss of peripheral pulses should be noted and checked carefully.

When a compartment syndrome is suspected, an *emergency* situation exists. Treatment is aimed at relieving the swelling and ischemia. Casts and bandages are removed, and the part is elevated. If improvement does not occur within a short time, fasciotomy and/or epimysiotomy is done. This means that the tough fascia enclosing a group of muscles is split longitudinally and, when necessary, the sheath (epimysium) covering individual muscles is divided. With this procedure, pressure on the nerve and blood supply is relieved. If the edema and muscle ischemia are not relieved, a permanent, disabling, unsightly contracture (Volkmann's) of the limb will develop. In time, atrophy and fibrosis of the muscle tissue will occur (Fig. 182), and, due to the nerve damage, motor and sensory functions will be absent.

Care of casts

Although care of the patient is the primary concern, the cast is also important. It has cost both time and money and is of considerable importance in the patient's recovery.

Supporting wet casts. Care of the cast begins before the patient is returned to the unit from the plaster room. It begins with the preparation of the bed. A firm mattress is a necessity. Boards spread, preferably lengthwise, under the mattress are essential when the cast encloses the legs and the body (body or hip spica cast). Pillows should be ready to support the wet cast (Fig. 100). These pillows need plastic covers to prevent dampness and mustiness that would result from absorption of moisture from the plaster. They also need to be pliable and easily adjusted to the contour of the patient's body. For the patient with a body cast, three pillows laid crosswise on the bed are usually satisfactory. For the patient with a hip spica cast, it is best to arrange one pillow crosswise at the level of the waist and two lengthwise for the

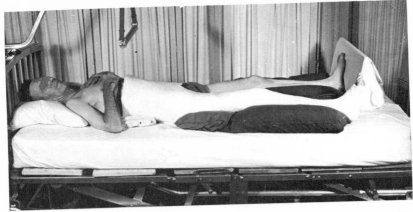

Fig. 100 Correct support for the patient in a hip spica cast in the supine position. The pillows beneath the limb enclosed in plaster provide support for the thigh and avoid pressure on the heel. The small pad that supports the lumbar region prevents the anterior portion of the cast from pressing on the abdomen, and the pillow for the head, placed well down under the shoulders, maintains good alignment of the cervical spine. Boards beneath the mattress provide a firm surface for the cast. Note the trapeze, which facilitates nursing care of the patient in a hip spica cast.

single leg in the cast. The latter should be arranged so that the leg portion of the spica cast is supported along its full length and no strain is imposed on the groin section, which is always vulnerable to cracking. If both legs are to be encased, two more pillows are needed for the second leg of the adult patient. A pillow for the head and shoulders is necessary unless the patient has had an anesthetic.

A common error is to elevate head and chest without providing for support under the back, with the result that an actual bending of the body occurs just above the body section of the hip spica cast. This causes the edges of the cast to press against the soft portion of the abdomen and frequently results in a feeling of fullness and pressure in the abdomen that is mistaken for distention. This troublesome feature usually can be eliminated by a pillow or pad placed beneath the lumbar region to support the body portion of the cast (Fig. 100).

The patient in a damp cast should not be lifted directly onto the hard bed when he is returned from the plaster room. The cast would become flattened over the bony prominences, particularly the back of the heel and the sacrum, and damage to the underlying soft tissues would be unavoidable.

The patient must be lifted carefully onto the bed that has been prepared with pillows. The nurse helping with this procedure should use the palms of the hands, not the fingers, to lift the cast. Fingers may make indentations in the soft plaster if it is not sufficiently set. This is particularly important in handling the foot and leg section of the cast.

Drying casts. If the patient has not been anesthetized, the cast usually is left uncovered for several hours. Many physicians prefer that casts be dried in this way —by natural evaporation. If quick drying is essential, as it often is when the patient is to leave the hospital shortly, it can be started as soon as the cast is set. Some form of external heat is usually satisfactory. Heat lamps or a cradle on which a low-watt incandescent lamp (preferably enclosed in a wire cage) is suspended at a safe distance from the patient and the cast may be used for this. A distance of at least fifteen inches from the cast to the light is usually considered safe. The cradle should not be covered with bedclothes because the moisture will be resorbed by the cast as the confined space under the bedclothes becomes saturated. Escape for the moisture-laden air is essential.

A hand dryer, such as that used for drying the hair, may be employed and is especially good for small areas of plaster that have become dampened through mishaps. Intense heat is never recommended because it tends to cause the outer layers to dry too swiftly while the underlying layers remain moist.

With the early setting and drying process, it frequently has been observed that during warm weather the cast becomes very hot. If the cast is left entirely uncovered, the air will greatly hasten evaporation and hardening, and the heat of the cast will be transitory.

It is necessary to understand the basic chemistry of plaster of Paris in order to know exactly what is happening in the cast as it sets and hardens. The plaster of Paris commonly used when a cast is applied is made from gypsum (calcium sulfate, $CaSO_4 \cdot 2H_2O$). When the gypsum crystals are heated, the water of crystallization is driven off, and the remaining calcined gypsum is plaster of Paris ($CaSO_4 \cdot \frac{1}{2}H_2O$). The finely powdered plaster of Paris is incorporated into a mesh bandage to produce the plaster-of-Paris roll or splint. When the plaster-of-Paris bandage is placed in water, preparatory to use, the reverse action takes place: water is absorbed and crystals of gypsum are formed. During formation of these gypsum crystals, the potential full strength of the plaster is determined according to the closeness with which the crystals interlock. The maximum strength is obtained only after all excess water has been evaporated from the cast's surface. When this is accomplished and the cast is wholly dry, it is strong and firm and able to withstand sudden stresses.

Finishing cast edges. When sheet wadding or similar material has been used to line the cast, it is impossible to pull the lining over the cast edge as is done with stockinet. However, adhesive tape may be used to cover the cast edges. If adhesive is used (without additional plaster of Paris to secure the outer edge), the cast must be thoroughly dry to prevent the tape from rolling. This usually requires from twenty-four to forty-eight hours, depending on the thickness of the cast and the humidity of the air. Petals of tape, cut round or pointed and about 1½ in long, are excellent for binding cast edges. When adhesive is applied to the dry cast, it is important that

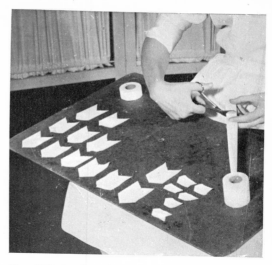

Fig. 101 Lapboard used in cutting petals for finishing the edges of a cast. Note the position of the tape strip. It is folded so that the sticky sides are out and then cut diagonally toward the center fold.

the edges be pressed securely against the plaster to prevent the tape from rolling and sticking to the bed linen. To prevent rolling, a plaster-of-Paris strip can be moistened and placed over the outer edge of adhesive tape; this will hold the petals in place and maintain a smooth, tape-covered cast edge. Likewise, the edges of the newly applied, damp cast can be finished with such petals if a plaster-of-Paris splint or bandage is used to secure their outer edges. The adhesive petals adhere nicely to the sheet wadding on the underneath side of the cast and are held in place on the outer aspect of the damp cast with a moistened plaster-of-Paris splint. This permits finishing the edges of a cast, lined with sheet wadding, immediately following application and trimming of the cast. Petals may be easily prepared by folding a strip of adhesive tape 1½ in or 2 in wide lengthwise (sticky side out) and cutting through it diagonally (at a 45° angle) toward the center fold (Fig. 101).

If stockinet has been used to line the cast, the ideal method of finishing the cast is to pull the stockinet over the edges and secure it with a moistened plaster splint. This can be done before the cast is completely dry, thus sealing off the edges and eliminating plaster crumbs.

Before the edges are finished, all rough spots or irregularities likely to cause pressure areas or irritation of the skin must be removed. Also, before the cast is finished around the buttocks, enough room for the patient to have proper care after voiding and defecation must be ensured. If the cutout space seems unnecessarily small, the physician should be consulted before it is bound. Since most physicians are eager to allow enough room for proper nursing care of these patients, an insufficient cutout usually is an oversight. An exception to this may occur in the case of patients in whom adductor tenotomies have been performed and whose incisions are very close to the perineum.

Protecting casts. The protection of casts from soiling and moisture is a point of considerable interest. The ingenuity of a generation of nurses has been taxed by this troublesome problem. The impossibility of properly protecting casts caused such men as Dr. Vittorio Putti and Sir Robert Jones to declare that plaster of Paris could be used for home treatment only with the greatest risks and danger. However, the modern nurse can devise many methods of protection that are also simple enough to make home care of patients in casts not only safe but also quite satisfactory.

The perineal region may be protected against body excretions by the use of a waterproof material. Inexpensive plastic materials provide excellent protection when they are properly applied (Figs. 102 and 103).

Waterproof material is cut in strips 4-5 in in width and tucked under the cast around the curved area at the buttocks. It is secured on the outside of the cast with adhesive tape, mending tape, or a single layer of plaster of Paris.

Casts cannot be washed, for water will soften them. The life of a cast that is frequently dampened will be shortened, its efficiency will be lessened, and mold will almost inevitably appear on its surface. It is usually considered permissible to remove very minor stains from casts with a cleanser (powder or cake) applied with a damp cloth. If the area is large, cleansing must be followed by some form of artificial heat or sunlight to dry the cast as quickly as possible. Shellac, varnish, or lacquer must not

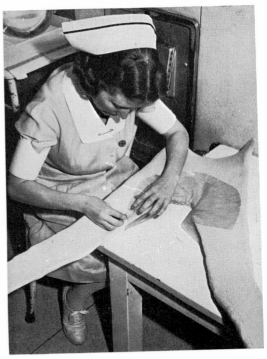

Fig. 102 Basting a waterproof pattern around removable shell of a hip spica cast. Pattern is a double semicircle of Pilofilm cut out to fit the cast opening and basted together on concave edges before it is applied to the shell.

be used to waterproof casts until they are thoroughly dried, preferably not until forty-eight hours after application. Waterproofing the entire cast before it is dry prevents the proper evaporation of moisture.

Old stockings may be used to cover casts in the home and provide excellent protection for leg casts on children. In some clinics all casts are covered completely with stockinet before the patient is discharged. The outer stockinet is sewed to that used as the cast lining. Unquestionably, this method does preserve the cast more satisfactorily than any other, but it entails a considerable amount of time, more than is usually available in the modern hospital.

It has been suggested that the waterproof material used to protect casts be applied in strips rather than in a solid piece. The reason for this is obvious because a curving surface is to be bound. The material is tucked under the cast so that it folds back, thus forming a dam against excretions, but too much material must not be used under the cast or it will become wrinkled. The plaster-of-Paris bandage or tape used to hold the outer edge should be applied in such a fashion that the waterproof material can be easily slipped out from under the cast without its being entirely detached.

Cleaning casts. The orthopedic nurse should take pride in keeping casts as spotless as possible. With the best of care, however, accidents do occur, particularly with small children. Knowing how to repair damage is a satisfying accomplishment and seems like nothing short of a miracle to the onlooker.

The outside of the cast may be cleaned easily. Superficial and small stains can be removed with a cleasner carefully applied with a damp cloth. For the larger areas of soilage, the pattern method of repair is recommended. A double thickness of plaster bandage of suitable width is cut to fit exactly over the soiled area. This pattern is swiftly immersed in water so that it is barely moistened through when it is lifted from the pan. Then it is applied directly over the soiled area and carefully rubbed into the cast. It must be well incorporated by rubbing, or it will peel off later like an onion skin. Some orthopedists advise that the cast be roughened slightly with a nail file or scissors before the pattern is applied. A sprinkling of talcum powder rubbed into the moistened plaster will help remove the odor that may accompany soilage.

A more troublesome problem is encountered when the inside of the cast becomes soiled. To remedy this, the stockinet lining of the cast may be carefully detached from the area around the buttocks or groin with either a razor blade or sharp scissors. It can then be pulled down and the soiled area trimmed off. Stockinet stretches to a considerable degree and is not at all difficult to manage. The clean stockinet edge is then pulled out over the cast edges and secured to the cast either with adhesive tape or a bit of moist plaster-of-Paris bandage. Repeated soiling and repair of this kind would, of course, deplete the available stockinet lining.

If sheet wadding instead of stockinet has been used to line the cast, small portions must be carefully pulled out, and the in-

side of the cast cleaned with a sparingly dampened cloth.

On the adult units, where all this elaborate precaution seldom seems necessary, protection may be managed by small disposable waterproof pads put in place only when the patient uses the bedpan. To risk such underprotection on a pediatric unit, however, is usually dangerous to the cast. Nor should too much confidence be placed in the adolescent girl in a spica cast. Any patient in a cast is relatively helpless in taking care of his toilet needs, and the orthopedic nurse must understand this from the outset.

Turning patients in casts

The time of the first turning of a patient in a new cast frequently depends on the physician's order, but in orthopedic hospitals usually there is a standing order that all patients be turned by the evening of the day the cast is applied. This is done primarily for the comfort of the patient and also to permit drying of the posterior surface of the cast. The first turning of a patient in a body cast or a hip spica cast requires more help than will be needed subsequently when the cast has become rigid and firm through drying. To turn a patient with a new cast without assistance endangers the cast and should not be attempted if it can be avoided.

With a crew of three people, an adult patient in a hip spica cast can be turned without much risk either to his comfort or to the integrity of the cast. The patient is gently pulled toward the side of the bed that corresponds to the leg in the cast. It is possible to effect this move by exerting a pull on the pillows beneath the cast. After the patient has been pulled to this side, two of the crew should go around the bed, where, if necessary, a fresh drawsheet can be started and the pillows arranged to receive the cast when the patient is turned (Fig. 103).

The pillowcases should be changed if they are damp. When they do not need changing, it is sometimes possible to pull the pillows partially through from under the cast without allowing the cast to drop from them.

Turning should always be done on the side not enclosed in plaster or toward the

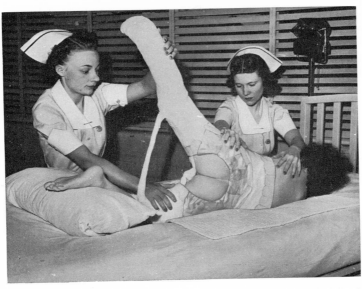

Fig. 103 Turning the patient in a hip spica cast. Note the pillow in place for foot support. The abduction bar should not be used as a handle when lifting or turning the patient. Strips of protective material have been applied to protect the cast in the perineal area.

side that has not been operated upon in the patient in a double spica cast. The patient is thus turned on his normal leg and toward the nurses who are assisting him. One nurse remains on the side of the bed toward which the patient has been pulled in order to overcome any sense of insecurity he may have from a fear of falling. The other two nurses turn the patient toward them from the opposite side. The patient is told exactly what is to be done, and he is instructed to place the arm on which he is turning above his head. With adults, it may be easier for the patient to keep his arms close to his sides. To avoid pressure on the arm on which he is turning, a folded towel should be placed between the arm and the cast. The pillow beneath the patient's head should be removed during the turning. In the turning procedure, the nurses must move in unison. One places her hands on the shoulder and hip of the patient while another supports the thigh and foot of the extremity in the cast. The nurse on the opposite side assists with the turning by pulling the shoulder through as the patient is gently eased onto his face.

Pillows along the entire length of the cast must be in readiness in order to avoid having to lift the patient after he is turned.

Not only is lifting exceedingly uncomfortable for the patient, but it also endangers the soft cast. In addition, it places an unnecessary and avoidable strain on the nurse's back. After the patient has been turned, the nurse should observe his position to see that the toes of the leg in the cast do not press against the mattress. A pillow laid crosswise on the bed, beneath the ankle, will provide support for the foot. If there is wide abduction in the cast, the toes of the foot in plaster may hang over the edge of the mattress. Another point to be observed is the position of the body section of the cast. If there are too many pillows under the patient's head and shoulders, the plaster may press into the back just below the ribs. If the pillow under the abdomen is not placed correctly, the cast edges may press into the soft tissues of the chest and abdomen (Fig. 104).

Later, when the cast is completely hardened, one or two nurses may turn the patient with a minimum of difficulty. Patients soon learn to assist with turning to such an extent that little help is needed from the nurse or attendant. When the cast is dry, pillows are needed only for the patient's comfort and may be dispensed with except at points of pressure. A support for the heel so that it does not rest on the bed

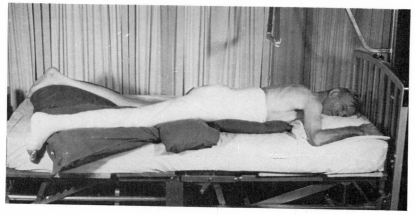

Fig. 104 Correct support for the patient in a hip spica cast in the prone position. The extremity enclosed in plaster is supported by pillows to prevent strain on the cast at the groin area. There is enough abduction to permit the foot enclosed in plaster to extend over the edge of the mattress. The thin pillow placed crosswise at top edge of the cast prevents undue pressure on the abdomen, and one pillow for the head maintains good alignment of the shoulders and neck. Note the position of the normal extremity.

is usually considered essential, and patients are generally more comfortable with a pillow beneath the body portion of the cast when they are in the prone position. When this pillow is in place, the patient's chest will be the forward portion of the body.

When the patient is turned the first time, the cast will still be damp on its posterior surface and will usually be rather compressed against the back. Some method of quick drying should be used at this time, and the patient's back should be given meticulous care. The buttocks will be blue and creased and will need particular attention. The skin around the cast edges and immediately beneath the cast can be reached with the fingers, and this area can be rubbed and gently stretched away from the cast to increase comfort and circulation. Any rough edges on the posterior surface of the cast must be cared for at this time. Insufficient room for defecation should be noted and reported.

After the cast has been trimmed, if necessary, the stockinet lining may be pulled over the cast edge and secured with a moistened plaster-of-Paris splint or bandage.

If the patient is a child, however, some thought must be given to the protection of the buttocks region. It is never safe to expect the child to get through the night without soiling the cast. Small strips of

waterproof material may be tucked under the cast and the outer edges secured with a plaster-of-Paris splint.

The patient should be urged to lie prone as long as he can. Encouragement from the nurse may often prolong this period to as much as forty-five minutes to an hour. When this rest period is completed, the patient is again turned with the precautions described.

If the surgeon has ordered a window cut over the abdomen or chest, it is usually wise to wait until the plaster is dry, for the cast may break or buckle if the window is cut too early. The surgeon, of course, should be consulted in this matter.

Placing patient in cast on bedpan

Even with the most artful padding and waterproofing, the nurse's worries are not over. Extreme caution must be taken when placing the bedpan so that the buttocks are not higher than the head and shoulders. Inevitably, this situation will cause urine to flow backward inside the cast, and the drying of the cast afterward is no small problem. Elevating the head of the bed slightly and placing another pillow under the patient's back while he is voiding will prevent this accident. Unless a patient is in shock or is hemorrhaging, it is almost always permissible to elevate the head and shoulders for use of the bedpan. Sharp

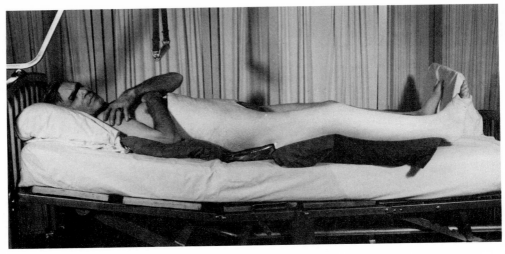

Fig. 105 Placement of the patient with a hip spica cast on the bedpan. To avoid strain on the cast at the groin area, pillows have been placed beneath the limb enclosed in plaster and beneath the lumbar and hip regions. The head of the bed has been elevated slightly to help prevent soiling or wetting the posterior aspect of the cast.

angulation at the groin must be avoided to prevent breaking the cast. In addition, a folded diaper or pad should be placed on the posterior aspect of the bedpan to absorb moisture and prevent the lining of the cast from becoming wet with urine (Fig. 105).

One of two methods is usually used to place an adult on the bedpan. One method consists of turning the patient on his uninjured side, placing the bedpan so that the fleshy part of the buttocks contacts the posterior section of the pan, arranging pillows or blankets to support the legs and back on the same level as the buttocks, and then returning the patient to the back-lying position. By the other method, with an overhead trapeze to support himself, the patient may be placed on the bedpan without turning. The nurse elevates the hips with one hand and slips the bedpan under them with the other.

Pillows should be used to support the legs of the patient in a long leg cast when he is placed on a bedpan. Otherwise, he will be insecure and uncomfortable with his legs unsupported in space as his body is elevated to the level of the pan. The groin area of long leg casts in children needs protection with a waterproof material.

The small child in a hip spica cast pre-

sents a more complicated problem. A Bradford frame hung on hooks in the crib or supported on boxes with the head end slightly higher than the foot end may be used. The frame is prepared with a two-piece covering, so arranged that an open space is left under the buttocks. A bedpan is kept constantly under this space. However, in recent years, with better methods of protecting the cast, it has been possible to care for the small child and to maintain a clean intact cast without the use of the frame. Plastic-covered pillows arranged to provide for a slight elevation of the head and shoulders are used to help prevent urine from running backward and inside the cast. As previously described, the perineal area of the cast must be protected with waterproof material. A folded disposable diaper, is used as a perineal pad and may be held in place by a regular diaper. In addition to applying the waterproof material, it is very essential that this child be checked frequently and that diaper changes be made as needed.

Care of patient's skin

Meticulous observation is essential in caring for the patient in a cast. All visible skin must be inspected daily for signs of abrasions or irritation. All areas that come in contact with cast edges must have particular attention, for cast sores are frequently encountered at these sites. Fingers moistened sparingly with alcohol should explore under the cast as far as it is possible to reach. If beginning abrasions or skin blemishes are noted, they should be inspected frequently. Nurses should also learn to inspect casts with the sense of smell as well as with the senses of sight and touch. It takes experience to learn to detect abnormal odors, but sometimes even an inexperienced nurse will be able to locate the exact position of a musty odor that may be the only evidence of a sloughing area beneath a cast. It is sometimes possible to detect an underlying pressure sore by the temperature of the cast, for the cast tends to become warmer over an area that is beginning to discharge. Eyes, nose, and fingers are of equal importance in cast care.

Each time the patient is given nursing care, the waterproof fabric around the groin and buttocks should be pulled out from beneath the cast and the cast inspected for soilage, dampness, and mold. Time should be taken to dry this portion of the cast, and the waterproof fabric should be washed with warm soapy water, rinsed, dried, and powdered before it is replaced neatly and smoothly under the edges of the cast. If this is done at least once a day, the life of the material will be greatly prolonged. It will also prevent the formation of small troublesome pimples on the skin that appear around the edges of the cast when the skin and cast are neglected.

Certain other areas of the patient in a cast are commonly vulnerable to pressure sores. The heel on the unaffected side may become sore because the patient habitually pushes himself up in bed with the uninvolved leg. The elbows sometimes become sore because the patient braces himself on them to see what is going on around him. These areas can be cared for more easily than those covered by casts and should never be allowed to reach the stage of skin breakdown.

The importance of providing support for the uninvolved extremity cannot be overemphasized. It should be in excellent condition to withstand the strain that will be put upon it when the patient becomes ambulatory. Support should be provided by footboards, boxes, pillows, or sandbags. In addition, bed exercises will do much to maintain muscle strength and joint range of motion.

Care of patients with arm and leg casts

The nurse responsible for the postsurgical or trauma patient with a newly applied cast needs to remember that immediate and continuous elevation of the limb (above the heart level) will help prevent edema and circulatory problems. She also knows that the application of cold lessens pain as well as edema and that care should be taken to place ice bags in positions that avoid weight and pressure on the involved limb. Encouraging the patient to move fingers and toes (unless contraindicated) will help prevent edema as well as stiffness and limitation of motion.

Elevation of the leg of a patient with a long leg cast usually requires three pillows (Fig. 106) or the use of an overhead frame with one crossbar and a hammock that may be suspended from the frame. The latter eliminates the use of pillows and ensures constant elevation of the limb. Pillows also may be used to support the upper extremity. However, continuous elevation of the part is more likely to be maintained if the arm can be suspended from an overhead frame. When a cast has been applied to the forearm, muslin bandage may be used for this purpose, and when a soft dressing has been applied to the hand, stockinet of the proper width and length may be slipped over the extremity. The proximal end of the stockinet is anchored to the upper arm, and the distal portion, which should extend beyond the fingers, can be used for suspending the extremity to the overhead frame. Holes will need to be cut in the stockinet to facilitate checking circulation in the fingers. When the forearm and hand are suspended in this manner, the flexed elbow and upper arm must be supported by the mattress or a pillow to prevent shoulder discomfort.

In the ambulatory patient, a sling may be used to support the arm in the cast. In this connection, the nurse should be reminded of the potential danger and discomfort of a sling tied in a hard knot over the back of the neck causing constant pressure on the cervical spine. The triangle

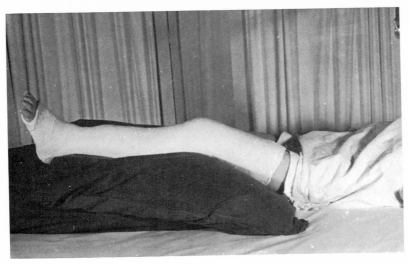

Fig. 106 Placement of pillows to support the leg of a patient with a long leg cast. Note that the support is continued along the entire limb in order to eliminate strain on any muscle group. The patient's foot extends beyond the edge of the top pillow, thus preventing pressure or weight on the heel. With some patients it will be necessary to place a sandbag or trochanter roll along the lateral aspect of the thigh to prevent external rotation of the extremity. To prevent edema, the foot is maintained at a level with or higher than the knee and hip.

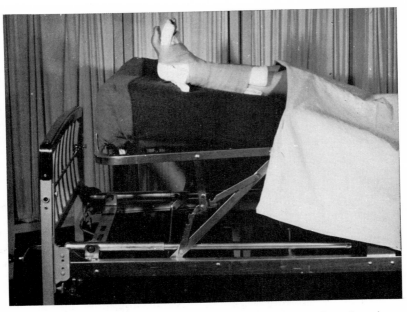

Fig. 107 With the type of bed illustrated, the leg of a patient with a short leg cast may be elevated by raising the knee roll and the lower portion of the springs.

sling is more comfortable if it is pinned in two places with safety pins to divide the stress of the weight. The three-cornered sling is applied so that the long bias edge encircles the wrist and the ends are crossed over alternate shoulders (Fig. 108). It should support the wrist and, in most instances, maintain the forearm at a right angle. With hand and wrist injuries, it may be applied in such a manner as to provide for some elevation of the hand.

The patient using a sling for an extended period of time should be instructed in range-of-motion exercise for the shoulder joint. Failure to use this joint due to hand or lower arm injury may be followed by

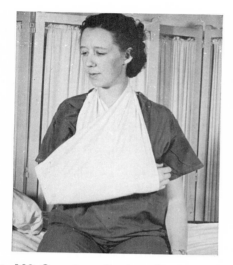

Fig. 108 Correct application of an arm sling. Note support of the wrist. The sling ends are crossed on the posterior aspect of the neck and pinned in two places.

tightening of the soft tissue around the joint and result in limited shoulder motion. Various types of slings made from durable material and in dark colors are available from surgical supply houses for the person who must use a sling for an extended period of time.

Short leg casts with an abduction bar as illustrated in Fig. 109 may be used to maintain the desired position of the extremities. When the patient is being turned, the abduction bar should not be used to lift or support the limb.

Cleanliness of toes and fingers in casts is frequently a point of neglect. The patient may be well bathed otherwise and the toes or fingers overlooked. Applicators moistened in alcohol can be used to clean, refresh, and deodorize unreachable fingers and toes. Cast crumbs in these areas are dangerous as well as annoying. They can be eliminated to a great extent by binding the edges of the cast around the toes and fingers with adhesive tape if there is no stockinet that can be pulled over these edges and taped.

Care of patients in anterior and posterior splints

Occasionally, hip casts and body casts are bivalved and made into removable

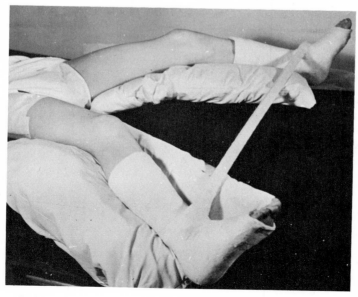

Fig. 109 Use of plaster to maintain the desired position of the lower extremity. The right limb is held in a position of abduction and internal rotation by means of bilateral short leg casts and an abduction bar.

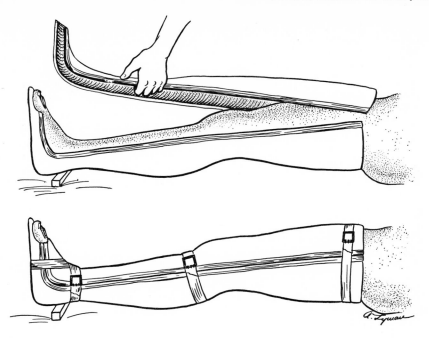

Fig. 110 The bivalved cast used frequently in convalescent care of patients with fractures, sprained ligaments, bursitis, poliomyelitis, arthritis, synovitis, and many other conditions, when protection is still necessary but access to the limb and joints is needed for daily treatments. Illustration also shows use of a heel bar to prevent rotation of the limb.

shells so that the patient may receive the benefits of skin care, massage, and/or exercises. If these casts have been on the patient for some time, considerable cleaning may be necessary in order to renovate them. A change of stockinet lining may be easily effected without disturbing the cast's padding. The cut edges may be bound with adhesive tape or the entire cast may be covered with stockinet that can be stitched on. Straps are used to hold the bivalved sections securely to the patient's body while he is being turned. If many such casts are in use on the units, it is a good policy to keep circular pieces of waterproof material on hand for protection of the gluteal region. These are made in various sizes, half-circle in shape, and stitched on the sewing machine around the concave section. They may then be turned inside out and neatly fitted into the curved area of the perineal buttocks region. Simple basting stitches will secure them nicely to the stockinet-covered bivalved shell, or they may be attached with adhesive strips (Fig. 102).

Frequently, posterior splints or bivalved casts are made to maintain the patient's extremities in good alignment. The splint illustrated in Fig. 110 is designed to maintain a neutral position of the foot and limb. The posterior shell provides support for the foot, preventing drop foot, and the bar placed at the ankle prevents external rotation of the limb. This type of support also may be worn to help prevent flexion contracture of the knee. It is held in place by an elastic bandage or figure-of-eight straps placed around the ankle and knee. Nursing problems, however, are not eliminated with the application of the bivalved cast. If it is not applied correctly, the patient may pull his foot up within the splint, and the foot is then held in a definite drop-foot position. The development of pressure areas at the heel may be a constant source of trouble, even though the cast is lined carefully. Sometimes this condition can be prevented by placing a small piece of padding, felt or sponge rubber, in the cast just above the heel space. This tends to lessen the amount of pressure on the heel.

Care of patient when cast removed

Nurses who have watched orthopedic surgeons apply casts have observed the comfortable support that such casts give the joints. Although casts are sometimes clumsy to handle, a well-applied cast is as perfect a fixation apparatus as can be devised for the human body. The patient himself may never realize this until he is removed from its support. Once out of his cast, he will become conscious of many aches and discomforts, and even minute changes in the position of the joints will cause him pain. Joint structures have become somewhat contracted, and muscles that have been immobilized are suddenly stretched. In addition, circulation is sluggish, and coldness, mottling, and swelling are often present. If the primary problem has been in the hip, the patient may become acutely alarmed because his greatest discomfort and stiffness now seem to be in the knee. This is a common occurrence and usually results from the fact that the quadriceps muscle group, which forms the bulk of the muscle at the front of the thigh, has suffered considerable disuse atrophy from the weeks spent in the cast. This muscle group is the main extensor of the knee and is absolutely essential in rising from the sitting position to the upright standing position. When attempting to rise, the patient will be much concerned with the weakness, instability, and pain he experiences in the knee. If he is told that the cause of his discomfort is merely the result of disuse and is not a permanent deformity, he will be able to bear it with much more fortitude.

To minimize the patient's discomfort, support to the joints is necessary immediately after the cast is removed. Slight relaxation rather than complete extension is usually the goal in applying casts, and it is important that this position of relaxation be maintained after the cast is removed. The normal curve of the lumbar spine should be supported with a firm narrow pillow are with a sheet folded to make a firm pad measuring about 6 × 20 in. Soft wide pillows do not give the correct anatomic support needed in this area. The knee should be held in a slightly relaxed position by placing a rolled towel beneath the head of the tibia. A foot support should be used to maintain the anatomic position of the feet—a 90°-angle leg position, with the toes pointing toward the ceiling. Frequently, outward rotation of the limb will be a troublesome feature that may need attention. Sandbags placed from the hip to below the knee may be used to overcome this, or a trochanter roll may be made of a sheet or bath blanket.

The boards that were placed under the mattress should not be taken out because the cast has been removed. A firm bed is necessary to protect the patient from the aches that a sagging bed could cause.

Some physicians feel that immediate support also should be given to the integumentary system when a cast is removed. If this is done, the edema that so often occurs after the removal of a cast can be somewhat lessened. All-cotton elastic bandages or elastic stockings may be used and must be applied immediately after the cast is removed to be effective. Other physicians believe that elevating the limb for certain periods of the day may be sufficient to reduce the edema. If elevation is ordered, nurses should see to it that support is given along the entire limb from the buttock to the heel and that the knee is not acutely flexed.

After a cast is removed, the patient usually is permitted to move freely about in bed, but certain precautions should be observed. Nurses should remember that considerable decalcification has occurred and that the bone is more brittle and vulnerable to stresses that would not affect it under normal conditions. Fractures brought about by minor stresses sometimes occur at this time and are sometimes disguised by the patient's general discomfort. In addition, muscles that are weakened need careful handling to eliminate unnecessary pain and discomfort. Nurses should be careful to lift a limb just out of a cast by providing adequate support at contiguous joints. Such a limb should never be lifted by grasping the muscle belly.

Upon removal of a cast that has been on a patient for a considerable period of time, the skin will be noted to be caked with a yellow exudate that is partly dead skin and partly secretions from the glands of the skin. It is generally conceded to be poor policy to try to soften the skin or forcibly remove the closely adhering exudate, particularly if a new cast is to be applied at once. If the patient is to remain out of the cast permanently or for a considerable period of time, the skin can be cleaned at the nurse's leisure and the patient's comfort, never forcing the caked matter in such a way as to cause bleeding or rawness. Since time is not a factor, no one will be accused of neglect if the process takes several days. Zeal in this matter is misplaced. Olive oil has been found to be the easiest and safest agent for removing the exudate.

Cutting casts

Casts in which windows or holes have been cut are usually considered to be hazardous because the flesh under the opened area bulges out alarmingly after an hour or so, exacerbating the patient's discomfort. It is customary for the physician to request the nurse to apply a felt pad over the window or hole and to use a snug bandage for eliminating this complicating edema. Sometimes a window is cut in the cast so that a surgical dressing may be applied, or the heel of a cast may be cut out to relieve pressure on a tender area. In any case the nurse must not discard the part of the cast that has been removed, for the pieces are nearly always put back and held in place by a new roll of plaster.

Every nurse should know how to cut a cast if an emergency arises. The short, curved-bladed plaster knife is not difficult to handle and the electric cast saw is fast and safe. However, use of the saw may be frightening to a small child. The saw blade, which vibrates, does not cut through the material used for padding but may feel very warm to the patient. If a cast knife or cast saw is not available, an ordinary shoe knife or a pruning knife may be used. Very heavy casts may be spread with household pliers. A spoon handle may be inserted under the cast to protect the patient's skin from the plaster knife. The spoon is advanced as the cast is cut. Vinegar or water is sometimes used to soften the cast before it is cut. The liquid is dropped on the cutting line with a syringe of the Asepto variety.

When an arm or leg cast is to be split to relieve edema, it should be cut along its entire length. Splitting the cast only part way will often add to circulatory congestion. It is always a mistake to attempt to prevent or overcome swelling of toes or fingers by cutting the edges of the cast. Usually, the more the cast is cut or trimmed back, the greater the area that will swell. When edema and circulatory problems are present, the cast is split along its full length and spread slightly. It is not enough to cut the plaster only, for frequently the underlying bandages or dressings may be the cause of the circulatory impairment or the pain. They should be loosened so that no constricting material binds the extremity. When a newly applied cast is split to relieve congestion, it may be taped together loosely until further instructions can be obtained from the physician.

It is never safe to postpone reporting circulatory congestion of an extremity in a cast. Night nurses sometimes feel that they can risk waiting until daylight or for the early morning rounds of the house physician. Although it is prompted by the best of motives, such a policy is dangerous. Irremediable damage may be caused by two or three hours of neglect.

Instructions for home care

What nurses have been taught or have learned through experience and the application of their ingenuity concerning the care of the patient in a cast is no sacred professional secret. It must be shared with all those to whom care of such patients is confided. Parents must be given adequate instruction before a child in a plaster-of-Paris cast is taken home from the hospital, and this includes instruction in all the details that have been mentioned: checking closely on circulation of the exposed body parts, giving attention to complaints of pressure and burning, detecting odors in casts, caring for the skin under the cast, and cleaning and protecting the cast. If possible, the parents should observe the patient's bath and cast care completely. They must be told that young children often make a game of hiding things in their casts, which may cause damage to the skin. They must understand why the patient is wearing the cast and must recognize when the cast has become inefficient for maintaining the position essential to correction of the

WRITTEN INSTRUCTIONS FOR HOME CARE OF PATIENTS IN HIP CASTS

Even though the plaster cast may seem extremely bulky and awkward, the patient has been placed in the cast for definite reasons—mainly to immobilize the hip joint and to maintain a corrected position. Consequently, if a definite position of the hip joint is to be maintained, the care of the patient must be such as to prevent softening or cracking of the cast. Equally as important, this care must provide for the general welfare of the patient and prevention of cast sores or bed sores.

Skin care

Special attention should be given the skin of the patient in a cast:
1 Cleanse the skin daily.
2 a Reach under the cast to remove plaster crumbs or foreign objects.
  b Feel and look for skin irritations at the cast edges.
  c Do not permit youngsters to poke crayons or other small objects down in the cast. Such articles may cause severe pressure areas.
3 a Turn the patient every four hours during the day and encourage him to lie on his abdomen several hours each day. Frequently, a patient will find it possible to sleep in this position.
  b If reddened areas appear on the sacral area, the patient must stay on his abdomen for longer periods of time.
4 Rub the back, especially around the edges of the cast and over the sacral area, with rubbing alcohol several times daily.

Check the following closely:

1 Is there swelling or discoloration of the toes?
2 Is the patient able to move his toes? Are they warm?
3 Does the patient complain of pain or numbness?
4 If the patient is a small child, does he fuss and seem unduly irritable?
(If for any reason you are in doubt concerning any of these things, consult your physician.)

Drying cast

If the cast becomes damp, it can be dried by exposing the area to the air or by using an ordinary hair dryer.

Cleaning cast

If the cast becomes soiled from stool, it may be cleaned with a cleanser applied with a damp cloth.

Finishing cast edges

To eliminate plaster crumbs in the bed and to provide a smooth nonirritating cast edge, the edges of the cast may be bound with adhesive tape. To prevent the tape from rolling, the cast must be thoroughly dry. This usually requires from twenty-four to forty-eight hours.

Protecting cast from urine

1 On the baby or small child, plastic waterproof material (cut in 4-in × 6-in strips) may be used to protect the cast around the perineum and buttocks.
  a One end of the strip is tucked under the cast in the area of the perineal opening and the material is folded back over the outer side of the cast.
  b The outer end of the material is secured with adhesive tape to the cast.
  c Six to eight strips of the plastic material are needed to protect both the back and front of a hip cast on a small child.
  d These strips may be pulled out at the perineum, washed, dried, and powdered daily. (The nurse will provide you with the plastic material and show you how to apply it.)

Continued.

Protecting cast from urine—cont'd

  2 In addition to the plastic material, a perineal diaper may be used on the child who is not toilet trained.

  a Fold a diaper in the form of a perineal pad and place it across the perineum, tucking it under the edges of the cast in the front and in the back. The ordinary diaper may be applied over this.

  b It is essential that this pad or diaper be changed as soon as it becomes wet or soiled.

  3 The small youngster or baby in a hip cast may be supported by placing plastic-covered or rubber-covered pillows so that the head and shoulders are slightly higher than the buttocks. This will aid in keeping the cast dry.

Placing patient on bedpan

  1 Elevating the patient's head and shoulders with pillows when he is on the bedpan will help to prevent urine from running backward and inside the cast.

  2 A folded diaper, soft cloth, or gauze pad placed on the back of the bedpan will absorb any moisture and will help to keep the cast clean and dry. It must be removed with the bedpan.

Turning patient

  If only one leg is enclosed in the cast, turn the patient toward the other leg. Turn the body simultaneously to prevent undue pressure on the cast at the groin.

---

child's deformity. They must be taught to look for signs that the child is outgrowing the cast. If the parent seems confused by the number of things to watch for instructions of this nature may be written down and sent home with the child. On the whole, patients in casts spend only a small portion of their convalescence in the hospital. It is but a short interlude, and the excellent care the child experiences in the hospital will be absolutely negated unless a follow-up of some type is provided for him when he returns to his home.

Plaster room technique

Several types of instruments are usually considered necessary for the application and removal of casts. Cast knives, cutters, and saws are needed for removing an old cast. Bandage scissors are necessary for removing bandages under the cast, and a heavy pair of shears are essential for cutting pieces of felt (Figs. 111 to 113).

Sheet wadding, a thin unabsorbent cotton web covered with starch to hold it together, is commonly used for padding. Piano felt, cut in suitable sizes, is used to provide additional protection against

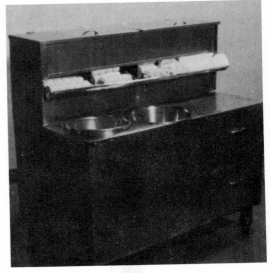

Fig. 111 The plaster cart may be taken to the operating room or to the bedside when a plaster-of-Paris cast is to be applied.

pressure on bony prominences. Sponge rubber occasionally may be used for this purpose. Material will be needed for reenforcing the cast at points of stress, and plaster splints, aluminum strips, yucca

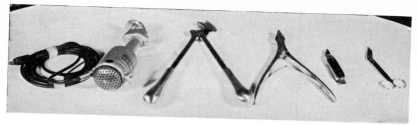

Fig. 112 Cast instruments: cast saw, cutter, spreader, knife, and bandage scissors.

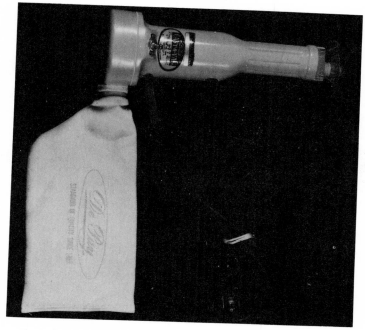

Fig. 113 Prevention of skin irritation caused by cast crumbs in the bed or inside the body cast is facilitated by the use of a cast saw with a vacuum bag in trimming the cast.

board, and plywood are among the most popular of these. Tubular stockinet, which comes in many different widths (from 2 in to 18 in), is used for a cast lining. A deep pail for soaking bandages, a pan of splints, and a waste water vessel, all lined with brown paper or old pieces of cloth to filter the waste plaster, will be necessary. Gloves and gowns should be at hand for the surgeon and assistants who are to apply the cast.

The temperature of the water used to soak the bandages should be between 95° and 105° F. Warmer or cooler water will delay the setting of the plaster.

Paper-wrapped bandages retain plaster satisfactorily when they are put on edge in water until the bubbling ceases. They may then be lifted vertically from the water with the ends firmly grasped in the palms. Bandages not so wrapped are usually submerged horizontally, with the nurse or assistant keeping her palm cupped over the end of the bandage to prevent loss of plaster. No compression of the bandage must take place at this time.

The bubbles of air in the water will rise until the bandage is completely saturated; i.e., until the water has penetrated every part of the bandage. When this is completed, the bandage should be removed immediately, because the crystallization (setting) process will have begun.

The bandage is lifted from the water and held horizontally with the ends secured in the nurse's palms. Water is expelled by

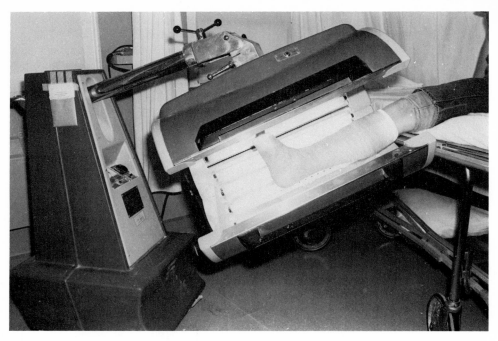

Fig. 114 The light energy generated by the Lightcast II pedestal lamp cures the cast to finished cast strength in three minutes. The lamp may be adjusted to accommodate patients in the sitting, standing, or lying position.

gently compressing the bandage in a short twist—no more than is necessary to supinate the right hand a single time, keeping the left hand in pronation. While the bandage should not drip when it is handed to the surgeon, it must not be wrung so dry that he will have difficulty incorporating it into a cast. The end of the plaster bandage is unrolled about two to four inches before it is handed to the doctor. Only a few bandages should be put in the water at one time. Change of immersion water may be necessary if a large cast is being applied. A waste basin lined with paper may be used to receive the plaster that is wrung from the plaster bandage when it is removed from the water.

By the time the cast application is completed, the plaster in the basins used for immersion will usually have settled to the bottom. The water above this plaster is poured into the sink, with the faucet wide open to assist in washing what plaster is still present in the water through the drain. If paper has been used to line the immersion basins, this is lifted from the container and deposited in waste containers. Caution

must be exercised in the care of all this equipment so that plaster is not allowed to gather in the sink and to clog plumbing fixtures.

Lightcast II

Recently, a casting system known as Lightcast II has been introduced and is being used for immobilization. This casting material consists of an open-weave knitted fiber glass tape embedded with photosensitive resin. It is available in various widths in a bandagelike roll. When this material is exposed to the light generated by a Lightcast II lamp, it becomes rigid. To provide a protective covering for the skin, Lightcast II stockinet is used. This stockinet, which appears similar to the stockinet used with the conventional plaster-of-Paris cast, is made of polypropylene and has water-shedding properties. Lightcast II web wrap, also made of polypropylene, provides padding for bony prominences. Usually, from three to five layers of the tape are applied and, as with plaster of Paris, the cast is rubbed to help laminate the layers. Prior to curing, the

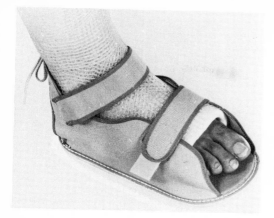

Fig. 115 Open-toe canvas shoe with Velcro closures features a patented rocker motion convex sole. The shoe is being used with a Lightcast II leg cast. (Courtesy Merck Sharp & Dohme Orthopedics Co., Inc.)

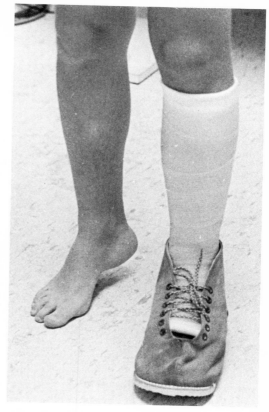

Fig. 116 A Lightcast II short leg weight-bearing cast and a closed suede model shoe with laces. (Courtesy Merck Sharp & Dohme Orthopedics Co., Inc.)

edges of the cast should be smoothed or rubbed together. If sharp or rough edges remain following curing, they may be smoothed with sandpaper. Care should be taken to prevent cast crumbs from getting under the cast. To cure the cast takes approximately three to five minutes and necessitates the use of a Lightcast II lamp (Fig. 114). These lights generate near ultraviolet light in the range of 3,200-4,000 Å. The cast is cured by light energy—not heat. The lamp remains cool.

During application, the cast material remains soft and pliable until the curing process is started. This necessitates that molding of the cast be completed during the first ten to fifteen seconds of the curing time and that the part being casted is maintained in the desired position for approximately one-half of the three-minute curing period.

The Lightcast II cast has the advantage of being lighter and thinner than the plaster-of-Paris cast, and consequently less bulky and cumbersome for the patient. Also, it is a porous cast that permits circulation of air to the skin surfaces. Bathing, showering, and use of the whirlpool bath are possible since water does not cause the cast to disintegrate. However, care must be taken to allow adequate time for drying (from two to three hours). Frequent repeated wettings of the cast could cause skin maceration. Use of a portable hair dryer hastens the drying process. Some objections to the odor of the newly applied cast have been voiced. This is caused by the vaporization of vinyl toluene, which is present in the tape, and disappears shortly after application.

To remove the cast, a standard cast saw is used. Special blades that facilitate cutting are available. The operator of the saw needs to remember that this cast material is harder and thinner than the regular plaster of Paris and thus exercise care.

The Lightcast II cast has been in use for a relatively short period of time, and it remains to be seen whether its advantages will outweigh its disadvantages and whether it can become a more acceptable means of immobilization than the conventional plaster-of-Paris cast.

7 The patient in traction

Modes of traction

The application of traction means that a pulling force is applied to an extremity or part of the body. Traction can be provided a number of ways: manually, through special bandages applied to skin, or transmitted directly to bone through special skeletal devices.

Skin traction is applied to the skin and soft tissues and thus indirectly to the skeletal system. Traction tapes made of various kinds of material with adhesive qualities for adherence to the skin surface are most commonly used for this type of traction.

Skeletal traction is applied directly to the skeletal system. The Steinmann pin or Kirschner wire is used in applying traction to an extremity, and Crutchfield or Vinke tongs and other devices are used to exert traction to the skull.

Manual traction means the application of traction to a part of the body by the hands of the operator. When assisting with the application of traction or a cast, the nurse may be asked to apply manual traction. This calls for a smooth firm grip on the extremity and the avoidance of sudden jerking movements. Occasionally, when nursing care is being given or when traction is changed, it is necessary to apply this type of traction to the extremity. Permission to substitute manual traction for the prescribed traction must be secured from the attending physician.

Purpose of traction

Perhaps the best way to begin studying the care of the patient in traction is to consider why the patient has been placed in this apparatus. Nurses caring for patients on an orthopedic service will discover varied reasons for the application of traction. Traction is frequently applied to the extremity of a patient with a fracture, first to lessen the muscle spasm and to reduce the fracture and then to immobilize and to maintain the corrected position. Traction also may be applied to correct or prevent flexion contractures of the hip and the knee in a patient with arthritis. In the child with scoliosis traction may be used as a form of treatment to lessen the deformity. Occasionally, the patient with back pain may be placed in traction to relieve muscle spasm, or traction may be applied to lessen muscle spasm around a joint.

Countertraction

Provision for countertraction must always be made if effective traction is to be maintained. Countertraction means a pull exerted in the opposite direction to the pull produced by the traction apparatus. This can be obtained by exerting the traction pull against a fixed point (such as the pelvis when a Thomas, Hodgen, or Keller-Blake splint is used) or by elevating the bed under the part that is being placed in traction; e.g., the foot of the bed is elevated for traction on the lower extremity, causing the body itself to exert countertraction in its gravitational pull away from the limb extension. The bed should be elevated from eight to twelve inches. Sufficient countertraction prevents the patient from sliding toward the foot of the bed when traction has been applied to the lower extremity. If a child or a thin adult is being subjected to many pounds of traction, this amount of countertraction may not suffice to keep the patient balanced against the traction being applied. Further elevation of the bed may be of assistance. Also, nurses must be most conscientious in aiding the patient to pull himself up in bed at frequent intervals during the day. Traction on an extremity will be entirely useless if the footplate or spreader is allowed to come in contact with the foot of the bed at any time.

Friction

Any friction created by ropes riding on the foot of the bed, ropes impinged by bedclothes, or heels digging into the mattress will lessen the efficiency of traction greatly. Orthopedic nurses must train themselves to observe these and other details that their experience and common sense tell them mitigate efficiency of the traction. A firm, thin pillow placed under the limb in extension does much to eliminate bed friction. Correct placement of the pillow also prevents pressure on the heel, a likely spot for a pressure sore.

Continuous traction

In caring for patients in traction a safe rule to follow is that traction cannot be released for any nursing procedure—that it must be continuous for twenty-four hours of the day. There are exceptions to this rule, however, but they must be given by the physician for a specific patient. Arthritic patients in traction for the prevention or correction of flexion contractures of the joints are sometimes an exception to the rule and frequently are allowed to be released from traction for a few hours during the day. From time to time there may be other patients who have this privilege, but it is given only on the explicit order of the physician in charge.

Traction equipment

Traction cart. In addition to the traction room, a traction cart is a useful piece of equipment for orthopedic hospitals or services and will save much time and effort when traction is to be applied. Any kind of wheeled carriage can be used for the purpose (Fig. 117). The cart may be stocked with various types of orthopedic equipment such as moleskin strips sewed or stapled to tape webbing, self-adhering traction strips, felt, stockinet, bandages,

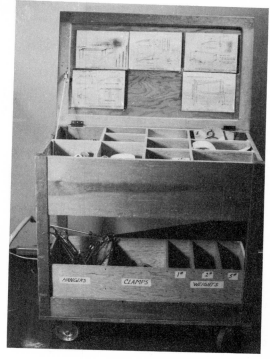

Fig. 117 The well-equipped traction cart is a time-saving device when traction is to be applied. Traction equipment can be taken to the bedside without delay or preparation.

and bandage scissors. A lower shelf or a drawer might contain various types of pulleys, weights, carriers, ropes, footplates or spreaders, sandbags, hammocks for limb suspension, pelvic girdles, and chin halters.

Type of bed. The patient in traction must have a firm mattress that does not sag under body weight. A bed that sags beneath the hips prevents the free play of the traction rope on the pulley and decreases the efficiency of the apparatus considerably. Furthermore, it may be the cause of a permanent flexion deformity at the hips of the patient who is in traction over a long period of time. The bed may be made firm by placing boards beneath the mattress. It is preferable that these boards extend lengthwise and that they be hinged at the backrest level.

It is not only desirable but in most types of traction also necessary to have a bed with overhead bars. In addition, the hospital bed equipped with a mechanism for lowering and raising either end of the bed

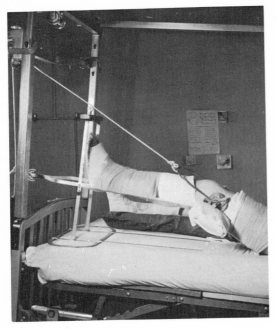

Fig. 118 The Braun-Böhler inclined plane splint may be used to support the limb after application of skeletal traction. Note that the splint supports the entire thigh and that the knee joint corresponds with the beginning of the inclined plane.

is helpful in positioning the patient and maintaining countertraction. If this type of bed is not available, shock blocks may be used to provide for countertraction.

The trapeze (unless contraindicated) should not be omitted from the patient's bed. If facilitates nursing care and enables the patient to do many things for himself.

Braun-Böhler inclined plane splint. The inclined plane splint (Fig. 118) may be used for patients with fractures of the lower end of the femur in conjunction with either skin or skeletal traction. Since this type of frame and traction rests on the bed, it does not maintain immobilization as automatically as a suspension apparatus. The physician should be consulted concerning the amount of motion allowed. As a general rule, it is permissible to turn the patient toward the splint for back care. In changing linen it is more convenient to use two folded sheets for the under part of the bed. One sheet rests under the splint, and the other reaches from the head of the bed to the level of the splint. It is thus possible to change the sheet under the patient fre-

quently without disturbing the sheet under the splint. Two or three rolls of 5-in muslin bandage may be used to cover the splint and to provide support for the affected limb. The bandage is started around the base and wrapped smoothly and tightly over the inclined plane.

Other splints. The half-ring or full-ring Thomas splint (Figs. 119 and 120), the Hodgen splint (Fig. 377), the Keller-Blake splint, and the canvas hammock are commonly used when traction and/or suspension is applied to the lower extremity. Suspension frequently is used with traction because it will permit the patient to move himself about in bed without disturbing the line of traction. Furthermore, suspension improves circulation and allows freer motion of the suspended part than would be possible if the patient had to lift the extremity against gravity.

Types of traction

Buck's extension, rubber surface traction, and Bryant traction may be described as straight or running traction that exerts a pull on the affected part but does not provide a balanced support by means of a hammock or splint (Fig. 122).

With suspension (Fig. 126), Dunlop (Fig. 162), and Russell traction (Fig. 163), the extremity has traction applied and is then supported by means of a hammock or splint held in place by balanced weights attached to an overhead bar.

Head, pelvic, and ankle traction is applied with some type of fitted apparatus, such as a corset (Fig. 127), head halter (Fig. 128), and anklet.

Skill in the nursing care of the patient in traction is an attribute that comes with knowledge and experience. Patients in casts present problems, but the problems are much simpler than those of the patients in traction. The patient in a cast may be moved as frequently as is necessary for the care of his back or for comfort. He may lie on his back, abdomen, or side without endangering the immobilization of the involved part. Patients in traction, on the other hand, usually have but one position in which to lie—the dorsal recumbent position. Good nursing care of these patients must include keeping the patient clean, comfortable, and free from pressure sores

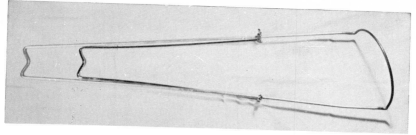

Fig. 119 The half-ring Thomas splint with Pearson attachment.

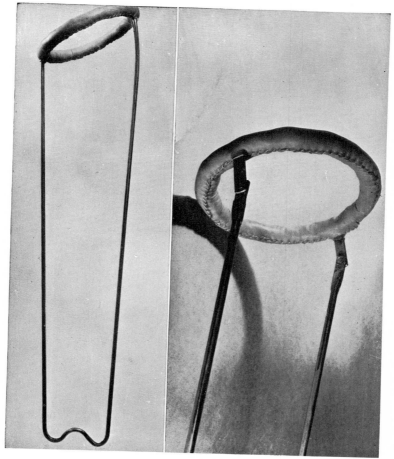

Fig. 120 The Thomas splint for the lower extremity and the modified Thomas splint with hinge for the upper extremity. (From Crenshaw, A. H., editor: Campbell's Operative orthopaedics, ed. 5, St. Louis, The C. V. Mosby Co.)

despite the handicap of his enforced and prolonged recumbency.

Buck's extension. Buck's extension (named after Gordon Buck, who described the apparatus in 1851) is perhaps one of the easiest types of traction to apply (Figs. 121 and 122). Also, it provides the basis

for most other types of skin traction and in an emergency can be applied with improvised equipment: two strips of 3-in adhesive the length of the patient's limb, a block of wood to be used for a spreader below the foot, some type of pulley, and a weight that may be a window-sash weight

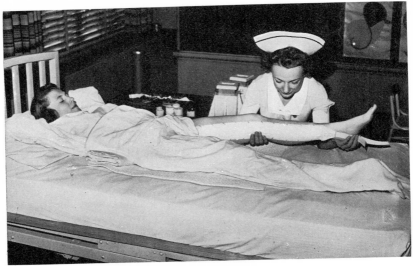

Fig. 121 Buck's extension. Moleskin tapes have been applied to each side of the limb. Sheet wadding or similar material is wrapped around the ankle to protect the malleoli and tendon Achilles, and an elastic bandage is applied over the traction tapes.

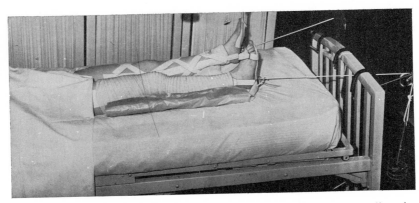

Fig. 122 Two types of adhesive traction for the leg. Note that a firm pillow has been positioned under the leg to eliminate friction and to free the heel of pressure. The left foot is supported by an adhesive strip to prevent drop foot. An aluminum footplate is used for the right leg. Traction is applied to the right leg with a single strip and is held in place with a spiral elastic bandage. The left leg has three-tailed adhesive strips wound obliquely over the leg and thigh. Note the bracelet of stockinet and cotton over the malleoli on the left ankle. Also, note the strips crossed high above the dorsum of the foot to prevent circulatory impairment. Both extremities are maintained in a neutral position. External rotation is to be avoided.

or a canvas bag filled with salt or sand. A chair may be used to elevate the foot of the bed to provide countertraction. Hospitals usually have more elaborate equipment for applying traction, but it is well for the nurse to understand how such traction can be applied and maintained satisfactorily with improvised equipment.

Some contraindications to the use of skin traction should be remembered and observed. This type of traction cannot be applied to the patient with a severely injured extremity with open wounds or to the patient who is allergic to tape. Circulatory disturbances, dermatitis, or varicose veins may prohibit the application of traction to the skin. The patient with diabetes may present a problem if skin traction must be maintained for a long period of time. Traction applied to the skin with adhesive type of tape may slip if a large amount of weight is applied.

The area to which adhesive tape is to be applied is usually shaved. However, some physicians advise against this because the epithelium is invariably removed in the shaved area and infection may occur under the tape. Clippers frequently are used instead of the razor. When a razor is used, shaving must be done very carefully, and accidental denudation or cuts of the skin should be reported before the tape is applied.

There are a few landmarks on the leg that must be given special consideration when traction tapes are applied. Strips of adhesive with tape webbing stapled or sewed to one end frequently form the basis of the equipment. Commercially prepared traction tapes also are available. With these, as with the adhesive or moleskin tape, some provision must be made for the traction tapes to adhere to the skin and thus provide for a "pulling force" (traction) on the extremity.

The traction tapes extend from the malleoli to the thighs, and many surgeons believe that these strips alone are sufficient for the pull. However, it is the custom in some clinics to use oblique strips of narrower adhesive tape to augment the lateral strips. These pass across the tibia and obliquely encircle the leg, crossing in the back of the calf and then above the knee. Although these strips add to the staying power of the traction as a whole, they present a distinct menace to the circulation of the foot if they are applied too snugly or are applied too near the dorsum of the foot. There is an inevitable amount of slipping of the adhesive tape when weights are applied, and oblique strips tend to be pulled down by the lateral strips and to cut into the flesh. An ischemia of the foot with resulting paralysis has been known to develop from the pressure on the dorsalis pedis artery, which lies beneath.

Another landmark of which the nurse should be conscious is the upper three inches of the fibula—i.e., the outer aspect of the calf just below the knee. It is here that the peroneal nerve lies close to the surface, and it can easily be compressed against the bone over which it passes. The result of this compression may be a peroneal paralysis. The paralysis prevents active dorsiflexion or eversion of the foot. This area should be well padded with felt or cotton before tape is applied. The foot should be observed daily for a tendency to turn toward the midline of the body. Any complaint of pain or a burning sensation under the tape must be carefully checked.

Although pressure upon the Achilles tendon will not cause paralysis, it must have special consideration. No tape should at any time pass directly over this tendon or very near above it. The tendon is exceedingly superficial and tends to become sore and denuded with great rapidity. Placing an oblong piece of felt over this area before applying bandage or traction will help eliminate danger to the area.

Oblique strips crossed on the tibia at any point are a threat to the underlying skin, and padding should always be applied at these points. Adhesive skin traction is not supposed to pull directly on bone. The pull is to be exerted on skin and subcutaneous tissues, and this fact should be borne in mind during application of the tape. Superficial bony points are to be guarded.

There are a few common errors in the use of apparatus that should be mentioned at this point. One of these is the use of a single pulley for more than one rope, a practice that greatly limits the efficiency of the pulley. Another error is the use of a foot spreader so narrow that the traction tapes connecting it to the leg contact the bony points of the ankle, always vulnerable spots for pressure sores. Still another error is the use of a foot spreader so wide that the traction tapes constantly pull away from the skin of the leg, thus adding unnecessary discomfort to the patient.

The skin frequently is painted with tincture of benzoin before the application of the adhesive with the idea that it serves as a disinfectant and gives the tape greater properties of adherence. However, such benefits are not routinely accepted, and some authorities do not think its use is always warranted. Its application is not always safe in infants because the adherence of the tape to the skin is so great that, upon its removal, bleeding points are almost invariably encountered on the baby's skin.

In any case, the skin should be dry and clean before tape is applied. Massaging the tape gently into the skin after its application will prevent much of the slipping that occurs when the weights are applied. Wrinkles or creases in the tape are to be avoided scrupulously since they may be the cause of pressure areas on the underlying skin.

Traction tapes should be applied with the knee in slight flexion to prevent hyperextension of the joint. The tape should cover a generous area of skin.

The tape should be started about one inch above the malleolus. It should never be applied directly to the malleolus but slightly above it. This is advisable, also, because space can be allowed for the tape to slip down as it inevitably will do for the first twenty-four hours. If a moderately large amount of weight is used, a downward slipping of the tape for one or two inches may be expected in twenty-four hours. It is advisable to clip the tape obliquely every inch or so, beginning from the top. These nicks should be no more than one-fourth inch in depth. They are to aid in fitting the adhesive tape more snugly and neatly to the contours of the leg.

The traction tapes are then applied to the leg on its inner and outer aspects. However, under no circumstances should the strips be allowed to pass over the patella or over the popliteal space; this may happen if the tape is hastily or carelessly applied. The tape is massaged gently into the skin and, if circumstances permit, some time should be allowed to elapse between the application of the tape and attaching of the weights. Slipping will be much less likely to occur if this is done.

As stated previously, the use of these two straps alone is preferred by a number of surgeons. This is particularly true in children's hospitals, where the delicate quality of the child's skin is a consideration and where only small amounts of weight are necessary to obtain traction.

With the straight longitudinal traction tapes unsupported by the transverse sec-

tions, a securely applied bandage is needed to maintain the position of the tape. In many clinics sheet wadding is applied over the adhesive in a simple spiral bandage, followed by an elastic bandage. In these cases the sheet wadding is brought under the tape webbing at the ankle to provide effective protection of the bony points. Some orthopedists feel that the upper ends of the tape should be visible at all times so that slipping may be detected without removing the outer bandage.

Temptation to apply the bandage very snugly to improve its appearance must be firmly resisted. Circulation in the foot should be inspected after the bandage has been in place for several minutes. Signs of mild cyanosis will be present if the bandage has been applied too tightly.

Pressure areas may form under traction straps with none but the mildest complaints on the part of the patient. Needless to say, every complaint from the patient in traction deserves prompt attention. With these patients, as well as with those in casts, the nose is of definite assistance in detecting the musty odor that may result from pus forming under the bandage.

Once traction tapes and bandage are securely applied, a footplate with buckles or a spreader is attached to the sole of the foot. The spreader must be wide enough to keep the traction tapes spread out somewhat from the malleoli. A small hook on the bottom of a footplate makes it possible to attach the rope.

The other end of the rope passes over a pulley secured at the foot of the bed. The weights attached to a carrier are suspended from this rope. The weights must be tied sufficiently high so that the patient's slipping down in bed will not permit the weight to rest on the floor. Also, traction weights must be attached in a manner that prevents their resting on the bed frame when the patient changes position. Canvas bags are sometimes used around traction weights to minimize noise and to prevent accidents from loosened knots. Weights must not be attached so high that the knot will rest against the pulley if the patient alters his position in bed. Rope should be of good quality and not be frayed or pieced together. When a large amount of weight is applied to an extremity, nylon rope should

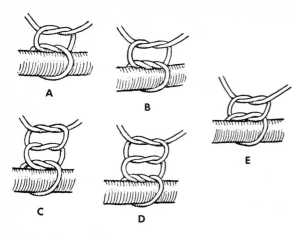

Fig. 123 A, Square knot. **B,** Surgeon's knot. **C,** Square knot reinforced. **D,** Surgeon's knot reinforced. **E,** Granny knot. (From Mobley, H. E.: Synopsis of operative surgery, ed. 2, St. Louis, The C. V. Mosby Co.)

be used. The added strength prevents sudden breaking of the rope and release of the traction.

All knots should be secure. The patient's comfort demands that no sudden release of knots occur to jar the leg in traction. All nurses should know how to tie a square knot (Fig. 123) and should make use of it in their orthopedic nursing. Narrow strips of adhesive tape may be used to make such knots additionally secure.

The amount of weight to be used depends upon the physician's order. For fractures, large amounts may be applied at once. A large amount of weight should be an indication to the nurse to be very solicitous in observing the patient so that injury to the skin does not occur at any point.

Orders regarding patients in traction are sometimes confusing to student nurses. For patients with scoliosis, for instance, it is occasionally the practice of surgeons to order a small amount of weight at the beginning with a substantial increase each day. In patients with fractures, the reverse may be true. A large amount of weight is frequently used during the first twenty-four to forty-eight hours, followed by a decrease in the amount after reduction is obtained. For patients with scoliosis, permission is frequently given to remove weights for short intervals during the day, but for those with fractures this would not be permitted.

The maximum amount of weight for reduction of the fracture is put on immediately, and once reduction has been obtained, only such weight as is needed to maintain the bone ends in good position is used. However, this remaining amount of weight is important and should not be disturbed without specific order from the surgeon.

A word should be said about the danger of tape constriction in patients with fresh fractures to which traction has been applied. Such traction should always be applied by the physician, but the nurse must realize that in trauma of this nature swelling inevitably occurs and an alarming degree of constriction may occur within the first three or four days. This must be watched for and reported to the surgeon immediately before any permanent damage is done to the extremity.

Rubber surface traction. Traction tapes are made from strips of synthetic sponge rubber backed with strong fabric. These are applied directly to the skin, as described for Buck's extension, and are secured to the leg by means of one or two 3-in cotton elastic bandages or Velcro straps. There is relatively little slipping when the weights are attached because of the suction of the rubber on the skin. The advantage of this type of traction is that the apparatus may be removed for physical therapy and hydrotherapy. Furthermore, it can be used on skin that needs more watching than would be possible if adhesive tape were applied.

There are dangers, however, that the nurse must not ignore. To prevent slipping, the elastic bandage or straps must be wrapped or fastened securely. This in turn may cause swelling and constriction of circulation, which is a real hazard with the older patient who has poor circulation.

Ankle traction. Ankle traction may sometimes be ordered as a temporary measure. It is obtained with a boot made of leather or canvas that is laced onto the foot and has straps extending below for rope and weight attachment. The shoe must be thoroughly padded over the dorsum of the foot as well as over the heel cord. Otherwise the skin will become denuded and the circulation impaired after a few hours in such traction. It is not the most satisfactory type of

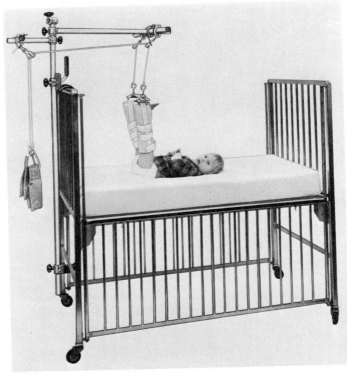

Fig. 124 Bryant traction used in fracture of the shaft of the femur in young children. A jacket restraint is usually necessary to maintain the desired position of the child. In this photograph, foam rubber strips fastened with Velcro are being used instead of moleskin tapes to secure the traction pull. (Courtesy Zimmer, Warsaw, Ind.)

traction, although occasionally its use is a necessity. Applying considerable weight to such a meager portion of the extremity is painful and dangerous. The nurse should release the laces over the dorsum of the foot frequently and rub the area with alcohol. Ridged blue areas across the top of the foot inevitably occur after a few hours in this type of traction. Deep fissures have been known to form at this area within twenty-four hours.

Bryant traction. Bryant traction (Fig. 124) has its foundation in bilateral Buck's extension and is used in the treatment of femoral shaft fractures in children under 6 years of age weighing no more than 25 to 30 pounds. For this type of traction two overhead bars, or similar apparatus, passing longitudinally over the crib or traction bed are necessary. Two pulleys are attached to each bar. The first set of pulleys is placed overhead at the level of the child's pelvis, making it possible to suspend his legs at

right angles to his body. The second set of pulleys is placed on the overhead bars near the foot of the bed and provide for attachment of the weights distal to the child's body. When the weights have been applied, the child's buttocks must just clear the mattress. This makes caring for his toilet needs much easier than when traction is applied in a horizontal direction.

Some form of restraint will be necessary to maintain the child in the correct position (Fig. 125). Bandages on the legs must be checked to see that they have not slipped in such a manner as to cause increased pressure over the dorsum of the foot or around the heel cord. Likewise, the feet should be checked at frequent intervals for circulatory disturbances. Discoloration, pallor, loss of motion, or loss of sensation must be reported to the attending physician. Immediate loosening of the elastic bandage, reduction of the traction force, or lowering of the limbs to a less than

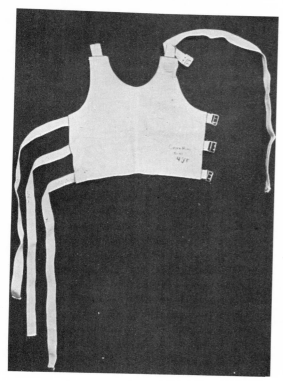

Fig. 125 Vest or jacket restraint for use with or without frame. (Courtesy University of Iowa Hospitals and Clinics, The University of Iowa, Iowa City, Iowa.)

vertical position is indicated to correct the circulatory problem. If the small child in Bryant traction is fussy and sleeps poorly, special attention must be given to the traction tapes to be certain that no neurovascular problem exists.

When callus formation at the fracture site is sufficient (three to four weeks), the child may be placed in a unilateral hip spica cast, which is worn for an additional three to four weeks.

Russell traction. Russell traction, when properly applied and in good mechanical working efficiency, is a comfortable device for the patient.

The equipment required is not elaborate (Fig. 163). A single section of the common Balkan frame can be attached to the bed, with the overhead bar directly above the injured limb. Four pulleys are used. These pulleys are arranged so that one is on the overhead bar at a level directly above the tubercle of the tibia of the fractured leg, another is attached to

the footplate or spreader, and two are attached to a crossbar at the foot of the bed and are placed at about the level of the mattress. A canvas hammock, which is used for the knee sling, and traction tapes form the basis of the traction.

In the original method, these strips were applied only to the knee. Russell believed that it was best to extend the tape only from the ankle to the knee because he wanted the pull exerted at the point of insertion of the large muscles of the thigh into the tibia and fibula—viz., the hamstring and quadriceps muscles. However, many modifications of this original method have been devised.

When the traction tapes have been applied, the hammock is slipped under the knee and a rope is attached to it. This rope passes to the overhead pulley and then to the uppermost of the two pulleys on the crossbar at the foot of the bed. It is then passed over the pulley on the foot spreader and back to the remaining pulley on the end of the bed. Weight is then attached. The amount usually ordered for an adult is eight to ten pounds (Fig. 163).

There are several important points in the nursing care of the patient in Russell traction. The knee sling should be smooth, and its edge must not cause pressure on the soft tissue over the peroneal nerve. The heel of the foot in traction should just clear the bed. Firm pillows should support the thigh and the calf along their entire length, leaving the heel free of the bed. The popliteal space must be watched for ridging and skin denudation. Elevation of the backrest is permitted, and few difficulties are encountered in giving nursing care because the fractured leg is not at the mercy of gravity and will not be altered in position during nursing care. Active dorsiflexion and plantar flexion of the feet should be encouraged. Because Russell traction includes suspension of the limb in traction, care of the back, making the bed, and giving the bedpan are much simplified. Other important features in nursing care are as follows:

1 A piece of felt should be inserted between the sling and the patient's skin to prevent wrinkling of the sling under the popliteal space. This will assist in eliminating pressure areas that sometimes form at this spot.

2 The heel should clear the bed. The ideal position for the heels of the patient in Russell traction is that of a person standing with his heels four inches apart. Abduction is to be avoided.

3 Two pillows are usually placed under the limb in traction: one under the thigh to maintain the desired angle and the other under the calf down to and including the Achilles tendon.

Suspension traction. When any type of ring splint or suspension apparatus is used in conjunction with skin or skeletal traction, the patient is usually allowed more latitude in moving about in bed. If the leg rests on the bed, as it does in Buck's extension, any movement the patient makes with his body will alter in some degree the position of the traction. When suspension is used, however, the slack occasioned by the patient's movement is taken up at once by the suspension apparatus and the line of traction remains unchanged. Suspension allows freedom of the body as a whole while efficient traction on the limb is maintained.

Thomas splint. We are told by Dr. Mc-Crae Aitken—historian for Hugh Owen Thomas who invented the Thomas splint—that Thomas invented the hip splint for a certain Sara McTurk in the year 1867. He had long disliked any type of traction apparatus that rested on the bed, because he noted the sagging of the limb that occurred when a bedpan was placed beneath the patient. The invention of the Thomas splint was an attempt to allow the patient to be moved for using the bedpan and for other nursing requirements without changing the position of the limb in traction.

Since the patient may be moved more safely, the problem of the sacral decubitus is not so troublesome as it is in patients with other kinds of traction. Furthermore, the splint usually is suspended or hung, and pressure on the heel of the leg in traction can easily be avoided. There are other nursing problems to consider, however, because of the pressure of the ring on the adductor and ischial area.

The ring of the Thomas splint is usually covered with smooth, moisture-resistant basil leather. It is usually considered advisable not to pad these rings with cotton or gauze.

When the daily bath is given, the area of skin that is contacted by the ring must have special care. Usually the patient may be tilted toward the leg in the splint for back care. The tendency for pressure sores to form in the adductors and the ischial region can be overcome by elevating the foot of the bed from twelve to eighteen inches. With sufficient countertraction, the patient will thus pull away from the splint somewhat.

A half-ring Thomas splint (Fig. 119) frequently is used in balance traction. The splint is placed with the half ring on the anterior aspect of the thigh. With this arrangement, the patient does not sit on the ring, there is less irritation in the groin area, and the difficulty and discomfort in using the bedpan are considerably lessened. The ring is not covered with padding and leather; consequently, there is not the nursing problem of keeping it dry and clean. Pressure in the groin and on the anterior aspect of the thigh is prevented by using a properly fitting splint, maintaining adequate countertraction, and placing a correct amount of weight on the rope suspending the ring. The weight lifts the ring slightly, and adequate countertraction keeps the ring from pressing in the groin area; thus need for padding of the splint is minimized (Fig. 126).

Position of extremity in suspension traction. The position of the extremity in suspension traction is determined by the physician, but the nurse should know that the limb usually is held in a neutral position or in a position of slight internal rotation. The amount of abduction may vary with the patient. However, the nurse must recognize that when only one leg is in traction, the position the patient assumes may greatly alter the amount of abduction being maintained. If the patient lies diagonally in bed, abduction is lost. Most patients with traction applied to the lower limb are encouraged to dorsiflex and plantar flex the foot at frequent intervals. Also, to maintain muscle strength, the patient may be taught to do muscle-setting exercises (quadriceps, gluteal, and abdominal). To prevent hip flexion contractures, a firm mattress is necessary and, in addition, it is desirable and usually necessary that the backrest be completely lowered several times daily. This provides for extension of

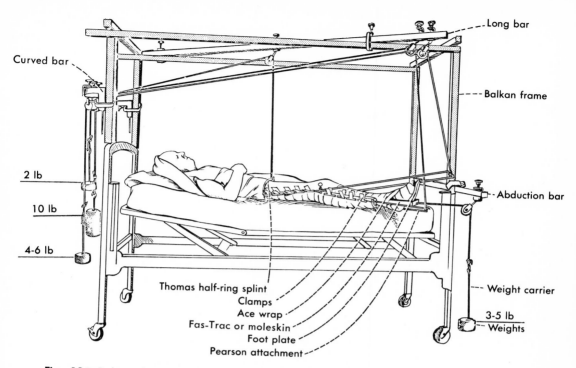

Curved bar

Long bar

Balkan frame

2 lb

10 lb

4-6 lb

Abduction bar

Weight carrier

3-5 lb Weights

Thomas half-ring splint
Clamps
Ace wrap
Fas-Trac or moleskin
Foot plate
Pearson attachment

Fig. 126 Balanced suspension with skin traction used with Balkan frame. (From the Orthopedic nursing procedure manual, University of Iowa Hospitals and Clinics, The University of Iowa, Iowa City, Iowa.)

the hip joints. A footboard for the uninvolved limb helps the patient to maintain the desired position; in addition, a bolster may be placed at the foot end of the bed to keep the mattress from sliding down.

With suspension traction, the patient's knee should correspond with the fastening of the Pearson attachment to the splint. Generally speaking, it is desirable to have the Pearson attachment (the part that supports the leg from the knee down) horizontal with the mattress and just high enough to swing clear of the bed. The position of the ring should be observed frequently. It should rest in the groin but not cause undue pressure or irritation.

Pelvic traction. The pelvic girdle customarily used to apply pelvic traction is made of canvas, darted to fit the shape of the body. It is more comfortable if it is lined with flannel, which may be quilted in several thicknesses. This girdle is not to be made to fit the waistline except in its upper border. It is a pelvic girdle and is to pull from the bony crests of the ilia, so that its lower border will be considerably

wider than the upper. It should fit snugly over the crests of the ilia and the pelvis, much as a girdle or garter belt does. On either side are tape webbing straps, usually two or three, joined together to form one strip at about the level of the midthigh. If possible, this strip should contain a steel ring for securing the rope for traction. The girdle is customarily fastened in front with Velcro straps or buckles (Fig. 127).

Because the girdle is exerting traction on bone, the crests of the ilia must have constant care, and padding over the crests frequently will be necessary for the thin patient. Weight in pelvic traction is usually increased gradually, and although it may be started with as little as five pounds on each side of the pelvis, it is usually increased conisderably. The hazards of this amount of pull to thinly padded bony prominences are readily understood.

Two pulleys about two feet apart are necessary at the foot of the bed. Ropes attached to the girdle extend through these and are attached to weight carriers and weights. It is the prerogative of the sur-

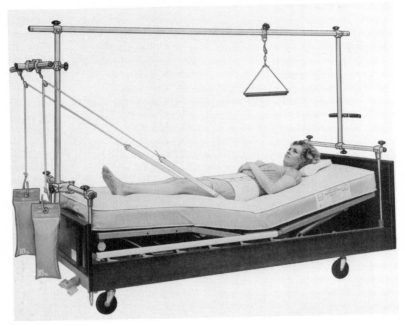

Fig. 127 Pelvic traction applied with a canvas pelvic belt. This type of traction may be used to relieve spasm of the back muscles. Slight elevation of the knee rest aids in the relaxation of the trunk muscles and provides some countertraction. (Courtesy Zimmer, Warsaw, Ind.)

geon to order the number of weights, but when this is left to the nurse's judgment it is better to begin with too little than too much. Discouragement on the part of the patient during the first few hours may make further treatment difficult. Weights are not lessened or removed without the permission of the physician who has given the order to apply them. Orders occasionally may be given to remove some of the weights at night to enable the patient to rest more comfortably. This type of traction may be applied to the patient with scoliosis to relieve pain and to gain some correction, or it may be applied to the patient with back pain to relieve muscle spasm.

The greatest complaint a patient in traction will have during his first twenty-four hours will probably have to do with pain in the lower part of the back, in the lumbar region. Usually placing a narrow firm pillow to support the lower back will provide relief from this discomfort. The pain is the result of a spasm of the extensor muscles of the back that occurs in conjunction with the pull upon the flexor muscles of the thigh.

Simple foot exercises carried out during morning and evening care help maintain muscle strength and range of motion.

Traction used in the treatment of fractures of the pelvis is discussed in Chapter 11.

Head traction. Various types of head halters may be obtained from orthopedic and surgical supply houses. These include soft disposable halters, as well as those made from leather or canvas (Fig. 128).

In addition to the halter, a spreader is needed. It should be wide enough to prevent pressure on the side of the head. The jaws and ears will become irritated if the spreader is too narrow. In addition to the halter and spreader, rope, weights, and a pulley attachment are needed for the application of head traction.

Too much emphasis cannot be placed on the necessity for conscientious care of the chin during the period of traction. Alcohol rubs are almost always permissible, except for patients with acute inflammation, and should be given at stated intervals during the day. Massage or oils should not be applied in the presence of acne, since in-

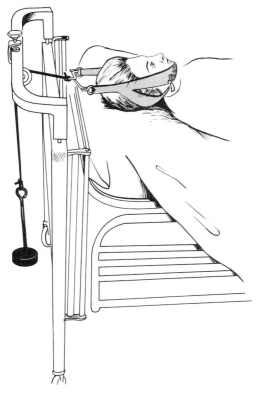

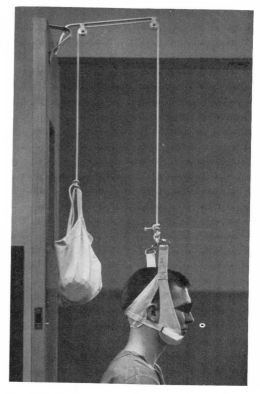

Fig. 128 This type of head halter is used to provide intermittent traction to the cervical spine. In some instances, it may be used as a temporary means of providing continuous traction until cervical tongs can be inserted. (From the Orthopedic nursing procedure manual, University of Iowa Hospitals and Clinics, The University of Iowa, Iowa City, Iowa.)

Fig. 129 Head traction that may be prescribed to be used intermittently in the home for the relief of cervical pain due to arthritis.

flammation is likely to follow. This is especially true in hot weather. Soft material such as sheet wadding or silence cloth, inserted into the chin cup and changed frequently, gives the patient considerable comfort. Frequent shampoos for the patient with any type of head traction are indicated to improve the circulation of the scalp and to lessen the danger of decubitus ulcers.

Head traction may be applied to relieve muscle spasm and pain caused by an injured cervical disc or a "whiplash" type of injury. The patient suffering with cervical arthritis may receive relief when this kind of traction is applied. Head traction is used to relieve pain caused by the presence of a cervical rib or a scoliotic condi-

tion. Frequently, some type of head traction is applied following surgical correction of torticollis. The traction helps to maintain a position of overcorrection. Head traction with a leather or canvas halter may be applied to provide temporary immobilization and support when fracture of the cervical vertebrae has occurred.

Intermittent head traction is sometimes used in the home for short daily periods for patients with dorsum rotundum, cervical arthritis, and other conditions requiring extension of the spine (Fig. 129).

When constant head traction is necessary for an extended period of time, skeletal traction is nearly always applied. However, to provide for adequate care of the chin and occiput, if constant head traction is being maintained with a halter, the surgeon *may* permit the nurse to remove the chin strap if manual traction is applied to the head. When manual traction is applied, the grip is more comfortable to the patient

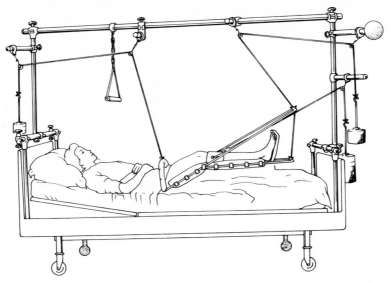

Fig. 130 Balanced suspension with skeletal traction (used with electric bed) applied to the proximal portion of the tibia. The limb is supported by means of a half-ring Thomas splint with Pearson attachment. The clips placed on the lateral aspect of the splint hold the canvas strips taut. The limb is in a neutral position and from the knee down is supported by the Pearson attachment. The position of the foot support can be adjusted to the patient's needs. Note the U-shaped clamp attached to the Kirschner wire. (From the Orthopedic nursing procedure manual, University of Iowa Hospitals and Clinics, The University of Iowa, Iowa City, Iowa.)

if the nurse's palms are placed against his cheeks with the fingers flexed under his chin. Increased flexion or hyperextension of the cervical spine must not be permitted. While the manual traction is being applied, a second nurse bathes (shaves male patient) and gently massages the skin and subcutaneous tissues of the lower jaw and chin.

Skeletal traction applied to extremity. Various types of surgical apparatus for applying direct traction to bone have been used in the past, but for the most part these have been supplanted by the Steinmann threaded or unthreaded rustless steel pin and the Kirschner threaded or unthreaded wire of chromic steel (Fig. 130). The latter is perhaps the most commonly used type of skeletal traction and is preferred to the Steinmann pin because it is smaller in diameter and the disturbance to the bone occasioned by its use is almost negligible. Skeletal traction may be applied to the lower extremity through the proximal or distal end of the tibia, through the heel,

and through the distal end of the femur. It also may be used in the upper extremity and in the skull.

The wire or pin may be inserted in the operating room or, if necessary, on the clinical unit. Either a general or local anesthetic may be used. Insertion of the wire or pin is a surgical procedure and requires the most scrupulous aseptic technique in its performance. Usually, the area in which the pin is to be inserted is prepared surgically in advance. The wounds made by the introduction of the wire may be dressed with sterile gauze sponges.

It is usually wise to have a Thomas splint and Pearson attachment prepared and sent to the operating room with the patient. If the wire or pin is to be inserted on the clinical unit, the splint should be ready to be put on the patient's leg before the skin area is surgically cleansed.

Equipment to attach the weight to the U-shaped clamp that will be attached to the nail or wire should be available. Much discomfort can be eliminated if the weights are attached before the patient becomes conscious or before the local anesthetic has completely worn off.

A cork or adhesive tape is usually applied over the sharp end of the wire or pin to protect the nurses and patient from injury. All handling of the U clamp, the rope, and the attached weights must be exceedingly careful to avoid causing pain and discomfort to the patient.

Skeletal traction may be used in fractures of the lower third of the femur when it is essential that the fracture be treated with the knee in flexion. The Thomas splint with a Pearson attachment generally is used with this type of fracture. The splint and attachment are prepared with wide canvas strips or slings to support the thigh and lower leg. These strips should be fastened securely with large traction clips or safety pins on the lateral aspect of the splint to make tightening them more convenient. An overhead frame with pulleys is necessary for suspending the Thomas splint. The splint usually is elevated at a 45° angle with the bed. The Pearson attachment is fastened to the Thomas splint at the knee joint. The knee is flexed to 45°, and the lower leg lies in the Pearson attachment, which is horizontal with the mattress (Fig. 130).

Equipment for preventing drop-foot deformity consists of an adhesive strip fastened along the sole of the foot and attached by rope to an overhead pulley. (Care must be taken not to exert pressure on the toes to avoid contracture of the toe extensors.) Also, commercial foot supports that clamp to the Pearson attachment are available.

Ropes are attached to the U-shaped traction clamp that holds the pin. This rope passes to a pulley at the end of the bed, where the weights are attached. The pull is in line with the Thomas splint and with the long axis of the femur.

The patient is allowed to move about rather freely in bed. He may sit up, or he may turn to his side as much as the traction will permit. The nurse must handle the apparatus with gentleness, however, for jarring movements are particularly dreaded by the patient. The rules applying to efficient skin traction also apply in skeletal traction, and nurses should be alert in their observations to see that the apparatus is mechanically correct and in good working order at all times.

When the wire or pin is to be removed, the skin is prepared as carefully as it was for the original procedure. The traction clamp and weights are removed from the limb, and the skin and wire on the lateral aspect of the leg are cleansed with an antiseptic solution. The skin is then pushed inward and the wire cut beneath the surface of the skin. The wire is pulled through from the opposite side. Small sterile dressings are applied to the pin areas until healing takes place.

Skeletal traction applied to head. Nursing care of the patient with skeletal traction applied to the head is included in the care of the patient with fracture of the cervical spine (Chapter 11).

Care of patients in traction

Bathing and bed-making. Patients in traction, like most other orthopedic patients, are bathed over the anterior surface of the body as the first step of their morning care. During the bath, the toes are carefully cleaned and the sole of the foot is massaged with alcohol or oil. At this time the area around the traction tapes or bandage should be inspected. Particular attention is given to the back of the heel and the Achilles tendon, which so often become sore when adhesive tape and bandage have been applied too snugly. The dorsum of the foot is inspected for signs of ridging or cyanosis. If the protective bandage over the traction tapes has become loosened either at the ankle or the groin, it should be reenforced or reapplied.

Without explicit permission from the physician, weights are never removed at any time during the nursing care given these patients. This is an axiom of such serious import that it can scarcely be emphasized too strongly. The damage that can be done in fractures of the extremity by this kind of thoughtlessness may, in some instances be almost immeasurable.

The nurse will frequently need assistance when giving back care and changing the bed linen of the newly operated upon patient who has been placed in suspension traction. Although, generally speaking, the patient in traction is not allowed to turn for this procedure, he can, with aid of a trapeze, learn to help with this aspect of his care. By grasping the trapeze and pulling, he is able to lift his shoulders off the bed, thus enabling the nurse to bathe and care for the upper portion of his back. To bathe the buttocks and the sacral area, the assistance of a second nurse is needed to help the patient lift his hips off the bed. The patient, by flexing his uninvolved hip and knee and pushing with his foot on the mattress as he pulls on the trapeze with his hands, is usually able with the assistance of a second nurse to lift his buttocks off the bed. This makes it possible for the first nurse to complete the back care and to change the bed linen. To change the bottom sheet, the clean linen is placed in position on the side of the bed beneath the patient's uninvolved limb. Then with the aid of the second nurse (on the opposite side of the bed), the patient's hips and shoulders are lifted as described previously, and the clean linen is pushed underneath the patient, replacing the solid linen (Fig. 388). The soiled linen is removed and the bed-making process completed. If the patient is a child, it is sometimes more convenient, to change bed linen from the bottom or the top of the bed. Many variations of bed-making and bathing procedures are necessary in caring for the patient in traction, and no one way can ever be set down dogmatically as the best for all patients.

An overhead bar, or trapeze, is almost indispensable for the adult patient in traction. With this device he can support himself for back care and thus spare the nurse much unnecessary lifting.

The following observations should be made when caring for the traction patient:

1 Neurovascular assessment—Note skin color, joint motion, and complaints of numbness, coldness, or swelling of the extremity. Avoid pressure in the popliteal space.

2 Condition of the skin—Check skin areas over the Achilles tendon, dorsum of the foot, heel, and sacral region.

3 Body alignment and position of the extremity—Is the purpose of the traction being accomplished?

4 Prevention of deformity—Have measures been taken to prevent drop foot and hip flexion contracture? Is the

backrest lowered several times daily to provide for complete extension of the hip joints?

5 Countertraction—Is countertraction sufficient or does the footplate frequently rest against the foot of the bed?

6 Slipping—Is there slipping of the traction tapes, and does the outer bandage need rewrapping?

7 Pressure—Is there pressure on the lateral aspect of the leg over the head of the fibula? Pressure in this area may result in a palsy of the peroneal nerve.

8 Patient's comfort—Traction should never be a source of undue discomfort for the patient. Listen carefully and heed complaints of discomfort.

9 Complication—Because of prolonged bed rest and minimal activity, hypostatic pneumonia is a constant threat, particularly to the elderly patient. Encourage coughing and deep breathing.

In washing the patient's back, close attention should be given to the sacral area, which is an extremely vulnerable spot that must have constant care to prevent breakdown of the skin. It should be emphasized that nurses caring for patients in traction should take the trouble to inspect this area. Since this part of the body is not in view, the nurse often washes and rubs it without sufficient inspection, thus missing any change in color such as the purplish redness of the skin that occurs in the early stages of pressure before skin breakdown has occurred. Further damage may be prevented at this time, and it is important to detect the oncoming trouble before it progresses further. If signs of pressure are present, the area should be massaged gently and covered with a thin coating of talcum powder. Squares of sponge rubber or acrylic fiber pads (artificial lamb's wool) may be placed under the sacral area. Most important of all, especially for the patient who cannot be turned, is frequent massaging of the part. This can be done, of course, without raising the patient each time. The nurse may slip her hand under the area and give an acceptable massage several times a day without changing the patient's position. Even moving the skin back and forth over a vulnerable spot for a short period may prevent undue pressure and will help to prevent skin breakdown.

In making the top of the bed, the efficiency of the traction and the warmth of the patient are the important considerations. The appearance of the bed is always secondary. Undersheets and drawsheets must be snug and tight, but the upper part of the bed may be made according to the patient's wishes.

The nurse's well-worn ingenuity comes into play when caring for the patient in traction, and no set rule can be laid down except that the comfort of the patient and the efficiency of the traction come before the appearance of the bed in orthopedic wards. Divided linen with ties may be helpful in some instances; however, this type of linen, also may interfere with the efficiency of the traction and with prescribed exercises. Many patients prefer that the top linen not be tucked under the mattress in the conventional manner but be tied loosely to the foot of the bed. Small blankets may be used to keep the limb and foot in traction warm.

Bedpans. Because a great majority of patients in traction lie in a bed in which the foot has been elevated for countertraction, some difficulty in the use of the bedpan may be encountered. In most instances, however, elevating the headrest is permissible and helpful. Also, the fracture bedpan with a tapering back can be slipped under the patient's buttocks without altering the position of the hips and with very little disturbance of the traction. With women patients, the use of a female urinal may cause less discomfort than use of the regular bedpan, plus the fact that less lifting is necessary to position the patient. Unless contraindicated the patient should be encouraged to use the trapeze and the uninvolved limb to assist in placement of the bedpan.

Prevention and treatment of pressure sores. The problem of preventing pressure sores on patients in traction is an extremely serious matter. Traction seems to predispose patients to this condition (1) because in many instances alteration of position is not allowed and (2) because a great number of patients in traction are elderly. It is very common for the older person in traction to have his back continuously elevated 30° to 45° as a safeguard against pulmonary congestion. This, of course, places a considerable portion of the body weight on the sacral area, and pressure sores tend to occur at that point with great frequency. In addition, the elderly patient often has dry tender skin, and the protective fat pads are gone from over bony surfaces. Often their nutrition is inadequate, particularly regarding protein and vitamin C, both of which are exceedingly important elements for promoting tissue health.

It is important that nurses recognize these hazards before trouble begins to occur. They should consult the physician in regard to proper diet and obtain his assistance and advice in meeting the problem. He will often be able to help them in planning for change of position. Usually, some latitude will be allowed the elderly patient who must be in traction over a considerable period.

The prevention of pressure sores is the responsibility of the nurse. It must be recognized that trauma of any nature that endangers tissue integrity is a great factor in the production of skin abrasion, and the trauma need be no more than that caused by a few crumbs in the bed. Trauma can occur to the skin from wrinkles in the undersheet, the plastic sheet, or the drawsheet and also from grit in talcum powder. A wet bed is a well-recognized cause of skin abrasion, and the necessity for keeping the bed dry and smooth can hardly be overemphasized. Patients who lift themselves on their elbows many times during the day may develop pressure sores at these areas. Another vulnerable site is the heel of the unaffected foot because the patient has a tendency to push himself up in bed with this foot.

Pressure areas go through certain rather well-defined stages. The first stage of redness usually will be accompanied by the patient's complaint of a hot burning pain at the site involved. After a day or so, the initial reddened area may cause the patient little pain because of the paralysis of the sensory nerve endings in the skin. The redness in the area may take on a purplish cast that will not disappear upon blanching. The skin may break, because of an almost undetectable vesicle formation. Unless this progression is checked, ulceration may follow, and the denuded area may become the source of secondary infection. Culture of these sores and appropriate antibiotics may be indicated in selected patients. Tissue nercrosis may cause deep craterlike holes in the skin and underlying soft tissues that may reach down to the bone.

Fundamental to all treatment for this condition is removal of pressure. Frequently, permission may be given to turn the patient to his side for short periods to relieve pressure on the sacral area. If this is done, the nurse should be careful to keep the legs in good alignment. The top leg should be supported with pillows to prevent sagging. A brisk rubbing to restore circulation to the threatened area can be given, but it should not be vigorous enough to endanger the skin. Alcohol may be used to toughen the skin, but it is advisable to use oil on the area occasionally to prevent excessive drying.

Small pressure pads placed around such points as the heel and the malleoli should be semilunar rather than circular in shape. Too often the circular pad with its dough-nut-like hole cuts off what little circulation is left to the part. A half moon that only partially closes the area accomplishes relief from pressure without the accompanying circulatory loss. Sponge rubber, cut into varying sizes and shapes, makes excellent pressure pads for heels, elbows, and other bony prominences.

Some physicians prescribe drying powders such as boric or zinc. Tincture of benzoin is sometimes beneficial in the early stages of denudation.

Treatment for the advanced pressure sore with its craterlike hole is a more difficult problem. If a culture taken from a decubitus ulcer grows a *Staphylococcus* organism, the patient should be isolated and precautions taken to protect other patients and personnel. Gloves and mask should be worn when dressings are changed. The physician may request that the ulcer be cleansed several times daily, depending on the amount of drainage. Sterile saline solution or solutions containing antibiotics are commonly used for such daily irrigation. Elase ointment, because of its action on necrotic tissue, may be placed on the ulcer. Packs of gauze impregnated with penicillin ointment or other antibiotics frequently are used. A and D ointment, granulated sugar, and many other drugs may be prescribed and are used with varying degrees of success. The physician frequently requests that dressings be omitted for certain periods of the day to permit drying of the area. Sunlight or treatment by the bactericidal lamp has been helpful in many cases. Dressings should be held in place with a minimum amount of tape, because adhesive itself can be a frequent cause of skin breakdown. With some patients cellophane or Blenderm surgical tape is advisable. These tapes are usually less irritating to the skin.

Surgical closure of a decubitus ulcer may be necessary to facilitate rehabilitation. Pressure sores treated conservatively heal slowly and, in some instances, the healing is superficial. The area breaks down when activity is resumed, revealing a larger underlying ulcer. It is necessary, therefore, to precede surgical closure of a pressure sore with several weeks of preparation. The patient must understand the importance of assuming positions that eliminate pressure on the involved area, and thus provide for a more adequate blood supply. Frequent cleansing and irrigation of the area are prescribed to lessen infection and to promote growth of healthy tissue.

Activity to prevent atrophy and stiffness of uninvolved extremities. It is always important that the parts of the body not in traction be kept in the best condition possible. No unnecessary stiffness or atrophy should be allowed to occur because of the immobilization of the injured part. Exercises for the uninvolved portions of the body should include flexion and extension of the hip and knee of the good leg, dorsiflexion and inversion of the ankle, static exercises to strengthen the quadriceps, gluteal, and abdominal muscles, exercises to develop the extensors of the elbows and wrists to facilitate future crutch walking, and breathing exercises. The patient with only lower extremity involvement is also encouraged to use his upper arms and shoulders freely, particularly in positions of outward rotation and abduction. Activities such as combing his hair, fastening his gown at the back of the neck, or lying with his arms out at the sides with elbows flexed and palms upward are beneficial and prevent shoulder restriction that often results from long periods of bed rest.

Diversional therapy. It is extremely important that the patient in traction be given something to do. He is confined so closely to his bed for such long periods that restlessness and depression occur rather easily. If available an occupational therapist will be able to suggest many crafts suitable for this type of patient. Otherwise, the nurse should provide some type of activity attractive to the patient, so that he will have the satisfaction of creating something with his hands while he is bedfast.

Wherever possible, schooling should not be interrupted.

Patients in traction may be moved without too much difficulty to recreational courts or porches to provide variation in their daily program. If swinging weights are attached to the bed, moving should not be done by one person. Someone should be responsible for holding the weights during the moving process so that they do not swing or become dislodged from the pulley.

8 Equipment frequently used to facilitate care of the disabled person

Alternating pressure pad or pneumatic mattress

The alternating pressure pad is made of air cells 1¼ in in diameter, running longitudinally to the bed. Every other cell is connected to an air tube that comprises the edge of the mattress. This arrangement provides for two systems of air cells. These air cells are alternately inflated and deflated by an electrically driven air pump. The air is shifted first into one system and then into the other. This means that the patient's body is alternately resting on the odd-numbered cells and then on the even-numbered cells. The cells are inflated and deflated at intervals of two to three minutes. This interchange of air in the cells is so smooth that it is barely perceptible to the hand. It produces a massaging effect to the cutaneous tissues and provides for a continuous change of pressure points. With improved circulation to the skin and changing pressure points, the danger of decubitus ulcers is somewhat lessened. This pad not only facilitates the care of the patient in the hospital but also may be used in the home to help prevent pressure areas (Fig. 131).

Lateral turning frame

The patient whose care necessitates immobilization of the spine and who needs to be turned at frequent intervals to prevent pressure sores is usually placed on a Foster frame (Fig. 132) or a Stryker frame (Fig. 133). This apparatus is similar to the Brad-

ford frame, except that both the anterior and posterior frames have been fitted on a standard that has a pivoting device. This pivoting device makes it possible in many instances for one nurse to turn an adult patient. Not only is it easier to turn the patient, but better immobilization also is secured; consequently, the patient experiences less pain in turning. The Foster and Stryker frames are used primarily in the treatment and nursing care of patients with various back conditions. The patient with spinal cord damage may be placed on this type of frame. Good position can be maintained, and it is possible to turn the patient frequently, thus changing the pressure points.

Canvas covers are used with these frames. They may be fastened with buckles or with lacings but must be firm and taut continuously. Divided covers frequently are used. Their use, however, depends on the diagnosis and the purpose for which the frame has been prescribed. The divided cover for the upper half of the posterior frame should extend from the top of the frame to the level of the patient's buttocks (gluteal cleft). A space of approximately four inches is left for the perineal opening. The lower half of the posterior cover extends to the end of the frame. The upper portion of the divided cover for the anterior frame will extend from the patient's shoulders to the symphysis pubis. Again, a space of four inches is maintained for the perineal opening, and the lower portion of the

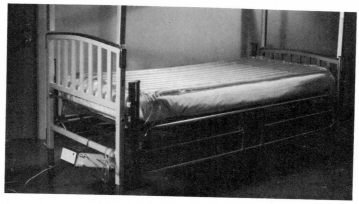

Fig. 131 Alternating pressure pad. The pad is placed on top of the regular mattress. Plastic material attached to each end of the pad is tucked beneath the mattress and maintains the pad in position. The smaller air cells or tubes, at the foot end of the pad, provide better protection for the patient's heels.

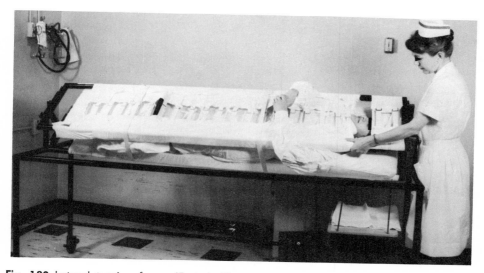

Fig. 132 Lateral turning frame (Foster). The patient is held snugly between the anterior and posterior frames. Two turning straps provide added security. The arm boards have been removed, the screw lock has been loosened, and the turning process has been started. Note ties of the muslin sheet covering the canvas frame cover and the narrow strip of canvas used to support the forehead when the patient is in the prone position.

anterior cover extends to the level of the patient's malleolus. This arrangement permits the patient's feet to extend over the frame cover when he is lying in the prone position. Some type of support must be arranged for the forehead or face. This usually consists of a narrow canvas strip buckled at the top of the anterior frame. When caring for a patient with incontinence on the frame, it will be necessary to protect the canvas covering around the perineal opening with waterproof material.

A narrow canvas strip is buckled across the perineal opening when the bedpan is not in place. This prevents the patient's buttocks from sagging and helps to maintain a good back-lying position.

The frame may be padded with strips of sponge rubber cut in the desired size. The outer linen covering is made to fit the frame and is held in place by tying the tapes on the underside (Fig. 132). When the patient is being turned from the supine to the prone position, a pillow should be placed crosswise above the dorsum of the feet. The top frame is fastened in place so that the patient is held snugly between the two frames. Two or three canvas turning straps are buckled around both frames and the patient. This gives the patient added security and will prevent the limbs from slipping during the turning process. The

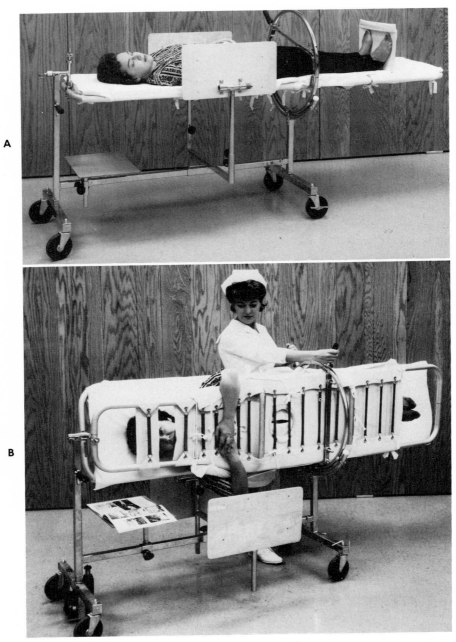

Fig. 133 A, Stryker's wedge turning frames—patient in the supine position. For added security in this position, the arm boards may be turned up as side boards and the ring closed over the patient. **B,** One nurse using the turning handles to turn the patient. The arm boards have been lowered, and the ring is closed over the patient. (Courtesy Stryker Corporation, Kalamazoo, Mich.)

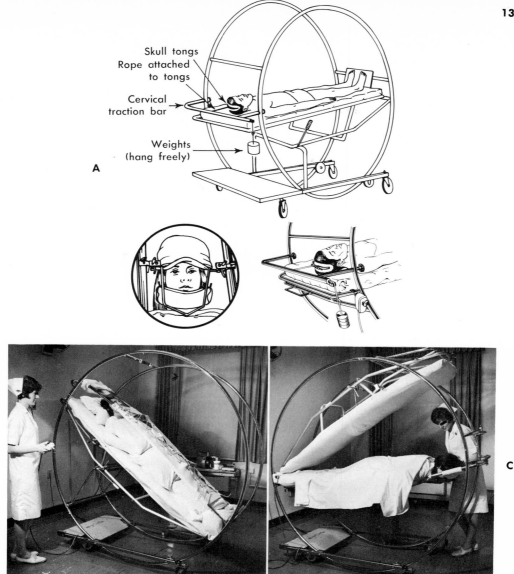

Fig. 134 The CircOlectric bed consists of an anterior and a posterior frame and provides for vertical turning as opposed to lateral turning of the patient. Thus, standing, Trendelenburg, and sitting positions also may be utilized. Since the bed is operated with an electric motor, even the very helpless patient may be able to adjust his position and assume a greater degree of independence. The many benefits (physiologic and psychologic) derived from frequent position changes and from self-dependence may be augmented with the use of this bed. In addition to hospital use, the CircOlectric bed can be used advantageously in the home to facilitate care of the disabled person. **A,** Use of the CircOlectric bed for the patient with skull tongs (cervical traction). The arrangement of the traction apparatus provides for the maintenance of continuous traction as the patient is turned vertically from the supine to the prone position or vice versa. Note close view of the adjustable face piece. Support for the head in either the prone or the supine position is an important factor in maintaining the desired position of the cervical vetebrae. **B,** The anterior frame has been put in position and turning of the patient is started. **C,** Prone position, with the posterior frame in the elevated position. (**A,** From the Orthopedic nursing procedure manual, University of Iowa Hospitals and Clinics, The University of Iowa, Iowa City, Iowa.)

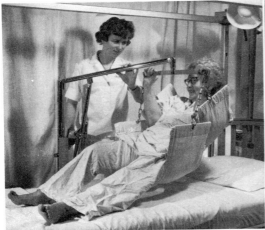
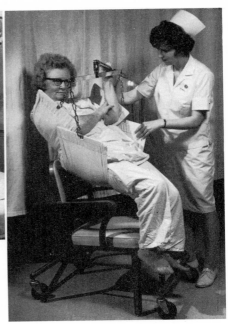

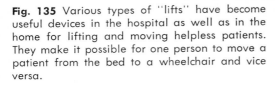

Fig. 135 Various types of "lifts" have become useful devices in the hospital as well as in the home for lifting and moving helpless patients. They make it possible for one person to move a patient from the bed to a wheelchair and vice versa.

arm boards are removed, and the screw or spring lock that keeps the frame from turning is released. The patient is instructed as to which way he will be turned. If he is being turned by one nurse, it is best that the nurse move to the side of the frame. The turning should be done quickly and smoothly. After the patient is turned, the screw or spring lock must be in place before the nurse's grasp on the frame is released. This screw or lock holds the frame firmly and prevents turning. The straps and upper frame are removed, and back care can be given. The covers and linen are changed when that half of the bed is not in use.

These frames may be used even when it is necessary for the patient to have traction applied. The frames are constructed so that traction can be applied to the patient's lower extremities or to the cervical region.

CircOlectric bed

A vertical turning frame may also be used when it is necessary to apply cervical traction (Fig. 134). The bed is equipped with a traction bar and pulleys that place the traction weight at the side of the bed (outside the circle). When the

bed is rotated, the weights hang free and thus provide for continuous traction. Nursing care given to the patient in a CircOlectric bed is usually adjusted to the turning schedule. When the anterior frame is being placed, the face support is positioned carefully. Change of position in the cervical region must not be permitted. A pillow may be placed over the lower limbs to help maintain proper body alignment, the footboard is positioned prior to fastening of the frame, and straps encircling the two frames will add to the patient's feeling of security during the turning process. The control button makes it possible to turn the patient slowly and without jerky movements. At the beginning of the turning process, the head end of the bed rises vertically while the foot end descends. The stop on the frame prevents the bed from turning too far. Adjustments in the patient's position, which facilitate feeding and diversional activities, can be made. When positioning the patient, the nurse should remember (if cervical traction is being used) that sufficient countertraction must be maintained to prevent the cervical tongs from resting against the pulley, resulting in a decrease in the traction force. Also, careful checking prior to the turning process is essential to prevent interference with the traction apparatus, which extends laterally to the bed.

The general nursing care of the patient is the same as for other bed patients. Skin care, change of position, prevention of deformity, and maintenance of normal joint motion are essential for his rehabilitation.

Lifting devices

Lifting devices (Fig. 135) facilitate caring for the disabled person and make it possible for one person to safely transfer the paralyzed or helpless or obese patient from his bed to a chair or, in some instances, to a tub. Canvas strips that are placed beneath the patient's shoulders and buttocks support the patient as the "arm" of the "lift" is raised. The "lift" is then moved so that the patient is positioned over the chair. The "arm" is lowered slowly, placing the patient in the chair. The canvas hammocks are detached from the "lift" and remain beneath the patient in readiness for his return to the bed.

9 Patients using braces, crutches, canes, and walkers

BRACES

During recent years, advances in the design and manufacture of braces and other orthotic aids have been responsible for increased functional activity for the handicapped individual. New synthetic materials such as polypropylene, polyethylene, and Plastazote are being used for splinting purposes. These new materials are water resistant, easy to clean, and cosmetically appealing. They also provide for strength and durability and have the advantage of being light in weight (Figs. 136, C, and 137). Braces, splints, and other supportive devices are prescribed for many reasons. They are frequently necessary to permit walking

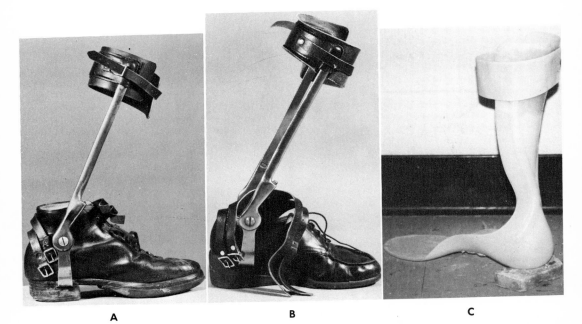

A   B   C

Fig 136 A, Klenzak inner upright brace. **B,** With inner and outer upright bars and outside T strap. The hinge has a built-in spring stop that prevents plantar flexion and is useful in the treatment of drop foot from muscle paralysis. The T strap stabilizes the foot against the varus position. **C,** This polypropylene brace can be used as a substitute for a drop-foot brace. It is light in weight and water and perspiration resistant. Also, it is more easily managed without attachment to a shoe and more cosmetically acceptable. Velcro straps are used to fasten the below-the-knee band.

without undue strain or fatigue. They also are used to prevent or overcome mild deformity or tendencies toward deformity. In other instances, they may be used to prevent motion in a joint or part of the body. The cock-up splint, which maintains the wrist and hand in a functional position, is often prescribed for the arthritic patient. Night splints also may be worn by the arthritic patient to help prevent or correct knee flexion contractures. The child with Legg-Perthes disease may wear an ischial weight-bearing brace or a modified Toronto orthosis (Fig. 273) to protect the hip joint. A spinal brace is frequently prescribed to provide support and immobilization for the patient with back pain. Various

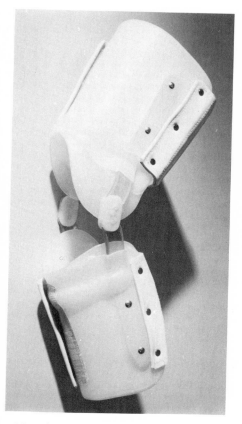

Fig. 137 The Iowa knee brace is an example of the use of new materials. This brace, worn to support unstable knees, even while the individual is engaged in athletics, contains a newly patented eccentric double-axis hinge joint made of plastic, which makes it more durable, more easily cleaned, and lighter than other braces. In addition, it can be worn while in water.

types of back braces also have been devised to help correct and prevent spinal deformity in the scoliotic child (Fig. 283). The Frejka pillow (Fig. 233) or the abduction brace (Fig. 234) may be used to maintain a congenitally dislocated hip in a corrected position, and long leg braces provide the support necessary to make ambulation possible when muscle weakness or paralysis is present in the lower extremities. The purpose of using a brace, as with other methods of treatment, is to help restore the patient to normal living. Braces are a step in this direction. However, when possible, the ultimate aim is to eliminate the use of braces either by further development of the patient's own remaining powers or by some type of reconstructive surgery.

Braces involve a considerable outlay of expense. A respect for the cost of the materials and the skilled labor going into their manufacture is a healthy virtue for the nurse to develop in the patient. Also, it is the nurse's responsibility to teach the patient and his family how to care for braces. Knowledge of their purpose and the correct way to apply them, with recognition of the purpose of each part and the necessity for keeping them intact, is essential. Nurses may encounter some resistance to the use of braces. Many persons honestly believe that to walk in any manner, however hazardously, without braces is preferable to walking with them. Nurses will need to be well informed about the reason for the prescribed brace.

Short leg brace. The short leg brace serves primarily to control motion of the ankle and foot (Fig. 138). Motion at the ankle joint (dorsiflexion and plantar flexion) may be controlled by a particular type of ankle stop. Prevention of plantar flexion (drop-foot position) can be accomplished with the posterior stop. This is frequently used when there is weakness or paralysis of the dorsiflexors of the foot. If the dorsiflexors are of normal strength and the plantar flexors weak, an anterior stop is used to prevent the patient from walking on his heel (calcaneus position). If the muscles that produce ankle motion are normal, the ankle joint in the brace is made without "stops," making free motion possible. If there is flaccid paralysis of all the muscles con-

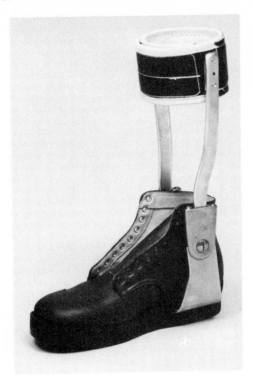

Fig. 138 Short leg brace with bichannel ankle. The main use for this brace is the prevention of drop foot from weakness of the dorsiflexor muscles. The anatomic ankle joint is aligned with the axis of the mechanical joint in the brace. A spring can be loaded to aid dorsiflexion or plantar flexion, whichever is required.

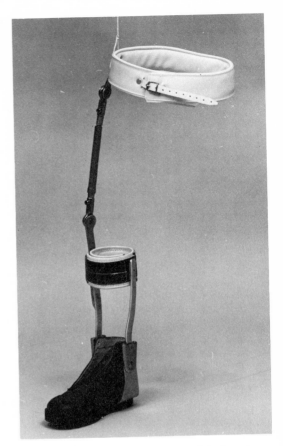

Fig. 139 This twister with a pelvic band can be added to the bichannel brace or to any shoe without other bracing to provide correction for in-toeing or out-toeing if such is part of the problem.

trolling ankle motion, the brace's ankle joint is made to provide only a few degrees of dorsal and plantar flexion. To control varus deformity of the foot, a leather T strap is attached to the lateral aspect of the shoe and buckled around the medial upright bar of the brace (Fig. 136, A and B). The reverse is used to control pronation (valgus deformity) of the foot.

Long leg brace. A long leg brace with knee pads or cuffs is necessary to prevent buckling of the knee and to permit weight bearing when there is paralysis or marked weakness of the knee extensor muscles (quadriceps). Knee pads worn over the anterior aspect of the knee indicate the presence of strong hamstring or flexor muscles around the joint combined with relatively weaker extensor muscles. Such pads are placed in front of the knee to prevent the patient's feeling insecure and fearful

of jackknifing as he walks. Knee pads on the posterior aspect indicate the presence of strong quadriceps (extensor muscles) that tend to pull the knee into a hyperextended position (genu recurvatum). Frequently these knee pads get lost because the nurse and the patient do not recognize them as an essential part of the brace. Also, to prevent hyperextension when there is paralysis of the hamstring muscles, padded metal cuffs are placed posteriorly on the long leg brace above and below the knee joint.

Various types of locks have been devised to permit flexion of the knee joint. Any such lock must function with a high degree of safety if buckling of the knee with weight bearing is to be prevented. Also, it

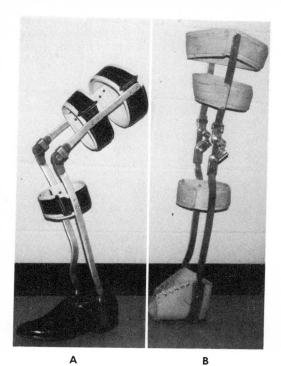

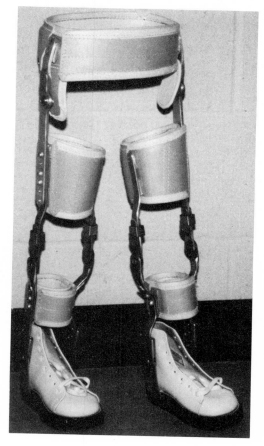

A   **B**

Fig. 140 **A,** Long leg brace with a "sleeve" lock at the knee and a stirrup attachment to the shoe. **B,** Long leg brace with a footplate and a special knee-locking device that permits straight knee support while bearing weight and a bent knee for sitting without the use of the droplock illustrated in **A.**

Fig. 141 Bilateral long leg braces with pelvic band. Note hip, knee, and ankle joints.

must be devised so that the individual wearing the brace can manipulate it without difficulty. The most common type of lock is known as the "sleeve" or "ring" lock (Fig. 140, *A*), which is placed on the lateral upright of the brace. This sleeve or ring slides up and down over the hinge joint.

The long leg brace constructed for a child is usually made with upright bars that overlap. This allows for frequent adjustment of the brace to meet the growth needs of the child (Fig. 141).

When there is paralysis of the hip and trunk muscles, a pelvic band or body brace may be added to the long leg braces (Fig. 141). This arrangement provides for control of hip motion and for good body alignment with correct support of the body weight. Pelvic bands should fit just below the iliac crests. The trunk part of the brace must be observed to be certain that the

fastening is in the midline of the body; any minute variation of this will make the fitting of the entire apparatus faulty.

Attachment of brace to shoe. The brace made for the lower limb may be attached directly to the shoe or may have a footplate that fits inside the patient's shoe (Fig. 140, *B*). The attachments commonly used to fasten the brace to the shoe are known as the caliper and the stirrup. With the stirrup attachment, the shoe cannot be separated from the brace. With the caliper attachment, the brace may be removed from the shoe, enabling the individual to attach the brace to more than one pair of shoes. However, the caliper attachment has the disadvantage of producing motion at the heel. The brace with the footplate that is placed inside the shoe enables the individual to wear different shoes, but when fitting shoes it is necessary to remember that space must be allowed for the foot-plate.

The selection and fitting of the shoe to be worn with a brace are significant factors. Many times adjustments such as arch supports or metatarsal pads are necessary. To provide proper weight bearing and position of the foot, the shoe may be altered with a metatarsal bar or with inner or outer wedges, or shoe lifts may be used to equalize leg lengths. When helping parents or a patient select a shoe to which a brace will be attached, the nurse must remember that the sole must be fairly thick and of a quality that will permit the brace maker to make the necessary alterations. For brace attachments a walking shoe with a low broad heel is preferable. If there is considerable spasticity of the ankle and foot muscles, it is desirable to have a shoe that opens over the toes. Care must be exercised when putting the spastic foot into the shoe to make certain that the toes are in the correct position. With a tight heel cord, it is difficult to keep the heel of the foot down in the shoe. The high-top, laced shoe may be helpful. If the individual has no sensation in the foot, a great deal of care must be taken to prevent the development of blisters and ulcers on the heels and toes. Frequent and careful inspection of the skin for reddened areas is necessary. In some instances, lining the shoe with sheep's wool has been helpful.

Arm splints. Arm splints should be inspected frequently to see that the splint is actually maintaining the arm in the position designed. Patients wearing arm splints have a tendency to lift the shoulder by contracting the strong upper trapezius muscle, thereby robbing the upper arm of the support of the splint. It may be necessary to take a little time to instruct the patient to relax the trapezius muscle so that the arm may rest in the splint as prescribed. If weakened shoulder or back muscles are present and no splint is worn, the weight of the arm in the splint should not be allowed to pull the shoulders downward in undesirable postural attitudes. Some provision to eliminate this pull may need to be devised. If the patient is bedfast, canvas hammocks may be suspended from an overhead bar that will support the arms

and prevent the pull on weakened shoulder muscles. If the patient spends considerable time sitting, the arms may be supported by armrests constructed of pillows or pads that may be placed on a desk or table top or on the arms of a chair. It is sometimes possible to improvise an upright support with an overhead bar to a wheelchair (Fig. 423). Hammocks or cuffs may be suspended to this bar to support the hands and arms for part of the day. It is usually permissible for the patient to use his hand and elbow functionally in eating, writing, or holding a paper if there is no involvement in these areas even though weakness is present in the shoulder muscles. Too constant use of the forearm, however, may put more strain than is desirable on the shoulder, and frequent periods of rest from activity are advisable.

Care of braces. All joints and locks on a brace should be oiled weekly with *3-in-1* oil or a similar lubricant, and surplus oil should be removed immediately so that it does not stain the surrounding leather. Lint should be removed from screws before they are oiled. Leather parts can be cleansed satisfactorily with saddle soap and small amounts of water. The leather should be polished after the use of saddle soap. This both refurbishes and imparts a certain amount of water resistance to the leather.

For the patient's comfort and for the cleanliness and long life of the brace, a cotton shirt may be worn beneath a body brace. Oils and lotions applied to the skin tend to stain leather portions of braces, and these stains are difficult to remove. If the patient is incontinent, the upper portion of the leather thigh cuff should be protected with waterproofing. Although desirable, it is not always possible to get bulky diapers and rubber pants beneath a brace, and when these have to be placed outside, the leather portions near the groin are exposed to frequent wetting.

All straps on braces should be securely fastened, but care should be taken, as the patient puts on weight or, if a child, grows, that constriction of circulation does not develop because of the straps. Nurses new to orthopedic services will need instruction in the application of each of the more complicated types of braces, particularly the

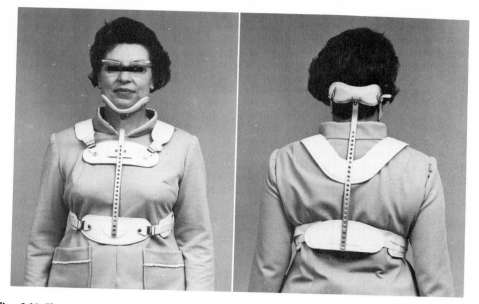

Fig. 142 The cervical brace (sometimes referred to as the SOMI brace—sternum, occiput, mandibular immobilizer) holds the cervical spine immobilized and is adjustable for any degree of flexion. There is considerable freedom of flexibility for the wearer to adjust to any position desired from the waist down while providing support for the cervical spine.

corrective scoliosis braces, the different kinds of clubfoot braces, and the Taylor spine brace. Automatic locks should be explained and their use demonstrated. The student nurse deserves to have this information from a clinical instructor rather than from a patient.

Lacings or shoestrings used on braces should be kept in good condition, without knots, and be changed as they become frayed. If the tips fall off, new ones can sometimes be constructed by the application of collodion in successive layers. Frayed straps and soiled or worn felt pads should be replaced by the brace maker.

Missing parts (screws, laces, hooks, straps, pads, or felt lining) should be reported as soon as noticed. The patient will learn respect for the apparatus by the nurse's prompt attention to such details. The shoes attached to braces, usually by caliper through the heel, must be inspected frequently for signs of wear and abnormal pressure. Children tend to outgrow shoes and braces with alarming rapidity. Points to be recognized as indications that a child is outgrowing the braces or shoes must be called to the attention of the parents when

correct application is demonstrated to them.

If elastic straps are attached to braces or shoes, inspection of the brace should include examination of this elastic for its resilience. These straps may go from the sole of the shoe to a point just below the knee to form a sort of external dorsiflexor to relieve drop foot caused by paralysis of the anterior tibial muscle.

Inspection of the skin when the brace is removed may reveal bruises, discolorations, skin abrasions, or dermatitis. Any deviation from the normal condition of the skin or underlying tissues should be reported. Suitable alterations usually can be made to overcome such friction.

In teaching parents and relatives, the nurse must constantly emphasize the necessity of periodic checkups for all patients wearing braces.

CRUTCHES

The orthopedic patient usually has ample time to anticipate the moment when he will be able to move about on crutches. It is a goal that he sets for himself and looks forward to with great eagerness because once again he will be able to get around and do things for himself. This is the aspect that usually appeals most to him. Sometimes, however, this same eager patient is considerably disappointed when he begins to use those crutches. He is weak, progress is slow, and many limitations of which he was previously unaware become apparent.

The nurse needs patience and foresight to manage such a situation. Many institutions have a physical therapy department to teach patients to walk on crutches. This, of course, is ideal for the patient, for he receives careful instruction and guidance from a physical therapist skilled in this procedure. In the smaller hospitals, however, no such assistance is available, and the nurse must assume responsibility for this part of the patient's treatment.

Measuring for crutches. Several methods of measuring for crutches may be found in the literature. Perhaps the most common is to have the patient lie on his back with his arms straight at his sides and to measure from the anterior axillary fold to a point six to eight inches out from his heel with a tape measure. If he lies with the arms elevated over the head, measurement is often inadequate, since contracture of the muscles in the axillae is essential for correct measurement. The patient should be measured in the shoes he will wear when learning to walk on crutches. Another method that may be used to determine the proper crutch length is to subtract sixteen inches from the patient's total height. In other instances, adjustable crutches may be used and replaced with the regular crutch when the correct crutch length is determined.

Crutches that are more than two or three inches too long should not be cut off to fit the patient without some provision being made for altering the hand bar, which will otherwise be too low. Placement of the hand bar is important and should provide for approximately 30° flexion of the elbow. As the body weight is taken on the hands and lifted off the floor, complete extension of the elbow is necessary. The types of ambulation aids most frequently used by disabled persons are shown in Fig. 143.

Crutch tips should be of good quality and be inspected from time to time for

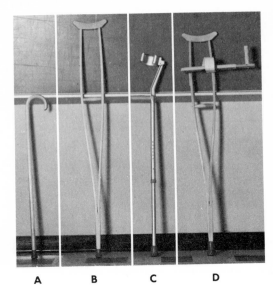

A   B   C   D

Fig. 143 Various types of ambulation supports. **A,** The cane with a half-circle handle is available in wood or metal. **B,** The underarm crutch illustrated is not adjustable but is lighter in weight than the adjustable crutch. This type of crutch is available in either wood or metal. **C,** Adjustable forearm crutch. **D,** An underarm crutch with a forearm adaptation platform. This type of crutch may be used for the arthritic patient who is unable to fully extend the elbow or who is unable to grasp the crutch hand bar. (Courtesy Physical Therapy Department, University Hospitals and Clinics, The University of Iowa, Iowa City, Iowa.)

wear. A worn crutch tip is a menace and must be recognized as such, since slipping is likely to result and may spell disaster for the handicapped person. The soft rubber suction crutch tip is most desirable. The entire tip has contact with the floor and is less likely to slip than the hard rubber tip.

Padding over the axillary bar is not necessary but frequently is used because the patient thinks it is more comfortable. Some authorities believe that such pads encourage the patient to lean on the crutches, thus bearing too much weight on the axillae. Since crutch paralysis is not an infrequent complication from too much pressure on the axillae, under which the radial nerves lie, it is well to reinstruct in the proper use of the crutch to avoid axillary pressure.

Preparatory exercises for walking on crutches. In hospitals or clinics in which intensive treatment of disabled persons is carried out, attention is first directed toward developing and strengthening the muscles of the shoulders, chest, arms, and back. The patient is helped to recognize the fact that he must have strong upper extremities and back muscles to support his weight when he becomes ambulatory.

To help the beginning crutch walker, specific exercises may be prescribed to strengthen the following groups of muscles:

1 *Finger and thumb flexors*—used to grasp the crutch hand bar. Exercises frequently used include squeezing a rubber ball, working with modeling clay, using a hand gripper, and lifting dumbbells.

2 *Wrist extensors*—maintain the wrist in dorsiflexion as body weight is taken on the hand. Exercises may include using the trapeze, lifting weights, and doing push-ups.

3 *Elbow extensors* (triceps muscle)— maintain the elbow in extension as the body weight is lifted off the floor. Exercises may include doing pushups and lifting weights.

4 *Shoulder depressors*—prevent elevation of the scapula as the body weight is supported by the hands and lifted off the floor. Exercises may include doing sitting push-ups or prone push-ups.

5 *Shoulder flexors*—used to move the crutches forward. Exercises may include dart throwing, etc.

An overhead trapeze is helpful in encouraging the patient to use his arms and shoulders to lift his weight from the bed. However, it should be remembered that the use of the trapeze does not help to strengthen the elbow extensor, an important muscle for the crutch walker. In some instances, it will be necessary for the patient to learn to balance himself in a sitting position. Standing exercises are started as soon as the patient's general condition permits. The tilt table or the CircOlectric bed frequently is used to help the patient adjust to the vertical position (Figs. 134 and 445). Prolonged lying in bed can lead only to loss of muscle tone and incipient deformities that will make standing and walking all the more difficult when they are finally undertaken.

During the time the patient is carrying out active and active-resistive exercises to strengthen the upper extremities, the weak legs are carried through the full range of joint motion several times during the day to prevent muscle contractures and to minimize joint stiffness.

For preparing the patient to use the parallel bars and crutches, push-up exercises from the prone position (Fig. 144) are useful in strengthening the triceps muscles. Sawed-off crutches that may be used in a sitting position in bed, or on the mat in the physical therapy department, will help the patient to become accustomed to the sensation of having crutches under the arms and will also give him the feeling of bearing his body weight on his hands (Fig. 145). He can be taught how to hold his shoulder girdle as he practices with these sawed-off crutches, so that he will avoid hunching and will keep the shoulders at a normal or slightly depressed level. He can learn to shift his weight on the crutches while he is still sitting in bed. These sideways shifts will enable him to transfer himself to the wheelchair when he is ready for that experience. Exercises may also include the use of weights. Push-ups also may be practiced when the patient is sitting in a wheelchair or a chair with armrests. He grasps the armrests and as he straightens the elbows, lifts the buttocks off the chair seat. Care should be taken to avoid hunching or elevating the shoulders. This type of exercise helps strengthen all the groups of muscles listed previously: the shoulder depressors and flexors, the elbow and wrist extensors, and the finger and thumb flexors. If the lower extremities are not paralyzed, tightening the quadriceps muscle by lifting the heel off the bed or performing straight leg–raising exercises will strengthen the knee extensors (Figs. 415 and 416). Lying in the prone position and lifting the leg off the bed (hyperextension) will strengthen the hip extensor muscles.

Crutch-walking posture. The standing postion is not attempted until the patient has mastered the bed exercises and has learned to transfer himself without help into a stabilized wheelchair. Standing with crutches may take a considerable time to master, for it is vitally important that the patient learn to balance himself on the

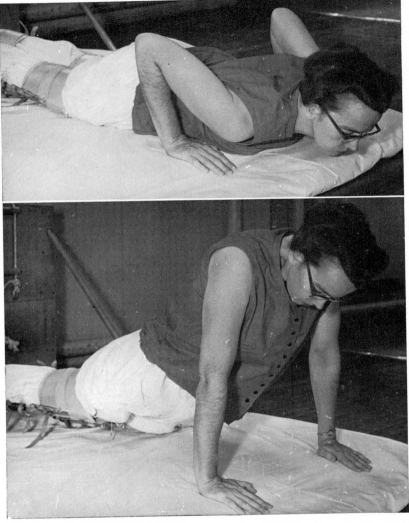

Fig. 144 Push-up exercises are done prior to walking on crutches. This activity is of special value in strengthening the triceps muscle (elbow extensor).

crutches (Fig. 146) before he undertakes any further activity. Parallel bars are used for exercises in balancing, standing, and walking (Fig. 147). Two hospital beds, placed with foot ends together and stabilized with wooden blocks, may be used as parallel bars.

Nurses usually are not required to teach the severely handicapped patient to walk on crutches. However, they must know what constitutes safe and efficient crutch walking for this type of patient if they are to supervise such activities on the clinical unit or in the home. They should

be able to recognize the patient's maximum degree of good crutch-walking posture and to encourage it at all times. The desirable stance is one in which the head is held straight and high, with the pelvis over the feet if the patient possesses sufficient muscle strength. The crutches are placed about four inches in front and about four inches at the sides of the feet, which makes a large standing base. As in all crutch walking, the patient should extend his elbows and carry his weight largely on his hands. He must not hunch his shoulders, and very little weight should be taken by the axillae

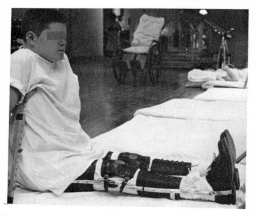

Fig. 145 Short crutches may be used in preparation for walking on crutches. Using the crutches to lift the body weight off the bed or mat is valuable in strengthening the shoulder depressors, elbow extensors, wrist dorsiflexors, and finger flexors.

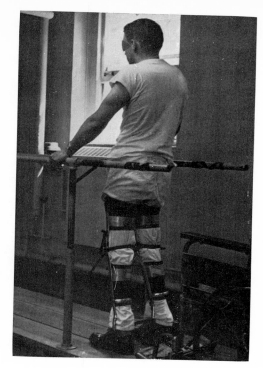

Fig. 147 Parallel bars are used for exercises in balancing, standing, and walking. They provide added security and safety for the disabled person.

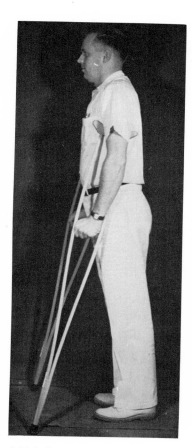

Fig. 146 Balancing in the tripod position.

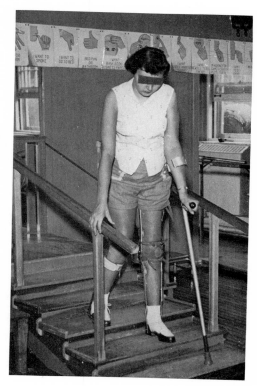

Fig. 148 Aluminum forearm crutch (Canadian type).

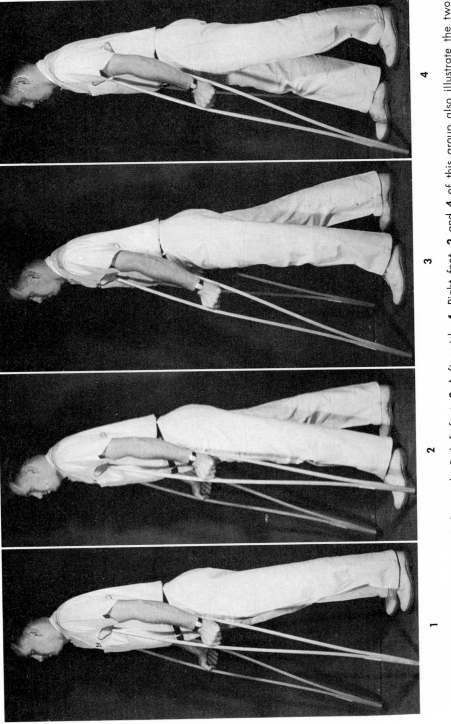

Fig. 149 Four-point crutch gait: **1**, Right crutch. **2**, Left foot. **3**, Left crutch. **4**, Right foot. **2** and **4** of this group also illustrate the two-point crutch gait: opposite foot and crutch are advanced simultaneously—i.e., the right crutch and left foot are advanced together, followed by the left crutch and right foot. With the four-point and two-point crutch walking gaits, weight is taken on each extremity.

at any time. When a crutch of the correct length is being used, it should be possible to place one or two fingers between the axillary bar of the crutch and the patient's axilla (adductor muscle).

If involvement is such that this position is impossible (i.e., when the patient has little or no use of the muscles of the hip joint, the back, or the abdomen), he is usually taught to balance himself in the tripod position. In this position the weight is forward from the ankles, with the hips forward and the crutches ahead and out at each side. It is important for patients with severe muscle involvement to keep the pelvis as far in advance as possible. They have little muscle power in the front of the body to support them if the pelvis is held too far behind the feet and so they must depend on anterior hip joint ligaments to stop them from going too far forward. The patient must, of course, always be assured of his own safety.

Attention to details of good posture is essential when the patient begins to walk. If he starts badly, he is likely to continue in the same attitude. Rounded shoulders, stooping back, slumping, flexion at the knees or hips, outward rotation of hips,

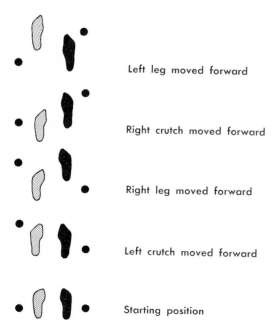

Left leg moved forward

Right crutch moved forward

Right leg moved forward

Left crutch moved forward

Starting position

Fig. 150 Four-point crutch gait with partial weight bearing on both limbs.

eversion of the feet are postural defects particularly common to the patient walking on crutches. Fatigue, overdetermination to make progress, and muscle weakness from prolonged bed rest may account for some of this. Discouragement also may play its part. Allowing the patient to see himself in a mirror sometimes produces amazing automatic improvement in posture.

Sitting either on the bed or in a chair with back and feet well supported should precede actual walking by several days for the patient who has been bedfast for a long time. This is followed by standing at the side of the bed in good position, hips and knees extended, back straight, chest forward, and head up. Contracting the abdominal and gluteal muscles will assist with later easy natural locomotion and good posture. As the patient stands at the bedside, he can be helped to shift his weight from one foot to the other without slumping provided his disability permits. Alternate knee flexion and extension and deep-breathing exercises may be used to prepare the patient for walking. This is the slow approach, and the patient may be impatient to start actual locomotion. The situation and reasons for the delay must be carefully explained. Getting a patient out of bed and allowing him to walk on crutches in the space of one day usually ends in tears and discouragement.

From the first day the patient should learn the proper way to balance on crutches as a safety measure and to give him a feeling of security. The starting position is a tripod formed by the patient's body and the two crutches. The patient stands with his feet slightly apart, and the crutches are placed forward and out from the body in such fashion that a line drawn between them would form the base of a triangle whose apex would be the patient's feet. All the factors of good standing posture must be observed. In teaching the patient to walk on crutches the aim is ultimately to enable him to walk without the crutches.

The patient is taught to extend and stiffen his elbow and to place the weight of his body on the wrists and the palms. He is taught to avoid bearing any weight at the axillary level, because the radial nerve passes under this area superficially. Injury to this nerve causes paralysis of the elbow and wrist extensors and is commonly referred to as "crutch palsy." Treatment of such nerve injury extends over a long period of time and necessitates that the individual stop using his crutches. For this reason, it may be advisable for the crutch walker to have the strength of these muscles checked periodically.

Persons beginning to walk on crutches have a tendency to try to lift a crutch when bearing weight upon it. Nurses should be alert to this tendency and explain the fallacy to the patient. The habit of taking a longer step with the weaker leg is another common mistake made by beginners. Patients should be instructed to take rather short steps of equal length with both legs.

The Canadian crutch (Fig. 148) without

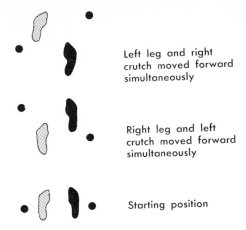

Left leg and right crutch moved forward simultaneously

Right leg and left crutch moved forward simultaneously

Starting position

Fig. 151 Two-point crutch gait with partial weight bearing on both limbs.

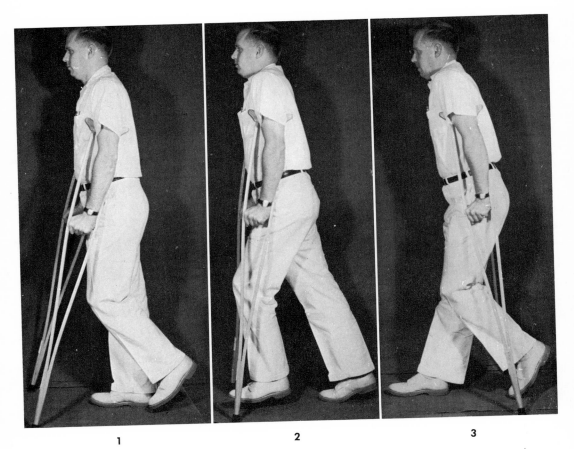

1   2   3

Fig. 152 Three-point crutch gait is used when there is involvement of one extremity. It may be used when no weight bearing has been ordered or when partial weight bearing is permitted. The affected extremity advances with the crutches, and the patient's weight is taken on the hands as the normal extremity comes forward.

axillary rest is preferred in some orthopedic clinics. One advantage in the use of these crutches is that there is more tendency on the part of the patient to make better anatomic use of the hips and pelvis in locomotion. In other words, the patient tends to depend on himself and his own muscles more than on the crutches, which are really not much more than canes. Absence of the axillary bar is considered to be advantageous also because likelihood of crutch paralysis is decreased greatly.

Canadian crutches are particularly useful for the patient who is likely to need them only for a short period, but the longer crutch with the axillary bar gives more adequate support. It usually is considered advisable to use the standard type of crutch for patients who have involvement in the trunk, hips, and arms.

Crutch-walking gaits. Walking on crutches is usually an ordeal for the patient who has been inactive over a period of time. Everything possible should be done to make the experience safe and comfortable. The patient will need instruction and constant encouragement if he is to learn to use crutches without undue fatigue.

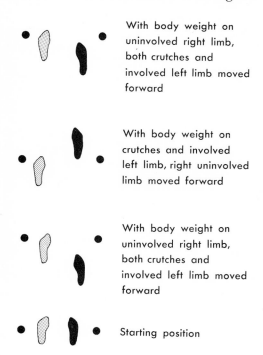

With body weight on uninvolved right limb, both crutches and involved left limb moved forward

With body weight on crutches and involved left limb, right uninvolved limb moved forward

With body weight on uninvolved right limb, both crutches and involved left limb moved forward

Starting position

Fig. 153 Three-point crutch gait with partial weight bearing on the involved limb.

The type of disability that the patient has determines the type of crutch walking he should be taught. When available, the help of a hospital physical therapist should be solicited in making the choice. In general, the following will apply to the most common types of orthopedic disability:

1 The patient who may bear some weight on each limb should be taught the four-point (Figs. 149 and 150) or two-point crutch gait (Fig. 151); e.g., patients with arthritis, cerebral palsy, etc.

2 The patient who must bear little or no weight on one extremity should be taught the three-point crutch gait (Figs. 152 and 153)—the method of advancing both crutches and the affected limb at the same time.

3 It is sometimes permissible to teach the swing-through crutch gait to patients whose lower extremities are paralyzed and who wear long leg braces (Fig. 154).

Modifications are recognized to be essential. For instance, although swinging between crutches is not recommended as a permanent practice for patients, it may frequently be necessary when speed in walking is essential. Also, the use of one crutch or cane is an advanced procedure. The crutch is used on the normal side, because it is put forward at the same time as the disabled limb, thereby taking the weight off that foot.

Four-point crutch gait. The four-point gait (Figs. 149 and 150) can be performed to a count of 1-2-3-4. The patient puts one crutch forward, followed by the opposite foot, the other crutch, and the opposite foot—left crutch, right foot, right crutch, left foot. This is hard for a normal person to do, although it approximates normal walking motions of arms and legs. However, with a little practice, its use becomes automatic to the patient.

Two-point crutch gait. The two-point gait (Fig. 151) is the same as the four-point gait except faster. With this gait, the patient advances the opposite crutch and limb simultaneously—left crutch and right limb, right crutch and left limb.

Three-point crutch gait. When no weight bearing has been ordered or when partial weight bearing is permitted on the affected extremity, the three-point gait (Figs. 152

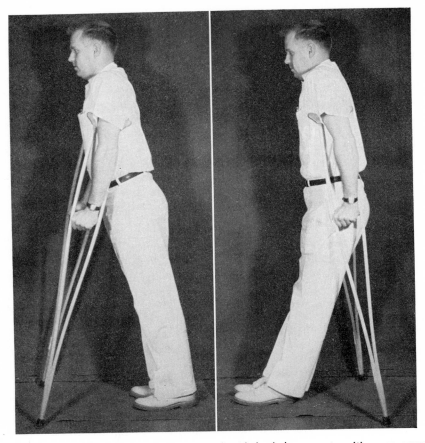

Fig. 154 The swing-through crutch gait is used with both lower extremities are paralyzed. The limbs are braced and swung forward together.

and 153) is usually considered preferable. The patient may be taught the mechanics of this gait by means of a diagram before he is out of bed. The affected limb and both crutches are advanced at the same time. Then, with the body weight balanced on the two crutches and the weak leg, the normal leg is advanced. The patient should be instructed to take steps of equal length; otherwise he will tend to take a long step when using the crutches and a very short one when advancing the unaffected extremity. Weight bearing, when permitted on the affected leg, should be started gradually.

Swing-through crutch gait. The swing-through gait (Fig. 154) is used by the patient with paralyzed lower extremities. The limbs are braced and swung forward together. This is a rapid gait but does not simulate normal walking.

Tripod crutch gait. The tripod gait may be taught to patients with severe involvement of the lower extremities. The right crutch is advanced first, then the left crutch, and the body is dragged up to the crutches. If the upper extremities and shoulders are strong, the patient can use the swing-to crutch gait. For this gait the crutches are placed together in front of the body. The patient then bears down on the crutches and lifts his body so that it is brought up to the crutches. The next step in advance of this method is the swing-through gait (described in the preceding paragraph), when both crutches are placed ahead and the body is lifted and swung beyond the crutches. This is more involved than the swing-to gait because the body is swung through the crutches and therefore comes to the floor ahead of the crutches.

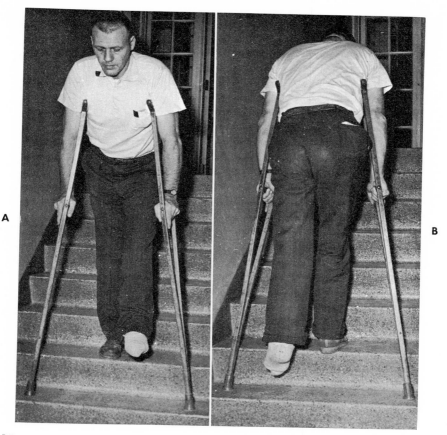

Fig. 155 A, Down the stairs with crutches. The crutch walker who is accustomed to the three-point gait will place his crutches on the lower step and his weight on his hands and bring the normal extremity down to the lower step with the crutches. Then with the body weight on the normal extremity, the crutches are placed on the next step and the procedure is repeated. **B,** Up the stairs with crutches. When going up steps, the body weight is taken on the hands and crutches and the normal extremity advanced to the upper step. The body weight is then taken on the normal extremity, and the crutches and involved limb follow. A safe rule to remember when teaching the three-point crutch gait is that the involved limb always goes with the crutches.

Other activities essential for crutch walker. One method of going up and down steps on crutches is shown in Fig. 155. Rising from and sitting down in a chair with crutches are illustrated in Figs. 156 and 157, respectively.

Hazards of walking on crutches. Everything possible should be done to ensure the patient's safety, for a fall is extremely hazardous after a long period of inactivity. Even a mild mishap may lead to a fracture. When the patient begins to walk, there should be one nurse or aide in front of and one behind him. He should not be encouraged to lean on his assistants, but he should feel confidence in their presence at all times. No wet spots, loose rugs, or other obstacles to safe walking should be in the patient's path. Crutch tips must be intact and should be replaced when there is any sign of wear (thinness in the rubber). Suction crutch tips, as the name implies, adhere to the floor surface and decrease the possibility of slipping.

It is advisable for the person learning to walk with crutches to wear a low-heeled walking shoe. Laces should be tied. With this type of shoe fastened securely to the foot, support for the arches is provided and accidents are less likely to occur. Flimsy,

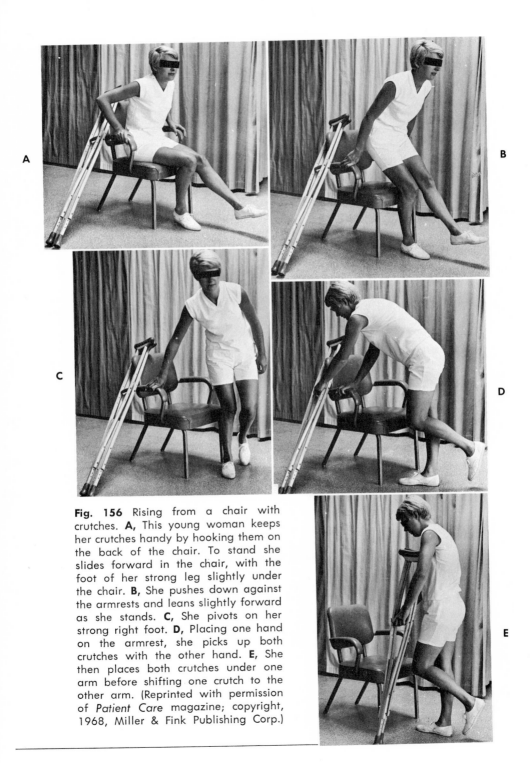

Fig. 156 Rising from a chair with crutches. **A,** This young woman keeps her crutches handy by hooking them on the back of the chair. To stand she slides forward in the chair, with the foot of her strong leg slightly under the chair. **B,** She pushes down against the armrests and leans slightly forward as she stands. **C,** She pivots on her strong right foot. **D,** Placing one hand on the armrest, she picks up both crutches with the other hand. **E,** She then places both crutches under one arm before shifting one crutch to the other arm. (Reprinted with permission of *Patient Care* magazine; copyright, 1968, Miller & Fink Publishing Corp.)

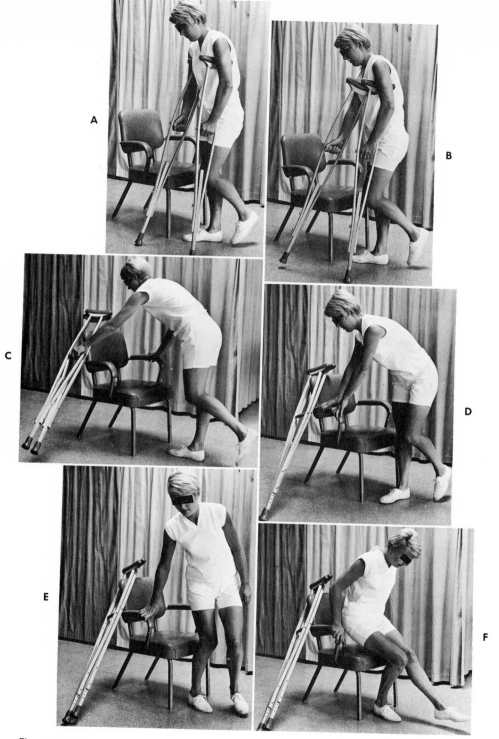

Fig. 157 Sitting down in chair with crutches. **A,** As the young woman approaches the chair, she moves her strong leg in close to the chair. **B,** She then places both crutches under her left arm. **C,** Placing her right hand on the left arm of the chair, she hooks the crutches on the back of the chair. **D,** Now she pivots on the right foot. **E,** Placing her right leg against the chair, she brings her left hand around to the left chair arm. **F,** She gently lowers herself into the chair. (Reprinted with permission of *Patient Care* magazine; copyright, 1968, Miller & Fink Publishing Corp.)

soft bedroom slippers should be avoided.

Errors commonly made by the patients and for which the nurse should be alert are (1) walking with the knee and hip flexed, the foot everted, and the hip in outward rotation, (2) a tendecy to walk with the weight on the ball of the foot and with the heel elevated, and (3) a sloughing posture, with the eyes fixed on the floor, the chin on the chest, and the shoulders and back rounded.

CANES

The cane is frequently prescribed to improve the patient's balance and to lessen the weight-bearing strain on an involved knee or hip. It probably provides the least amount of support of any of the walking appliances. However, it does widen the base of support and, by so doing, helps to maintain the patient's feeling of confidence and sense of balance. When one cane is used, it is held in the hand opposite the involved limb and is advanced with the involved limb. Thus the body weight is taken partially on the cane and the involved limb as the uninvolved limb is moved forward. The height of the cane should permit 15° to 30° of flexion at the elbow joint. As weight is taken on the hand, the elbow is extended. A rubber tip with a wide flat surface for contact with the floor is desirable. Canes that have three or four small legs are also available and are helpful to the elderly person who walks slowly and has poor balance.

WALKERS

The use of a walker may be preferable to crutches, particularly for the elderly individual. The walker has a wide base of support and consequently provides more security for the person fearful of falling. The pick-up walker is most commonly used. Different types of hand grips to accommodate hand and finger disabilities, as well as an attachment that facilitates use of the walker on stairsteps, are available. However, it should be remembered that most elderly individuals using walkers need assistance when going up or down steps. With the patient standing straight with the elbow flexed 15° to 30°, the correct height of the walker may be determined by measuring the distance from the junction of the thumb and index finger to a point on the floor five to six inches to the side of the forefoot. Walkers have some disadvantages such as being difficult to maneuver in small places and on stairsteps. They provide for a slow pace and do not encourage a normal walking sequence. To help prevent loss of balance, the person using a walker should be instructed to pick the walker up with his arms (this tends to keep his weight forward). Another important point is that he should remember to use the chair armrests for body support rather than the walker when sitting down or rising from a chair.

• • •

Unit II has dealt with some of the orthopedic apparatus used by the individual with a physical disability. Frequently the nurse must assume responsibility for teaching the patient and/or the family about the brace, cast, etc. This includes helping them to understand explanations they may have had from other members of the health team. If braces are to accomplish the intended purpose, they must be applied correctly. A responsible person needs to understand that a child may outgrow his brace, that a missing strap or part may make it ineffective, and that worn shoe lifts and soft casts are useless. The skin beneath cast edges and braces must be inspected daily for signs of irritation, and frequent assessment of motor and sensory functions is necessary. The nurse who has a keen interest in helping the patient understand the purpose of the apparatus, the care it needs, and the signs and symptoms to which he should be alerted is truly motivating the patient not only to accept the apparatus and his disability, but also to assume responsibility for helping himself.

Unit II STUDY QUESTIONS

THE PATIENT IN A CAST

Nursing care of the patient in a cast must provide for patient comfort and safety as well as for the maintenance of a clean intact cast. Discuss the following factors as they relate to the care of the patient in a cast:

1 Neurovascular assessment of the extremity in a cast
2 Sensory and motor functions of the following nerves:
  a Median   d Peroneal
  b Radial   e Tibial
  c Ulnar
3 The meaning of compartment syndrome and the symptoms that occur when this is a problem
4 Method(s) of turning a patient in a hip spica cast
5 Placement of the patient with a hip spica cast on the bedpan
6 Methods that may be used to finish the cast edges and why such finishing is necessary
7 Provision for protecting the perineal area of the cast
8 Instructing parents in the care of the small child in a hip spica cast
9 Skin care and positioning of the extremity following removal of a cast

THE PATIENT IN TRACTION

Many adaptations in the application of traction have been devised to provide proper treatment for the individual patient. However, if the nurse has an understanding of the basic modes of traction and principles involved, she will be able to meet the nursing needs of the traction patient, regardless of the variations that are necessary.

1 There are three basic modes of applying traction to a part of the body. These are referred to as skin, skeletal, and manual traction. Explain each.
2 A variety of material is available that may be used to apply traction. List and describe equipment available in your hospital for the application of:
  a Skin traction
  b Skeletal traction
3 The following types of traction usually refer to skin traction: Buck's extension, Russell traction, Bryant traction, and balance suspension traction. Review the equipment needed for each type and nursing implications.
4 Skeletal traction involves the use of head tongs, Kirschner wire, Steinmann pin, or other apparatus. Review nursing care of a specific patient pertaining to:
  a Application of this type of traction
  b Care of the patient wearing Crutchfield tongs
  c Care of the patient with skeletal traction applied to the femur
5 Discuss the following aspects of nursing care as they pertain to the traction patient:
  a Neurovascular assessment of the extremity
  b Prevention of skin irritation or development of pressure sores
  c Factors that may interfere with maintenance of continuous traction
  d Provision for correct body alignment
  e Exercises that may be prescribed for the patient with lower limb traction
  f Maintenance of countertraction for:
    (1) The patient in head traction
    (2) The patient with traction applied to the upper extremity
    (3) The patient with traction applied to the lower extremity
  g Changing the bed linen and placing the bed covers to provide for warmth and coverage of the patient

THE PATIENT USING CRUTCHES

1 Discuss several methods of measuring a patient for crutches.
2 What nerves and muscles are involved when "crutch paralysis" develops?
3 List the most important muscle groups used in crutch walking. Explain the various types of exercise that may be prescribed to strengthen these muscles.
4 Demonstrate the following crutch gaits:
  a Two-point gait
  b Three-point gait
  c Four-point gait
  d Swing-through gait
5 For what type of orthopedic disability is each gait most likely to be prescribed?

Unit II REFERENCES

1 Alves, R., and Martin, T. A.: An overview of orthotics and prosthetics, ONA J 4:231-235, Sep 1977.
1a Anderson, M. G.: Orthopedic traction and nursing care, ONA J 2:304-307, Dec 1975.
2 Anderson, M. I.: Physiotherapeutic management of patients on continuous traction, Physiotherapy 58:51-54, 10 Feb 1972.
3 Bailey, J. A.: Tractions, suspensions, and a ringless splint, Am J Nurs 70:1724-1725, Aug 1970.
4 Beaumont, E.: Product survey: wheelchairs,

Nursing (Jenkintown) 3:48-57, Nov 1973.

5 Bonner, C., Hofkosh, J., Jebsen, R., and Neuhauser, C.: Tips on choosing and using crutches, canes and walkers, Patient Care 2: 17-54, Oct 1968.

6 Bradley, D.: Checking a plaster—how and why, Nurs Times 70:1190-1192, Aug 1974.

7 Brown, S.: Orthopedic nursing. Part 1. Easing the burden of traction and casts, RN 38:36-41, Feb 1975.

8 Bunch, W. H., and Keagy, R. D.: Principles of orthotic treatment, St. Louis, 1976, The C. V. Mosby Co.

9 Day, B. H.: Orthopaedic appliances, London, 1972, Faber & Faber, Ltd.

10 Dison, N.: Clinical nursing techniques, ed. 3, St. Louis, 1975, The C. V. Mosby Co.

11 Eaton, R. G., and Green, W. T.: Epimysiotomy and fasciotomy in the treatment of Volkmann's ischemic contracture, Orthop Clin North Am 3:175-186, Mar 1972.

12 Foss, G.: Breaking the architectural barriers with crutches, wheelchairs, and walkers, Nursing (Jenkintown) 3:17-31, Oct 1973.

13 Glancy, G. L.: Compartment syndromes, ONA J 2:148-151, Jun 1975.

14 Gordon, J.: CircOlectric beds: circumventing the trauma of positioning, Nursing (Jenkintown) 7:42-47, Feb 1977.

15 Hogberg, A.: Orthopedic nursing. Part 2. Preventing orthopedic complications, RN 38: 34-37, Mar 1975.

16 Hrobsky, A.: The patient on a CircOlectric bed, Am J Nurs 71:2352-2353, Dec 1971.

17 Jebsen, R. H.: Use and abuse of ambulation aids, JAMA 199:63-68, 2 Jan 1967.

18 Kamenetz, H. L.: Selecting a wheelchair, Am J Nurs 72:100-101, Jan 1972.

19 Kamenetz, H. L.: The wheelchair book; mobility for the disabled, Springfield, Ill., 1969, Charles C Thomas, Publisher.

20 Kennedy, J. M.: Orthopaedic splints and appliances, Baltimore, 1974, The Williams & Wilkins Co.

21 Kerr, A. H.: Orthopedic nursing procedures, ed. 2, New York, 1969, Springer Publishing Co., Inc.

22 Knapp, M. E.: Orthotics (bracing), Postgrad Med 43:241-246, Mar 1968.

23 Knapp, M. E.: Orthotics: bracing the lower extremity, Postgrad Med 43:225-230, Apr 1968.

24 Knapp, M. E.: Orthotics: bracing the upper extremity, Postgrad Med 43:215-219, Jun 1968.

25 Lane, P. A.: A mother's confession—home care of a toddler in a spica cast: what it's really like, Am J Nurs 71:2141-2143, Nov 1971.

26 Law, J.: Nursing care study: use of Dunlop traction, Nurs Times 71:537-539, 3 Apr 1975.

27 Licht, S. H., and Kamenetz, H. L., editors: Orthotics etcetera, New Haven, 1966, Elizabeth Licht, Publisher.

28 Lowman, E. W., and Klinger, J. L.: Aids to independent living; self-help for the handicapped, New York, 1969, McGraw-Hill Book Co.

29 O'Brien, J. P., Yau, A. C., Smith, T. K., and Hodgson, A. R.: Halo pelvic traction, J Bone Joint Surg [Br] 53:217-229, May 1971.

30 Owen, R.: Indication and contra-indications for limb traction, Physiotherapy 58:44-45, 10 Feb 1972.

31 Peltier, L. F.: A brief history of traction, J Bone Joint Surg [Am] 50:1603-1617, Dec 1968.

32 Powell, M.: Application of limb traction and nursing management, Physiotherapy 58:46-51, 10 Feb 1972.

33 Powell, M.: Limb traction—some aspects of nursing management, Nurs Mirror 137:26-32, 27 Jul 1973.

34 Ranalls, J.: Crutches and walkers, Nursing (Jenkintown) 2:21-24, Dec 1972.

35 Raney, R. B., Sr., and Brashear, H. R. Jr.: Shand's Handbook of orthopaedic surgery, ed. 9, St. Louis, 1978, The C. V. Mosby Co.

36 Rose, G. K.: Total functional assessment of orthoses, Physiotherapy 63:78-83, Mar 1977.

37 Rusk, H. A.: Rehabilitation medicine, ed. 4, St. Louis, 1977, The C. V. Mosby Co.

38 Sarno, J. E., and Lehneis, H. R.: Prescription considerations for plastic below-knee orthoses, Arch Phys Med Rehabil 52:503-510, Nov 1971.

39 Schmeisser, G.: A clinical manual of orthopaedic traction techniques, Philadelphia, 1963, W. B. Saunders Co.

40 Schneider, F. R.: Handbook for the orthopaedic assistant, ed. 2, St. Louis, 1976, The C. V. Mosby Co.

40a Schoen, D. C.: Compartmental syndrome, ONA J 4:208-210, Aug 1977.

41 Shafer, K. N., Sawyer, J. R., McCluskey, A. M., Beck, E. L., and Phipps, W. J.: Medical-surgical nursing, ed. 6, St. Louis, 1975, The C. V. Mosby Co.

42 Smith, D. W., and Gips, C. D.: Care of the patient; medical-surgical nursing, ed. 3, Philadelphia, 1971, J. B. Lippincott Co.

43 Spiegler, J. H., and Goldberg, M. J.: The wheelchair as a permanent mode of mobility. A detailed guide to prescription. I. Frame, armrests and brakes, Am J Phys Med 47:315-326, Dec 1968.

44 Spiegler, J. H., and Goldberg, M. J.: The wheelchair as a permanent mode of mobility. A detailed guide to prescription. II. Upholstery, leg supports, wheels and accessories, Am J Phys Med 48:25-37, Feb 1969.

45 Stewart, J. D. M.: Traction and orthopaedic appliances, Edinburgh, 1975, Churchill Livingstone.

46 Stolov, W. C.: Progressive ambulation (mobility), Postgrad Med 47:229-235, May 1970.

47 Synnestvedt, N.: The dos and don'ts of traction care, Nursing (Jenkintown) 4:35-41, Nov 1974.

48 Warner, T. F., Shorter, R. G., McIlrath, D. C., and Dupree, E. L., Jr.: The cast syndrome; an unusually severe case, J Bone Joint Surg [Am] 56:1263-1266, Sep 1974.

49 Wiley, L., editor, Hohf, R., Epler, T., Haskell, M., and Otto, W.: The threat of thrombophlebitis, Nursing (Jenkintown), 3:38-43, Nov 1973.

Unit III
ORTHOPEDIC NURSING IN TRAUMA TO BONES, JOINTS, AND LIGAMENTS

10 Injuries

THE ACUTELY INJURED PATIENT

Accidental injuries constitute one of the most important health problems facing the nation today. Injury is the leading cause of death in the first half of man's life-span and ranks fourth among causes of death at all ages. One of each eight beds in general hospitals throughout the United States is occupied by the victim of an accident. The needed attention therefore becomes a very important problem to nursing, both in care of the trauma to the musculoskeletal system and in care of the patient with multiple injuries.

Triage

Triage means sorting or putting first things first as the needs of a patient are surveyed upon his arrival in the hospital emergency room. Hospitals have provided accident rooms for the first-line care in surgical emergencies. A surgical emergency is a sudden unexpected medical crisis that requires rapid action, and today most of these are sustained through violence. The location of the emergency rooms must be readily and quickly accessible to all modes of transportation so that the injured person can receive immediate attention. Furthermore, these emergency rooms, to fulfill their purpose, must provide all the tools necessary to save life. Most importantly, the personnel must be on standby alert and ready for triage as a patient enters the emergency room.

A team captain must be in charge of the patient who has been acutely injured. While this leader is usually a general surgeon or the general practitioner with the widest experience, he uses all available specialists immediately as the needs indicate. The captain must have the authority to assign diagnostic and therapeutic priorities. This is the essence of triage.

Treatment priority

In any patient with multiple injuries, treatment priorities must be rapidly assigned.

1 Restoration of the cardiorespiratory physiology is of first priority.
2 Then comes the treatment for injuries of hollow viscera such as intestines and bladder.
3 Laceration of the soft parts, head injuries, and closed fractures can await treatment until after the preceding have been managed.
4 Injuries of the bone are next in importance.

For example, in a patient with a combination of skull fracture, femoral fracture, and rupture of a hollow viscus, shock is treated immediately. External bleeding is controlled by pressure or ligature, and the fractured extremity is simply splinted. As soon as the vital signs are stable, the patient may be transferred quickly to the operating room for laparotomy to repair the visceral injury and prevent peritonitis. Coma, unlike shock, does not interdict needed operation. (See also Chapter 5.)

Nursing responsibilities

Obviously of first importance is the patient's breathing, which can be determined at a glance (see discussion of assessment of respirations, p. 81). Lack of aeration, evidenced by blueness, means an obstructed airway, especially in the face of gasping efforts to breathe. If an adequate passageway cannot be obtained by proper use of suction and the usual insertion of an airway, more drastic measures may be required. It is important, therefore, to make certain that proper instruments and airways are readily available in the emergency room so that the doctor may proceed with tracheotomy. Syringe and needle may be required for pleural aspiration or the relief of pressure pneumothorax. If the chest is flail, from multiple fractures through the rib cage, mechanical assistance to respiration becomes necessary. As a temporary measure, sometimes a sandbag placed against the flail chest can give some support.

In the presence of obvious external bleeding, the size and location of any wound from which the blood comes is noted, and control is instituted by the application of pressure with a gauze pack held firmly by hand or a bandage. Only rarely is a tourniquet indicated. (See discussion on control of hemorrhage, p. 85.)

Once respiration is established, bleeding controlled, and blood volume replacement initiated, further evaluation of the extent of injury is then more systematic. At this time, the patient can be questioned about identification and the circumstance of the injury, and the more subtle injuries, such as internal bleeding and bowel ruptures, can be dealt with properly.

NURSE'S ROLE IN PREVENTING INJURIES

It would be illogical to outline ways in which nurses may assist in preventing such conditions as tuberculosis, poliomyelitis, and back strain and then to omit emphasizing their part in the prevention of fractures. Their role as health teachers demands that they recognize some of the commonest causes of accidents, particularly those in the home, and know how they may be eliminated.

Studies have shown that the greatest number of injuries result from falls; indeed, falls are responsible for almost one-half of all injuries in the home.

Because falls play a large part in the etiology of fractures, home hazards that frequently cause falls should be recognized by nurses. Many grave accidents occur in the course of going up and down stairs. Waxed stairs and waxed landings are always dangerous. Stairs should have handrails. If they do not, a cord or rope adequately supported by firm uprights should be stretched along the stairs at a suitable level. In homes with young children, gates at the top of stair flights are essential to prevent falls.

Steps should never be cluttered with stray objects, as cellar stairs, for instance, are so likely to be. They should be kept clear for traffic, and all members of the family, young and old alike, should recognize that running down steps is distinctly hazardous. All outside steps should be covered with coarse salt or sand during icy weather.

Children and adults should be alert for such objects as marbles, clothespins, pencils, and toys left about on stairs, landings, and floors. Every child and adult should recognize the great danger and threat to balance that a round rolling object, like a marble or pencil, presents to the unwary walker. All should be taught to pick them up from the floor or sidewalk whenever they are observed.

Small scatter rugs can be very treacherous. They must be well anchored to prevent slipping. This may be done by rug fasteners or by the use of rubber floor mats. Scatter rugs should never be placed at the top or bottom of stairs.

To assist in preventing some of the hundreds of bathroom accidents that take place each year, a rubber mat in the tub is advisable. A railing on the wall near the tub will give more confidence and provide safety for the elderly person.

Another common cause of home accidents is standing on rocking chairs or on old frail kitchen chairs to reach high shelves or to put up curtains. A small firm ladder should be available for all such household jobs.

If the household includes an elderly person who must get up at night to go to the toilet, it is important that a clear, unobstructed lane be left between his bed and the bathroom. Also, an easily available bedlight should be provided to discourage nocturnal journeys in the dark, which are fraught with so much hazard for the elderly person.

These are only a few of the more obvious

pitfalls in the home from which many severe fractures originate. The alert and observing nurse will be quick to notice others.

In addition to the prevention of accidents in the home, it is also very important for the nurse to aid in the prevention of injuries to hospitalized patients. The commonest causes of injury in hospitals are falling from the bed, rolling off carts, and slipping on waxed floors. Side rails on the bed are mandatory in some hospitals for all patients and should certainly be put to use for those patients who are medicated, feeble, or confused. Transport carts are commonly equipped with straps and side rails for holding the patient to the cart, and these should be utilized. Slippery floors should be avoided when patients are walking with crutches or just beginning to ambulate.

SPRAINS, STRAINS, DISLOCATIONS, AND FRACTURES

This discussion will deal with the damage to bones, joints, and ligaments that is produced by external forces such as a blow, twist, pinch, fall, or crush. The skeletal system has a certain resilience for resisting such forces until the force from the outside becomes greater than the strength of the bones, at which point bone will yield and break. The individual bones have differences in strength, depending mostly on their shape and size, to resist these forces. They also vary in shape, size, and strength from one person to another and from one age to another. For example, the bones of children are more flexible and less brittle than those of adults. In the elderly person, the strength of the bones diminishes as it does in disease states, such as osteoporosis, so that less external force is required to break them. These external forces will be referred to as trauma. Tissues of the body exposed to external violence or insult can be damaged. The bones, joints, and ligaments of the body are vulnerable to injury, and the effects therefrom can cause serious disability. Therefore, an understanding of the effects of trauma to the body is essential.

Injuries resulting from accidents on the highways, in industry, in the home, on the farm, and in sports are increasing each year. Constant attention to the prevention of injury has become a national theme. Safety belts in automobiles, safety guards on machinery, nonslip floor materials in homes and public places, and improved protective gear for football players are examples of the emphasis on prevention. Plans for the care of mass casualties are a part of hospital organization today and indeed are carried out on a national scale through the Emergency Medical Services under the Health Services Administration.

Sprains and strains

Sprains and strains are terms used to describe the damage done to ligaments by an injury. Each joint in the body is protected by ligaments, and each is subject to injury.

The nurse on the orthopedic unit will seldom have occasion to care for a patient with a sprain. The nurse in the doctor's office or in an outpatient area, however, frequently may be called upon to assist in the application of support to a sprained ligament (Figs. 158 to 160) and to instruct the patient in the care of the injured area.

A sprained ankle is the most common joint injury and occurs when the foot is inverted forcibly. Normally, the lateral ligament of the ankle is a dense fibrous structure with a set length. One end is fixed to bone at the tip of the fibula (Fig. 161) and the other to the astragalus. When the foot is inverted, this ligament becomes taut and stops further inversion. If the force acting to invert the foot is greater than the resisting force or strength of the ligament, the ligament must tear. This tear is a *sprain*. Should the tear be incomplete or, in other words, microscopic in extent, it may be called a *strain*. If the ligament holds and the giving way occurs at the fixation site to bone with a small fragment of bone attached to the ligament, this would be called an *avulsion fracture*. Any ligament thus damaged will repair by scar tissue if the torn ends are approximated and held in place for three or more weeks, which is the usual healing period.

Treatment consists of providing support and protection of the ligaments until healing can occur. Support is provided by strapping the foot and ankle with adhesive tape or an Elastoplast bandage. To prevent swelling, the extremity should be elevated

Shave ankle.

Cover lacerations with sterile dressing before applying tape.

Paint skin with tincture of benzoin or tincture of rosin.*

Select tape size to fit contour of ankle (1-2 in wide).

Hold foot in neutral position in regard to inversion or eversion.

Keep foot as near right angle as pain will allow.

Avoid constrictive circular taping.

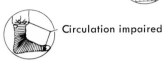

For subject sensitive to tape:

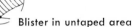

Use stockinet or wrap with gauze
before taping.

Circulation impaired

Cover skin with cotton or gauze where tape edges cross; pre-

vents blisters and lacerations.

Leave no small areas of exposed

skin between strips of tape.

Blister in untaped area

*Tincture of rosin: 1 lb rosin + 1 gal
alcohol (any alcohol can be used, even
rubbing alcohol)

Fig. 158 Rules for adhesive taping used for prevention as well as treatment of sprains of the ankle. (From Paul, W. D., and Allsup, D.: Prevention and treatment of ankle sprains, The University of Iowa College of Medicine and Department of Athletics, Iowa City, Iowa.)

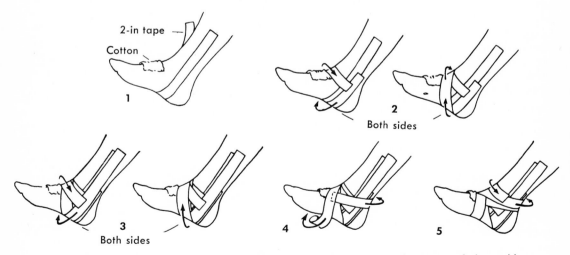

Fig. 159 Western wrap used in the prevention and treatment of sprains of the ankle. This wrap is easy to apply. It prevents inversion and eversion but allows flexion and extension. It protects ankle mortise. (From Paul, W. D., and Allsup, D.: Prevention and treatment of ankle sprains, The University of Iowa College of Medicine and Department of Athletics, Iowa City, Iowa.)

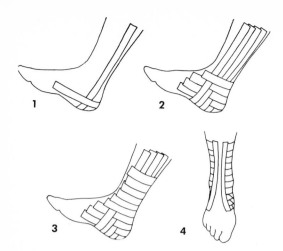

Fig. 160 Basket weave used in the treatment of ankle sprains. This support is used only in the acute stage to allow swelling but does not protect ankle mortise. (From Paul, W. D., and Allsup, D.: Prevention and treatment of ankle sprains, The University of Iowa College of Medicine and Department of Athletics, Iowa City, Iowa.)

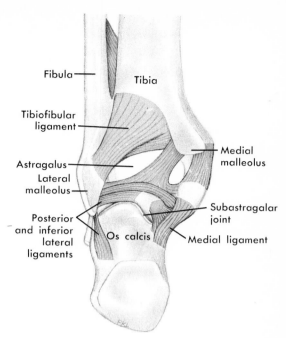

Fig. 161 Posterior view of the ankle joint.

much of the time for the first two or three days. Also, the application of an ice bag during this time is helpful in minimizing hematoma formation. Although only a minimum of weight bearing is permitted at first, the amount is gradually increased as the soreness diminishes. After such an injury, the physician usually will reorder a roentgenogram to rule out the possibility of a fracture.

At the end of a two-week period, the Elastoplast support is removed, and, if the tenderness has disappeared sufficiently, an elastic bandage or support may be applied. This bandage is worn to prevent swelling of the ankle, and its use is gradually discontinued as the patient's condition warrants.

Occasionally, the torn ligament ends will curl just enough that the ends cannot be kept together. In such a case there is a chance that healing will be incomplete. An unstable joint or easily recurring sprain of the joint will be the outcome. Recourse to external support or surgical repair of such a ligament is occasionally necessary.

Dislocations

Traumatic dislocation of any joint occurs when the force of the injury is greater than that which would cause a sprain. A joint is protected by more than a single ligament, and if all the ligaments yield or tear under pressure of the force, the entire joint can separate so that the surface of one bone making up the joint no longer meets or opposes the surface of the other bone making up the joint. This is called a dislocation and is ordinarily described in terms of which way the acting force displaced the distal portion of the joint; e.g., posterior dislocation of the hip, which means that the head of the femur comes to lie outside of and behind the acetabulum. In order for any dislocated joint to function properly again, the dislocated portion of that joint must be relocated to its original anatomic relation with its articulating member. Usually, an anesthetic is required to relax the muscles which, in their spasm, tend to hold the bones in the dislocated position. On rare occasions, the dislocation cannot be reduced by simple manipulation because a portion of the torn tissues or some associated soft tissue such as tendon becomes wrapped around the dislocated part in such a fashion as to prevent relocation. In this event, a surgical operation (open reduction) is necessary.

Once the dislocation is reduced, whether by open or closed reduction, the damaged joint must be immobilized for three or more weeks to allow the torn ligamentous and capsular tissues to heal.

Fractures
Mechanical forces in causation and treatment of fractures

An understanding of the causes of fractures and their management requires some knowledge of forces and how they act. This is a subject that is urgent, as judged by the rapidly increasing accident rate, if we consider the question of the type and magnitude of stresses and strains the human body can safely tolerate. Crash injury research groups are collecting data on the speed of vehicles at the time of crashing, the position of the injured persons in the vehicles, the direction the persons faced, and the structural parts of the vehicles believed to be responsible for the injuries. One of the common injuries in survivors is fracture of one or more bones.

The study of stress-strain phenomena in bones is a problem in biomechanics. During movement, as well as during rest, the bones are subjected to a variety of forces that are primarily the result of muscle action and body weight.

A *force* is simply a push or a pull. There are three kinds of force: *tensile* (pulling apart, like a rubber band), *compressive* (pushing together, like an accordion), and *shearing* (a force acting perpendicular to long axis to produce a twist).

When forces act on a body, there is internal resistance to absorb or transmit that force. The internal resistance, which cannot be seen nor measured, is called *stress*. *Strain*, on the other hand, can be seen and measured as a deformation or change in shape.

If force continues to act on a bone in a longitudinal direction with sufficient magnitude, the bone will bend (strain); if the force continues, the internal resistance (stress) will fail to absorb more force and the bone will break. The force has exceeded the capacity of the bone to absorb it. Practically all materials including bone, have an *elastic limit* or point of maximum stress beyond which they will not return to their original shape.

Another important concept is the relation of force to energy (energy is the capacity to do work). The importance of the idea of work lies in the fact that a body upon which work is done thereby acquires the capacity to do an equal amount of work in returning to its original state. For example, work is done when the mainspring of a watch is wound and the spring acquires energy, which can be measured by the work it does as it unbends. To raise a 10-lb weight 100 feet above the ground, 1,000 ft-lb of work (energy) are required. Once raised, it has gained the power to do that same amount of work in returning to its original position. At 100 feet above the ground, the weight has potential energy. When it falls to the ground, it retains the energy it had but it is now energy of motion. When it reaches the ground, it has lost all its advantage of position but still has power to do work by virtue of its motion, which is called kinetic energy.

Translated into practical terms, this discussion points out that a person riding in an automobile has kinetic energy received from the forward velocity of the automobile. If the automobile comes to a sudden stop (e.g., by bumping into a stone wall), the person not wearing safety belts or straps continues to move in the same forward direction until another force alters that direction. As the person goes forward and strikes the windshield, the velocity of forward motion becomes zero. If the windshield does not break, the kinetic forces still present in the body are absorbed into each segment of the body until the forward motion of each segment becomes zero. One such segment is the head, which strikes the windshield as though thrown like a baseball. The weight of the head brought to a sudden stop transmits the kinetic energy to the skull. This energy is rapidly absorbed by the internal stress resistance of the bones of the skull. If the amount of stress exceeds the elasticity of the bone, there will be strain failure to return the shape of the skull to normal. This failure will result in a break of the bone in the form of a depressed skull fracture. Any kinetic energy remaining after that spent to produce the fracture can either depress the fracture further or enlarge the fracture, depending on the amount of energy available. If the occupant of the automobile had been wearing a shoulder strap, the continued forward motion of the body (kinetic energy) would have been transmitted to the strap, imparting to it a push force. Because the stress resistance of the harness is more elastic than the bone, the strap would absorb all the remaining kinetic energy without exceeding its elastic limit, therefore decelerating the body to zero velocity without injury.

If the occupant is asleep with the knees resting on the forward dash compartment, the forces would act in a different direction on the body. The center of gravity of the body would be in the same longitudinal plane as the thighs; therefore, forward momentum of the body would be directed to the dashboard through the femurs, and the kinetic energy would be absorbed by the internal stress resistance of the thigh bones, and one of the two events, or both, could occur. The stress in the femur could exceed the limits of strain deformation (the elastic limit of bend), and the bone would break. The break would allow a gradual deceleration of the remaining energy as the bone fragments angulate or shorten the bone. The other possibility would be a failure of the elastic limit of strain at the hip, resulting in a dislocation of the hip.

In these examples, the dissipation of kinetic energy can be compared to a rubber ball thrown at a pile of rocks. As the ball bounces from one rock to another, the distance it bounces becomes less and less as the kinetic energy is dissipated or used up in each bounce. The ball finally comes to rest when all forces acting on the ball are in equilibrium.

Similarly, an injured body will come to rest when the kinetic forces have been dissipated and gravity has neutralized body weight, whether it be by the support of the ground or the floor of the car or part of each. The center of gravity of each body segment may have altered as a result of the injury. A fracture in the femur, for example, will have added a new center of gravity of the thigh since the fracture has, in effect, created two thighs out of one. The upper half of the thigh will rest independently on the lower half; thus one could be rotated inward and the other outward. One segment could rest in line

with the body and the other at a right angle yet still aligned with the lower leg. Whatever the position, whether with or without deformity, the injured limb very quickly gains equilibrium and remains at rest until shifted by a new force. Any attempt to move the injured limb will create muscle spasm, which becomes a new internal force. The muscle spasm occurs from a nerve reflex whose stimulus is initiated by any tension or compression of the injured periosteum. This reflex also is accompanied by acute pain. Therefore, both pain and muscle spasm can be controlled by immobilization of the injured part. Obviously, first-aid immobilization disregards proper reduction of the fracture but does control pain and muscle spasm while the injured person is transported to a hospital.

In the hospital, the decision for "setting" the fracture is made. Restoration of the fractured bone to its original length and alignment constitute a reduction. Because any manipulation causes pain and muscle spasm, the injured patient must have adequate anesthesia, whether general or local. In some fractures, such as in the femur, the powerful muscles continue spasms even in a cast and the reduction cannot be maintained. In this instance, a better means of reducing the fracture and maintaining the reduction is by traction.

Traction is the act of pulling by external force. The force must have proper direction and proper magnitude to accomplish a reduction of the fracture as well as to maintain the proper length and alignment of the injured bone until it is repaired and healed. The nurse should understand the forces that act on the body when traction is applied. As a reminder, Newton's third law states that "with every force there is an equal and opposite reaction force." If the injured person is to remain at equilibrium in bed and the fractured extremity is to be pulled by a force, there must be an equal and opposite force to neutralize the pull. The bed will neutralize the force of gravity. The internal force of muscle spasm will be neutralized by the force of the traction. Obviously, none of these forces is acting in the same direction and therefore is not exactly opposed. Any two or more forces acting on a body and not exactly opposed are known as *vectors* of

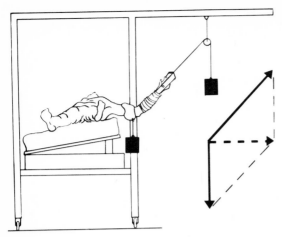

Fig. 162 Dunlop traction. The humerus is fractured just above the elbow. The traction is applied to pull the humerus to its proper length (reduce the overriding of the fragments) and to restore the proper longitudinal alignment of the humeral shaft. One weight pulls the forearm up and out. Another weight pushes the humerus downward by means of a sling. The parallelogram shows one solid-line arrow parallel to the line of pull on the forearm and the other parallel to the downward push on the humerus. These are the vectors of force, whereas the broken-line arrow (the diagonal of the parallelogram) indicates the direction and amount of the resultant force.

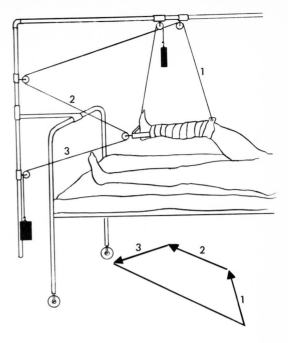

Fig. 163 Russell traction. The pull is applied through adhesive strips to the skin over the leg. The limitation for uses of this skin traction is the tolerance of the skin to tension stresses over a period of time. This traction illustrates the vectors of force and the *resultant* direction and amount of pull in the long axis of the femur. The single weight suspended at the foot of the bed provides the total energy, while the pulleys determine the directions of pull provided through one weight. The weight at the top of the bed simply prevents drop foot and has no relationship to the original traction. If a 5-lb weight were pulling at the foot of the bed, there would be, in effect, a 5-lb pull at **3** as well at **2** and, therefore, a total of 10 lb pulling on the leg. A single force of 5 lb would be lifting the knee at **1**. An irregular polygon can be drawn to unit scale with the forces connected by representative lines each parallel to the force it represents. In the diagram, **3** corresponds to **3** etc., leaving the unmarked line as the direction and amount of *resultant* force acting nearly in line with the femoral shaft.

force. If the direction and amount of each force are known, their combined action becomes known as the *resultant* force (Figs. 162 to 164). The nurse must understand the vectors and the resultant force in order to deal expertly with the patient in traction.

Vectors. A *force* may be defined as that which tends to cause or alter the motion of matter. It can be a push or a pull. Many forces may act on a body to cause motion, and any motion that occurs will be the result of the combined action of all the forces. If the forces act in the same direction, their sum will be the strength of a single force acting in one direction. If there are two forces acting in exactly opposite directions, the amount of resulting single force will be the difference between the two, whereas the direction of that force would be the same as the larger of the two. If the opposing forces were equal, no motion would occur since the sum of the forces is equal to zero. When the sum of the

forces acting on a body equals zero, the body is said to be in equilibrium.

Any two or more forces not exactly opposed or not exactly in the same direction are designated vectors of force—only a part of one force may neutralize a part of another, while the direction of the final force will be different from either.

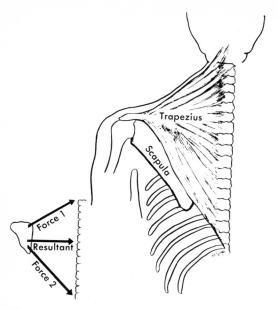

Trapezius

Scapula

Force 1

Resultant

Force 2

Fig. 164 The action of the trapezius muscle on the motion of the scapula provides another example of force vectors as they relate to bodily functions. **Force 1** is the direction of pull when the upper fibers of the trapezius contract, and **Force 2** is the direction of pull for the lower fibers. The *resultant* force indicates the direction the scapula will move when the upper and lower fibers contract essentially equally.

Vectors may be added geometrically to determine both the amount and the direction of the *resultant* force acting on the body.

In actual practice, the precise amount of force is seldom, if ever, computed. With experience and awareness of the objectives of a given traction, both the direction and amount of weight can be estimated. Furthermore, there is a daily change in the demands on the traction as muscle spasm subsides and the muscles actually fatigue; this, combined with the patient's shifting position in bed, makes correction a somewhat trial-and-error proposition until the situation stabilizes after a week or so. During this unstable period, the direction and amount of pull on the traction can be adjusted according to need indicated by repeated roentgenographic or other examination findings. Particular care must be exercised to prevent overpull, since this will distract the fragments in the case of fracture.

Types of fractures

A fracture is a break in the continuity of a bone. To understand fractures, it is necessary to know terms that describe type (Fig. 165), location, and other pertinent features.

Each bone in the body is highly developed to carry out a specific purpose. It is logical, therefore, that each bone has its own characteristics. In general, the long bones (femur, tibia, humerus, radius, and ulna) are tubular with variations relating to internal stress patterns of trabeculae as well as variations in cortical thickness from one end to the other. These variables are explainable on the basis of stress, since nature provides the necessary strength (resistance) when it is needed to bear weight, resist muscle pulls, etc. The cortex of the tibia in a football player or a weight lifter will be thicker than that in a man of similar size in a sedentary occupation. If such tibias were tested by strain gauges and breaking points determined, more force would be required to break the tibia with the thicker cortex. Nonetheless, every bone has a point at which it can no longer resist applied force without breaking. This is the basis of all fractures. Because bones are adapted to ordinary stresses of day-to-day living, it would take a stress greater than ordinary to produce a fracture. Most fractures are the result of instances in which there is no control of the amount of force involved.

Since injuries are not deliberately sustained, they occur when least suspected and when one is not prepared to resist them. Consequently, the forces that occur come from any direction and in variable amounts. This accounts for the fact that of the thousands of fractures that occur, no two are exactly alike. Another variable factor is that of the muscle pulls in effect at the time of the fracture. An example of the latter accounts for the gymnast who can dive over a bar to a hard floor and absorb enough of the shock by well-timed muscle relaxation to break the impact. The type of fracture sustained in this instance would be by indirect force and could be located at any point from the wrist to the shoulder. The direction of the line of fracture would most likely be long oblique.

Direct force, such as that supplied by a

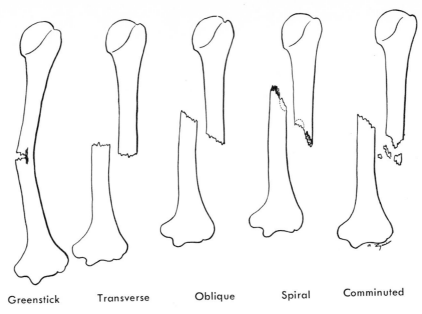

Greenstick   Transverse   Oblique   Spiral   Comminuted

Fig. 165 Fracture types.

lead pipe falling across the forearm, allows more accuracy in the prediction of a transverse fracture line exactly at the point of impact of the lead pipe.

When a bone is fractured, it means that a single unit becomes two units, and each unit is spoken of as a fragment. The fragment nearest the cephalad end of the body is referred to as the *proximal* and the other as the *distal* fragment. These two fragments ordinarily become separated at the site of the fracture in various ways. Imagine a piece of bamboo two feet long with a strong rubber band stretched from one end to the other and fastened and with another but weaker stretched rubber band placed on the other side. If the bamboo were cut transversely in its middle, it would bend immediately from the overpull of the stronger elastic. This is the mechanism of a *transverse* fracture. The angle at the fracture site will furnish the identifying description for this particular fracture; e.g., a transverse fracture in the middle third with lateral angulation (if the apex of the angle points away from the midline of the body) of 30° (or whatever angle the distal fragment has moved from the original bone alignment).

To construct another possibility, return to the bamboo and this time cut the bamboo on a four-inch diagonal instead of transversely. Upon completion of the cut, the two fragments will slide by one another until the original length of the bamboo becomes shortened enough to release the tension in the elastic bands. Because one band was shorter than the other, the stronger side will also angulate similarly but less than it did with the transverse cut. This fracture will be described then as an *oblique* fracture of the middle third with a two-inch overriding (or whatever amount the total length has been shortened) and lateral angulation of 10°.

These two examples will account for the majority of fractures, but because minor variations are possible, additional descriptive terms are needed. The fracture site may be splintered, in which case there may be multiple fragments. In this case, the fracture would be called a *comminuted* rather than a transverse or an oblique fracture. Should the fracture line be oblique and follow a spiral course as it involves a tubular bone, it is referred to as an *oblique spiral*, followed by the usual description of location, overriding, and angulation.

Occasionally, when a long bone is fractured, the fractured end of one fragment

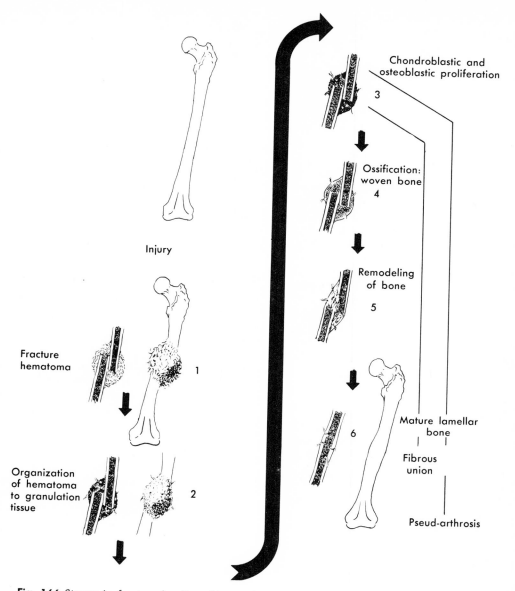

Fig. 166 Stages in fracture healing. (From Schneider, F. R.: Handbook for the orthopaedic assistant, ed. 2, St. Louis, The C. V. Mosby Co.)

near the fracture site in an attempt to improve the circulation. In some instances, the extremity may be braced and activity increased in order to improve the blood supply to the part. Bone grafting to the affected area may be necessary. Bone from the tibia or the iliac crest is placed across the fracture site. This is known as an onlay graft. In another method of bone grafting the graft is inserted directly into the medullary canal.

Malunion. With the complication of malunion, union of the bony fragments takes place but does so in a position of deformity. Numerous factors, such as inadequate reduction, an improperly applied cast, or a cast that has softened and permitted movement of bony fragments, may cause this.

Infection. Infection is always a possibility in a compound fracture. Also, with open reduction of a fracture, there is some risk that infection can occur and complicate the healing process.

Nerve damage. Nerve damage may be caused by the sharp edges of the bone fragments or by the injury that caused the fracture. Motor power of the muscles of the extremity and the sensitivity of the skin should be checked carefully. Damage to the peroneal nerve may result in drop foot, or injury to the radial nerve may result in wristdrop.

Circulatory disturbance. Circulation in the part distal to the fracture should be checked carefully. This is particularly important with fractures around the elbow. Volkmann's contracture may result from a disturbance of the circulation in the elbow region. Nail beds of the fingers of the affected extremity should be observed, and the radial pulse should be taken at frequent intervals.

Epiphyseal damage. If the fracture causes damage to the epiphysis of a child, growth may be arrested in that extremity or in a portion of the extremity. This, of course, results in deformity as the child grows.

Posttraumatic arthritis. When an intra-articular fracture causes damage to a joint surface, a painful posttraumatic arthritis may result. In some instances, an arthroplasty or an arthrodesis may be performed to alleviate the pain.

Kidney stones. Kidney stones can occur when total body immobilization is carried out. They result when disuse causes excessive loss of calcium from the bones. Maintaining a high fluid intake is helpful in eliminating the calcium, but maintaining prophylactic muscle activity is better treatment.

Emboli. Occasionally in compound fractures or in simple fractures in which clotting has taken place in a vein, a portion of the clot may break off and be carried throughout the circulation to various parts of the body. Air emboli also occur. If an embolus makes its way to a vital organ, such as the lung, heart, or brain, there may be disastrous consequences, even death.

The patient usually develops a rapid pulse and evidences of shock that come on abruptly. Death may occur within a few minutes or within a few hours after the onset of symptoms. Those patients with emboli in the less vital areas may have the symptoms and signs in a milder degree and yet recover. The emboli are most frequently found in the lung and may occur as late as six to eight weeks after the injury (see Chapter 5).

Evaluation of injured part

The trauma from a single force, such as a blow to the forearm, results in a single injured part. Such a direct blow can be expected to break the bones at the site of impact and produce an angulation like a bent twig. Landing on both feet in a fall from a height, however, produces indirectly transmitted forces that can injure bones and joints at a distance from the point of impact, such as the collapse of a vertebral body in the upper lumbar spine. Crushing injuries from cave-ins increase areas of damage further because they involve both direct and indirect forces. Crushing injuries commonly involve tissues, such as internal organs in addition to bones, and thus internal hemorrhage can occur and produce shock that demands immediate detection and treatment. An associated head injury may render the victim unconscious, which complicates the picture of shock. The forces on the chest might have fractured enough ribs to produce paradoxical breathing that interfers with proper ventilation. When poor ventilation, unconsciousness, and shock are present simultaneously, the evaluation and treatment of the injured bones and joints are of secondary concern. Any patient with multiple injuries requires immediate evaluation by a physician well versed in all aspects of trauma, and seldom in medicine does the situation call for more astute, careful, complete, yet quick analysis to institute proper treatment in proper sequence to ensure first things first.

First aid and fractures. In first aid, any contaminated open fracture should be dressed and splinted in the exact position in which it was found so that proper precautions can be taken when the patient reaches a hospital or other point where he can receive adequate surgical attention. Some surgeons contend that because a thorough debridement is necessary in any open fracture, the additional amount of contamination occurring when the bones are pulled into line when first seen does not materially increase the chances for infection of the compound wound. This contention is doubtful.

It is preferable that a clean dressing, handkerchief, or sheet be applied at the site of injury and that the limb be splinted in the position of the existing deformity. The use of strong irritating antiseptics such as iodine, Lysol, or carbolic acid is contraindicated. Alcohol, Mercurochrome, Mercresin, or Scott's solution may be used with little chance of local damage or coagulation of the tissues.

If the patient is in shock, all possible attention should be given to its treatment. Intravenous saline infusions, transfusions, or blood plasma may be necessary.

Following are a few simple rules that apply to first aid in fractures.

1 Keep the patient at rest in a horizontal position as long as he is unconscious or until the extent of his injury can be determined.

2 If the patient must be transported while still unconscious, keep him in the horizontal position until consciousness is regained sufficiently for him to signify points of pain and tenderness.

3 In the patient with a back injury, every precaution should be taken to avoid motions of the spine, particularly such as would occur if the person were brought into a sitting position, because this may lead to damage to the spinal cord by fragments of bone protruding into it or pressing upon it.

4 When there is injury to the spine or to the limbs, it is of particular importance that the surgeon know definitely whether or not any paralysis was present immediately after the injury. This cannot be determined in the unconscious patient with a head injury, but it can be determined in other patients.

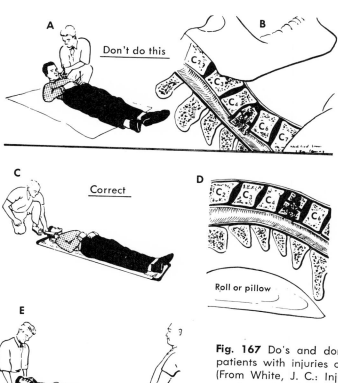

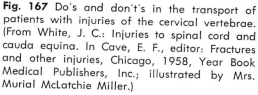

Fig. 167 Do's and don't's in the transport of patients with injuries of the cervical vertebrae. (From White, J. C.: Injuries to spinal cord and cauda equina. In Cave, E. F., editor: Fractures and other injuries, Chicago, 1958, Year Book Medical Publishers, Inc.; illustrated by Mrs. Murial McLatchie Miller.)

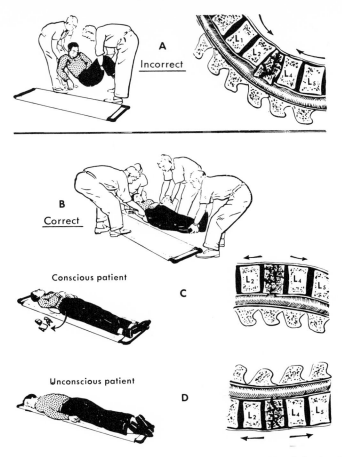

Fig. 168 Do's and don't's in the transport of patients with injuries of the lumbar and lower thoracic vertebrae. (From White, J. C.: Injuries to spinal cord and cauda equina. In Cave, E. F., editor: Fractures and other injuries, Chicago, 1958, Year Book Medical Publishers, Inc.; illustrated by Mrs. Murial McLatchie Miller.)

The knowledge of this fact may decide the ultimate recovery or loss of function in a limb or limbs. This is also true in compound fractures. Written records of what has been found and done should accompany each patient to the hospital or surgeon's office.

5 There is considerable debate at present as to the advisability of using a tourniquet, since the prolonged use may lead to death of the tissues in the extremities beyond its point of application. In open fractures it is preferable to use a piece of sterile or clean bandage or string to tie off the bleeding vessel if it is exposed or to apply local pressure to the vessel by means of a pad of sterile gauze and a sterile bandage. If a tourniquet must be used on a patient with violent bleeding, it should be removed every 20 to 30 minutes and the bleeding should be observed. If coagulation has occurred in the vessel, the tourniquet may be left loosened but there should be constant observation for return of bleeding.

6 Emergency immobilization and transportation depend on the anatomic location of the injury (Figs. 167 to 172) as follows:

a In injuries of the spine or head, the recumbent position is essential. If a rigid stretcher such as a plank, door, ladder, or two poles and a blanket cannot be obtained, it is advisable to roll the patient horizontally onto his face and transport him in the arms of two or three persons to a truck or the back seat of a car. He should never be brought into a position that will flex the spine.

b In injuries of the clavicle, ribs, shoulder, and elbow, splinting can best be done by bandaging the arm to the side of the chest. This may be done with any materials obtainable, such as a torn sheet, shirt, or other clothing. Two triangular slings work well if obtainable.

c In fractures around the elbow and

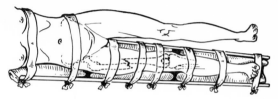

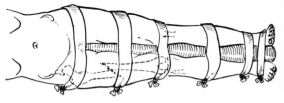

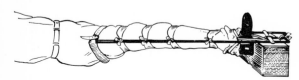

Fig. 169 Keller-Blake splint for first-aid immobilization of a fractured femur. The ankle is carefully padded, and the leg is supported in the splint by encircling strips of cloth. The shoes and clothing are not removed in order to avoid unnecessary painful movement of the damaged extremity. Traction is maintained by means of a strip of cloth that is secured around the ankle, tied over the end of the splint, and twisted taut by means of a stick. The distal end of the splint is supported to give some elevation. (From Brown, T.: Fractures of the femoral shaft. In Cave, E. F., editor: Fractures and other injuries, Chicago, 1958, Year Book Medical Publishers, Inc.; illustrated by Mrs. Murial McLatchie Miller.)

Fig. 170 Improvised splint, made of boards or sticks, for fracture of the femoral shaft. The lateral splint extends distally from just below the axilla and is secured to the trunk; the medial splint extends distally from the groin. All splints are padded to avoid pressure over bony prominences. (From Brown, T.: Fractures of the femoral shaft. In Cave, E. F., editor: Fractures and other injuries, Chicago, 1958, Year Book Medical Publishers, Inc.; illustrated by Mrs. Murial McLatchie Miller.)

Fig. 171 Improvised immobilization for fracture of the femoral shaft when no splints are available. The legs are secured together with padding in between. The feet also are bound together in order to control rotation. (From Brown, T.: Fractures of the femoral shaft. In Cave, E. F., editor: Fractures and other injuries, Chicago, 1958, Year Book Medical Publishers, Inc.; illustrated by Mrs. Murial McLatchie Miller.)

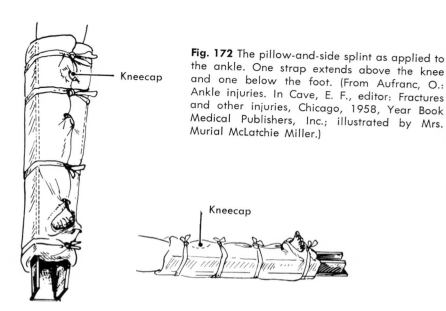

Kneecap

Kneecap

Fig. 172 The pillow-and-side splint as applied to the ankle. One strap extends above the knee and one below the foot. (From Aufranc, O.: Ankle injuries. In Cave, E. F., editor: Fractures and other injuries, Chicago, 1958, Year Book Medical Publishers, Inc.; illustrated by Mrs. Murial McLatchie Miller.)

forearm, one or two wooden splints from the axilla to the fingertips may be tied to the arm with handkerchiefs or strips of clothing.

d In injuries of the hip, thigh, knee, and leg, immobilization may be obtained by narrow boards placed on either side of the leg and held together by a bandage or strips of clothing. When the hip is injured, the splinting should extend from the heel up to the side of the chest and the bandage should encircle the chest and the leg. All injuries of the bone should, if possible, be immobilized to include the joint above and below the injury. If no splinting material is available, fairly adequate immobilization can be obtained by tying the injured leg to the uninjured one with a series of bandages from the thigh to the foot.

e For fractures of the ankle and the lower leg, the most satisfactory temporary splint is the pillow bandage. The limb is laid longitudinally on a pillow so that the heel is just above the edge. The lateral edges of the pillow are then brought together over the limb and pinned. When the ankle is reached, the lower ends of the pillow are crossed under the foot, brought upward, and pinned so that a compact splinting effect is obtained. In all splinting of fractures, the bony prominences should be protected by cotton batting if obtainable or by any soft material.

f The Thomas splint for the leg and the Jones splint for the arm are easily applied and give good immobilization for transportation. They are carried by almost all first-aid stations and ambulances.

7 Shock is the result of a disturbance in the vasomotor system that allows relaxation in the peripheral circulatory system, thereby decreasing the amount of blood returning to the heart. The heart pumps from an empty system and is unable to fulfill the requirements for blood exchange to itself and other parts of the body. Shock may be the result of hemorrhage or of a complete temporary disarrangement of the nervous system as a result of the injury. Fear may be an element in its production. It may be fatal. The blood pressure is greatly lowered, and the pulse is rapid and weak. The skin becomes pale, and the injured person may become listless or even unconscious. If hemorrhage is the cause,

it should be stopped as promptly as possible and fluid should be administered in replacement. Stimulants such as coffee or tea may be used. Morphine and its derivatives tend to restore the balance between the peripheral and central circulations. Complete rest must be given in a recumbent position. As soon as infusions and blood or plasma transfusions are available, they should be given. Shock usually is caused by pain due to movement at the point of fracture and from hemorrhage rather than from malposition.

Hospital treatment in open fracture. To prepare an open wound for operation, soap and water should be used. A brush or sponge will help the effectiveness of this. Benzine is used to dissolve greasy materials. The skin and wound are then painted with a noncoagulating antiseptic, and draping is applied. The wound is flushed clean with several quarts of saline solution under low pressure. This is done with an elevated bottle and a glass nozzle on the end of rubber tubing. All loose, bruised, or contaminated portions of tissue are then removed with knife or scissors. Bone should be preserved if possible.

The antibiotic drugs have aided greatly in lessening the fight against infection. They are placed directly into the wound after the cleansing and debridement. In addition, a specific antibiotic is given orally, intramuscularly, or intravenously over a period of three to seven days after the injury. This practice has served to lessen the occurrence of infection tremendously. It should be noted, however, that the use of antibiotics should not be considered a substitute for but rather an adjunct to adequate debridement.

Antibiotics do not eliminate the necessity of giving both tetanus antitoxin and gas bacillus antitoxin as prophylactics to all patients with compound fractures. Immobilization after open reduction of open fractures is an essential part in the avoidance of infection and other complications. All patients with open fractures who arrive at the hospital for treatment within six hours after injury are considered clean and are treated by debridement, flushing with quantities of sterile saline solution, instillation of an antibiotic, reduction, closure, and the application of a cast.

Open fractures sustained more than six hours before the patient gains admission are considered primarily infected in spite of the most careful debridement and other precautions, including antitoxins. In these patients, drainage is instituted and, if necessary, because of pain and elevation of temperature for a twenty-four–hour to forty-eight–hour period, the cast should be bivalved or a window made and the wound inspected. Otherwise, the open wound is left undressed within the cast.

The odor of gas bacillus infection is characteristically sweet and pungent, and air bubbles may be seen exuding from the wound. The presence of air in the tissue also may be demonstrated roentgenographically. The pulse is rapid, and the temperature is variable. Removal of the cast may be necessary, since the fracture is now of secondary importance. Multiple incisions into the tissue for adequate air penetration and drainage may be needed. In addition to the administration of gas gangrene antitoxin, the complication may call for hyperbaric oxygen therapy. This therapy consists in administering 100% oxygen in an environment (hyperbaric chamber) that provides for an increased atmospheric pressure.

11 Fractures and dislocations

FRACTURES AND DISLOCATIONS OF FACE, JAW, SKULL, CLAVICLE (COLLAR BONE), AND SHOULDER

Fractures of the skull are problems for the neurosurgeon and require special instruction from him concerning nursing care. Similarly, serious injuries to the face involving the nose and sinuses are problems for the nose and throat specialist, whose ingenuity often is taxed in devising methods and apparatus capable of restoring and maintaining the position of misplaced fragments.

Fractures involving the jaw usually call for the special attention of an oral surgeon. However, certain principles in their treatment can be mentioned. Loose teeth near the fracture line should not be removed unless absolutely necessary. Sometimes the alignment of the teeth and jaw may be obtained by using wires or rubber bands to hold together the teeth of the upper and the lower jaw. Occasionally the fragments of the jawbone may have to be held together by wires through the bone. Sometimes metal bands may be required to supplement wiring, and sometimes plates fastened along the teeth, attached to a plaster-of-Paris headgear by means of wires and elastic bands, may be used for adequate correction.

Dislocations of jaw

Cause. Dislocation of the jaw usually is caused by violent yawning or yelling or by blows against the chin.

Anatomy. Dislocations of the jaw may be unilateral or bilateral and usually consist of the forward or inward displacement of the condyles of the mandible from their articulating surface on the skull.

Symptoms and signs. Forward protrusion of the chin and inability to close the mouth are symptoms of dislocation of the jaw. If the dislocation is unilateral, the chin is displaced away from the dislocated side. There is usually rather severe pain and muscle spasm, and the lips and tongue become dry.

Treatment. Simple dislocations of the jaw usually can be reduced without anesthesia. With his thumbs swathed in gauze and bandage to prevent being bitten, the surgeon exerts pressure against the mandibular molars with increasing force downward and backward until reduction is accomplished. Following reduction, the upper and lower jaws should be held together by bandages around the head (Barton four-tailed bandage) for a period of two to three weeks so that habitual dislocation does not develop.

Fracture of clavicle (collar bone)

Fracture of the clavicle is one of the commonest of fractures. It may occur in any part—inner, middle, or outer. Treatment may be different for each type.

Cause. A fall on the shoulder or outstretched hand with the entire force exerted on the clavicle and occasionally a direct blow may cause a fracture of the clavicle.

Anatomy. The pectoral muscles and weight of the arm bring the shoulder downward, inward, and forward, with overriding of fragments. The clavicle is the only bony connection between the chest and shoulder girdle.

Problem. The length of the clavicle must be maintained by keeping the shoulder up

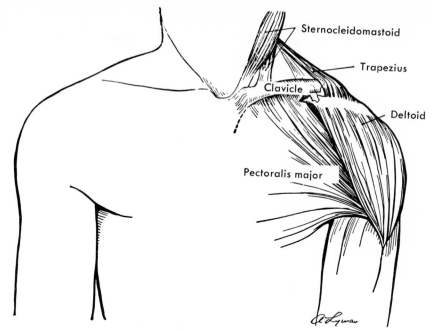

Fig. 173 Muscle mechanics of fracture of the clavicle. The sternocleidomastoid pulls upward on the proximal fragment while the weight of the shoulder pulls down, and the pectoral muscles pull inward and forward, tending to override the fragments.

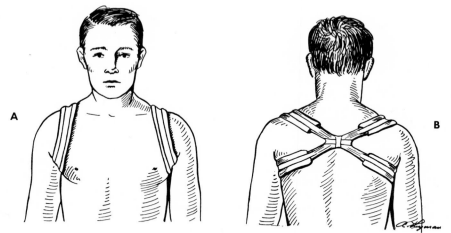

Fig. 174 Figure-of-eight dressing. **A,** Front view. **B,** Back view. Felt, bias flannel bandage, and adhesive tape are used. The dressing should be changed every week or ten days for cleanliness.

and held backward during healing (Fig. 173).

Healing period. A healing period from four to eight weeks is usually required for fractures of the clavicle. Children under 10 years of age heal rapidly.

Treatment. In children, the figure-of-eight dressing (Fig. 174) usually will suffice for the full treatment until union is shown to be present clinically and roentgenographically. The dressing is changed for cleanliness only.

In adolescents and adults, it is usually preferable to use a Velpeau dressing (Fig.

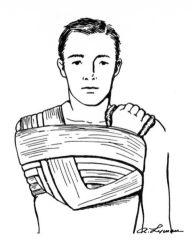

Fig. 175 The Velpeau bandage is used temporarily to immobilize the clavicle, shoulder, humerus, elbow, or forearm. A protective pad should be inserted wherever skin comes in contact with skin.

175) for ten days to two weeks. This can be followed by a figure-of-eight dressing.

In obstinate cases, adolescent or adult, and especially in girls, when perfect alignment is necessary, side traction should be used for three to four weeks, followed by a figure-of-eight dressing.

Occasionally, when proper alignment cannot be obtained conservatively, an open reduction may be performed. Wiring with stainless steel or the use of a Kirschner wire inserted into the medullary canal can, except for the scar, give perfect results.

Fracture-dislocations and dislocations of acromioclavicular joint

Fracture-dislocations and dislocations of the acromioclavicular joint are the result of the same type of injury as that causing fracture of the clavicle. Roentgenograms frequently do not show the extent of the injury.

Problem. The shoulder must be kept upward and backward.

Treatment. A figure-of-eight bandage with adhesive strapping from the chest to the back and a pad over the clavicle is frequently employed in treatment of these fractures. Adhesive tape is changed often to prevent skin irritation. Immobilization must be maintained long enough to allow complete healing (six to ten weeks).

Patients with severe injury may require operative repair of the acromioclavicular joint as well as the ligament between the clavicle and the coracoid process.

In chronic painful dislocations, the resection of the outer inch of the end of the clavicle usually leads to relief of symptoms and restoration of function. Recovery occurs in about three weeks. Metallic fixation by a nail or Kirschner wire may be used in some instances.

Dislocations of head of humerus

There are several types of dislocation of the head of the humerus, but the most common is a forward and downward displacement.

Cause. Dislocation of the head of the humerus usually is caused by a fall on the outstretched arm. Abduction of the shoulder joint is possible to only 90°. At this point, the humerus presses against the acromion process. This levers the head of the humerus downward or forward. The capsule of the joint is torn either anteriorly or at its attachment to the glenoid fossa. The head of the humerus enters the space below the glenoid fossa and rests under the coracoid process.

Symptoms and signs. The major symptom is pain. The arm cannot be brought against the side of the body, and there is a depression under the acromion process where the head of the humerus should be. The dislocation may be accompanied by fracture of the tuberosity (Figs. 176 and 177).

Reduction. Reduction should be performed with the patient under complete anesthesia to prevent further damage to the head of the humerus and to allow free movement so that the capsule will again close over the head, allowing it to fall back into its normal position.

Problem. It takes about three to four weeks for ligamentous structures to heal. However, motion that does not put strain on the healing area in the torn capsule maintains flexibility and does not retard healing. Therefore, with a simple dislocation of the joint, it is desirable to begin motion within a few days. In dislocation of the shoulder, the problem is to keep the elbow constantly forward to the shoulder plane on the affected side. If there is a de-

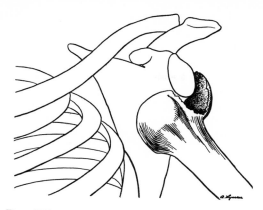

Fig. 176 Fracture-dislocation of the shoulder. The greater tuberosity is torn off (subglenoid type).

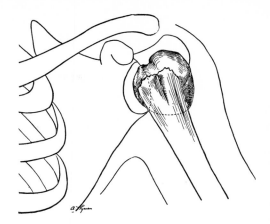

Fig. 178 Fracture of the neck of the humerus showing anterior and upward displacement of the distal fragment. The fracture line of the head is angled forward.

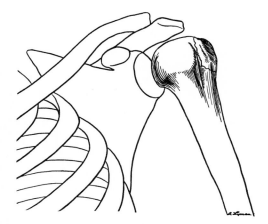

Fig. 177 Dislocation of the shoulder reduced. The tuberosity has resumed normal position.

tached fragment from the head to the humerus, it usually falls back into position during the reduction.

Treatment. Frequently a Velpeau dressing is used for a few days after reduction and then may be replaced with a neck-wrist strap. This strap must keep the wrist close to the chin so that only forward flexion and forward rotation can be accomplished. As more complete healing occurs, this distance between the neck and wrist can be increased.

When habitual dislocations occur from placing strain on the healing capsule too early or from repeated dislocation, operative repair is needed. This may be done by suturing the capsule and labrum to the anterior inferior lip of the glenoid fossa (Bankart).

Fractures of neck of humerus

Cause. Usually a fall directly against the shoulder with the arm against the chest or incompletely abducted is the cause of fracture of the neck of the humerus.

Anatomy. The pectoral muscles pull the distal (controllable) fragment inward and forward (Fig. 178), and the deltoid pulls it upward. They are the strongest muscles of the shoulder girdle group. The three types of fracture of the neck of the humerus are transverse, oblique, and comminuted.

Reduction. In all patients except those without displacement, an immediate attempt should be made to restore perfect anatomic replacement under general anesthesia. With the transverse type this usually can be accomplished. In the other types, however, reduction may be difficult or impossible by this means.

Problem. The elbow must be kept close to the midline of the body to relieve the pull of the pectoral muscles. Some form of traction that will relax the deltoid and thereby prevent overriding and anterior angulation, the two salient factors necessary to reduction, must be provided.

Treatment. In fractures within or in close proximity to the shoulder joint, early motion is of great importance. Whenever anatomic reposition can be accomplished, motions can be started ten days or two weeks after injury. In some instances, however, reductions are difficult to obtain and main-

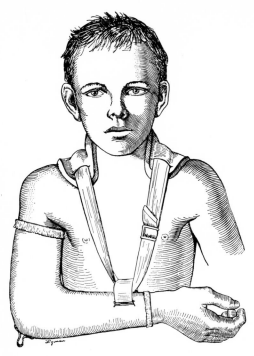

Fig. 179 The pendulum method of treatment of fractures in the region of the shoulder or shaft of the humerus; this is the so-called hanging cast. Frequently, the cast is not essential, and efficiency depends on the neck-wrist strap combination. The loop at the elbow is for night traction.

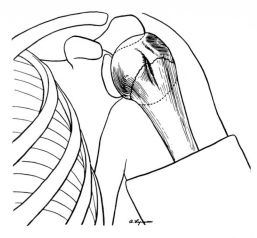

Fig. 180 Fracture manipulated under anesthesia and a pendulum cast applied. For additional traction along with a neck-wrist band, a 3-lb lead weight was incorporated in the cast at the elbow.

tain, and it may be necessary to use a Velpeau dressing for three to four weeks or a lateral traction apparatus that maintains forward flexion and traction.

As soon as gluing of the fracture is present after the most nearly perfect position has been attained, active motion is started. This may require two to four weeks, depending on the appearance of the primary and subsequent roentgenograms and the estimated mechanical difficulties.

Usually a cast extending from the axilla to the wrist with a neck-wrist strap can be applied early (Figs. 179 and 180). The weight of the cast (which can be augmented by sheet lead at the elbow) will give the necessary traction, and the neck-wrist strap can be adjusted to give the required anterior flexion of the shoulder. In this way, early motion without strain in the fractured area may be started.

Healing period. The healing period is from six to ten weeks.

Stiff shoulder

In all kinds of fractures of the shoulder, arm, elbow, forearm, or wrist, delayed return of function frequently is caused by adhesions about the shoulder joint as a result of disuse. It is best, therefore, with the approval of the surgeon in charge, to begin shoulder motion early in all patients with fractures of the upper extremity. This should consist of external rotation and forward flexion of the arm two or three times daily.

FRACTURES OF ARM, FOREARM, ELBOW, AND WRIST
Fractures of shaft of humerus

Cause. Direct violence, such as a blow from the side, or indirect violence, such as a fall on the outstretched hand, may cause fracture of the shaft of the humerus.

Anatomy. There is usually overriding, especially when the fracture is above the attachment of the deltoid muscle. There is also a tendency toward outward bowing. If the fracture is in the middle third of the humerus, special observation is indicated at once because of the proximity of the radial nerve to the bone (Fig. 181). If the radial nerve is injured, it may be in one of three ways, which may be recognized as follows:

1 Severance of the nerve may be indi-

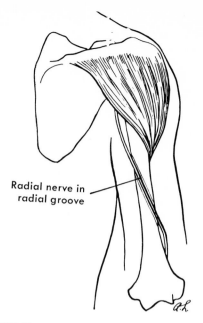

Fig. 181 Diagram showing the proximity of the nerve to the bone, with accessibility to injury.

cated by immediate inability to extend (raise) the hand at the wrist. Prognosis is poor for recovery without suture.

2 Contusion at the site of injury may cause edema and sufficient pressure on the nerve to produce a gradual paralysis of the wrist (drop wrist). Prognosis for recovery is good with rest.

3 Paralysis as a result of bony overgrowth in healing is evidenced by the gradual development of wristdrop two to three months after injury. Prognosis is good with removal of bony overgrowth, freeing the nerve.

Problem. Maintaining traction and restoring the best alignment of the fragments are usually the chief problems in treating this type of fracture. There is often a tendency toward outward bowing that can be overcome either by more traction or by a pad placed between the elbow and the body.

Treatment. If transverse, fracture of the shaft of the humerus may be treated by immediate reduction with the patient under anesthesia, or in a few instances, it may be plated or wired. Usually, a cast from the axilla to the wrist (with the elbow flexed) is most satisfactory to the comfort of the patient and adds to the simplicity of treatment in all fractures in the shaft of the humerus. A loop of webbing or tape may be incorporated at the elbow so that traction by weights and pulleys can be maintained when the patient is lying down (Griswold) (Fig. 179).

Those fractures that occur a few inches above the elbow must have special consideration, since there is a great tendency to angle outward as a result of the combined pull of the biceps and triceps muscles. This causes a loss in the carrying angle at the elbow if it is uncorrected. The tendency may be overcome to some extent by applying a cast from the axilla to the fingers with the forearm in a position of extreme and forced pronation (palm down).

Healing period. Fractures of the shaft of the humerus may be slow to heal. In about 10% of the patients, either delayed union or nonunion occurs. Ordinarily, however, a fracture of the humerus will heal sufficiently for elbow motion in about four to eight weeks. Complete recovery may occur in eight to ten weeks. In delayed union, it may take as long as three to six months. In nonunion, a bone graft operation is usually the most satisfactory way to obtain union.

When patients are in casts, usually little nursing care is required except to watch for complications. The nurse should attempt, however, with the consent of the surgeon, to maintain freedom of motion in as many of the neighboring joints as possible by means of massage around the joints and assisted active motions.

Fractures near elbow

Cause. Fracture near the elbow is most common in two forms of injury: in falls with the elbows extended (children) and in direct violence exerted against the elbow (adults). There may be an impact from a passing car when a person's elbow is extending out of the window of the car in which he is riding, or there may be a fall on the elbow. The type of fall that would likely cause a dislocation of the elbow in an adult as a result of leverage of the olecranon process in the olecranon fossa would cause a supracondylar fracture in a child.

Anatomy. The elbow cannot normally

extend beyond 180°. Forcing beyond this point will cause either a dislocation of the joint or a fracture just above the joint. The ulnar nerve runs downward just behind the inner posterior side of the joint, and the medial nerve runs just in front of the joint. Either is likely to be damaged at the time of injury or in reduction. With ulnar injury there may be an immediate or a delayed loss of sensation in the little and ring fingers, and with medial injury there may be an immediate or delayed loss of sensation in the index and middle fingers (Fig. 99). Any swelling or edema occurring within the firm capsule of the joint or within the aponeurosis (muscle covering) may cause great tension to be exerted from within. This may lead to (1) paralysis of the median, ulnar, and radial nerves, causing disturbance of motion and sensation in the forearm and hand, and (2) extravasation of blood into the fibers of muscle tissue so that they go through a stage of swelling and, later, scar formation (Volkmann's contracture; Fig. 182). There is frequently much swelling after fractures and other injuries near the elbow joint, and symptoms of constriction of vessels and injury to muscles may be apparent within four to forty-eight hours after injury. Patients with injuries around the elbow joint, therefore, should be under hourly observation for at least forty-eight hours whether the fracture has been reduced or not. During this time, notation by the nurse of any excessive swelling or loss of sensation should be made constantly. If such should occur, there should be immediate release of tension by complete freeing of any pressure caused by the cast or by incision of the superficial tissues by operation. The fracture should be disregarded until a circulatory balance is reestablished. (See discussion of compartment syndrome in Chapter 6.)

Some of the most severe and complicated fractures the surgeon has to deal with occur in the elbow sideswipe injuries. They are usually compounded, and the humerus, the ulna, and the radius may be shattered. Nerves and tendons are frequently damaged. The repair is tedious and consists of thorough debridement, suture of nerves and tendons, and restoration of bone and joint alignment. The latter frequently requires internal fixation with wires, screws, or plates. Some patients, however, may be treated after repair by lateral traction in recumbency.

Treatment. Supracondylar fractures (Fig. 183) and dislocations should be reduced with the patient under anesthesia. It is usually necessary to place the elbow in a position of flexion to maintain reduction.

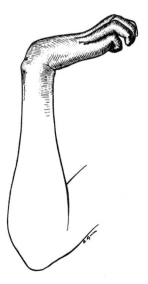

Fig. 182 Well-established Volkmann's contracture with clawhand and flexion of the wrist and fingers. Note atrophy of the forearm.

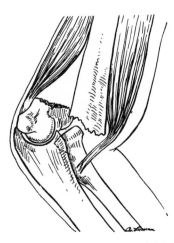

Fig. 183 Supracondylar fracture of the humerus. There is posterior displacement of the distal fragment with tension on nerves, tendons, and vessels. The fracture is within the capsule of the elbow joint.

The amount of flexion must be determined by the ability of the circulation to tolerate it. In fractures in young children, the flexed position may be necessary for only two to three weeks. This is true of dislocations in young and old, but older persons may need a longer period for complete bone healing. If swelling is severe in patients treated early, or if reduction has not been accomplished to a satisfactory degree after seven to fourteen days, lateral traction by either adhesive traction or skeletal traction through the olecranon process should be instituted. In the majority of patients it will be successful provided the surgeon and nurse are vigilant in the application of forces to correct the deformity.

Healing period. Motion should be begun within three to six weeks, depending on the stability at the time of reduction. Complete healing of the fracture requires approximately eight weeks, but return of complete motion may require three to six months.

Fractures of olecranon process

Cause. Fracture of the olecranon process (Fig. 184) usually is caused by a direct blow.

Symptoms and signs. Pain, swelling, and

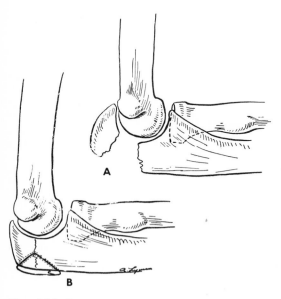

Fig. 184 Fracture of the olecranon process, which always requires open reduction if the fragments are separated. **A,** Fracture. **B,** Wire suture, which should be fairly superficial for best results.

inability to extend the elbow forcibly are symptoms of fracture of the olecranon process. Before swelling has occurred, a groove may be felt between the fragments.

Treatment. Open reduction is the treatment of choice in all patients who manifest any perceptible separation of the fragments. Reduction may be obtained by wiring or nailing, or it may be maintained by a removable beaded screw.

Forearm fractures

Cause. Forearm fractures may be caused by either direct or indirect violence, usually the latter.

Anatomy. Pronation and supination are the essential functional motions in the forearm. To preserve these after fracture, the bones must be replaced so that they will be parallel to each other and of equal length. There must be no obstacle or obstruction between them. The width of the interosseous space varies according to the tension or relaxation of the controlling muscles that rotate the forearm from pronation to supination (Fig. 185). Therefore, when the fracture occurs near the elbow, in the mid-arm, or near the wrist, the governing factor determining the position in which the controllable distal portion of the fractures is placed in relation to the uncontrollable or fixed proximal fragments depends on the location of muscle attachments and the various tendencies of their pull.

Treatment. In fractures above the pronator radii teres, there is outward rotation of the upper fragment of the radius by the biceps tendon. Therefore, the forearm must be placed in outward rotation (supination). In fractures below the pronator radii teres, the forearm must be placed in a position of inward rotation (pronation) to match the muscle action above.

The radius, probably because it has a better blood supply, usually heals faster than the ulna, but nonunion in the bones of the forearm is not uncommon and may require bone graft operations to stimulate bone union. Some irreducible fractures may be treated by bone plating or by intramedullary nailing.

Problem. Rotatory motion of the forearm must be restored as soon as sufficient union to tolerate the strain has been dem-

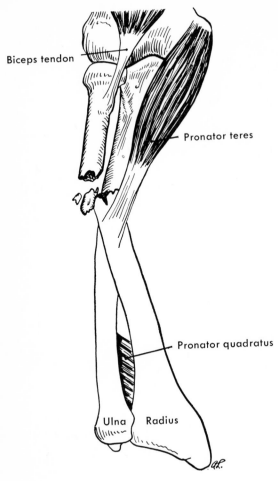

Fig. 185 Anatomy of the muscles of the fore-arm that influence pronation and supination. In fractures above the pronator teres, the un-controllable upper fragment is rotated outward (supinated). In fractures below the pronator teres, the upper fragment is rotated inward (pronated). Fractures are placed in the fixed position to meet the upper fragment accord-ingly. The pronator quadratus always has a tendency to pull both bones together.

onstrated roentgenographically. The cast must extend from the fingers to the shoulder. The nearer the fracture is to the wrist, the sooner the cast can be cut to below the elbow. Daily full ranges of mo-tion of the shoulder and, as soon as possi-ble, of the elbow should be carried out to prevent adhesions.

Healing period. The healing period varies considerably with the amount of soft tissue damage at the time of the injury, the age of the patient, and the individual speed of healing. Solid union cannot be expected (except in children) in less than eight to twelve weeks. In some patients in whom there is delayed union, immobilization must be maintained for three to four months. This causes considerable delay in the re-turn of motion and function in the joints and muscles.

Fracture of wrist (Colles' fracture)

Colles' fracture is one of the most com-mon and classic fractures (Figs. 186 and 187).

Cause. Colles' fracture is caused by a fall or by breaking a fall with the outstretched hand.

Anatomy. The far end of the radius is broken off and displaced backward. The typical silver fork deformity results. Mus-cles play no particular part except to cause overriding by spasm. With the posterior displacement of the end of the radius, sev-eral other complications usually occur, such as (1) shortening of the forearm, which tends to make the ulna impinge on the carpal bones, (2) fracture of the styloid process of the ulna, and (3) posterior fac-ing of the wrist joint, which interferes with action of the flexor tendons.

Problem. Reduction may be maintained by the use of one of the following:

1 The circular cast
2 Anterior and posterior splints that are molded and held in the correct posi-tion by bandage, preferably bias flan-nel or elastic
3 Commercial splints, which as a rule are not dependable except in a few pa-tients with fractures in which frag-ments are not much displaced and

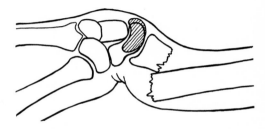

Fig. 186 Colles' fracture. Lateral view showing overriding and posterior displacement of the controllable fragment (silver fork deformity).

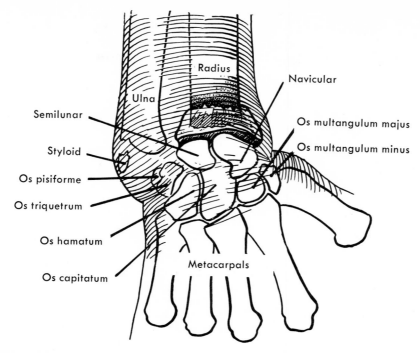

Fig. 187 Anteroposterior view of Colles' fracture showing shortening of the radius, posterior facing of the joint, and fracture of the styloid process.

forcible maintenance of corrective position is not necessary

4 Skeletal traction, which may be essential to good reduction with some patients with comminuted fractures; a Kirschner wire may be passed through the olecranon and another through the metacarpal bones of the hand and are incorporated in the cast after reduction (this method also may be used when both forearm bones are broken)

Anesthesia. One of several types of anesthesia may be used: (1) local injection of procaine HCl (Novocain), 1% to 2%, into the area of hemorrhage within the fracture site, (2) intravenous injection of thiopental (Pentothal) sodium, and (3) general anesthesia.

In the few patients who are given treatment immediately, reduction may be performed without anesthesia because of nature's temporary anesthetizing effect.

The aforementioned types of anesthesia may be employed in the reduction of all fractures and may be selected according to the condition of the patient. The blood pressure level, age, and length of anesthesia time must be taken into consideration.

Treatment. In reduction it is important that the lines of the deformity be the determining factor in the application of the traction force. The flexed elbow offers a satisfactory means of countertraction when a nurse or assistant applies a firm grip there. Traction on the fingers and hand must be exerted first in the line of the deformity. When sufficient traction has been obtained to overcome muscle spasm and to free the impacted serrated bone ends, correction of the deformity will be easy if the distal portion is brought into a position that meets the proximal portion of the fracture. It is essential to proper reduction that these three requirements be fulfilled:

1 Restoration of the length of the radius
2 Restoration of forward facing of the joint surface of the radius
3 Ulnar deviation of the wrist to restore reposition of the styloid process and ensure adequate space in the ulnocarpal region.

Convalescent treatment, combining exercise, heat, massage, and splinting (Fig. 188), hastens the return of function.

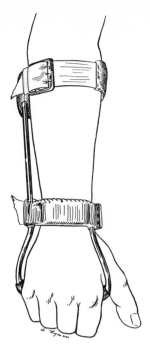

Fig. 188 Three-point splint for wristdrop; also used for protection of the wrist after fractures of the carpal bones on the lower end of the radius. This splint allows free use of the fingers and thumb.

Nursing management

As a general principle, cold applications or ice caps should be used in all injuries (fractures and sprains) within the first twenty-four or thirty-six hours to lessen swelling and relieve pain. After this, heat is more soothing.

In most patients with bone and tissue injury, aspirin or some form of salicylate is effective for relief of the aching pain. When muscle spasm is present, however, some of the morphine derivatives may be used fairly freely at first. This is particularly true when the injury is associated with shock.

Fractures occurring through the neck or upper third of the humerus that are reduced by traction offer some perplexing problems to the nurse. For traction the bed must have a firm mattress, and some method of countertraction must be devised. Usually, elevating the bed by shock blocks under the head and foot of the affected side will provide sufficient countertraction, although occasionally some type of restraint jacket secured to the unaffected side also may be necessary. The traction is applied in two parts with the arm flexed. Two adhesive straps that extend to a board and pulley ex-

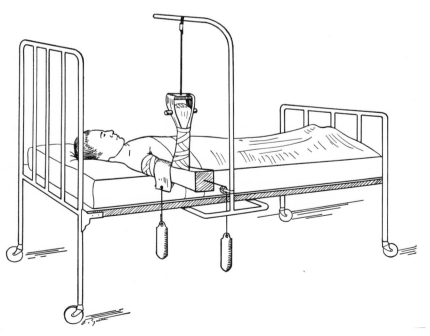

Fig. 189 Side-traction apparatus, which is adaptable to fractures of the clavicle, the head and neck of the humerus, and the shaft of the humerus and supracondylar fractures.

tending from the side of the bed are used for the upper arm. Another set of adhesive straps is applied to the forearm and attached to a spreader that is a considerable distance beyond the ends of the fingers. From this spreader a rope extends to an overhead pulley and then to the weights. Some type of padded handle suspended from this spreader is useful, inasmuch as it enables the patient to flex his fingers and hand over it. Extension on the forearm is used to eliminate its dependent weight as well as to relax muscle spasm in the upper arm (Fig. 189). See Chapter 7 for a complete discussion of nursing intervention for the patient in traction.

Fractures above the condyles of the humerus (the elbow fracture of common parlance) are very common in active youngsters. Such patients do not often remain long in the hospital. They frequently are brought in for reduction and dismissed in a few hours. It is essential that the parents be warned of the danger of circulatory impairment from subsequent swelling and that they be told how to detect such a complication. They must understand that the fracture itself should not occasion severe discomfort for the child and that continued crying or repeated complaints may indicate that there is an obstruction in circulation. A small boy with such a fracture was taken to his home after reduction of a supracondylar fracture in the hospital outpatient department. The child complained bitterly for twenty-four hours before the parents realized this was not the normal sequence of events after a fracture. When he was brought back to the hospital, a fully developed ischemic contracture of the kind described and named by Volkmann had occurred, and ten months of constant treatment were necessary to bring back even partial use of the child's hand.

A good test for circulation is the blanching sign that determines patency of blood flow. The nail of the thumb is momentarily compressed, and the return of blood to the nail is observed. If the return is immediate, circulation is thought to be adequate. Sluggishness in the return of the blood to the part is indicative of some degree of impairment and should be reported to the physician. One authority warns in huge letters in his textbook on fractures:

"WATCH THE HAND FOR SWELLING AND BLUENESS OF THE NAILS. CAUTION ALL CONCERNED THAT IF THIS OCCURS THE FIXATION APPARATUS SHOULD BE REMOVED AND THE ARM BROUGHT INTO EXTENSION. THE FRACTURE CAN ALWAYS BE REDUCED THE SECOND TIME BUT A VOLKMANN'S CONTRACTURE IS A PERMANENT DISABILITY."*

Surgeons make it a rule to disregard the fracture in any circulatory emergency.

Elevation of the arm by pillows or by suspending the arm in an overhead sling may sometimes reduce the swelling considerably. With the first evidence that circulation is not normal, however, the nurse should be on guard. No excuse can possibly be made for delay in reporting the condition to the surgeon, and this means at night as well as during the day. When no doctor is available, the nurse may have to split the cast throughout its entire length. (See discussion of compartment syndrome in Chapter 6.)

Occasionally, the surgeon will order a small window cut out over the radial artery before the patient is brought back from the plaster room after reduction of fractures of the elbow. This allows the nurse caring for the patient to check frequently on the circulation in the extremity. It is of great importance that the pulse rate be carefully taken and recorded at stated intervals, perhaps as often as every fifteen minutes. A faint disappearing pulse may indicate pressure on the artery and should be reported. Comparison with the pulse of the unaffected arm will be of assistance in gauging the seriousness of the constriction. Nurses notifying physicians of circulatory impairment should chart the notation and the time at which the physician was called.

FRACTURES OF HAND
Fractures of carpal scaphoid

Fracture of the carpal scaphoid, encountered alone or in combination with dislocations of the wrist, deserves special comment. The disabling possibilities are often underestimated, and treatment is often insufficient or lacking.

*From Magnusson, Paul, B.: Fractures, Philadelphia, 1949, J. B. Lippincott Co.

Cause. Falling on the outstretched hand is usually the cause of fractures of the carpal scaphoid.

Anatomy. The bones of the wrist are peculiar in that the greater part of their surface is covered with articular cartilage. This means that the supply of circulation is correspondingly limited.

An interruption of the circulation by fracture or loss of continuity means starvation to one or another portion of the injured bone with resulting disintegration or death of bone (aseptic necrosis).

Diagnosis. Diagnosis is based on roentgenographic findings. Four views should be taken. Sometimes the fracture line does not show up for two or three weeks. There are pain and tenderness in the "snuffbox."

Treatment. Complete reduction by adequate manipulation is the first requirement. Adequate and prolonged immobilization in a cast or splint is next. If nonunion should occur, drilling holes through the fracture line or a bone graft may lead to healing, or the removal of one or both of the fragments may improve function and relieve pain.

Healing period. A fracture of the carpal scaphoid requires immobilization in a cast or splints for eight to ten weeks for union to take place.

Fractures of metacarpals

Cause. Fractures of the metacarpals are caused by direct violence or crushing injuries and indirect violence, such as striking a blow with the closed fist.

Anatomy. Most of the muscle power in the hand is on the palmar surface—the interosseous and lumbrical muscles. These muscles act to bow the metacarpal bones backward in the event of fracture.

Problem. The metacarpals must be immobilized adequately in a position that will overcome the tendency toward posterior bowing.

Reduction. Manipulation under anesthesia is often necessary to restore normal position. To maintain this, one of two methods is used.

A plaster cast may be employed to apply pressure posteriorly along the shaft and anteriorly on the palmar surface under the head, or the metacarpophalangeal joint.

Skeletal traction is another method used to maintain reduction of the fracture. By passing a small pin through the phalanx or by using the miniature ice-tong apparatus, sufficient traction may be applied through elastic bands and the banjo splint to maintain proper position of the fragments. This is particularly adaptable to the overriding oblique or spiral fracture.

At the critical time of about three weeks, roentgenograms must be made to check whether proper reduction has been maintained.

Healing period. The healing period is four to five weeks.

Fractures of phalanges

Fractures of the phalanges comprise two types: the transverse and the oblique fractures of the phalanges and the chip fractures of the posterior surface of the distal fragment of the distal phalanx.

Transverse and oblique fractures

Anatomy. The lumbrical muscles tend to cause palmar angulation of the fragments.

Treatment. The problem of reduction, as well as treatment, is to keep the fingers in flexion until the critical time has passed. This may be done by binding the fingers over a rolled bandage. When bandages are removed, motion should be reestablished.

Chip fractures of posterior surface of distal fragment of distal phalanx

Anatomy. The tendon of the long extensor is attached to the posterior surface of the distal fragment of the distal phalanx. Injury causes an inability to extend the distal phalanx and grave loss of an important function. A stiff joint or an amputation is less disabling than this deformity (baseball finger).

Treatment. Complete, exaggerated, and prolonged (four to six weeks) hyperextension of the distal joint of the finger is the treatment of choice. As a rule, this gives sufficient time for complete reattachment of the tendon and a return of function. Suture by operation occasionally is necessary.

FRACTURES AND DISLOCATIONS OF SPINE AND PELVIS
Fractures of cervical, thoracic, and lumbar spine

Fractures or dislocation of the spine are divided into the following groups in order of severity:

1 Fractures or dislocations with extensive displacement and immediate paralysis of the nerves below the point of fracture

2 Fractures or dislocations with displacement and delayed paralysis below the point of fracture

3 Fractures with compression of the vertebrae but with no neurologic disturbance

4 Fractures of the accessory processes (such as spinous or lateral processes) without any evidence of nerve pressure

Cause. Fractures of the spine are caused by (1) a fall in the sitting or stooped position, (2) a jackknife type of injury such as occurs when force is exerted against the shoulders and pelvis at the same time, (3) a direct blow against the back or flank, and (4) certain diseases that cause softening or disintegration of the bones of the spine, such as hyperparathyroidism and malignant metastasis. In the latter condition, the break may occur spontaneously or with minimal strain.

First aid. There is a great lesson to be learned in the treatment of acute injuries, which is particularly exemplified in fractures of the spine. Usually, such injuries occur in auto accidents, in athletics, as the result of falls in construction work, or under similar circumstances. Treatment should be started at the scene of the injury. Obviously, the victim of such an accident may have spicules of bone that could cause damage to the tissues of the spinal cord if he is improperly transported.

Anatomy. The spinal cord is encased in a tube or channel of bone. The abnormal position of the vertebra may cause complete shearing severance of the cord at the time of injury, or the cord may be subjected to damage from spicules of bone or the pressure from surrounding hemorrhage and congestion. If severance occurs, paralysis is immediate below the fractured vertebra. If the damage results from pressure alone, the paralysis is delayed in its development.

Problem. If paralysis occurs but is not immediate or complete, laminectomy (decompression of the spinal cord) and the removal of bone fragments are sometimes indicated. In complete immediate paralysis,

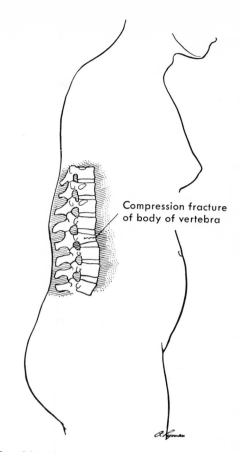

Compression fracture of body of vertebra

Fig. 190 Compression fracture of the spine. Angulation or gibbus may occur over the spinous process of the fractured vertebra or the one above.

laminectomy has no value. In uncomplicated compression fractures, the problem is to restore the normal contour of the spine.

After injury to the spine (Fig. 190), there is almost invariably a shock to the sympathetic nervous system. With this shock comes disturbance of intestinal and bladder activity, and the most serious immediate problem of the patient with spine fracture often directly results from these factors.

The presence of pain often requires morphine sedation, which exaggerates internal stasis and sluggishness of bladder muscles to such an extent that enemas and catheterization are frequently necessary for several days. Strong cathartics should not be given because they may cause increased discomfort. The use of a rectal tube and gastric suction is advocated. An indwelling catheter is occasionally necessary for five to seven days.

Treatment. Providing for and maintaining extension of the spine may be accomplished in several ways. A frame or Gatch bed may be used in the treatment of these patients. Its angle is gradually increased within four to fourteen days (Fig. 199). Maintenance of reduction is checked roentgenographically. After reduction, a body cast is applied (Fig. 200).

Early reduction under anesthesia is accomplished with the patient suspended by his feet and shoulders, face down. Pressure is exerted on the spinous processes at the point of fracture until correction has been obtained. Roentgenographic examination may be used to confirm the reduction before the cast is applied. The cast should extend from the hips to the neck to maintain correction. The higher the fracture in the spine, the more difficult it is to maintain the correction. In fractures above the fifth dorsal vertebra, it is necessary to carry the cast on up to the head and chin.

Some spine fractures that have healed with persistent pain need internal fixation by some form of bone fusion or graft or other apparatus to stabilize the spinous processes and laminae in the correct position (see Chapter 20).

Fractures or dislocations of the cervical spine are best treated by the use of the Crutchfield tongs (skeletal traction). These allow the use of 30-lb to 40-lb weights for reduction.

Treatment in the extension cast is usually necessary for three to six months, according to the severity of the fractures. This is followed by use of an extension brace such as the Taylor back brace (Fig. 191) for an additional four to six months.

Healing period. The healing period of vertebrae is from six to twelve months.

Nursing intervention for patient with fracture of spine without cord injury. Upon arrival in the emergency room, and prior to being moved from the ambulance cot, the patient with a possible back injury and/or cord damage should have a preliminary evaluation of his injuries. Specific instructions pertaining to type of bed and needed equipment make it possible to avoid unnecessary transfers of the patient. In some instances, to facilitate turning and maintenance of desired position, the patient is placed on a lateral or vertical turning frame. If the regular hospital bed is to be used, a fracture board is placed beneath the mattress to secure a firm surface or, if increased extension of the spine is desired, a second mattress may be needed.

When transferring the patient with back injury from the cot to the x-ray table or the bed, it is advisable to use a "three-man lift" (Fig. 192). By keeping the patient's pelvis and shoulders in the same plane, flexion and rotation of the spine are avoided. If there is a cervical injury, a fourth person is needed to support the patient's head. Sandbags placed at either side of the head will help maintain the desired position. When removing the patient's clothing, it frequently is necessary to cut garments to avoid motion at the site of injury. All of these efforts are directed toward preventing possible trauma to the spinal cord, which could affect the ultimate outcome.

Upon admission, the patient's vital signs are checked and recorded. The rate and

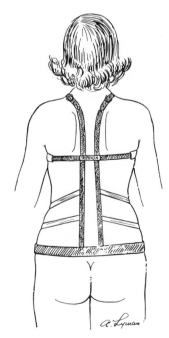

Fig. 191 Taylor back brace used for support of the spine in many conditions; e.g., during the convalescence of patients with fractures or tuberculosis and in patients with epiphysitis, arthritis, malignancy, and round-shoulder deformity.

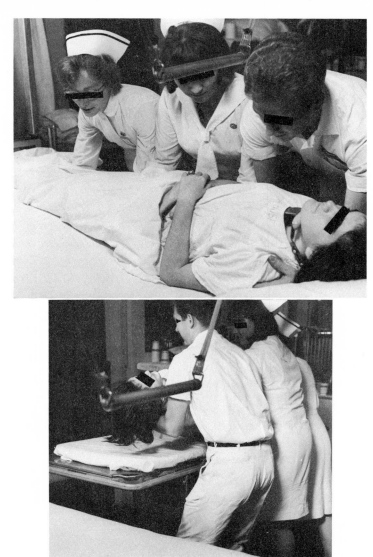

Fig. 192 When immobilization of the spine is necessary, the "three-man lift" may be used to transfer a patient from the bed to a cart or vice versa. If immobilization of the cervical spine is necessary, a fourth person should support and control the position of the head. Note that all the "lifters" assume positions at the same side of the bed. The first nurse slips his arms beneath the patient's shoulders and chest region, the second nurse places her arms beneath the patient's lumbar and buttocks areas, and the third nurse supports the patient's lower limbs. The cart usually is placed at a right angle to the foot end of the bed (this may vary depending on the situation). With the "lifters" working in unison, the shoulders, hips, and lower extremities of the patient's body are moved simultaneously to the edge of the bed. As the second step in the transfer process, and again in unison, the "lifters" raise the patient's body from the bed and move in a circular direction to place him on the cart. (Before starting the procedure, it is advisable to lock the bed and cart wheels.) In some instances as the patient is lifted from the bed, it may be permissible to roll his body toward the "lifters." Carrying a weight close to the body provides for more efficient use of muscles. However, if immobilization of the patient's vertebral column during the moving process is essential, omitting this step may be desirable. Another point to remember is that the use of good body mechanics by the workers is an important aspect in preventing back strain.

type of respirations and the presence of any cyanosis should be noted. If the injury is in the cervical region, respiratory embarrassment caused by involvement of the phrenic nerve may be anticipated. For this reason, equipment for tracheostomy, as well as for administering oxygen, must be available for immediate use. Frequently, suction is necessary to maintain a patent airway and to prevent aspiration of secretions. Equipment and facilities for giving intravenous infusions or blood transfusions are necessary items; drugs for combating shock, such as ephedrine or phenylephrine hydrochloride (Neo-Synephrine), must be administered as directed by the physician. Pain medications that depress the respirations and those that tend to mask neurologic signs are usually withheld.

Hyperthermia apparent a short time after a cervical cord injury may be of central origin. Intracranial involvement may be detected by checking pupillary reaction of the eyes to light. Signs of confusion or amnesia denoting the patient's level of consciousness should be recorded. The patient with a fracture of the vertebral column must be checked for bladder distention. Usually the physician asks that a Foley catheter be inserted and secured in place. The amount and appearance of the urine should be noted and a specimen saved. The physician may wish to do a spinal puncture, either to determine if there is bleeding into the subarachnoid space or to determine whether there is a block of the cerebrospinal fluid.

Fracture or dislocation of cervical spine

Skeletal traction, applied by tongs inserted in the parietal eminences of the skull, usually is used for reduction of fractures and dislocations of the cervical (Fig. 193) vertebrae. In some instances, it may be necessary to use rather large amounts of weight to reduce the fracture. Progress of reduction is checked roentgenographically. When complete reduction has been obtained, the amount of weight is decreased.

The stab wounds through which the tongs are introduced into the skull are usually dressed with small circular sponges. Very little danger of infection exists, although occasionally it does occur. Inspection of the wound dressings should be made

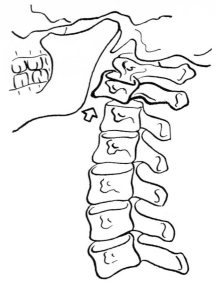

Fig. 193 Dislocation of the cervical spine. (From Kenney, W. C., and Larson, C. B.: Orthopedics for the general practitioner, St. Louis, The C. V. Mosby Co.)

each day, but the dressings should not be disturbed without order of the surgeon. Tightening of the tongs is usually done by the surgeon or his assistants.

Although such emergencies are not common, skeletal traction in the skull has on occasion become loose, in which case the tongs may actually slip out. For this reason, a set of alternate equipment that the nurse may apply until the physician can be reached should be kept on hand. A chin halter, a spreader, some rope, and a few sandbags will suffice to maintain the desired position until the tongs can be replaced in the skull.

With the Crutchfield skull traction (Figs. 194 and 195), careful turning of the patient for back care may be permitted. Permission and instruction pertaining to turning, however, must be obtained from the attending surgeon. The patient must be watched for signs of cyanosis during the process and for dyspnea, which might indicate damage to the cord.

Body alignment should be carefully maintained during the turning process, and the patient should be turned as though he were a log and would not bend. Head, shoulders, and pelvis must be turned simultaneously. Flexion of the cervical spine is

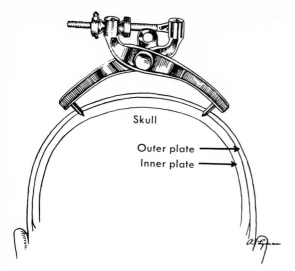

Fig. 194 Crutchfield tongs apparatus.

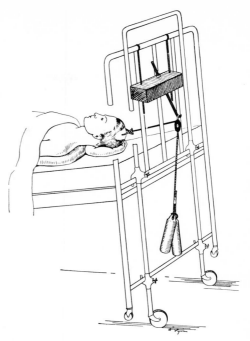

Fig. 195 Crutchfield tongs. The head should be low and the shoulders high. The upper end of the bed should be elevated. Traction weights of 25 lb to 35 lb may be used safely and comfortably.

not permitted. A pillow should be placed in front of the patient's chest to support the shoulder and arm, and another should be placed between the thighs and legs to prevent sagging of the hip. Either of these conditions, sagging of the hip or of the shoulder in the side-lying position, will inevitably alter the position of the spine and should be avoided.

When longitudinal traction is maintained by skeletal tongs, it may be necessary to adjust the position of the cervical spine to accomplish alignment—especially in extension. This may be accomplished by several methods. Two mattresses may be placed on the bed—one in the usual position and the other (the upper one, which may be a youth mattress) positioned so that it reaches only to the patient's shoulders (Fig. 195). A thin pillow or pad may be used under the head to help provide the desired position. The same effect can be obtained by placing a sponge rubber mattress on top of the regular mattress (Fig. 196). If *only* longitudinal traction is necessary, the patient may be placed on a bed frame that provides for lateral (Foster or Stryker frame) or vertical (CircOlectric bed) turning (see Chapter 8).

The patient with a cervical fracture being treated by head traction will be dependent upon the nurse for many of his needs. If cervical extension is being maintained, soft foods that are easily chewed will be less likely than liquids to cause choking. Liquids should be taken slowly until the patient becomes accustomed to swallowing in this position. As a precautionary measure, since the patient's head cannot be elevated or rotated, suction equipment should be available at the bedside. The patient will have to be fed since he will not be able to feed himself. In some instances, he may have a poor appetite. Consequently, a relaxed unhurried atmosphere at mealtime is desirable. Adequate intake of needed nutrients is important.

During the first few days, the patient with compression fracture of the spine or injury to the cord is likely to have a troublesome stasis of the gastrointestinal tract due to a paralytic ileus. The abdomen may be ballooned to drumlike tenseness by distention of the bowel, and respiratory embarrassment is present because of pressure on the underside of the diaphragm. Relief may be gained by the insertion of a rectal tube, and neostigmine (Prostigmin) may be prescribed to help produce peristal-

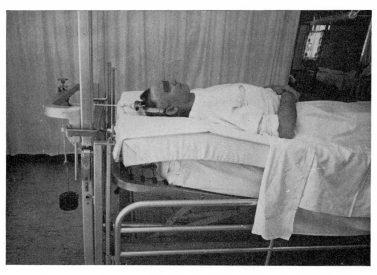

Fig. 196 Vinke tongs applied to a patient with cervical fracture. Note arrangement of the mattresses to provide for extension of the cervical region.

sis. However, it frequently is necessary to use a nasogastric tube and suctioning to provide relief for the patient. During the time that suction is being used, the patient is maintained on intravenous feedings.

Careful observation for change in skin sensation and for loss of motion or muscle strength (handgrip) is an essential aspect of the care needed by the patient with a fracture of the spine without cord damage. Such symptoms can be indicative of pressure on the cord and should be reported to the surgeon. The pressure may be caused by increasing edema or by a change in the position of the bone fragments. Surgery may be indicated to relieve pressure and to prevent permanent cord damage.

Because of the traction apparatus and the injury, turning may not be permitted, and positioning of the patient is more difficult than with most patients. Thus, frequent encouragement of the patient to breathe deeply is helpful in removing secretions and preventing hypostatic pneumonia. Likewise, skin care and the prevention of pressure sores become a challenge. To prevent skin breakdown, it is usually desirable and necessary to use such aids as sponge rubber pads, acrylic fiber pads (artificial lamb's wool), or perhaps an alternating pressure mattress. Use of these "aids," however, does not lessen either the need for maintaining a wrinkle-free and

crumb-free bed or the need for massage to vulnerable spots. Even though turning may be limited, massage to the back can be given at frequent intervals. Pressure placed on the mattress with one hand enables the nurse to slip her other hand beneath the patient's back and give massage to the sacral and scapular areas, likely spots for pressure necrosis.

Placement of the patient on the bedpan presents additional problems. The fracture bedpan, which has a low tapering back, usually can be slipped under the buttocks if pressure is placed on the mattress at each side of the buttocks. Two nurses can do this with less discomfort for the patient than one nurse alone.

Changing the bed linen is easier if two drawsheets are used instead of one full-length sheet. Pillowcases or towels may be placed at either side of the head. When these are soiled, they can be changed without disturbing the head position. During this period of bed rest, active or passive exercise of the arms and legs (as prescribed by the surgeon) is necessary to ensure maintenance of normal joint motion.

Time passes slowly for the patient with a cervical fracture. The use of prism glasses makes it possible for him to read, to watch television, or to observe other activities in the area (Fig. 197).

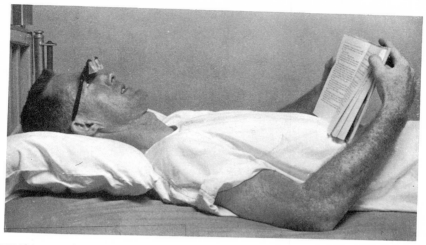

Fig. 197 The use of prism glasses makes reading and watching television possible for the patient who cannot have the backrest elevated.

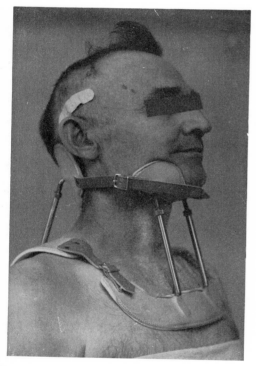

Fig. 198 After removal of the Crutchfield tongs, the patient is fitted with a brace designed to provide support and immobilization of the cervical vertebrae.

When roentgenograms indicate that sufficient healing has taken place to permit ambulation, the patient is fitted with a neck brace (Figs. 142 and 198). When traction has been removed and a brace

applied, the brace must be worn continuously until permission for its removal is given by the surgeon. Ambulation for this patient must be a slow and gradual process. Assistance with walking is necessary until danger of falling is past.

Fracture of dorsolumbar spine

A wedge compression fracture (Fig. 190) of one or more vertebral bodies of the dorsolumbar spine is not an uncommon injury and usually is caused by a vertical force on the long axis of the vertebral column. On examination, the area is tender to palpation, muscle spasm limits motion, and the posterior spinous process of the involved vertebral body may be prominent. If the injury has not disturbed the supporting ligamentous structure of the spine, particularly the posterior ligaments, the fracture is considered to be a stable fracture. Early treatment for this type of injury (when there are no neurologic deficits) consists of bed rest on a firm mattress. Elevation of the headrest, standing, and sitting usually are not permitted, since these positions cause increased pressure on the injured vertebra. However, turning from side to side is often permissible and does provide for changes in body position and added patient comfort. Due to the spinal shock accompanying this type of injury, an ileus frequently develops, peristaltic sounds are absent, and the patient has severe abdominal distention. To provide relief, gastric

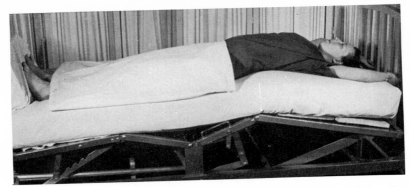

Fig. 199 The spine is maintained in a position of extension by use of the three-crank Deckert bed. The amount of extension can be increased or decreased according to need. The same position can be secured with the ordinary Gatch bed by placing the patient's head at the foot and then elevating the knee rest.

suction may be necessary, oral intake is restricted, and parenteral fluids are administered. When the patient has recovered from the acute phase and is not having bowel or bladder problems, plans are made for mobilization. This necessitates immobilization of the spine with a body brace or cast (Figs. 200 and 201). Use of the tilt table may be indicated to overcome hypotension. With the spine immobilized, ambulation (with assistance) is started and gradually increased as tolerated, and the patient is instructed in exercises designed to maintain and strengthen the trunk muscles. Strong trunk muscles are necessary to permit removal of the external support when fracture healing has taken place. Support for the spine is usually needed for ten to twelve weeks.

Spinal injuries that result in a subluxation or dislocation of one vertebra on another are likely to cause cord damage, as well as injury to the ligamentous support of the spinal column. Treatment is aimed at reduction of the dislocation, and rigid immobilization is necessary to prevent further damage to the spinal cord. Careful and continuous assessment of the patient for motor and sensory changes is essential. The nurse should seek specific instructions from the attending surgeon pertaining to immobilization, activity permitted, turning procedures, etc. Frequently with this type of patient, the horizontal or vertical turning frames are used to provide immobilization of the spine. Fracture-dislocation with loss of the posterior ligamentous support results in an unstable fracture and usually

necessitates operative fixation—spinal fusion (Fig. 202), Harrington rod (Fig. 361), etc.

Fractures of sacrum and coccyx

Cause. Fractures of the sacrum and coccyx usually are caused by direct violence and are very painful. Falling on ice in a sitting position is a common cause.

Symptoms. Pain that is aggravated by sitting down or getting up and tenderness over the sacrum or sacrococcygeal joint are symptoms of fracture of the sacrum and coccyx.

Treatment. After the patient has spent a period of rest in bed with the affected area supported on a rubber ring and much time lying prone, low adhesive strapping or a low girdle may be used to relieve muscle pull. Sitting on hard surfaces should be avoided. Repeated massage of the piriformis muscles (rectally) often gives relief. Occasionally, as a last resort, the coccyx may be removed.

Fractures of pelvis

Cause. Fractures of the pelvis usually result from crushing between two forces with considerable violence.

Anatomy. The pelvis is a ring composed of the sacrum posteriorly, the ilia on either side, and the symphysis pubis in front. The weakest spots in this ring are the rami of the pubis. Most of the pelvic fractures occur in the rami (Figs. 203 and 204), but they may occur in the ilia with displacement of the pelvis.

Complications. At the time of injury,

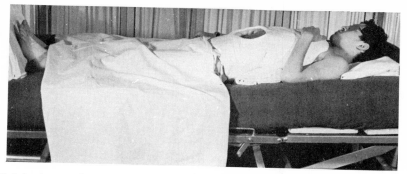

Fig. 200 A body cast that had been applied to maintain the spine in an extended position.

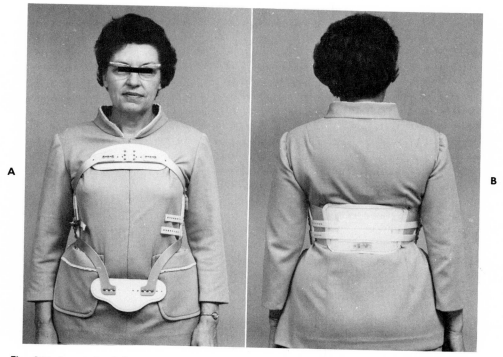

A

B

Fig. 201 Jewett back brace. This brace is designed to maintain the spine in extension. It is particularly adapted for the ambulatory treatment of compression fractures of the vertebral bodies. It applies the three-point pressure principle—pressure backward on the sternum and pubis and pressure forward on the midback.

there may be damage to the pelvic organs as a result of the direct force or spicules of bone. The urethra is most frequently damaged; the bladder is next. There may be damage to the rectum. If the bladder is full at the time of injury, damage is more likely.

There are two main reasons for restoration of the symmetric ring of the pelvis: (1) to avoid future abnormal strain on the sacroiliac joints and (2) to restore the normal birth canal in women.

Treatment. Overriding of the fragments may be overcome by the use of Buck's extension or skeletal traction on the leg of the fractured side. Traction automatically causes abduction and pull at the same time, although side traction also may be necessary.

When sufficient correction has been ob-

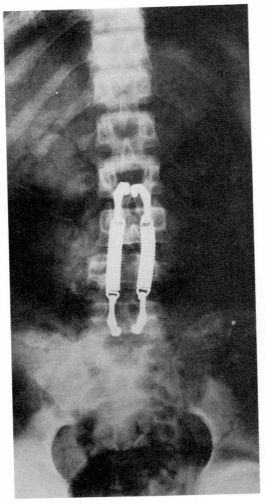

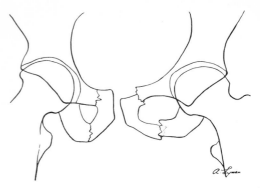

Fig. 203 Fracture of both rami of both sides of the pubis. Note the asymmetry of the pelvis. Abduction of both thighs is necessary for correction.

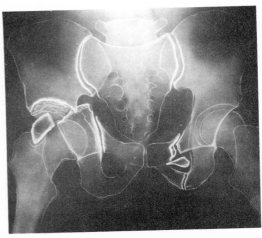

Fig. 202 Weiss spring clamp to aid in stabilizing the spine following open reduction for fracture-dislocation of the spine.

Fig. 204 Severe fracture of the pelvis. Note the break of continuity of the ischium and the pubic bone on the left. Note the fracture through the acetabulum on the right, with posterior dislocation of the hip. The large fragment near the trochanter is the posterior wall of the acetabulum.

tained through traction, a plaster-of-Paris hip spica cast is applied with the hip in abduction. It usually is necessary to apply it only down to the knee.

Healing period. Healing usually takes place in six to eight weeks. Weight bearing on the affected side should be avoided during that time. Crutches may be used. Patients with this injury are likely to have persistent difficulty in the sacroiliac joint. It is wise to use some form of pelvic girdle for protection during the early months of weight bearing to prevent permanent damage to the sacroiliac joint.

Nursing intervention. Under the classification of pelvic fractures are fractures of the ilium, pubic bone, sacroiliac, and acetabulum. They are of varying degrees of severity, but in all of these fractures the nurse should be aware of the danger of internal injuries, particularly to the bladder, urethra, or rectum. A urine specimen by catheterization usually is ordered immediately. A soft rubber catheter should be used—never one made of metal. A rectal

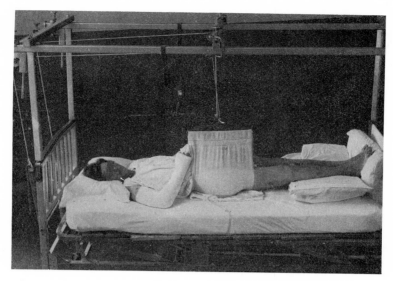

Fig. 205 Pelvic sling used in the treatment of fractures of the pelvis.

examination is carried out by the physician to rule out injury to the lower bowel.

The most common fracture of the pelvis is that occurring in the pubic bone, and it is often caused by a compression between two solid objects or a fall in which the patient lands on the hip.

If there is separation of the fracture fragments, the patient may be placed in a canvas sling attached to an overhead frame (Fig. 205). Buck's extension is usually applied to the leg of the injured side. Compression of the pelvis is obtained by fastening the ends of the canvas sling together over the front of the patient. If compression is not desired, the canvas sling may have wooden spreaders at either side and be supported by separate ropes and pulleys on the overhead frame. The hammock should be about five feet long and two feet wide. It should extend from the upper border of the lumbar vertebrae to midthigh. Just enough weight to keep the pelvis off the mattress is used, and for nursing care the hammock may be pushed or folded back over the buttocks. This type of hammock-sling accomplishes lateral compression on the sides of the pelvis, forcing the separated pubis together at the symphysis. It is usually continued for about six weeks.

To care for the toilet needs of a patient who is wearing a pelvic sling presents problems. With the female patient, the doctor may prescribe the insertion of a Foley catheter for use at least during the first portion of the time that traction is necessary. If a catheter is not inserted, a female urinal may be used. For bowel movements, the use of a small flat pan or a child's fracture pan will cause the least discomfort to the patient, and the least disturbance of the traction apparatus. In some instances, the physician may permit partial release of the traction to provide for adequate bathing of the buttocks and perineal areas.

When there is no separation of the fragments, the patient may be placed on a firm mattress, with Buck's extension applied to the legs. Unless orders are specifically given to turn the patient, back care is given by elevating the patient either with the aid of an overhead trapeze or with the assistance of another nurse.

Scultetus or abdominal binders are sometimes used instead of hammocks, particularly if there has been no involvement of the acetabulum. The binder should extend from the iliac crest to two or three inches below the pubis. If the binder is made of canvas, it is wise to insert a lining of flannel cloth or other soft material between the skin and the binder. Instructions usually given for the application of the binder in different types of pelvic fractures are listed at the top of the next page.

1 For fracture of the iliac bone, the binder is applied without snugness.

2 For fracture of the ischium or pubic bones, the binder is applied snugly.

3 If there is separation of the symphysis pubis, the binder is applied as tightly as possible.

FRACTURES AND DISLOCATIONS OF HIP
Femoral neck fractures

Cause. Fractures in the upper end of the femur may be near the head. These are called intracapsular. Those occurring farther out in the neck of the femur are called extracapsular, and those occurring still farther out, in the region of the trochanters, are called trochanteric or intertrochanteric fractures (Fig. 208). To the laity all of these are broken hips, but to the orthopedic surgeon they are very different in regard to treatment and prognosis.

Anatomy. The hip is a ball-and-socket joint. To allow free range of motion, the capsule that surrounds the joint is quite flexible and extends a considerable distance out along the neck. This means that the blood vessels that supply nutrition must enter outside the point of attachment of the capsule. Unfortunately, the ligament between the head and the acetabulum (ligamentum teres) carries little or no circulation to the head. Most of the circulation enters the neck of the femur through nutrient foramina and reaches the head inside the bone. Fractures of the neck cause a tearing of these vessels, and the head within the capsule may be left with little or no circulation. This anatomic fact is the chief cause of the percentage of nonunions that occur in spite of perfect reduction (20% to 25%). This is also the cause of the necrosis and disintegration that may occur in the head of the femur. When the fragments have been separated by the injury, the strong gluteus medius muscle pulls the distal portion upward. The iliopsoas tends to rotate outward, as does the gluteus maximus. Immediately after the accident, therefore, the leg usually is found in the position of helpless eversion. There are both some shortening of the extremity and considerable pain and muscle spasm on any attempt to move the patient.

Reduction and treatment. Because of the injury, the patient has, in most cases, been forced abruptly from an active to a completely inactive existence. Reduction may be accomplished by the use of traction or by manipulative procedure. Reduction and immobilization by traction take a longer period of time, and the patient is confined to bed rest and is subject to the many complications caused by inactivity. Surgical procedures that provide for closed reduction with internal fixation of the fracture or replacement of the femoral head with a prosthesis offers many advantages.

Reduction by the manipulative method of Leadbetter means that manual traction is applied with the hip and knee in the flexed position and then the limb is slowly extended, rotated internally, and abducted. Following reduction, the type of internal fixation is determined by the proximity of the fracture to the head of the femur. When there is a fair amount of neck connected with the head fragment, fixation of the fracture site may be accomplished with a compression screw, Smith-Petersen flanged nail, or other device (Figs. 206 and 207).

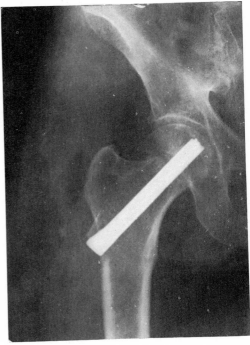

Fig. 206 Smith-Petersen flanged nail used for internal fixation of fractures of the neck of the femur.

With internal fixation of the fracture, the patient may be permitted to sit in a chair for well-tolerated intervals on the first postoperative day. If his general condition warrants, he is encouraged to stand on his uninvolved extremity and pivot to sit in the chair. The use of crutches or a walker is encouraged in a few days if the patient's general condition warrants it. However, weight bearing should not be allowed for three to five months, and then only if the roentgenographic examination shows sufficient healing.

When the fracture is very near the head of the femur or when circulatory damage appears to be severe, it may be advisable to treat the fracture by the insertion of a femoral head prosthesis (Fig. 215).

Intertrochanteric fractures (Fig. 208) almost invariably heal. However, with the strong pull of the muscles, they tend to heal with a loss of the normal angulation between the shaft and the neck of the femur. This tends to create deformity. Shortening, external rotation, and adduction often result. To prevent deformity, the fracture must be held by an apparatus that will overcome these tendencies until solid union is present. Several types of apparatus for internal fixation of intertrochanteric fractures have been devised (Fig. 209). Following the surgical procedure, the patient usually is permitted to sit in a chair the first postoperative day and essentially goes through the same routine of convalescence as those patients with internal fixation of fracture of the femoral neck. In recent years, the danger of surgery on the aged person has been minimized and the number of postoperative deaths greatly reduced.

Nursing intervention. Since fracture of the upper end or neck of the femur (commonly called hip fracture) presents more nursing problems than any other type of femoral fracture, emphasis will be placed

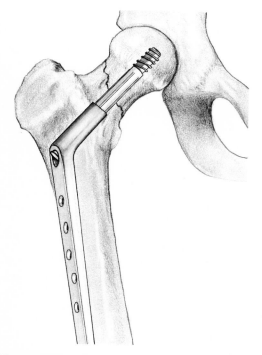

Fig. 207 The coarse threads of the sliding nail have good purchase on the head of the femur. As the bone at the fracture site resorbs, the head can move toward the distal fragment to close the gap at the fracture site. The sliding nail will project through the hole in the side plate to permit gap closure yet maintain alignment. Failure to permit gap closure leads to nonunion.

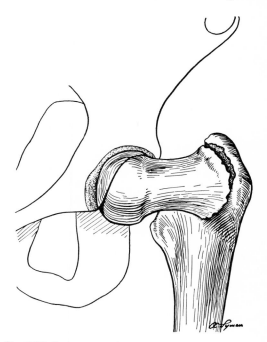

Fig. 208 Fracture at the base of the neck of the femur (intertrochanteric type). Note the decrease in the angle of the neck and eversion. The lesser trochanter shows up prominently, denoting outward rotation.

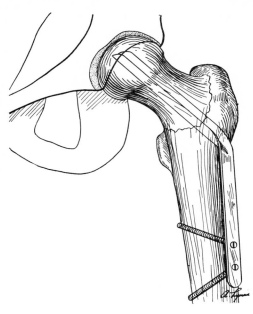

Fig. 209 Open reduction of an intertrochanteric fracture with Neufeld nail inserted into the neck and head and down the shaft of the femur with divergent screws. This nail is a one-piece stainless steel nail with V-shape flanges into the neck and head.

on the nursing care required for this condition. The operative procedure usually performed (closed reduction with internal fixation) is not considered a serious threat unless the patient is in very poor physical condition.

Preoperative nursing care. The patient with this type of fracture will complain of pain in the hip region, and any movement of the involved limb causes increased pain and spasm of the thigh muscles. Also, the nurse may note that the involved limb is slightly shorter than the other limb and is held in a position of external rotation.

Pain and discomfort can be lessened if unnecessary transfers from ambulance cot to x-ray table to bed, etc., are avoided. As the patient is moved, the application of a small amount of manual traction to the involved limb lessens the pain by immobilizing the bone fragments.

Most of the patients will have other chronic health problems. The hip fracture is complicated by or perhaps complicates an existing cardiac condition, a diabetic problem, or other health deficit that fre-

quently accompanies the aging process. In some instances, reduction and internal fixation of the fracture is delayed twenty-four to forty-eight hours to permit a complete medical evaluation and treatment of any existing health problems. If surgery is delayed, the application of skin traction (Buck's extension or Russell traction) will lessen muscle spasm and the patient is more comfortable with the immobilization produced by the traction. When the muscle spasms have been relieved an attempt should be made to gently roll the limb to a neutral position. A trochanter roll or sandbag is then used to maintain the correct alignment of the limb.

Pressure sores are a constant threat to the elderly person confined to bed. The heel of the involved limb is a particularly vulnerable site. If pressure is not relieved, a blister or reddened area indicating a beginning pressure sore will develop within a few hours.

Provision for activity and change of position will result in increased patient comfort, as well as the prevention of pressure areas and hypostatic pneumonia. If the bed is equipped with a trapeze, the patient can be taught and encouraged to frequently shift his position. By flexing the hip and knee of his uninvolved limb and pushing with his foot as he pulls with his hands, the patient finds that he can assist with his own care and have a small degree of independence. The activity provides for active exercise of the uninvolved extremities and encourages self-care. These are aspects of his care that the nurse will want to foster throughout his hospitalization. Bed positions can be altered by raising and lowering the headrest, and in some instances (when Buck's extension has been applied) the physician may ask that the patient be turned to his well leg side. Maintaining a correct "line of pull" can be accomplished by moving the traction pulley (in the same direction the patient is turned) and by supporting the involved limb as the patient is rolled onto his well leg side. As the patient is turned, the involved limb is maintained in the same relationship to his body and is supported in a neutral position with pillows.

Encouraging and teaching the elderly patient to cough and to breathe deeply should

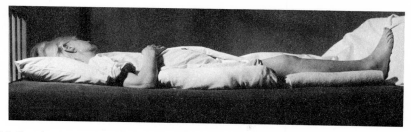

Fig. 210 Good supine position for the postoperative patient with internal fixation of a hip fracture. The footboard provides support for the feet, and heel pressure is relieved by a small pad beneath the calf of the leg. Neutral position of the limb is maintained with a trochanter roll, and full extension of the hip joint is encouraged by lowering the headrest. It must also be remembered that continuous pressure over the head of the fibula, on the lateral aspect of the leg, may cause paralysis of the peroneal nerve, resulting in an inability to dorsiflex the foot. This pressure may be caused by permitting the leg to remain in a position of external rotation or by pressure from sandbags, casts, or traction.

be included in his preoperative care. This will help prevent hypostatic pneumonia by removing secretions and mucus from the lungs and bronchial tubes.

Accurate intake and output records will help the nurse to know if the patient is drinking sufficient fluid. Assisting and encouraging the patient to take fluids is frequently necessary to prevent dehydration. Also, it is not uncommon for the patient with a fracture of the hip to have bladder distention with overflow incontinence. Early detection of this problem is necessary to prevent additional complications. The use of a fracture bedpan that can be slipped under the buttocks with little or no elevation of the hip region will cause less discomfort than the regular bedpan. When the patient is placed on the pan at frequent intervals, incontinence may be prevented. Needless to say, any nursing care that will prevent the need for insertion of a catheter is desirable. The catheter is a source of worry to the older person and may contribute to urinary tract complications.

Postoperative nursing care. Care of the patient following internal fixation may vary considerably. The amount of activity permitted is determined and ordered by the attending physician. If the hip is considered unstable, Buck's extension or some type of suspension traction in combination with a half-ring Thomas splint may be applied for a brief period. The traction provides for temporary immobilization, helps overcome muscle spasm, and increases the patient's

comfort. If the hip is considered stable, the patient usually is given much latitude with regard to movement in bed (Fig. 210), and as early as the first postoperative evening he may be turned to the side-lying position for back care. The patient with an internal fixation of a hip fracture may be turned to either side. However, the patient usually prefers to be rolled toward the uninvolved limb, with the limb that has been operated on kept uppermost. Good body alignment can be maintained with the use of pillows. Two nurses working together can turn the patient to the side-lying position, causing him a minimum of discomfort. He is moved in the bed toward the side operated on; one pillow is placed between the thighs and a second between the legs and feet. The side rail is raised, and the nurses go to the opposite side of the bed. The first nurse places her hands on the patient's far shoulder and hip (using care to avoid the operative site), and the second nurse slips one hand beneath the knee of the leg that has been operated on and the other hand beneath the patient's ankle. As the patient's body is rolled toward his well leg side, the operated limb is rolled on the pillows that have been placed between his legs. Careful handling and control of the involved limb are necessary to prevent pain and discomfort. If the patient desires further support when he turns, he may steady himself by placing his upper hand on the nurse's shoulder. Adjustment of the patient's hips and the pillows between his legs will provide for a comfort-

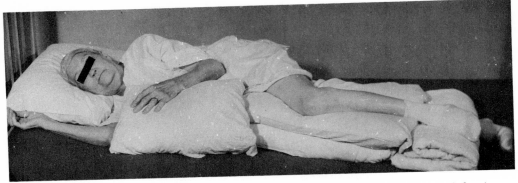

Fig. 211 Good side-lying position for the postoperative patient with an internal fixation of a hip fracture. The entire length of the uppermost limb is supported with pillows. The hip and knee are maintained in the same plane, and pressure on the lower limb is avoided.

able position and good body alignment. To prevent strain on the fracture site in the side-lying position, it is necessary to maintain the hip and knee in the same plane. Frequently, additional support in the groin area will increase the patient's comfort (Fig. 211).

Helping patient to be ambulatory. Postoperatively, if there are no contraindications, the surgeon usually requests that elderly patients be up in a chair the morning after surgery, with no weight bearing on the affected extremity. If the patient is able to stand on his uninvolved leg and pivot to sit in a chair, this method should be used in preference to lifting him out of the bed. Not only does standing provide exercise for the muscles and joints of the uninvolved limb, but the older patient's morale is given a "boost" when he learns that he is able to stand at the bedside and to sit in a chair. However, the nurse should remember that the patient's endurance has been somewhat lessened by the surgical procedure and that several short periods of time spent in a sitting position are better than one long period, which may completely exhaust the patient. Assisting the patient to a chair (preferably one with armrests) after hip surgery should be an unhurried activity. Adequate explanation of the procedure will help allay some of the fears and doubts the elderly person may have about his ability to get out of bed. In addition, he should understand that his weight should not be placed on the involved limb. The patient should wear his

shoes if they are available. Following surgery, support stockings or elastic bandages are applied to both extremities. This support helps to prevent dependent edema and phlebitis.

When permission has been given for the patient to be up in a chair, he should first roll onto the side of the uninvolved leg. When this has been accomplished, the knee and hip of the uninvolved leg should be flexed to a right angle, approximating the sitting position of the body. If the patient is able to partially flex the hip and knee of the affected side, this should be done, but it must be remembered that this leg will require the most gentle handling at all times and that the joints should never be forced beyond the point of pain.

To bring the patient to the sitting position (Fig. 212), place one arm under his shoulder and the other under the knees, gently swiveling him to the sitting position. If the fractured leg is extremely sensitive, another nurse may be needed to support it. Check your own body mechanics carefully for this procedure, being sure to assume the foot-forward position with knees and hips flexed and back straight. Considerable strain and torsion may be placed on the back if resistance from the patient is encountered, and you should be prepared for this before beginning the procedure. When the sitting position has been obtained, continue to support the patient's back until he is steady. Permit him to sit on the side of the bed for several minutes, and at this time instruct him to lift the chest, to practice breathing

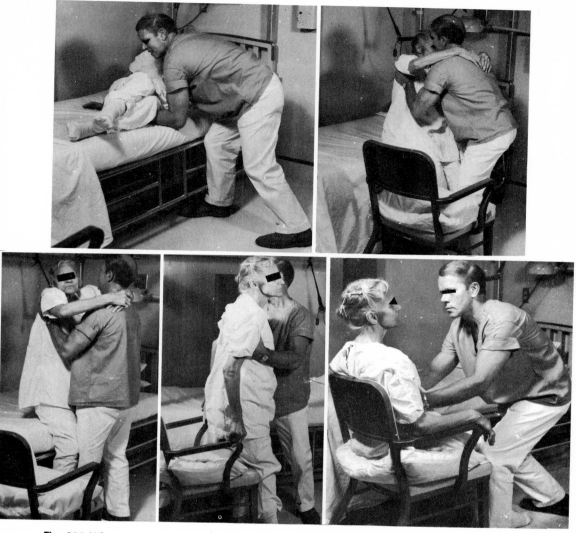

Fig. 212 When an elderly patient is being assisted from the bed to a chair, a low bed will be helpful to the patient but may pose a hazard for any nurse who uses poor body mechanics. As the nurse assists the patient to a sitting position on the side of the bed, strain to his own back muscles is minimized if he assumes the foot-forward position and flexes his hips and knees. The nurse shown is in a position to give an unstable patient considerable support and assistance in assuming the standing position, without strain to his back. The patient pivots and may place her hands on the armrest preparatory to sitting in the chair.

exercises, and to contract the gluteal and abdominal muscles. If there are no signs of dizziness or weakness, assist the patient to the standing position.

Place your hands under the patient's axillae and ask him to place his hands firmly on your shoulders. In this way he is assured of adequate support for his first

standing experience. The chair is placed parallel to the bed, and the patient turns or pivots on his uninvolved limb so that his back is toward the chair seat. Flex your knees and hips, ask the patient to reach for the armrests, and then assist him in lowering himself slowly into the chair. If placement of the bed and chair is such that the patient is pivoting and moving toward his uninvolved limb, the body's center of gravity is maintained over the supporting limb and balance is maintained more easily.

When constant attendance with the elderly person is not possible, it is frequently advisable to apply a restraint or "safety belt," which will prevent the patient from falling from the chair or attempting to walk by himself. While in the sitting position, the patient should be encouraged to comb his hair and care for his teeth. If being up in a chair can be arranged at mealtime, eating becomes a much more pleasurable event. Remember also that the elderly patient needs more than physical care. Nursing care that shows understanding and respect for the individual as a person and that supports the older person's self-esteem will help stimulate a desire for independence and recovery. This is very necessary when caring for the older person.

The patient can be taught to come to a standing position from the chair without too much difficulty, and his confidence in his ability will be greatly increased once he has accomplished this. The chair must be steady, propped against the bed or wall. The patient is instructed to bend forward from the hips, to place the unaffected leg backward until an acute angle of the knee is formed, and to have the knee on the affected side flexed as much as possible with the foot flat on the floor. The patient places his hands on the armrests of the chair with the elbows slightly flexed to assist in elevating himself. Weight is taken entirely by the uninvolved foot as the patient comes to the erect position.

Complications. Problems that commonly occur in the elderly patient need special attention.

Contractures. Prevention of contractures is accomplished by supporting the body in good alignment and by encouraging activities that enable the patient to exercise his extremities. The deformities to be guarded against are flexion and adduction of the hips, flexion of the knees, and an equinus position of the feet. Full extension of the hip and knee joints should be encouraged by lowering the backrest and by discouraging the use of pillows beneath the knees. Sandbags or a trochanter roll can be effective means of preventing ex-

ternal rotation of the leg, and encouraging the patient to dorsiflex his foot several times daily will prevent the development of a drop-foot deformity.

Pneumonia. A high percentage of the patients with fractured hips are elderly. The nursing problems involved in their care are geriatric as well as surgical in nature. Many complications of advanced age may be present. Hypostatic pneumonia is always a threat if the patients are confined to bed even for short periods. For this reason, prophylactic antibiotic therapy is sometimes instituted after fractures and continued for a week or longer. The patient does not feel the development of lung complications. The cough may be painful and the patient will resist the coughing mechanism, but the accumulation of mucus in the bronchi may still be present in the form of increasingly solid masses. The longer the process goes on, the more difficult it is to get rid of the plugs by coughing. Change of bed position, elevation of the head of the bed, maintenance of fluid intake, protection from drafts, and solicitude in keeping the patient well covered during bathing and turning are essential nursing measures. This patient must be encouraged to breathe deeply and to cough up mucus. Frequent assessment to detect evidences of beginning lung congestion is essential.

Thrombophlebitis. Another common cause of death after fracture of the femur in elderly patients is thrombophlebitis with embolus. As a prophylactic measure against this, an anticoagulant medication may be prescribed. (See Chapter 5.)

Decubitus ulcers. Skin care for the elderly patient is of the utmost importance. A daily bath and the use of strong soaps may increase the dryness of his skin and tend to cause discomfort. A complete bath every other day or twice a week is usually sufficient. Frequent cleansing of the hands, however, and of the perineum and buttocks region is essential. The use of baby oils or lotions will aid in preventing dryness and irritation of the skin. If evidences of chronic malnutrition are present, or if there is circulatory impairment as a result of arteriosclerosis, the fight to prevent pressure areas must be particularly vigilant. It must be begun the moment the patient enters the hospital. The responsibility for seeing that decubitus ulcers do not develop is completely in the hands of the nurse. (See Chapter 4.)

Gastrointestinal disturbances. Obstinate constipation is almost invariably present in elderly patients. Its management can be extremely troublesome if strong cathartics have been used too frequently during the early course of immobilization. Distention is not infrequent, and rectal tubes may sometimes be necessary to correct this. Careful attention to the patient's diet for roughage, and vitamins and the elimination of foods that cause distress will help to overcome constipation. Fecal moistening agents usually are prescribed. Enemas or suppositories may be necessary occasionally, and a laxative may be ordered as needed. Attention to regularity is, of course, essential.

Nutritional problems. A large number of the patients will have eating problems. They may have no teeth and may be unable to see or hear well. Often, they have definite food likes and dislikes, and it is difficult for them to understand hospital routines and methods. The thoughtful nurse can help to make mealtime a pleasant occasion for these older patients.

Because the rate of repair in fractures has been shown to be greatly influenced by the deficiency diseases and malnutrition so often present in elderly patients, considerable thought must be given to the diet to include the necessary food elements. Sufficient vitamin and protein intake is particularly important. To build tissue resistance and hasten repair, protein supplements may be given. Protein hydrolysates and amino acid mixtures are procurable for this purpose when the patient is unable to eat sufficient foods containing these substances. Vitamins B and C also are considered important in fracture healing. If the patients are unable to ingest a sufficient diet orally, supplementary feedings containing the essential proteins and vitamins may be given in a formula through a polyethylene tube. The polyethylene tube is a small plastic tube that is inserted through the nostril into the stomach. This tube is taped to the nose and is left in place.

It must be remembered, also, that anything that affects the patient's general condition will be likely to affect the healing of the fracture. Age, of course, plays a large part in the rate at which a fracture will heal. A fracture of the femur in a very young baby will heal firmly in four weeks, whereas in a person 50 years of age or older the time required may be three or four months or longer. Deficiency diseases, cachexia, and senile osteoporosis definitely will retard the rate of bone union. Blood chemistry determinations may be ordered by the physician when the progress of healing is slow. Serum calcium of 10-12 mg/100 ml of blood and phosphorus concentration of 3.5-4 mg are considered normal. Milk and a calcium medication or a parathyroid solution and synthetic vitamin D are sometimes ordered.

Urologic complications. Elderly patients are particularly prone to develop urologic complications during a period of immobilization. This is sometimes caused by an unwillingness to take sufficient fluids and by an already existing renal impairment. Scantiness of output, discomfort on voiding, concentrated urine, suppression, incontinence, and/or edema should be reported to the physician. Intake and output should be recorded accurately.

All patients, whether young or old, are in danger of developing renal stones if they are inactive for a considerable period of time. Good nursing care can play an important part in diminishing this danger (see Chapter 4).

Mental aspects in nursing care of patient with hip fracture. Frequently the elderly patient with a fractured hip becomes disoriented. The pain and shock, coupled with a strange environment, are sufficient to cause mental confusion. This confusion may not be apparent in the daytime, but at night the patient may attempt to get out of bed and his speech may be incoherent. The nurse must realize that this can be expected, and side rails or other protection should be provided. Preventing dehydration, controlling pain, providing items that help the patient determine time and place, and the presence of a family member are factors that help to eliminate or minimize the patient's confusion.

Elderly patients with fracture of the hip rarely escape serious mental depression. The prospect of inactivity is, in itself, a heavy burden to bear, and when it is accompanied by financial worry, it is extremely difficult to prevent depression and melancholy. Furthermore, these patients frequently have a pessimistic outlook regarding their own recovery. The nurse caring for them needs to develop considerable understanding and sympathy for their problems. Good mental hygiene demands that the patient be given something to do. Although the services of a trained occupational therapist are highly desirable in assisting with the daily program of the fracture patient, the bedside nurse can help by urging the patient to do as much as he can for himself, even though he is confined to a chair. If the nurse makes it clear to the patient that the desire to have him do things for himself stems from interest in his progress, he will be much more likely to cooperate and less likely to feel neglected when he is urged to care for his own wants as far as it is possible for him to do so. Many physicians order a series of gentle bed exercises to be carried out under the nurse's direction several times during the day to prevent loss of muscle tone and to prepare the patient for successful ambulation at as early a date as possible.

Problems in preparation for weight bearing. The amount of time that elapses before a patient is permitted to bear weight varies according to the progress of union. It may be from twelve to sixteen weeks or longer. As has been stated, exercises frequently are prescribed. These include muscle-setting exercises for the abdominal, gluteal, and quadriceps muscles, dorsiflexion and inversion exercises for the feet, rhythmic breathing exercises, and exercises to strengthen the arms and shoulder muscles. Explanation of the importance of these exercises may need to be repeated at frequent intervals.

Unexpected weaknesses and stiffness of many parts of the body that were not involved in the fracture may be present. These will alarm and depress the patient. The nurse who can help the patient understand that the weaknesses and the stiffness in his joints are the natural outcome of his fracture and inactivity and not a permanent sequela to it will aid greatly in bolstering his failing courage. Nothing should be done that will make him more apprehensive.

Any rough or hurried movement while carrying out the prescribed exercise for increasing motion in hip or knee or any enthusiastic increase in the range of motion beyond which the patient has previously gone also will be conducive to much loss of courage. Furthermore, acute muscle spasm around the hip will make it impossible to do anything further in the way of mobilization at that time.

Instruction in crutch walking for this age group is usually delayed until partial weight bearing can be permitted. Then the three-point gait is taught. This delay is necessary because the danger of falling and of weight bearing on the affected extremity is too great. Frequently the use of a walker (Fig. 213) is preferred to crutches. The elderly patient feels more secure with the walker and is less likely to fall.

Need for home care after fracture of hip. After a fracture of the hip there is one

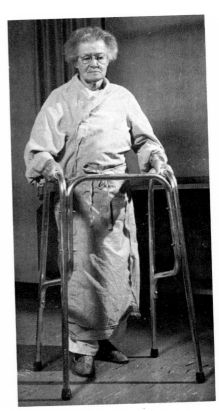

Fig. 213 A lightweight adjustable aluminum walker may be used by the elderly patient when ambulation is permitted.

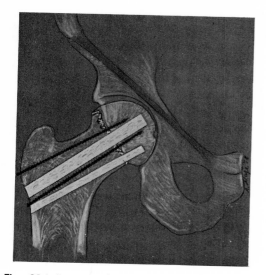

Fig. 214 Bone graft with threaded Steinmann pin fixation may be used in the absence of union after nailing procedure. (From Ziffren, S. E.: Management of the aged surgical patient, Chicago, 1960, Year Book Medical Publishers, Inc.)

question that always seems to arise and that causes the patient much worry: "Where am I to go when I leave the hospital?" With the increasing number of elderly persons in our population, the need for adequate convalescent care has become a major problem. The patient with a fractured hip can no longer take care of his needs, and often his elderly mate is physically unable to assume any added responsibility. Barring complications, it will be ten or twelve weeks before weight bearing is possible. Good care is essential during this convalescent period if the elderly person is to maintain his strength and the desire to walk again. Will the family be able to provide the needed care, or will plans for care in a nursing home or an extended care facility be necessary? Whatever plans are made for convalescent care, the assistance that the public health nurse is able to provide the family and patient at this time may mean the difference between failure and success—a patient who later

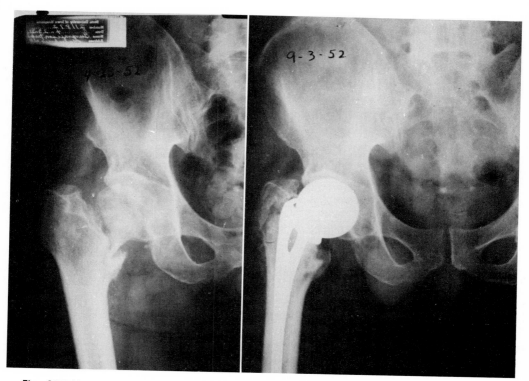

Fig. 215 Hip prosthesis. When aseptic necrosis of the head of the femur occurs after a fracture of the neck of femur, a prosthesis may be inserted, thus making weight bearing possible.

is able to walk, care for his own needs, and live an independent life.

Nonunion and aseptic necrosis. It is necessary that provision be made for adequate follow-up care for the patient with a fractured hip. Early detection of loss of position, nonunion, or aseptic necrosis makes it possible to institute corrective measures (Fig. 214). When nonunion persists after adequate reduction, the surgeon may wish to insert a tibial bone graft in the freshened nail tract. Or when aseptic necrosis has taken place, he may wish to replace the head of the femur with a Vitallium prosthesis. The ball part of the prosthesis (Fig. 215) fits into the acetabulum.

Nursing care following insertion of hip prosthesis. To help prevent dislocation following the insertion of a hip prosthesis, the involved limb is usually maintained in a neutral position with slight abduction. If the hip is unstable, suspension traction or a hip spica cast may be used to maintain the desired position. However, at other times the patient is returned to his bed following surgery with no supportive apparatus. In such a patient, sandbags or a trochanter roll may be helpful in maintaining the desired position of the operated limb. If turning to the side-lying position is permitted, slight abduction of the involved limb is maintained by placing pillows between the thighs and lower legs, and the turning is accomplished in the same manner as that described for the patient with a hip nailing. If the side-lying position is not permitted, the patient is asked to use the trapeze and his uninvolved limb to assist in lifting his hips off the bed (Fig. 388) and thus facilitate back care and linen changes.

During the first few postoperative days, frequent positioning is necessary and good nursing care is of the utmost importance if the complications so common to elderly patients are to be prevented. Also during this period the patient is instructed and encouraged to do upper extremity exercises preparatory for crutch walking. Abdominal, quadriceps-setting, and gluteal muscle-setting exercises may be included. When ambulation is permitted, it should be a relatively slow process, allowing time for the patient to adjust to the sitting and standing positions. When dizziness and weakness are overcome, the three-point crutch gait with "touch" weight bearing is usually prescribed (a walker may be substituted for the crutches). As the individual progresses with crutch walking, he is encouraged to resume normal activity. The elderly person may find it necessary to use the crutches or a cane for an extended period of time and follow-up care should include periodic examination by the orthopedic surgeon.

Traumatic dislocations of hip

There are several types of hip dislocations, but the most common are posterior dislocation with or without fracture of the acetabulum and anterior or obturator dislocation.

Posterior dislocation with or without fracture of the acetabulum is caused by force against the knee with the hip flexed and adducted (dashboard dislocations). There may be damage to the sciatic nerve.

Anterior or obturator dislocations are caused by forced abduction of the thigh with the hip in flexion. The head of the femur is displaced forward and enters the depression of the obturator foramen. There may be damage to the obturator nerve with weakness or paralysis of the adductor muscles.

Characteristic of the posterior upward dislocation is the patient's inability to abduct, extend, or externally rotate the limb. This is in contrast to fractures near the hip joint. There is a mass (the head of the femur) palpable on the ilium. With the obturator dislocation, the mass is felt in the groin, and the patient is unable to abduct or internally rotate the limb before reduction. Both conditions are very painful during the period of dislocation because of muscle spasm.

Reduction and treatment. In posterior dislocation, general anesthesia is necessary. Reduction can be accomplished by placing the patient on his back and exerting manual traction with the hip in full flexion (surgeon's shoulder under patient's knee). Relaxation is essential. If this method fails, the method of Lorenz for congenital dislocations may be successful—i.e., extreme flexion and abduction to bring the head into the catyloid notch and then further abduction combined with a decrease in flexion to force the head upward into the acetabulum.

In obturator dislocation, exertion of forceful traction in the line of deformity and then adduction as the head engages in the acetabulum accomplish reduction. All reductions of dislocations of the hip usually are accompanied by relaxation of the muscles, freedom of movement, and great relief of pain. A thud usually can be heard and felt as the head enters the acetabulum. The clinical signs should not be relied upon to indicate adequate reduction. Evidence should be established by roentgenograms taken in two directions.

Hip dislocations are comparatively easily treated after reduction. It is comforting to the patient with ligamentous injuries to have Buck's extension (with about 5 lb to 10 lb of weight) for two or three weeks—long enough for ligamentous healing. During this time, daily exercises of all joints should be carried out as soon as the patient is able to tolerate them.

In fractures of the acetabulum, the same treatment is used, but traction should be prolonged for two to three additional weeks. A wheelchair, crutches, and gradual weight bearing with crutches and then a cane follow over a period of six to ten weeks.

Attention has been drawn to the possibility of permanent damage to the head of the femur as the result of ligamentous tearing and disturbance in the blood supply to the head. Aseptic necrosis may occur if the damage is great. Such necrosis may manifest itself after several years by degenerative change in the joint. There may be degeneration of the cartilage and partial or complete ankylosis. Patients with dislocations uncomplicated by fracture, however, usually recover in six to eight weeks without further difficulty.

FRACTURES OF FEMUR
Fracture of femur below trochanters

Anatomy. Fracture of the femur below the trochanters is one of the most difficult fractures to treat successfully. The fracture occurs above the stabilizing attachment of the adductor muscles so that the upper fragment is controlled entirely by the intrinsic muscles of the hip (Fig. 216). The proximal fragment is brought into acute flexion by the action of the iliopsoas,

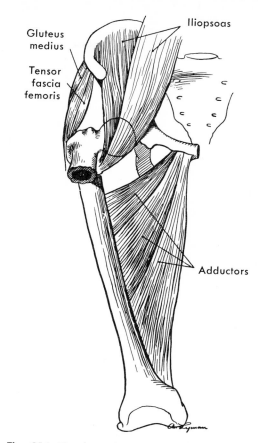

Fig. 216 Muscle action in subtrochanteric fractures of the femur.

into abduction by the gluteus medius, and into external rotation by both the iliopsoas and the gluteus maximus. Consequently, it tends to project forward at a right angle to the body and to abduct and rotate outward.

Problem. The problem is to bring the controllable distal fragment into a position that will meet the position of the uncontrollable proximal fragment in flexion at about 80° and abduction and external rotation.

Reduction. Reduction often can be accomplished with skeletal traction and suspension of the limb in a half-ring Thomas splint with a Pearson attachment. Lateral traction of 5 lb to 10 lb may be necessary to bring the distal fragment outward to engage the proximal fragment. Alignment may be obtained and demonstrated in anteroposterior and lateral views roentgeno-

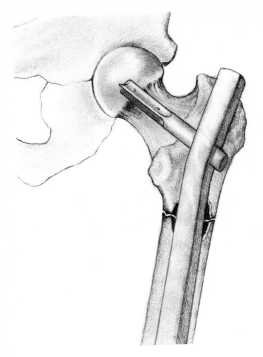

Fig. 217 Use of the Zickel nail. This is very helpful for stabilization of subtrochanteric fractures, especially pathologic fractures secondary to metastatic lesions in the upper third of the femoral shaft. This provides more rigid fixation than most any other apparatus. However, it is technically somewhat more exacting for the operator to apply.

graphically. If not, additional changes in the apparatus may be made.

If alignment does not take place this way, however, some means of internal fixation may be used, such as properly arranged and fixed steel pins, Vitallium or stainless steel plates, or intramedullary pins (Fig. 217).

Healing period. Healing is slow. Solid union usually does not occur in less than ten to twelve weeks. We are, again, frequently confronted with a hospitalization problem. Internal fixation does not always obviate the necessity of immobilization but may make the treatment of the fracture a more flexible one in regard to hospitalization and the necessity for bed treatment.

Fracture of shaft of femur (middle third)

Cause. Direct or indirect violence is the cause of fracture of the middle third of the shaft of the femur.

Anatomy. The action of the gluteus medius has some tendency to pull the upper fragment outward, and the strong pull of the adductor muscle group tends to cause outward bowing at the point of fracture. In this fracture there is a general tendency to develop inward rotation of the lower fragment and outward bowing. This, if allowed to develop, constitutes an awkward deformity and is quite disabling.

Treatment. Fracture of the femur may be treated by traction, a cast-brace, or surgery.

Traction. Some form of traction is required that will maintain pull. Russell or suspension traction usually fulfills the requirements. Abduction and external rotation of the distal fragment must be maintained. Roentgenograms should be taken frequently to check the position. If there is anterior or posterior angulation or if there is inward or outward bowing, the apparatus must be adjusted with proper slings and weights to counteract and correct the tendency toward deformity. Here, again, the critical period is important before the callus has developed so firmly that it cannot be molded into correct alignment. Necessary correction must be made before this state occurs. Skeletal traction obtained by use of a Kirschner wire or Steinmann pin may be used to secure the desired position of the fragments and to provide for immobilization. Skeletal traction and suspension applied by means of the Thomas, Hodgen, or Keller-Blake splint are frequently used. Skeletal traction is preferred to skin traction because a considerable amount of weight must be applied to overcome spasm of the thigh muscles. When reduction of the fracture has been secured, the amount of weight is reduced to prevent separation of the bone fragments. Traction must be continued until sufficient healing has taken place to permit crutch walking or until sufficient callus has formed to permit the application of a hip spica cast.

The child under 6 years of age with fracture of the femur is usually placed in Bryant traction for approximately six weeks. After this, a hip spica cast is applied and is worn until roentgenograms show that there is solid union at the fracture site. Care of the patient in traction has been described previously (Chapter 7).

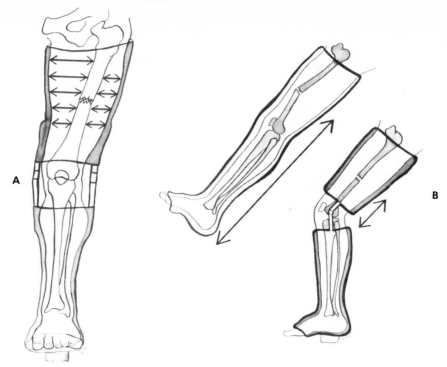

Fig. 218 A, The three components of the cast-brace. **B,** The comparative lengths of the lever arm distal to the fracture site with a long leg cast and with the cast-brace.

Cast-brace. The ambulatory treatment of lower extremity fractures is not a new concept. Dr. H. H. Smith reported great success with this form of treatment in seven patients with femoral shaft fractures in 1855.

However, the concept of weight bearing during fracture healing was not revitalized until the post-World War II era. Dr. Dehne popularized the concept of early weight bearing in patients with tibial fractures in long leg walking casts. The rate of nonunion of tibial fractures decreased markedly, and the time required for solid bony union to occur was significantly shortened.

The idea of early weight bearing in patients with femoral shaft fractures could not be successfully revived until the mid 1960's. The success of the treatment was the result of the new techniques and principles developed in the care of amputees.

The appliance designed for early weight bearing in patients with femoral shaft fractures is the cast-brace. This is made up of three components:

1 The thigh cuff with its quadrilateral opening superiorly, which controls the rotation of the proximal fracture fragment and creates an increase of the thigh soft tissue hydrostatic pressure to dynamically immobilize the fracture fragments

2 The short leg walking cast that provides support for the thigh cuff and controls leg edema

3 The polycentric hinges at the knee level joining the thigh cuff and short leg cast, which serve two functions: allow active motion of the knee and decrease the length of the lever arm distal to the fracture whose forces could prevent healing (Fig. 218)

Weight bearing in patients with tibial fractures in long leg walking casts is started as soon as the initial soft tissue swelling has subsided. This is also true for those with femoral fractures. The patient is treated in balanced skeletal traction for the first two or three weeks to allow soft tissue healing and resolution of swelling. The cast-brace is then applied without anesthesia. The patient is instructed on quadricep exercises and weight bearing with crutches.

The cast-brace immobilization of the fracture to produce solid bony union usually requires from six to eight weeks. By the end of that time, the patient usually can walk without crutches and has at least 90° of active knee flexion in the appliance. Consequently, after the removal of the cast-brace, the extremity is readily rehabilitated to a functional level.

Surgery. Other satisfactory methods of treatment are those requiring operation. The ones most commonly employed are reduction and insertion of an intramedullary nail, reduction with internotching of the fragments so that they cannot slip off, and plating with slotted stainless steel or Vitallium plates and screws.

Insertion of intramedullary nail. Fracture of the shaft of the femur may be treated by the insertion of an intramedullary nail. After open reduction the metal pin is inserted distally through the greater trochanter and across the fracture site (Fig. 219).

Postoperatively, support for the limb usually is provided by means of suspension traction. The traction helps to prevent rotation of the limb until the patient is able actively to control the position of his leg. If traction is not applied postoperatively, sandbags placed along the lateral aspect of the limb will help to prevent external rotation. During the time that the patient is in suspension traction, quadriceps-setting and gluteal muscle–setting exercises are performed. These exercises help maintain muscle strength, prevent distraction, compress fragments, and stimulate callus formation. When the postoperative pain has lessened and the patient has developed sufficient muscle power to control the position of his limb, partial weight-bearing (three-point gait) crutch walking usually is permitted, but crutches should be used until roentgenograms show bony union at the fracture site.

Internotching of fragments. In reduction with the internotching of the fragments, stainless steel wire may be used to prevent slipping. Open reduction may be followed by the application of a hip spica cast extending from the chest to the toes of the affected side with the leg in abduction and external rotation.

Plating. In plating with slotted stainless steel or Vitallium plates and screws, it must be remembered that muscular and mechanical stresses are great and that it may be necessary to have plates on two sides of the bone, preferably at right angles to each other. The screws should penetrate both cortical surfaces of the bone.

Healing period. Femoral shaft fractures heal quickly in children. There is frequently solid union in three to four weeks. In adults, solid healing sufficient to avoid deformities from constant muscle pull may not take place in less than ten to sixteen weeks. The likelihood of deformity must be judged clinically according to the age of the patient, the type of the fracture, and the speed with which the individual produces callus. The callus is not only visible in the roentgenogram but is also recognized clinically by its tendency to shrink and solidify.

It should be remembered that whatever

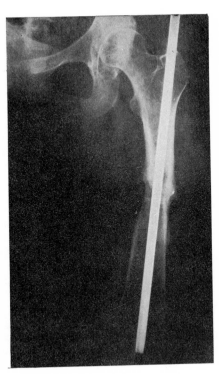

Fig. 219 Treatment of fracture of the femur by means of the intramedullary nail. Following reduction of the fracture, the nail is driven down through the shaft of the femur across the fracture site. This type of internal fixation permits increased activity and earlier ambulation.

the method used, the speed of healing is not changed, and whatever apparatus chosen by circumstances for the individual case must be kept functioning until complete healing has occurred.

Fracture of lower end of femur (supracondylar)

Cause. Direct or indirect violence causes fracture of the lower end of the femur.

Anatomy. Fracture of the lower end of the femur (Fig. 220) is distinctive because there is always a tendency toward deformity. It may be serious and permanent if the mechanical principles are not recognized. The gastrocnemius group of muscles is attached above the knee joint and between the condyles of the femur in the popliteal space. The only other muscles that influence the position of the lower fragment in this fracture are the thigh muscles, which cause overriding. Therefore, flexion occurs. This varies according to the distance of the fracture above the joint. Flexion may approach 90°.

Problem. Traction on the leg must be applied with flexion of the knee joint (to release gastrocnemius pull).

Reduction. Usually reduction is accomplished by means of adhesive or skeletal traction with the knee in a flexed position.

If the fracture is of the transverse type, reduction may be accomplished immediately with the patient under anesthesia and

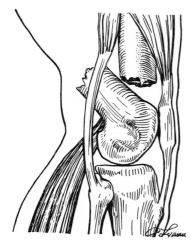

Fig. 220 Supracondylar fracture of the femur (transverse). Note the pull exerted by the gastrocnemius.

maintained by a plaster cast with the knee in flexion. This applies also to young persons in whom there is an epiphyseal separation of the lower femoral epiphysis rather than a fracture.

Healing period. These fractures heal rather rapidly. Complete immobilization is usually necessary for only four to six weeks. Physical therapy is often valuable in restoring free motion in the joint. Full development of union and function usually takes place in six to ten weeks.

Fractures into knee joint (femoral condyles)

Cause. Direct force either against the inner or the outer side of the knee joint usually causes fractures into the knee joint.

Anatomy. Such fractures may involve either condyle of the femur or may be of the plateau type involving either of the articular surfaces of the tibia. They are characterized by a tendency to produce a knock-knee (genu valgum) or bowleg (genu varum) deformity of the leg. Muscle pull plays very little part in the treatment, but the lateral and internal ligaments of the joint play a considerable part.

Problem. The contour of the joint must be restored as nearly perfect as possible, and the tendency toward deformity must be slightly overcorrected. Wherever there is damage within a joint as a result of fracture, the prognosis should be guarded, because the healing process in itself may be the surface of irregularities that can lead to future irritation and disturbance of joint function.

Reduction. In some instances, reduction may be accomplished spontaneously by manipulation with or without anesthesia and the position maintained by a plaster-of-Paris cast. If the fracture is badly comminuted, the cast may need to be extended from the waist to the toes. Usually, however, it need not extend above the thigh.

Knee joint fractures heal better in traction with adhesive tape from the knee down. Often lateral traction is used to correct any tendency toward lateral deformity in the knee. This treatment has the advantage of allowing active motion of the joint during healing of the fracture, but of course it adds to the number of hospital days.

Open reduction is used in patients with severe fractures. This usually consists of the removal of small fragments that prevent apposition of the main fragments. Fixation by the use of nails or threaded wires may be necessary to hold the fragments together during healing.

Healing period. These fractures usually heal rapidly, but strength and stabiilty are lacking for three or four months. Early motion is important in the knee joint, but protection from the development of knock-knee or bowleg deformity using a long leg brace may be necessary during the healing period of three to four months.

FRACTURES AND DISLOCATIONS ABOUT KNEE, ANKLE, AND FOOT
Fracture of patella

Causes. Direct violence is usually the cause of fracture of the patella. Muscle action is another cause.

Types. The three types of patellar fracture are transverse, comminuted (stellate), and linear.

Anatomy. The action of the quadriceps may separate the fragments as much as several inches when the injury occurs. It is important to recognize the significance of this in considering the damage to the capsular ligaments of the knee joint. The repair of lateral tears should be an important part of the treatment.

Treatment. Only linear fractures or stellate fractures without separation of the fragments should be treated conservatively. Conservative treatment can be accomplished by immobilization in a cast in extension for three to six weeks.

When there is separation of the fragments with tearing of the capsule, open reduction is always indicated. It is preferable in open reduction around joints to delay the operation three to six days to allow the traumatic reaction to subside and to permit tissue resistance to develop. This lessens the chance for infection. Open fractures may need to be treated immediately.

As a rule, it is best to remove small fragments of the patella and leave only one main fragment to which the patella or quadriceps tendon is sutured (Fig. 221). There is no longer a fracture to heal, but only the ligamentous attachments. Therefore, immobilization time is greatly re-

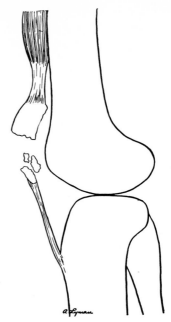

Fig. 221 Fracture of the patella with comminution of the lower fragment. This was removed.

duced. When severe comminution with separation occurs, the entire patella is removed, with restoration of good function.

Acute and habitual dislocations of patella

Causes. Acute dislocation of the patella is usually caused by direct force against its inner side when the knee is flexed.

Habitual dislocation may start from the same mechanism, but there may be other factors, such as too shallow a groove in the femoral condyles, ball-like shape of the patella, and knock-knee. Here, the pull transmitted from the quadriceps tendon to the attachment of the patella tendon on the tibia is not in a straight line, and therefore it places abnormal tension on the ligamentous structure of the inner side of the knee.

Symptoms and signs. The patella can be seen displaced to the outer side of the knee. There are severe pain and muscle spasm, and the knee cannot be actively extended.

Treatment. Reduction occurs automatically when the knee is extended, but sometimes an anesthetic is necessary to accomplish reduction.

When reduced, primary dislocations are immobilized in a well-molded plaster cast from the ankle to the groin. This cast should be worn about four weeks. After this, an elastic support with stays should be worn for another two or three weeks.

In the habitual type, some form of operative fixation is necessary. The commonest methods are (1) transference of the patella tendon and its bony attachment inward on the tibia to create a direct-line pull, (2) osteotomy and wedging to deepen the femoral groove if it is shallow, and (3) tendon or fascia lata fixation of the patella to the inner condyle of the tibia.

Fracture and dislocation of tibia below knee (bumper fracture)

Cause. Usually direct violence is the cause of fracture and dislocation of the tibia below the knee. They are frequently caused by a person stepping between two cars that are in motion toward each other and are commonly known as bumper fractures. Sometimes they are compound. The section immediately below the knee usually is involved.

Anatomy. The tibia is composed of two plates or surfaces that articulate with the two condyles of the femur. The knee joint has four important ligaments and two semilunar cartilages. The lateral ligaments protect the knee joint from any instability when it is completely straight. When it is extended, both lateral ligaments are tight and prevent any lateral motion of the knee joint.

The internal cruciate ligaments are those in the center of the knee joint and are designed to prevent the leg from displacing itself either forward or backward on the femur. To become acquainted with the direction of these ligaments, remember the direction of the anterior cruciate ligament by placing your right hand, with fingers spread, directly over the right patella when the knee is in flexion. The index finger will give the direction of the anterior cruciate ligament that goes from behind forward and is attached to the anterior tibial spine. The posterior ligament goes in the opposite direction—i.e., from the inner condyle of the femur backward to the posterior spine of the tibia. These four ligaments are responsible for the stability of the knee joint in all directions.

The test for injury or tearing of the

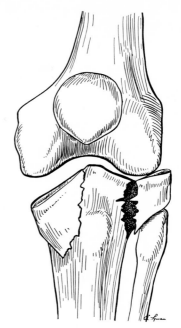

Fig. 222 Fracture of the condyles of the tibia into the knee joint. Open reduction was done.

anterior cruciate ligament is to force the knee completely straight into extension. The anterior ligament becomes tight, and hyperextension is not possible when the ligament is intact. If the ligament is torn, however, the joint may be carried to a position beyond 180°.

If the posterior ligament is damaged or torn or if there is a detachment of the ligament with a small amount of bone from the posterior spine of the tibia, the knee joint, when it is placed in a position of 90° flexion, may be displaced forward on the femoral condyles to the extent of one-half to three-fourths of an inch. Rotary motions are also increased.

The tendency for deformity is toward the collapsed or fractured side of the tibial condyles (Fig. 222). Should it be the outer condyles, there is a tendency toward the development of a knock-knee (genu valgum) deformity. Should it be the inner condyle, there is a tendency toward the development of a bowleg (genu varum) deformity. Both of these are preventable.

Problem. The deformed leg must be maintained in proper alignment to the normal leg, and normal joint motion must be reestablished at the earliest possible time.

Restoration of the most perfect contour of the joint surface is another important problem with which to deal.

Treatment. In most instances when there are fractures of the upper end of the tibia involving the knee joint, conservative treatment is best.

Conservative treatment consists first in the use of moleskin adhesive traction from the knee down, with 5 lb to 8 lb of weight. If there is a tendency toward knock-knee deformity, a sling may be arranged so that lateral traction may be applied at the inner side of the joint, using 5 lb to 8 lb of weight over the outer side of the bed. The side traction is flexible, as is the traction in the vertical line. Therefore, during the process of healing and repair, the patient is able to carry on motions that will greatly facilitate the speed of recovery of joint motion. In all fractures involving any joint, the patient or his relatives should be advised of the possible difficulties in reestablishing joint motion.

In spite of the fact that the knee joint is a weight-bearing joint, the results of fractures into the knee joint are often more favorable than might be expected from the severity of the fracture affecting it.

It is sometimes necessary, because of the interposition of small fragments between the main fragments of the condylar fractures of the tibia, to perform an operation in which the area is approached, the fragments are removed, and the condyles are brought together in the best possible alignment of the joint surface. Occasionally, it may be necessary to employ a threaded bolt that penetrates both condyles and buckles them together by means of nuts properly arranged and properly designed to exert their pressure. The semilunar cartilages that are frequently mentioned in the literature as a source of trouble in these fractures seem rarely to be the cause of any serious trouble. The scar developed during healing usually anchors them sufficiently to assure future stability.

In some types, hospitalization time may be shortened by the application of a cast in an overcorrected position; e.g., if the inner condyle is fractured and there is a tendency toward the development of bowleg deformity, the cast can be applied in a position of knock-knee. If the opposite is the case, then the cast

must also be applied from high in the groin to the toes in a slightly exaggerated position of bowleg. In either case, the cast should be bivalved at an early period with daily motion of the knee joint. Throughout the course of treatment, positive active motion and a slight range of assisted passive motion should be practiced.

Healing period. In cancellous bone, such as that found in and near the joint, there is a stage of rapid primary healing, but the stability of the callus so formed is insufficient to withstand much strain in less than three or four months. This allows the early establishment of motion in the joint, but there is not strength enough for early stress, strain, or weight bearing without danger of the development of deformity.

Condylar fractures of the tibia may heal sufficiently within three or four weeks for guarded motion with a split cast. Weight bearing on crutches should not be undertaken until the roentgenogram shows a fair amount of union.

It is desirable at times, particularly when early weight bearing is necessary, to use a brace that extends from the ischium to the heel of the shoe with a strap on the inner or outer side of the knee joint (depending on the tendency toward deformity) to prevent abnormal strain.

From the industrial standpoint, it usually takes from four to six months for patients with this type of fracture to recover sufficiently to return to their normal occupations. The amount of permanent disability is variable. Many patients with severe fractures may return to their normal occupations without any permanent disability. In some, however, whether mildly or severely affected, there may be partial permanent disability and the development of traumatic arthritis.

If the ligaments of the knee joint are sufficiently damaged to create permanent instability of the joint and interfere with the normal function, it may be necessary to operate, using ligamentous structures, such as tendons or tensor fascia lata (from the outer side of the thigh), to stabilize the joint. The procedure requires hospitalization of a patient for 3 to 6 weeks.

Fracture of shaft of tibia

Cause. The cause of fracture of the shaft of the tibia may be either direct or in-

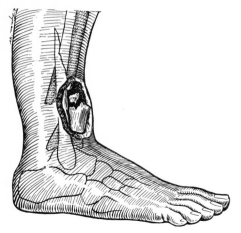

Fig. 223 Open fracture of the tibia and fibula at the junction of the middle and lower thirds.

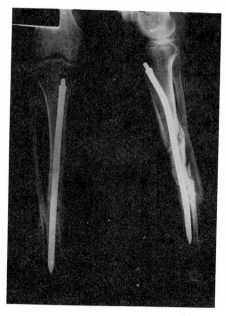

Fig. 224 Roentgenograms showing internal fixation of fracture of the tibia by insertion of an intramedullary nail (Lottes nail). Fracture of the distal third of the tibia is frequently complicated by delayed union or nonunion.

direct violence. When there is direct violence, the fracture may be open (Fig. 223). A twisting injury may cause a spiral fracture. Fracture of the tibia is one of the most common fractures occurring in automobile accidents, and the percentage of open fractures is greater than in almost any other region of the body. Fractures that occur in automobiles, industry, and war are most often caused by direct violence. The tibia may be broken by the direct impact of the penetrating force or may be broken in such a way that the points of the fracture penetrate the skin.

Anatomy. The tibia is the main weight-bearing bone of the leg. It is well covered with muscle tissue in the upper and middle parts, except over the shin, but sparsely covered with subcutaneous tissue and skin in the lower third. For this reason, circulation is poor and healing is slow. Nonunion is relatively frequent in the middle and lower portions. The relation of the planes of the knee joint and those of the ankle are important in reduction. The injured leg should be compared with the uninjured leg before reduction is attempted so that the proper position in regard to rotation may be obtained.

Problem. The problem depends largely on the nature of the fracture—whether transverse, oblique, or comminuted. The problem is to reduce the fracture and maintain reduction by the simplest possible means. Any deviation in alignment must be avoided.

Treatment. With the patient under anes-

thesia, simple transverse and many oblique fractures may be manipulated into position and treated in a long leg cast. Roentgenograms should be taken at frequent intervals during the first few weeks to see that slipping does not occur. If severe swelling should occur shortly after reduction, the cast should be split its full length and spread sufficiently to relieve circulatory embarrassment. It can be brought together again after swelling subsides.

If fractures of the tibia are difficult to hold in position, they may be treated by intramedullary nailing (Fig. 224), plating, or skeletal traction. In the oblique type, two or more screws may maintain reduction by transfixing the fracture site. In either case, a cast is used for immobilization during the healing period. The fixation apparatus is incorporated.

When nonunion occurs, bone grafting will usually stimulate union. The onlay full-thickness graft held in place by metal screws seems to be the most popular method.

Pott's fracture

Cause. A blow against the outer side of the ankle when the foot is in contact with

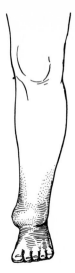

Fig. 225 Pott's fracture showing posterior and outward displacement of the ankle joint. Ordinary joint contours disappear.

the ground or twisting the ankle when slipping or falling may cause Pott's fracture (Fig. 225).

Anatomy. The ankle joint forms a mortise with the internal and external malleoli acting as stabilizing forces to prevent lateral motion. The astragalus acts as a gliding hinge against the lower articular surface of the tibia, allowing only plantar movement and dorsiflexion. All lateral movements occur in joints below the ankle joint. The classic Pott's fracture, frequently called trimalleolar, consists of a fracture of the internal malleolus and of the lower end of the fibula combined with a backward and outward displacement of the astragalus. Frequently, the posterior lip of the tibia (posterior malleolus) is also broken.

Problem. Proper alignment and contact of the various fragments must be restored by manipulation with the patient under anesthesia. The ease or difficulty with which this reduction may be performed depends on two main factors:

1 If the inner malleolus is fractured near the tip rather than at the base of the malleolus, the proximal portion can serve as a barrier against overcorrecting the fracture inwardly.

2 If the fracture of the posterior malleolus involves as much as one-third or one-half of the posterior surface of the tibial part of the joint, the difficulty in maintaining the forward reduction of the dislocation is very great and some form of open fixation is usually necessary.

Reduction. In addition to an accurate interpretation of the roentgenograms of Pott's fracture, a comparison between the fractured and unfractured sides should be made. In some persons the ankle joint and the knee joint work in the same plane, whereas in others the ankle joint may be outwardly or inwardly rotated. If reduction is attempted without taking this into consideration, the internal and external malleoli may not come in close contact at the points of fracture.

Treatment. Under fluoroscopic control, the fragments are manipulated into a position that gives the closest contact. This usually consists of forced inversion, dorsiflexion, and lateral pressure through the ankle to restore accurate contact of the internal malleolus with the astragalus and of the external malleolus with the tibia. A circular plaster-of-Paris cast is applied to maintain this position and must extend from the toes well up on the thigh with the knee moderately flexed in order to maintain the corrective amount of rotation. When the fracture line of the internal malleolus is at the same level of the joint surface or above it, fixation of the internal malleolus by nailing may be necessary.

Healing period. Healing usually requires from eight to twelve weeks. As a rule, the portion of the cast above the knee may be removed at the end of eight weeks, and frequently the lower portion of the cast may be bivalved for daily motion at the same time.

When the fracture is the stable type, weight bearing with the use of a walking iron or similar device incorporated into the cast may be begun as early as four to six weeks. There may be some permanent disability as a result of traumatic arthritis in the ankle joint.

Nursing intervention in fractures of bones of lower leg

Nursing care of a simple fracture of either or both bones of the lower leg after reduction has been obtained and a cast applied presents no very troublesome fea-

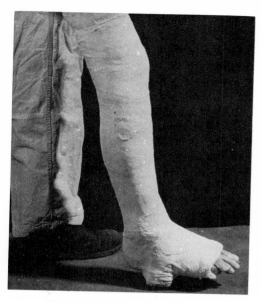

Fig. 226 Long leg walking cast.

tures to the nurse. If there is considerable swelling, the patient may be admitted to the hospital for a short period before reduction is attempted. Ice bags frequently are used to reduce edema. These bags should not be too heavily filled with ice, and air should be eliminated before the bags are closed. The pressure of several very tightly filled ice bags on a swollen and painful ankle has been known to cause great discomfort to the patient as well as considerable interference with circulation. Attention to the underlying skin to eliminate the danger of ice burns is important. Ice bags should not be applied without some material between the patient's skin and the rubber, even in an emergency. Heat usually is substituted for the ice after twenty-four to thirty-six hours.

Walking casts (Fig. 226) sometimes are applied for simple fractures of the leg in order to allow the patient to continue his normal activities. The manner of applying these casts varies somewhat in different clinics. Reinforcements on the sole either with additional layers of plaster or with some type of flexible wood may be used. Stirrups or walking irons of metal may be incorporated into the plaster on the plantar surface of the cast. The patient should wear some type of protective sock or cast shoe to keep the cast and foot clean.

Complications of open fractures

Tetanus and gas bacillus infection are two complications of open fractures with whose symptoms every nurse should be familiar. Gas gangrene will first be noted at the site of infection as local edema, discoloration, and puffiness. Increase of the pulse rate is a constant systemic manifestation. The complete clinical picture is one of severe localized pain, increase in the size of the limb, rise in temperature, continued acceleration of the pulse rate, and a general picture of severe illness. The coppery color of the skin, which caused Velpeau to name the disease bronze erysipelas, is a characteristic of a very advanced state. Crepitation, which is caused by gas bubbles beneath the skin, is usually present. After some trauma has broken the patient's skin, any of these symptoms is extremely grave and demands immediate surgical attention.

Fracture of astragalus

Cause. Usually indirect violence, such as landing on the foot in a fall, is the cause of fracture of the astragalus.

Anatomy. The astragalus articulates with several bones, and a large portion of its surface is covered by articular cartilage. The area in which the blood supply may reach it is therefore small. In many instances fractures will damage the blood supply to such an extent that healing is delayed. Disintegration of the bone through aseptic necrosis is not infrequent, or there may be nonunion.

Treatment. Perfect reduction of the fracture is essential. To maintain reduction, nailing or bone graft may be required. Occasionally, removal of the astragalus is indicated.

Immobilization in a plaster-of-Paris cast is advocated. The ankle should be placed in a right-angle position so that, if ankylosis should occur, the best function will ensure.

Healing period. Healing is slow, and weight bearing cannot be allowed until union is demonstrated roentgenographically. However, the cast may be bivalved in six to eight weeks, and some motion, heat, and massage may be started for the restoration of joint function. When the cast is discarded, the arch should be supported for weight bearing. Total healing may not occur sooner than ten to fourteen weeks.

Fracture of os calcis (calcaneus)

Cause. Direct violence, usually from falls in which the victim lands on his heels, is the cause of fracture of the os calcis. Frequently, these injuries are bilateral and may be associated with compression fractures of the spine.

Anatomy. The os calcis (or calcaneus) is composed almost entirely of spongy bone. When the outer surface is broken, the inherent strength of the bone is lost.

Displacements that occur from the injury are usually in three directions. Lateral compression shoves the fragments out under the external malleolus and tends to cause a flatfoot deformity. Upward displacement of the posterior portion tends to exaggerate the flatfoot tendency. This is increased by the pull of the Achilles tendon. Outward rotation also occurs.

In the usual anteroposterior and lateral roentgenograms of the foot and ankle, the true degree of displacement is not shown. This has led to disastrous undertreatment of these fractures. Because of their disabling effect, they are usually much more formidable than they appear. Therefore, roentgenograms should be taken from behind the leg at a 45° angle so that a true picture of the lateral displacement and outward rotation of the fragments will be shown. For this view, the foot is in complete contact with the x-ray plate.

Treatment. There are several methods of treatment, but the essential factor of all is that the bone be restored to as near its normal shape as possible. This requires lateral impaction of the fragments and downward displacement of the heel. The latter can be accomplished through lengthening of the Achilles tendon and downward replacement through leverage in skeletal traction. The arch must be restored and all corrections must be maintained by the proper application of a plaster-of-Paris cast.

Healing period. Weight bearing cannot be allowed in less than six to eight weeks and then only with the arch well supported to prevent weight being exerted on the os calcis. The degree of permanent disability is usually determined by (1) the extent of involvement of the subastragsloid joint, (2) the amount of residual lateral displacement under the external malleolus and against the peroneal tendons, and (3) the residual flattening of the longitudinal arch.

The rule in many clinics is that, if the pain persists beyond the six-month period, the accumulation of bone under the external malleolus should be removed and the subastragaloid joint, and possibly others, should be ankylosed by operation.

Fractures of metatarsal bones and toes

Cause. Usually, fractures of the metatarsal bones and toes are caused by direct violence.

Anatomy. The metatarsal heads comprise the anterior arch and one of the main weight-bearing surfaces of the foot. The muscles and tissues here are sparse. Restoration of length and alignment, therefore, particularly in the anteroposterior plane, are the main problems of reduction and treatment because a prominence of bone on either the plantar or dorsal surface of the foot could lead to irritation from weight bearing or shoes. The treatment following the necessary amount of reduction is usually the application of a plaster-of-Paris cast from the calf to the end of the toes. Skeletal traction may be necessary occasionally.

Healing period. These bones usually heal in about four weeks. After the removal of the cast, protection must be maintained for several weeks by the use of an arch support within the shoe and a metatarsal bar on the outside.

PHYSICAL THERAPY IN TREATMENT OF FRACTURES

Physical therapy after any type of fracture is recognized to be of great importance regardless of what type of reduction has been used. Although nurses will not be required to carry out these treatments as a rule, it is important that they have a good concept of the treatment and its purpose.

The main purposes of physical therapy after fractures are (1) to encourage absorption of traumatic hemorrhage and exudate, (2) to relax muscle spasm and thereby eliminate discomfort and possible deformity, (3) to promote normal circulation in the part and thus to hasten the healing process, and (4) to restore muscle tone and flexibility so that normal functioning is possible.

Muscle stimulation to encourage muscle contraction is usually part of the physical therapy program. This may be done through electric stimulation or through the patient's own voluntary effort (voluntary effort is usually considered preferable). Although this voluntary effort is possible even though the patient is encased in a plaster cast, many orthopedists provide some type of fixation that allows guarded use of contiguous joints while controlling the fracture site. Traction, hinged splints, or bivalved casts are particularly useful for this purpose.

Active or active assistive exercises with gentle stretching are frequently prescribed for the patient in traction or splints. It is exceedingly important during the first few weeks after fracture. Development of muscle power is recognized as essential if normal function is to be regained. The method of DeLorme, known as the heavy-resistance, low-repetition method, has worked well in the hands of experienced physical therapists.

Some type of apparatus to assist the patient in active exercise of the hip may be attached to the bed. This may consist of an overhead frame, skin or ankle traction, and a series of ropes or pulleys that permit the patient to exercise his leg in adduction, abduction, flexion, and extension. The patient is taught to do this by himself, although supervision of his activities is repeated at frequent intervals.

Unit III STUDY QUESTIONS

Mrs. S., a 77-year-old woman, has been admitted to the hospital following a fall in her home. She complains of pain in the hip region, and roentgenograms reveal a fracture of the neck of the femur.

1 Describe the typical position of the limb after fracture of the neck of the femur.
2 Moving this patient from the ambulance cot will cause increased pain at the fracture site. Describe the method of transferring the patient that will cause the least discomfort.
3 Traction may be applied to the involved limb.
   a What type(s) of traction will most likely be applied? Explain.
   b Describe desirable position of the limb following application of the traction.
4 Surgical treatment of this type of fracture usually consists of a closed reduction with internal fixation. Explain.
5 Review preoperative and postoperative nursing care of the elderly patient with a fracture of the hip pertaining to:
   a Prevention of pressure sores
   b Prevention of hypostatic pneumonia
   c Bowel and bladder problems
   d Bed positions and activity
   e Prevention of joint contractures
6 Explain or demonstrate method(s) of helping the postoperative patient from the bed to a chair.
7 a What is meant by "aseptic necrosis"?
   b If aseptic necrosis occurs, what surgical procedures may be performed to provide the patient with a functional hip?
8 Review the problems associated with providing continuous care for the patient after her discharge from the hospital. This may include provisions for care in a nursing home, an extended-care unit, her own home, or other available facilities. What financial assistance is available to the elderly individual pertaining to health needs?

Unit III REFERENCES

1 Anderson, H. C.: Newton's Geriatric nursing, ed. 5, St. Louis, 1971, The C. V. Mosby Co.
2 Attenborough, C. G., and Reynolds, M. T.: Lumbo-sacral fusion with spring fixation, J Bone Joint Surg [Br] 57:283-288, Aug 1975.
3 Bradley, D.: Fractures of the patella, Nurs Times 67:1531-1534, 9 Dec 1971.
4 Bradley, D.: Fractures of the ankle joint, Nurs Times 68:1115-1119, 7 Sep 1972.
5 Bradley, D.: Fractures of the pelvis, Nurs Times 68:376-378, 30 Mar 1972.
6 Bradley, D.: Fractures of the upper end of the femur. 1. Clinical features, Nurs Times 66:1523-1525, 26 Nov 1970.
7 Bradley, D.: Fractures of the upper end of the femur. 2. Treatment, Nurs Times 66:1552-1555, 3 Dec 1970.
7a Cave, E., Burke, J., and Boyd, R. (editorial board): Trauma management, Chicago, 1974, Year Book Medical Publishers, Inc.
8 Clissold, G. K.: The body's response to trauma: fractures, New York, 1973, Springer Publishing Co., Inc.
9 Connolly, J. F., and King, P.: Closed reduction and early cast-brace ambulation in the treatment of femoral fractures. J Bone Joint Surg [Am] 55:1559-1580, Dec. 1973.
10 Crenshaw, A. H., editor: Campbell's Operative orthopaedics, vol. 1, ed. 5, St. Louis, 1971, The C. V. Mosby Co.
11 Devas, M. B.: Stress fractures in athletes, Nurs Times 67:227-232, 25 Feb 1971.
11a Deyerle, W. M., and Crossland, S. A.: Broken legs are to be walked on, Am J Nurs 77:1927-1930, Dec 1977.
12 Farrell, J.: Nursing care of the patient in a cast brace, Nurs Clin North Am 11:717-724, Dec 1976.
13 Francis, Sister M.: Nursing the patient with internal hip fixation, Am J Nurs 64:111-112, 1964.
14 Henderson, J.: Emergency medical guide, ed. 3, New York, 1973, McGraw-Hill Book Co.
15 Hogan, K. M., and Sawyer, J. R.: Fracture dislocation of the elbow, Am J Nurs 76:1266-1268, Aug 1976.
16 Holdsworth, F.: Fractures, dislocations, and fracture-dislocations of the spine, J Bone Joint Surg [Am] 52:1534-1551, Dec 1970.
17 Laros, G. S.: Fracture healing; compression vs fixation, Arch Surg 108:698-702, May 1974.
18 Law, J.: Symposium on current surgical nursing: the fat embolism syndrome, Nurs Clin North Am 8:191-198, Mar 1973.
19 Lindh, K., and Rickerson, G.: Spinal cord injury: you can make a difference, Nursing (Jenkintown) 4:41-45, Feb 1974.
19a Louther, S.: Nursing care study: internal fixation of intertrochanteric fracture with complicating thromboembolism, ONA J 4:293-301, Nov 1977.
20 Marcus, N.: Fractures and dislocations of the spine, ONA J 1:94-95, Nov 1974.

21 Michele, A. A.: Principles of fracture care, Am J Orthop 9:34-37, Feb 1967.

21a Molyneux-Luick, M.: The ABC's of multiple trauma nursing, Nursing (Jenkintown) 7:30-36, Oct 1977.

22 Mooney, V., Nickel, V. L., Harvey, J. P., Jr., and Snelson, R.: Cast-brace treatment for fractures of the distal part of the femur, J Bone Joint Surg [Am] 52:1563-1578, Dec 1970.

23 Murray, D. G., and Racz, G. B.: Fat embolism syndrome (respiratory insufficiency syndrome), J Bone Joint Surg [Am] 56:1338-1349, Oct 1974.

24 Ryan, J.: Compression in bone healing, Am J Nurs 74:1998-1999, Nov 1974.

25 Sarmiento, A.: Functional bracing of tibial and femoral shaft fractures, Clin. Orthop. 82:2-13, Jan-Feb 1972.

26 Schneider, F. R.: Handbook for the orthopaedic assistant, ed. 2, St. Louis, 1976, The C. V. Mosby Co.

27 Slater, R. R.: Triage nurse in the emergency department, Am J Nurs 70:127-129, Jan 1970.

28 Sproul, C. W., and Mullanney, P. J. (editors): Emergency care, St. Louis, 1974, The C. V. Mosby Co.

29 Stauffer, E. S., and Kelly, E. G.: Fracture-dislocations of the cervical spine, J Bone Joint Surg [Am] 59:45-48, Jan 1977.

30 Stein, A. M., Mandell, D., and Ferguson, J.: Multiple fractures: look out for those pulmonary complications, Nursing (Jenkintown) 4:26-32, Nov 1974.

31 Thomas, J. E., and Ayyar, D. R.: Systemic fat embolism, Arch Neurol 26:517-523, Jun 1972.

32 Todd, R.: Fractures of the femur, Nurs Mirror 144:62-63, 17 Mar 1977.

33 Tronzo, R., editor: Symposium on fractures of the hip. Part I, Orthop Clin North Am 5:477-665, Jul 1974.

34 Wagner, M. M.: Assessment of patients with multiple injuries, Am J Nurs 72:1822-1827, Oct 1972.

35 Webb, K. J.: Early assessment of orthopedic injuries, Am J Nurs 74:1048-1052, Jun 1974.

36 Wells, L. B.: Seven steps to take in orthopedic emergencies, RN 37:OR14 passim, Oct 1974.

37 Whitehead, D. J.: Emergency care in orthopedic injuries, Nurs Clin North Am 8:435-440, Sep 1973.

38 Wray, G.: Injuries of the spinal cord: primary nursing management, Nurs Times 70:663-666, 2 May 1974.

12 Congenital deformities

Deformities that are present at birth are considered congenital. They may follow hereditary patterns or be the result of embryologic defects.

It is estimated that 2% of newborn infants have congenital malformations. Only 25% of the cases are of genetic origin, whereas 75% are the result of external factors influencing an originally healthy ovum. The importance of these external factors became evident when it was found that a woman who develops rubella in the fifth week of pregnancy may give birth to a child with cataracts. Rubella contracted in the ninth week of pregnancy may lead to lesions of the inner ear, and if the disease is contracted between the fifth and tenth weeks of pregnancy, the infant may be born with cardiac deformities. The administration of Thalidomide, a sedative, to pregnant women resulted in many of their children being born with multiple congenital deformities, especially phocomelia.

Congenital malformations resulting from external factors do not depend merely on the nature of the causative agent but more on the stage of pregnancy at which the agent acts on the embryo and on the vulnerability of certain cells in the embryo. Poisons or parasites, such as in toxoplasmosis, can produce ocular and/or neural lesions. Roentgen rays or irradiation from radioactive substances can cause anencephaly, exencephaly, hydrocephalus, and ocular anomalies. Irradiation late in pregnancy may cause spina bifida, velum palatinum fissures, and limb malformations of all types. Avitaminosis, particularly a deficiency in vitamins A, E, or B_2 (pantothenic

acid deficiency)—whether caused by a lack of supply, a lack of absorption, or the presence of substances that impede normal utilization—can result in malformations. Many of the progesterones (4-pregnene-3, 20-dione) can lead to virilization in female fetuses. They may cause total or partial fusion of the labia majora, hypertrophy of the clitoris, or opening of the ureter into the vagina. More than four hundred drugs are known to have teratogenic effects in animals, but only a few of these drugs can cause malformations in human beings. It is important when treating a pregnant woman to prescribe only those drugs that are imperative to her well-being, such as insulin, cortisone, and isoniazid.

The types and variations of deformity are almost limitless. Many deformities, however, are not disabling. Those encountered frequently will be described in this chapter.

The nurse's function in detecting and reporting congenital anomalies is an important one. Whether a hospital nurse working with newborn infants, a public health nurse giving instructions to a new mother, a nurse in the pediatric ward, or a school nurse, she will have opportunities to assess and evaluate for congenital abnormalities. To do this intelligently, a clear understanding of what is normal in the structure, function, and development of the child is required. In addition, a knowledge of the symptoms of the common orthopedic conditions found at birth is necessary. Abnormal conditions such as limitation of joint motion, excessively free joint motion, limpness or a disinclination to move a part, tendency to lie in one position constantly, alteration of body contours, or asymmetric folds in the skin should alert the nurse that something is wrong. Although most congenital deformities cannot be prevented, certain birth injuries sometimes can be averted by proper care during the prenatal period and delivery.

Advancement in medical science during recent years has provided knowledge about some of the external factors that influence the developing fetus and result in malformation. Again, with proper prenatal care, the known hazards can be avoided. Amniocentesis makes it possible to detect some genetic defects that may be present in the developing fetus. This procedure may be indicated when there is a history of birth defects in one of the parents. Health workers should use their influence to see that all pregnant women are given good care.

Not all congenital anomalies are detected in the newborn infant or very young child. The child may have reached school age before an abnormality is noted. Sometimes the condition will be manifest only when the child is tired, and then a slight limp or alteration in gait will be detected.

The importance of early recognition, of course, is that it makes early treatment possible. Early treatment is paramount in the management of these patients. Delay may make any attempted treatment only palliative. The nurse should realize this factor in order to help the family understand the necessity for securing immediate treatment. Strong emotional reactions often accompany this kind of condition. Parents may experience shame, pride, despair, or bewilderment. The nurse should appreciate their feelings and lend them support through sympathetic understanding and informed commonsense.

Congenital dislocation of hip

The term congenital dislocation of the hip implies that the head of the femur is outside the confines of the acetabulum at birth. Actually, there are degrees of dislocation, from incomplete to complete, and these are identified by definite terms.

Subluxation, or *predislocation,* is an incomplete dislocation. This is more common than dislocation and is more difficult to detect. If untreated, however, many sub-

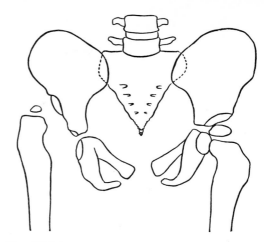

Fig. 227 Line tracing of a roentgenogram of congenital dislocation of the right hip. There is upward and backward displacement of the head of the femur, as well as thickening at the base of the acetabulum (prenatal). Note on the involved side that the femoral head is small and that the acetabulum is shallow with a sloping roof.

luxations eventually result in complete dislocations, and for this reason their early recognition assumes importance.

The exact cause of congenital dislocation is unknown, but the defect is primarily improper development of the acetabulum. This does not cause symptoms. However, the condition should be suspected when certain signs are present (Fig. 227) and then verified by a roentgenogram. Limited abduction of the hip in the flexed position and/or a click sign (Ortolani sign) when the hip is being abducted are the most useful objective findings. A positive Ortolani sign means that the dislocated femoral head can be relocated in the acetabulum easily and without pain or discomfort to the baby. As the head of the femur slips into the acetabulum, a click is audible or palpable. Treatment by means of a Frejka pillow splint should be instituted immediately.

Congenital dislocation refers to those cases in which there is an actual complete dislocation. This can occur during intrauterine life or result from an untreated subluxation sometime after birth. In either case, it demands early recognition and treatment to obtain a satisfactory result.

The signs of congenital dislocation vary

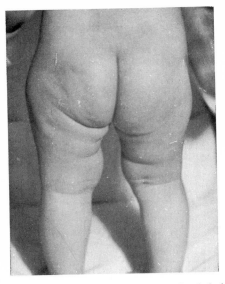

Fig. 228 Congenital dislocation of the left hip. Note the prominent trochanter on the affected side and asymmetry of the gluteal folds.

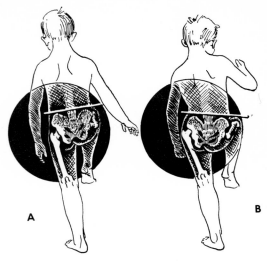

Fig. 229 A, Negative Trendelenburg sign. When the body weight is placed on the normal limb (stable hip) and the opposite limb is elevated, the pelvis rises on the side of the lifted limb. B, Positive Trendelenburg sign. When the body weight is placed on the unstable hip (as in congenital dislocated hip) and the opposite limb is elevated, the pelvis drops on the side of the lifted limb.

with the age of the child. Walking is often delayed, and the mother may have noted an extra gluteal fold on the affected side. Occasionally it is brought to attention by a shortness of the leg, an unusually broad perineum (especially in bilateral cases), or an unusually prominent trochanter (Fig. 228). Should dislocation be unrecognized until walking begins, the most obvious sign will be a Trendelenburg gait. On examination it is usually apparent that the affected leg is shorter, the range of hip motion is freer than normal, there is lack of stability on the push test, and the trochanter is higher than normal. When standing, the child will demonstrate a positive Trendelenburg test, which is indicative of an unstable hip joint (Fig. 229). When the body weight is put on the normal or stable hip and the affected limb is elevated, the pelvis on the side of the dislocated hip rises (this is true with normal hip joints). However, when the body weight is taken on the dislocated hip and the normal limb is elevated, the pelvis drops on the side of the normal limb. To compensate for the pelvic drop, the body shifts to the opposite side to maintain balance.

Treatment must be started immediately after the diagnosis is made. The aim is to reduce the dislocation to a normal posi-

tion. This is ordinarily accomplished by a closed manipulation while the patient is under anesthesia. The reduction must then be maintained for sufficient time to allow the acetabulum to develop to a point at which it will maintain reduction. This may require months, during which time the hip will be immobilized in a plaster spica cast. The surgeon in charge will vary the position to obtain proper placement of the femoral head within the acetabulum. Various splints are available as substitutes for plaster casts and have the advantage of being removable. These are more applicable in the later stages of treatment.

Operative reduction is necessary when closed manipulation has failed to correct the dislocation. The after treatment is similar to closed reduction, both in time required and in type of fixation apparatus.

When treatment is begun early (within the first eighteen months of life), the outcome usually will be excellent. A few patients treated early and many treated late will show degenerative changes of the hip by the time they reach middle age. These degenerative changes cause painful disabil-

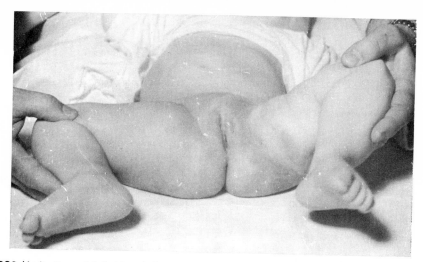

Fig. 230 Limitation of left hip abduction in an infant with congenital left hip dislocation.

ity sufficient to require further treatment. For the details of treatment at this stage, as well as for unreduced dislocations found in adults, see under arthroplasty in Chapter 20.

Nursing intervention. It is hardly possible to overestimate the importance of early recognition of congenital dislocation of the hip joint. In the newborn infant, there is more cartilage in the joint area, and the joint structures, including muscles, ligaments, and joint capsule, are more pliable. These factors make reduction easier. Early reduction (placement of the femoral head in the acetabulum) provides for deepening of the acetabulum and molding of the head of the femur as the infant's activities increase and growth takes place. These processes are important for the development of a normal hip joint. If reduction is not accomplished early, the acetabulum and the femoral head and neck become malformed. This makes later treatment more difficult and lengthy. The possibilities of a perfect result diminish rapidly as the child grows older.

When examining an infant's hip joint for dislocation, careful evaluation of hip motion is important. Limited abduction is of particular significance. To evaluate abduction motion, the baby is placed in the supine position and the hips flexed to approximately a right angle (Fig. 230). With the extremities in this position, gentle traction can be applied to abduct the thighs.

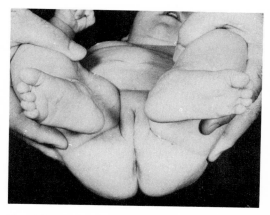

Fig. 231 Position of the examiner's hands for detecting the Ortolani sign (in a subluxated hip). As the thighs are abducted and upward pressure is placed against the greater trochanter, the femoral head is reduced and a click may be felt.

Normally the hips will abduct to 70° to 90° and the infant's thighs will almost rest on the table top. If limited abduction is present in either hip joint, additional diagnostic studies should be done to determine the position of the femoral heads.

With the baby in the position just described, the Ortolani sign may be detected. With gentle abduction of the thighs and upward pressure against the trochanter (Fig. 231), a click may be felt. The click indicates the head of the femur has been replaced in the acetabulum. Following this,

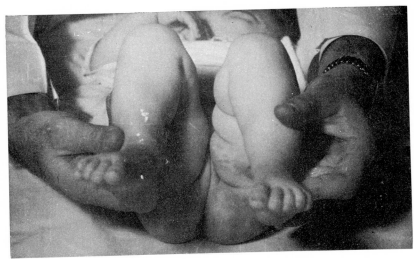

Fig. 232 Apparent shortening of the left thigh as the result of left hip dislocation. The left knee appears lower than the right, and two extra skin folds are present in the left thigh.

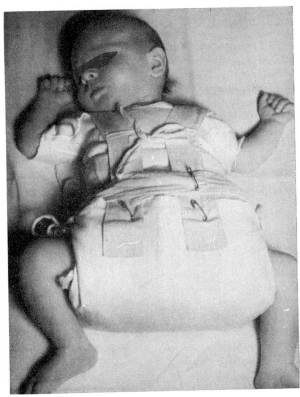

Fig. 233 Correct application of the Frejka pillow splint. The pillow maintains the thighs in flexion, abduction, and external rotation. It frequently is used for patients with mild hip dislocation or tightness of the adductors.

greater abduction of the involved limb is usually possible. (Gentleness when maneuvering the hip joint is imperative to prevent damage to the growth center.) The Ortolani sign is usually positive when subluxation of the femoral head is present. However, if a congenital dislocation is present, the Ortolani sign is negative. This means that reduction of the head of the femur in this manner is not possible.

When examining the hip joints, careful comparison of the leg lengths is helpful. Placing the infant in the supine position and flexing the hips and knees makes it possible to compare knee levels (Fig. 232). The apparent shortening of the limb is due to the fact that the involved head of the femur is not in the acetabulum but displaced both lateral to and upward on the ilium. The dislocated position of the head of the femur also may cause a discrepancy in the number or the depth of the thigh folds and can result in uneven gluteal folds. In addition, the greater trochanter may appear more prominent and higher on the involved side (Fig. 228). In bilateral dislocation, a wide perineum and broad buttocks may be apparent due to the position of the femoral heads.

When subluxation of the hip joint is diagnosed during the first few months of life, it is usually treated with a pillow splint (Fig. 233). This splint, which is held in place by a "romperlike" garment, is available in several sizes and consists of a square pillow (filled with kapok). Hospitalization usually is not necessary. The infant is fitted in the outpatient clinic with a pillow of the proper size, and the mother is taught the correct application of the splint. The pillow maintains the limbs in an abducted position, with the femoral head in the acetabulum. This position of the femoral head deepens the hip socket and promotes development of a normal hip joint. The splint is applied over the diaper and must be removed and reapplied each time the diaper is changed. The infant should wear plastic pants to protect the pillow from wetting and soiling; however, it is advisable that the mother have a second cover for the pillow to permit change and laundering. Care of the infant wearing a pillow splint is somewhat easier than that of one in a bilateral hip cast. The baby

can be picked up and moved with greater ease and, generally speaking, the mother is not so apprehensive as the one who must care for her infant in a hip spica cast. The splint must be worn until roentgenograms show a normally developed hip joint—possibly for a period of seven to ten months. The splint is worn continuously at first and then gradually discontinued for increasing periods of time. This should be carefully controlled by the orthopedic surgeon.

If the Ortolani test remains positive during treatment with a pillow splint, use of the splint will be discontinued and the baby may be fitted with an abduction brace (Fig. 234). This brace maintains the hip joint in an abducted and flexed position. It is worn continuously and, with the limbs fixed in this position, the femoral head is held in the acetabulum. The infant's skin must be cleansed beneath the splint and checked for signs of irritation. Plastic material may be used to provide some protection for the leather parts of the brace. However, frequent checking and keeping the child in a clean dry diaper are necessary to maintain healthy skin and a clean brace. The brace is worn several months. As with the pillow splint, the length of time must be carefully controlled by the orthopedic surgeon to ensure the desired result—a normally functioning hip joint.

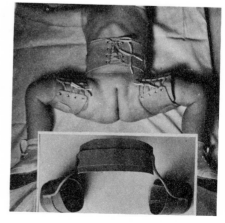

Fig. 234 Anterior and posterior views of the abduction brace used in the treatment of hip subluxation and dislocation.

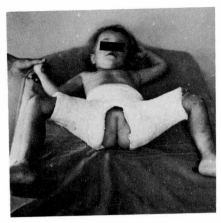

Fig. 235 Hip spica cast used in treatment of hip dislocation or subluxation.

When congenital dislocation of the hip (as opposed to subluxation) is diagnosed, closed reduction is the preferred method of treatment. Reduction is performed with the patient under anesthesia. The manipulation and manual traction used to reduce the congenital dislocated hip is gentle and involves little force. Prior to reduction, the child may be placed in traction for ten days to two weeks. The traction helps to stretch the hip muscles, places the femoral head in a better position for reduction, and makes manipulation of the hip easier, with less likelihood of trauma to the femoral head.

Following reduction, the hip is held in a position of 90° flexion and 60° to 70° abduction by means of a plaster cast. Abduction of the thighs beyond 70° tends to increase pressure on the head of the femur and thus endanger the blood supply. Subcutaneous tenotomy of the adductor tendon also frequently is done to decrease pressure on the femoral head in the reduced position. The cast is very carefully applied and well molded to maintain the reduction. With the head of the femur well centered in the acetabulum, the hip joint is considered stable, and the cast is not extended to include the knee joint on either side (Fig. 235). However, the cast edges need to be trimmed carefully to prevent pressure in the popliteal region. If the hip is in an unstable position, the cast is extended to below the knee on the involved side (Fig. 236). It is not necessary to include the feet and ankles in the plaster cast.

The small child who has had a closed reduction usually is hospitalized twenty-four hours or less. Prior to discharge, the edges of the cast are trimmed and finished with tape and plaster splints (see Chapter 6). If this is the first time the infant has been placed in plaster, the parents will need considerable reassurance and help pertaining to his care. They should be carefully instructed in the care of both the patient and the cast. Such instruction cannot be given hurriedly if the child is to have adequate care.

The parents should have an opportunity to observe the nurse as she finishes the cast edges and applies protective material to prevent wetting or soiling of the cast. An additional supply of the waterproof material should be sent home with the family. A perineal pad made from a folded regular or disposable diaper is tucked under the cast anteriorly and posteriorly. A second diaper is used to anchor the pad and to provide cover for the child. The mother should understand that prompt changing of the wet or soiled diaper is very important in the maintenance of a clean and intact cast. A urine-soaked cast not only is foul smelling, but also may become soft, and thus provide inadequate immobilization for the hip joint. A hair dryer can be used to dry a damp cast. The parents should be instructed to return the child to the hospital or clinic immediately if the cast is broken and not wait until the next appointment date.

The first twenty-four to forty-eight hours following application of the cast is usually an unhappy time for the small child. Restriction of movements, which the patient does not understand, is frustrating to him. He reacts by crying. This is upsetting to the parents, who already are bewildered by the thoughts of caring for their baby in a cast. However, after the first several days, the small child should be quite comfortable in the cast, and normal eating, sleeping, and play activities should be resumed. Nurses should bear in mind that most mothers tend to be afraid of damaging the cast. It is essential that they realize that it is possible to give the child wholly adequate care. Methods of keeping the

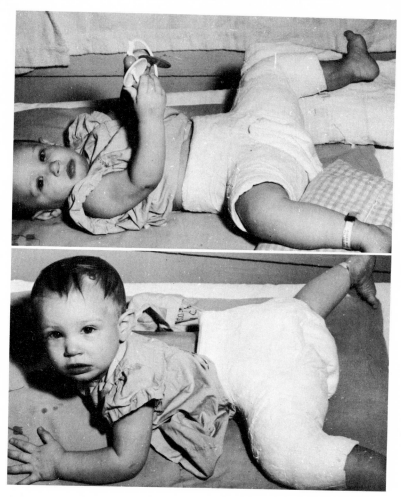

Fig. 236 Anterior and posterior views of a 9-month-old infant with hip spica cast applied after reduction of congenitally dislocated left hip. The cast maintains the hips in positions of flexion and abduction. Edges of the cast have been covered with tape. Strips of protective material will be applied about the perineal and buttocks regions prior to the patient's discharge from the hospital.

cast clean and dry and of caring for the skin beneath the cast should be demonstrated. The necessity of using the fingers to clean under the cast must be particularly emphasized. Many times sores near the edges of the cast, where they should be discovered without difficulty, are overlooked. The mother must be instructed to observe signs that the child is growing too large for his cast, and the freedom the child is to be allowed should be discussed. Most surgeons permit the child to stand or even walk in the crib if he so desires. Sitting astraddle a chair or some kind of

kiddy car usually is permitted (Figs. 237 and 238).

Proper placement of pillows to provide correct support for the limbs and to prevent pressure from the cast edges should be explained. In the supine position, placing the pillows so as to support the child's shoulders and back slightly higher than the pelvis will help maintain a dry cast by preventing urine from running under the posterior aspect of the cast (Fig. 239). Observations to detect swelling, discoloration, or lack of motion are important. Active use of the joints not immobilized is

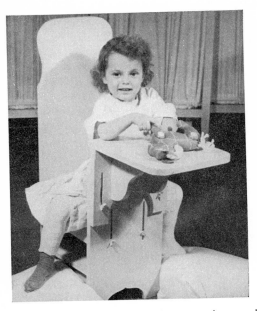

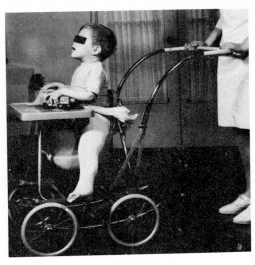

Fig. 237 Adjustable chair that can be used by a child in a hip spica cast after reduction for congenital dislocation of the hip.

Fig. 238 Use of a go-cart equipped to support the child in a hip spica cast in an upright position. In addition to facilitating his care, this position permits him to do many things that would be impossible in a horizontal position.

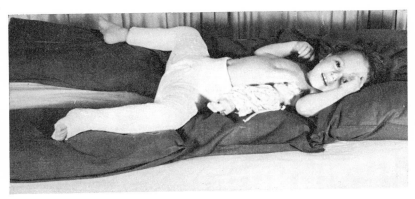

Fig. 239 Arrangement of rubber-covered pillows to support the patient in a hip spica cast. Note the space left for the bedpan and for a folded diaper across the perineum. The head of the bed may be elevated slightly to help prevent wetting of the cast.

encouraged. Normally the small child will use all joints not restricted by the cast. With the surgeon's permission, simple exercises to prevent atrophy and loss of function in the feet can be taught. Usually, dorsiflexion and inversion exercises will be prescribed.

When possible, a public health nurse should be notified of the homecoming of a child who has had a hip reduction in order to be able to assist the mother dur-

ing the first daily bath and to answer any questions that may arise.

After approximately one month, the child is returned to the clinic and roentgenograms are taken (through the cast) to check the position of the femoral head. If the position is satisfactory, the cast is worn for another two or three months. If the knee was enclosed in plaster, the cast may be cut to allow for knee motion. Crawling and active use of the limbs, within limitation of the cast, are encouraged. When the cast is removed, an abduction brace usually is prescribed (Fig. 234). This brace maintains the hip in the same position as the plaster cast and is worn full time until roentgenograms show good acetabular development. At this time, the brace is removed for several hours daily, permitting the child free use of his limbs. The time without the brace is gradually increased, and within several months the child will be able to stand and start walking. An abduction brace frequently is ordered to be worn at night for several years to help maintain a well-developed acetabulum and to prevent a subluxation of the femoral head. The child should be examined by the orthopedic surgeon at frequent intervals to permit early detection of undesirable changes in the hip joint.

If the anomaly of the hip is not detected during the first couple of years of life, other symptoms, with which the nurse should be familiar, become apparent after weight bearing is established. Walking usually is delayed for two to three months, and the gait of the child with a unilateral dislocation is that of an asymmetric limp, while the child with bilateral dislocations has a symmetric limp known as a waddling gait. The limp and the waddling gait are due to the instability of the hip joint(s) and the altered function of the hip abductor muscles (see Trendelenburg sign and Fig. 229). Even a slight asymmetry of gait in the small child should be evaluated carefully and roentgenograms of the pelvis obtained to rule out the possibility of a dislocated hip.

In addition to the abnormal gait, the buttocks and perineum may seem abnormally broad, and there will be lumbar lordosis accompanied by a protuberant abdomen (Figs. 240 and 241). By the time the child is 10 or 11 years of age, the lordosis usually has become very marked and unsightly; also, scoliosis may have developed if the dislocation is unilateral. There will be shortening of the limb and often an adduction deformity of the leg. When this stage is reached, great difficulties stand in the way of treatment, but much can still be done to ensure the child a fairly stable hip and to reduce the possibility of arthritis and allied conditions in later life.

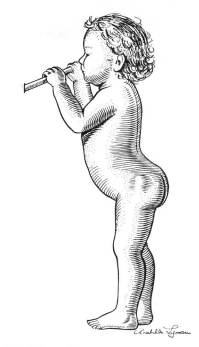

Fig. 240 Bilateral congenital dislocation of the hip in the older child. Note prominence in the gluteal region and swayback. The swayback position compensates for the backward displacement of the hips.

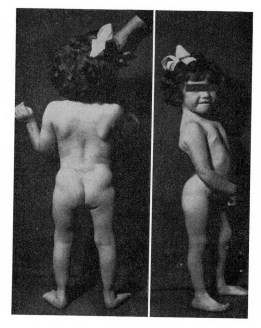

Fig. 241 Bilateral dislocated hips in the older child. Note the marked lumbar lordosis, protruding abdomen, wide perineum, and prominent trochanters.

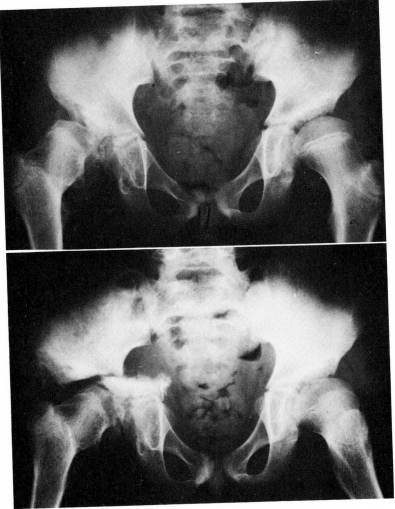

Fig. 242 Preoperative and postoperative roentgenograms of a congenitally dislocated right hip in an older child treated with a Chiari osteotomy of the ilium.

Treatment of congenital dislocation of the hip in the older child varies somewhat according to the age at which the diagnosis is made and the kind of dislocation present.

Open reductions are frequently necessary to supplement the closed reduction. Palliative operations, such as shelving operations and the various types of osteomies (Chapter 20) may be necessary if both closed and open reductions fail.

Traction frequently is used preparatory to open reduction or other surgery on congenital dislocation of the hip in the older child. It has been found that this proce-

dure will shorten the time necessary for reduction while the child is under anesthesia and often will eliminate the use of undue force in placing the head of the femur in the acetabulum. The purpose of traction is to bring the head of the femur down to the level of the acetabulum.

Open reduction of the hip and osteotomies (Figs. 242 and 370) or other reconstructive surgery may be attended by a certain degree of shock during the first twenty-four hours after surgery. Replacement of lost blood and the administration of intravenous fluids are usually needed, and careful monitoring of the vital signs is important. Immobilization usually will involve the use of a hip spica cast, and the nursing care the child receives may do much to determine the success or failure of the treatment. Following surgery, the cast must be worn for several months, and careful instruction of the parents pertaining to the home care of the child is important. Follow-up visits from the public health nurse are important to the family caring for a child in a hip spica cast.

Congenital clubfoot

Congenital deformities of the foot are of many kinds and are primarily hereditary since they can frequently be traced through several generations. The typical clubfoot (Fig. 243) is composed of three main elements of deformity, i.e., equinus, varus, and forefoot adduction, and is known by the common term "talipes equinovarus," which was derived from the Latin.

Intrauterine positions of the foot can easily be mistaken for true clubfoot deformity, but examinations will reveal the difference. A true clubfoot cannot be passively corrected to a neutral position in all elements of deformity, whereas an apparent positional deformity corrects itself quite readily. Treatment should begin immediately after a true clubfoot is known to exist, whereas no special treatment is necessary for a positional clubfoot. The same holds true for other foot deformities, such as pes adductus and talipes calcaneovalgus (Figs. 244 and 245).

True clubfoot may be unilateral or bilateral and occurs not infrequently in association with other defects such as spina bifida and arthrogryposis. In any patient with clubfoot, therefore, other defects should be carefully looked for during examination.

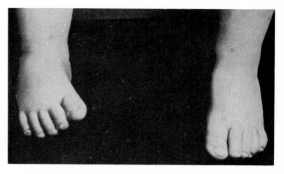

Fig. 244 Forefoot adduction (pes adductus) of the right foot.

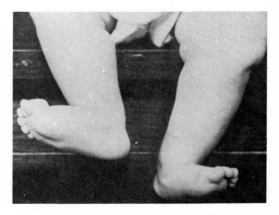

Fig. 245 Calcaneovalgus deformity of both feet. (From Kenney, W. C., and Larson, C. B.: Orthopedics for the general practitioner, St. Louis, The C. V. Mosby Co.)

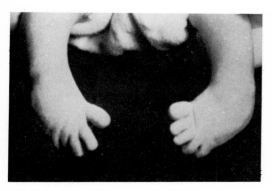

Fig. 243 Bilateral clubfoot (talipes equinovarus).

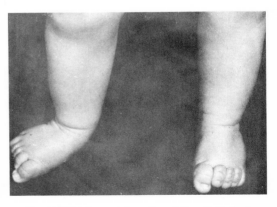

Fig. 246 Valgus deformity of the right foot.

Treatment and nursing intervention.
Treatment of a clubfoot is quite successful in most instances. The principle of treatment is to attain correction of all elements of deformity by manipulation and to maintain correction throughout the early growth years. This has been accomplished by various techniques, ranging from simple adhesive strapping to manipulation under anesthesia. Time and experience have taught us that excessive force can be harmful to the growing centers. The most common technique is the use of repeated manipulations and plaster casts. By this method the foot is stretched gently into a corrected position, and a cast is applied to hold the gain. This is repeated at intervals of a few days until correction is attained. Ten or more manipulations over a period of several months may be required. Weight bearing plus some type of retentive apparatus at night will usually maintain correction.

Many variations may be made in an effort to accommodate prolonged treatment to specific needs in each case. Frequently one element of deformity (viz., equinus) will be more resistant to treatment and will require special effort, even to the point of operative correction, Achilles tendon tenotomy or lengthening. In other instances, muscle imbalance will prevent maintenance of correction so that operative transfer of tendons, such as shifting the anterior tibial pull to a more lateral position, will be indicated.

In addition, it is important that these patients are followed until growth is complete to be certain that the deformities do not recur.

In no other congenital orthopedic condition are early recognition and treatment more important than in clubfoot. There is much cartilage in the foot of the newborn baby, and the soft tissues (tendons, ligaments, and muscles) are pliable. This means the foot can be manipulated and molded much more easily the first few months of life than later. The number of manipulations needed will be fewer and the prognosis for a normal functioning foot is much better when treatment is started in the first few weeks of life.

Although severe clubfeet are not likely to be overlooked at delivery, a mild involvement is sometimes not noticed for periods of weeks or months. Nurses in the delivery room and nursery should be especially observant of exaggerated attitudes in the infant's feet. It is not abnormal for an infant to lie with the feet slightly inverted; i.e., turned inward with the soles of the feet toward the midline of the body. The normal infant can easily assume and maintain the opposite position if slight manipulation is used. An infant with talipes equinovarus cannot maintain the everted position. Any indication, however mild, that the baby's ability to change the position of his feet is limited should be reported.

A few years ago considerable persuasion was sometimes necessary to convince parents that the baby with a clubfoot needed immediate attention. Although understanding is now more prevalent, the nurse occasionally will encounter parents who are extremely reluctant to begin early treatment. It will be necessary to help these parents understand the necessity for prompt treatment. Clubfoot is a condition of which control has been definitely established; i.e., the treatment is known, its results are almost certain, and the risk attending it is very minor. The orthopedic specialist talking to parents of infants with clubfoot first and foremost insists upon early treatment but also emphasizes continued treatment. Too often, following prompt early treatment and dismissal with apparently satisfactory feet, the doctor's insistent demand that the child be seen at frequent intervals for several years afterward is ignored. The deformity, like most congenital deformities, tends to recur. The child is then brought back to the clinic three or four years later with a badly deformed foot for which radical treatment is necessary. The watchword, therefore, is early treatment and prolonged observation by the specialist.

Forms of treatment include (1) manipulation and casting, (2) the Kite method, (3) the Denis Browne splint, and (4) braces and shoe corrections.

Manipulation and casting of clubfoot.
Correction of a typical clubfoot deformity (talipes equinovarus) by means of manipulation and casting follows an orderly plan. The forefoot adduction is corrected first, the heel (os calcis) varus next, and

the equinus position last. The latter usually entails a subcutaneous tenotomy of the tendon Achilles. Correction of each aspect of the deformity separately is necessary to prevent the development of a "rocker bottom" deformity of the foot, a position difficult to remedy.

The very young baby in the plaster cast (Fig. 247) should always have close attention. The danger or circulatory impairment is so important that it should never be overlooked. The foot should be inspected frequently for swelling and discoloration, as well as for motor and sensory changes. All toes should be visible. Sometimes the little toe is difficult to see. The cast is usually applied with the knee in a position of flexion, which prevents it from slipping downward—a complication that was common when it was applied only to the knee. Parents are warned about the necessity of closely observing the circulation when the infant in a clubfoot cast is taken home and are advised to call the physician if any question should arise about the circulation in the baby's foot.

Prior to leaving the clinic, some kind of waterproofing should be applied around the

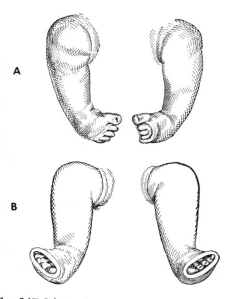

Fig. 247 Bilateral talipes equinovarus in the infant. **A,** Before correction. **B,** Undergoing correction in plaster casts. (From Raney, R. B., Sr., and Brashear, H. R., Jr.: Shand's Handbook of orthopaedic surgery, ed. 8, St. Louis, The C. V. Mosby Co.)

thigh edge of the cast. The edges must be carefully smoothed and taped to avoid irritating the soft skin of the thigh. Failure to protect this portion of the cast lessens its life considerably. A diapered child inevitably will wet the cast each time he voids (see discussion on care of casts in Chapter 6). An older child's parents must be warned that if the foot part of the cast gets soft and thin from wear, much of the correction so far attained may be lost.

Kite method. The Kite method consists of gradual correction that systematically deals with the different aspects of talipes equinovarus deformity. It is done by cast with a series of wedging maneuvers that seek to correct the adduction deformity of the forefoot first, then the inversion deformity, and finally the equinus deformity. From the standpoint of the nurse, the cast may seem simple enough. However, it should be kept in mind that each wedging is a threat to the patient's circulation. Night nurses especially should be solicitous about inspecting the child's foot after such wedgings. Considerable strain is placed on tendons, blood vessels, and ligaments after the equinus correction, which forces the plantar-flexed foot into a position of dorsiflexion. Undue pain or circulatory impairment should be reported at once.

Denis Browne splint. The Denis Browne splint works on the mechanical principle that it is possible to correct the position of one foot by means of the other. In this treatment, the muscles of the leg and foot may be used and strengthened while the deformity is being corrected, thereby eliminating some of the atrophy and joint stiffness that often occur when casts are used for correction. Many modifications of the original splint have been made, but the general principle remains the same. The splint is composed of a flexible horizontal bar attached to a pair of footplates. A device under the plates allows for rotation of the footplate on the horizontal bar. The apparatus is constructed so that each footplate is manipulated by means of the other (Fig. 248). Various means of securing the splints to the feet are used. Sponge rubber or felt is used to cover the footplates on the surface contacting the foot.

The technique of strapping the foot to the plate varies somewhat in different

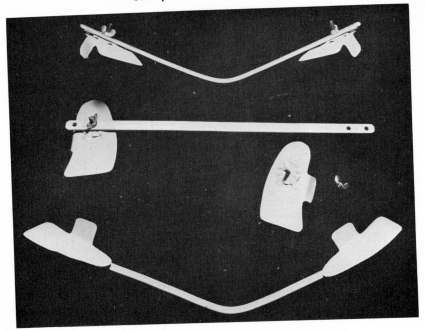

Fig. 248 Details of construction of Denis Browne splints.

clinics, but certain basic principles must be observed to assure the success of the treatment.

1 The skin of the foot must be inspected carefully to see that it is clean and free from abrasions. For the original strapping, the skin is prepared by washing and drying and may be painted with tincture of benzoin. For subsequent strapping, however, most surgeons prefer that the skin be left as it is.

2 There should be careful apposition of the foot to the footplate. The heel and sole must be held firmly to the plate; the sidepiece should contact the infant's ankle.

3 No wrinkles that might be the cause of pressure areas are allowed in the tape.

4 There should be no open spaces between the strips of tape, or window edema may occur.

During the period of correction, which may take from six to eight weeks, strapping is changed frequently, usually every five or six days. The child may be cared for at home if the parents can bring him to the clinic at the desired time for change of strapping.

After one or two strappings, the con-

necting bar may be straightened to the horizontal position. The feet will follow the position of the bar, and adduction and inversion will gradually be corrected until a neutral position is obtained.

In order to secure a valgus position, some orthopedists prefer to angulate the bar into a true V shape at the time the foot has reached the neutral position.

As treatment proceeds, effort is made to stretch the calf muscles. This may be done by increasing the V angle of the bar when the foot is in 90° of outward rotation. If the deformity is unilateral, the bar on the normal side is bent horizontally so that the normal foot is held in physiologic position at all times.

The more vigorous the infant's activity, the greater will be the correction; as he flexes one leg and extends the other, the foot on the flexed side is forced into a valgus position, which, of course, is the corrected position for varus deformity. Furthermore, with the foot in the valgus position, flexion of the knee will cause the foot to go into dorsiflexion, thereby stretching the posterior calf muscles. This is necessary for correcting the equinus deformity. It can readily be seen that with this treatment the infant provides his own correc-

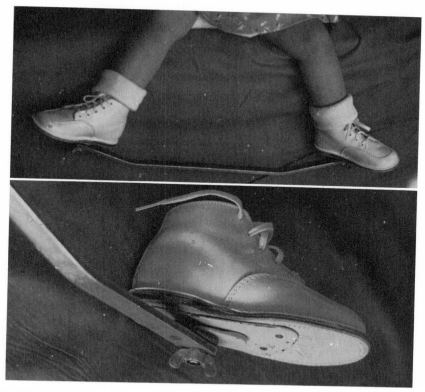

Fig. 249 After correction of clubfoot deformity, the modified Denis Browne splint may be prescribed to maintain correction. The splint is worn continuously at first and is gradually discarded as the child's activity increases and as muscles of the foot and leg become stronger. The desired position of the foot is controlled by positioning the abduction bar and by the screw mechanism that attaches the shoe to the bar.

tive manipulation by his normal activity. As little as five or six weeks of this activity may be sufficient to obtain correction, but maintenance of correction will require a far greater length of time. The splint may be used as described for five or six months, after which time shoes may be attached to the plates. After the child reaches walking age, alterations frequently are applied to the walking shoe. An outside wedge or patch of leather 3/16 in thick may be placed on the sole. This alteration aids in overcoming any tendency the child may still have toward adduction or varus. The physician sometimes prefers that the child wear a shoe without a heel in order to continue stretching the Achilles tendon. The night splint usually is continued for a year or longer even after the child begins to walk.

It cannot be overemphasized that the skin of a baby upon whom adhesive tape

is being used for any reason must be carefully watched for signs of swelling, excoriation, or blueness.

When the child is discharged from the hospital in the Denis Browne splint, some physicians instruct the parents to remove the plates from the bar once or twice daily in an effort to prevent pressure areas. The parents also are instructed to check the position of the baby's heel at frequent intervals. If the heel is found to be slipping up, the instructions usually are to remove the foot from the plate and to return the child to the clinic.

Braces and shoe corrections. When an overcorrected position of the clubfoot has been attained by the use of casts, the child is fitted with a splint designed to maintain the correction. This splint may be worn continuously at first and then discarded gradually as the leg and foot muscles be-

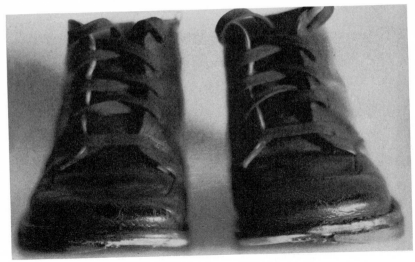

Fig. 250 Shoe corrections for clubfoot deformity. The elevation on the lateral aspect of the shoe sole helps prevent recurrence of the varus deformity. The importance of maintaining these shoe corrections cannot be overemphasized if recurrence of the deformity is to be prevented.

come stronger. The Denis Browne splint may be used for this purpose (Fig. 249). The footplates and abduction bar are fastened to the child's shoes. The position of the feet is controlled by the abduction bar and by the mechanism used in fastening the bar to the shoes. The feet usually are held in a position of abduction, eversion, and dorsiflexion.

Exercises may be prescribed by the physician and demonstrated to the parents at this time. Experience has shown that follow-up exercises are a most neglected feature of home care. These exercises, however, are important. They are not difficult to perform, and parents should be urged to continue them faithfully for the welfare of the child. A little time given to explanation will pay surprising dividends.

Shoe corrections (Fig. 250) may consist of an elevation to the outer border of the sole and heel. This will place the foot in a slightly everted position and aid in the maintenance of overcorrection. Here, again, the parents must be warned that the child should be brought to the clinic when the shoe corrections are worn down. It is disheartening to observe children returning to the clinic in shoes with run-over heels and worn-down corrections after a long and costly series of treatments by the orthopedist.

Treatment and nursing intervention for older child. The older child with recurrent or neglected clubfoot usually will require some type of operation. It is never possible to reconstruct the foot to perfect contour and function by surgery, but a good weight-bearing foot that will minimize the deformity usually can be obtained. In order to eliminate chances of disappointment after surgery, the parents and the patient should be given a realistic understanding of what the operation will accomplish. Only a careful explanation of the expected result, given before the operation is performed, will prevent disappointment.

Soft tissue procedures, such as tendon lengthenings, stripping of the plantar fascia, or capsulotomies, are performed for neglected clubfoot. Surgery on the bone may be required for maximal correction in some patients. These operations may be wedge resections, osteotomies, or astragalectomies.

On a busy orthopedic unit where major surgery is being done daily, the problems of this patient may seem of only minor importance. The risk is not minor, however, and the danger of congestion and hemorrhage is great. The patient usually will be immobilized in a cast extending to the thigh. To minimize swelling, continuous elevation of the extremity with pillows or a hammock is necessary.

The nurse should be alert for seepage of blood at the site of surgery and also at the thigh where the cast ends; frequently hemorrhage may be detected there. An overhead frame with a hammock to support the cast is the preferred apparatus for the support of the leg. Pillows may be used but are not so stable. Elevation is maintained usually about forty-eight hours but may be continued longer if congestion or pain is excessive. The nurse must heed complaints of the patient and interpret them intelligently. Knowledge of the line of incision is necessary in order to detect pain at other points where pain should not be present. A complaint of pain at the heel, the patella, or the dorsum of the foot is not an expected aftermath of such surgery and should be reported. When the surgeon has given an order to have the cast cut over any of these points, the cutting should be done at once—not at the end of the day, when it is easier to secure an orderly.

The three principal causes of failure in the treatment of clubfoot are (1) delay in beginning treatment, (2) imperfect nerve supply to muscles, as in conditions such as spina bifida, and (3) failure to obtain and maintain complete overcorrection of the deformity. Nurses will readily recognize their part in helping to eliminate at least two of these causes of failure—the delay in beginning treatment and the failure to continue medical supervision after correction has been obtained. Parents should be guided to the realization that follow-up treatment in clubfoot is as important as the active correction. They must have a clear understanding of their responsibility in this matter.

Torticollis (wryneck)

Signs and symptoms. At birth or shortly after, the child with wryneck may have a tendency to hold the head to one side. On palpation of the neck, a mass may be felt in the sternocleidomastoid muscle. There is limitation of motion in attempts to move the head away from the affected side.

Cause. The cause of wryneck is considered to be an engorgement of the muscle as a result of overstretching during the passage through the birth canal. Some observers hold to the theory that the affected muscle was inherently weak before birth.

Anatomy. When tearing occurs in the muscle, hemorrhage and extravasation of blood into the fibers take place. During the healing process, this undergoes organization and development of scar tissue. The scar so completely involves the muscle

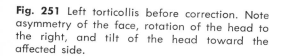

Fig. 251 Left torticollis before correction. Note asymmetry of the face, rotation of the head to the right, and tilt of the head toward the affected side.

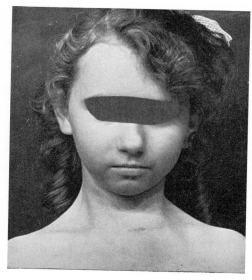

Fig. 252 Left torticollis after surgical correction. Same patient as shown in Fig. 251.

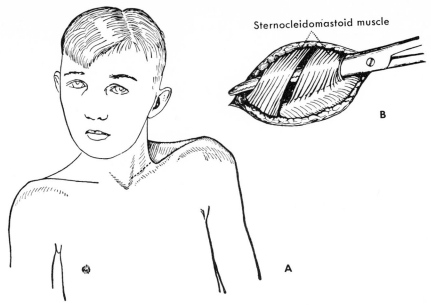

Sternocleidomastoid muscle

Fig. 253 Operation for torticollis. **A,** Line of skin incision. **B,** Clavicular and sternal attachments of the sternocleidomastoid muscle withdrawn from wound and divided. (From Crenshaw, A. H., editor: Campbell's Operative orthopaedics, ed. 5, St. Louis, The C. V. Mosby Co.)

fibers that elasticity is lost and contraction occurs. As the child grows older, this also leads to the development of a facial asymmetry (Fig. 251).

Treatment and nursing intervention. In most cases of congenital wryneck discovered shortly after birth, correction and cure can be assured within a month or two by the daily use of heat, massage, and carefully regulated stretching of the affected muscle.

In cases that have gone untreated or unrecognized, fibrosis takes place in the muscle and permanent deformity develops. Operative treatment is necessary (Fig. 252). This consists in the resection of the tendon of the muscle from both the sternal and the clavicular attachments (Fig. 253). Usually, about three-fourths of an inch of the tendon is removed.

There are various methods recommended for maintaining correction after operation, but probably the safest is the application of a plaster-of-Paris cast that covers the chest, neck, and head in an overcorrected position. This requires that the chin be brought high above the shoulder of the affected side.

The cast should be left on for approximately six weeks. After its removal a Thomas collar may be worn, and massage and stretching may be continued for several weeks.

Early recognition and treatment of torticollis are essential. It is now generally recognized that much facial and postural deformity can be prevented if conservative treatment is begun early. The deformity may be so mild at birth that it is unobserved or, if observed, may be considered something that, with function, the child will outgrow. As time goes on, however, the ligaments on the affected side become so shortened and twisted that facial deformity becomes pronounced. Very early in the child's life an elongated swelling may be noted in the lower half of the sternocleidomastoid muscle. It is quite tender at this time, and the child will cry if the swelling is touched or if the neck is stretched. Since the swelling and tenderness eventually disappear, the mother usually decides that there is nothing further to fear. Later, however, it can be observed that muscle tenseness exists. A band of fibrous connective tissue develops and, by contraction, pulls the head into the characteristic attitude: the ear on that side seems to be pulled downward toward the clavicle, and the face itself is turned in the opposite direction. When this condition is left without treatment, a slowly developing atrophy of the side of the face near the affected muscle will occur and become very apparent as the child grows older. This, of course, is followed by tissue changes. The soft tissues on the deformed side will become adaptively shortened. This is followed by certain definite bony deformities in accordance with Wolff's law.[*]

The nurse caring for a young baby should be alert to any signs of limitations of movement in the head or neck. Frequently, when the stage of tumor and tenderness is missed, the deformity may escape notice because there are no marked symptoms except this limitation.

In mild cases, after the stage of tumor and tenderness has passed, manipulation and exercise usually are instituted; often these alone will suffice to overcome the deformity. These manipulations should be prescribed and demonstrated to the nurse by the surgeon for each patient, and progress should be checked frequently by the surgeon to ensure proper results from the treatment.

Surgery usually is indicated if the manipulative treatment fails or if the child is not seen until he is 2 years or more of age. In severe cases, surgery is sometimes performed on the young infant, in which case one of the foremost nursing problems is to care for the baby properly in the traction apparatus.

When the child with torticollis is being prepared for surgery, it is necessary to shave above the hairline on the affected side. Specific instructions should be obtained as to the extent of the area to be shaved. When a young girl undergoes a tenotomy of the sternocleidomastoid tendon, it is possible to part her hair low on

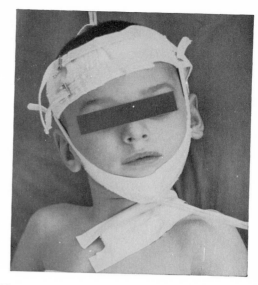

Fig. 254 Traction apparatus designed to maintain a position of overcorrection after surgical correction of left torticollis. Note that in the overcorrected position the chin points toward the incision and the back of the head is pulled upward.

the affected side, comb it to the opposite side, and braid it tightly.

Casts are not always applied immediately after surgery. Postoperative nausea and the possibility of respiratory embarrassment make it safer to apply the cast the following day. Some type of retentive apparatus may be used in the interval (Fig. 254). Head traction is difficult to apply and can be dangerous if it is done inefficiently, particularly in a young child. A flannel sling for the chin may be devised to exert head traction, but it must be inspected frequently lest it slip and impair the child's breathing. The amount of weight used will be ordered by the physician, but it is usually very little. Sandbags may be used to control the position of the head.

Traction of this nature may be worn for a week or two, after which a brace is often applied. This brace is usually one that comes well down over the spine and may be a Taylor body brace with some type of corrective chin apparatus.

If the cast is applied in surgery before the patient becomes conscious, considerable care must be exercised to prevent aspiration of vomitus. Suction apparatus must be available. The area around the

---

[*]Wolff's law: Every change in the form and the function of bones, or in their function alone, is followed by certain definite changes in their internal architecture, and equally definite changes in their external conformation, in accordance with mathematical laws. (Julius Wolff, 1868.) Briefly, the law may be remembered as "form follows function."

chin and mouth should be protected with pieces of waterproofing that may be tucked in until the cast is dry enough to finish the edges.

After the cast is dry, the scalp section of the cast will usually be cut out to permit care of the head, and constant attention to this area will be necessary to prevent itching and irritation from plaster crumbs. At feeding time it will be necessary to protect the cast with a towel or napkin to prevent food from falling inside. The ears must be inspected frequently to see that no plaster crumbs or pieces of food are lodged in them. The scalp and ears become sore easily when this type of cast is worn. These patients are soon ambulatory and are often left to care for themselves, but it must be remembered that careful supervision will be necessary daily to detect signs of skin irritation, pressure areas, or cracking and softening of the cast.

The cast may be kept on from six weeks to several months, according to the severity of the condition (Fig. 255). After it is removed, physical therapy will be ordered,

consisting of massage, manipulation, and exercises. These treatments may need to be continued over a considerable period, particularly in the older child. The parents should understand that torticollis cannot be completely corrected by surgery alone. A period of follow-up care under the supervision of the physician will be necessary. If the child is dismissed from the hospital soon after the cast is applied, the mother will need careful instruction in the details of caring for the patient and his cast.

Congenital elevation of scapula (Sprengel's deformity)

Symptoms and signs. In Sprengel's deformity (congenital elevation of the scap-

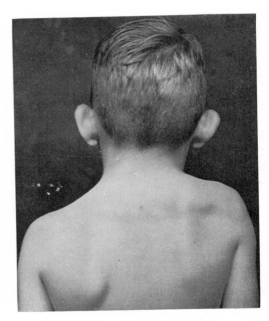

Fig. 256 Sprengel deformity.

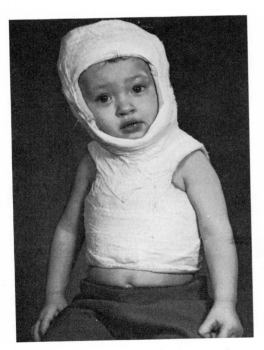

Fig. 255 Left torticollis. The position of overcorrection is maintained four to six weeks postoperatively.

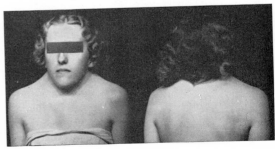

Fig. 257 Klippel-Feil syndrome. (From Kenney, W. C., and Larson, C. B.: Orthopedics for the general practitioner, St. Louis, The C. V. Mosby Co.)

ula; Fig. 256), one or both shoulder blades are high, and there is usually some limitation of the movement in the shoulder joints.

Anatomy. It is the opinion of most authorities that the term congenital elevation is a misnomer. The scapulae normally are high during the period of development but descend and rotate before birth. This deformity is, therefore, a failure of descent of the scapulae. It may be associated with other congenital deformities, such as abnormalities in the shape of the vertebrae, webbed neck or Klippel-Feil syndrome (Fig. 257), and possibly other deformities.

Treatment. The treatment of choice for congenital elevation of the scapulae is that recommended by Schrock. This consists in the complete subperiosteal and submuscular release of the scapulae, followed by rotation of the bone within this compartment to its normal position. Immobilization for a period of a few weeks follows, allowing reattachment of the periosteum. The scapulae are now in their normal position. In properly selected cases in younger children, this treatment gives complete correction of the deformity.

Absence of bones (tibia, fibula, radius, fingers, toes, etc.)

Clinical picture. A child may be born with whole extremities or parts of the extremities missing or with various bones missing. Extremities or digits may be partly missing, and there may be constricting bands or circular creases.

Causes. Absence of bones seems to be caused by the arrest of development during the early stages of embryonic growth.

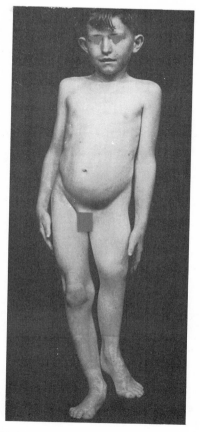

Fig. 259 Congenital shortening of the left femur.

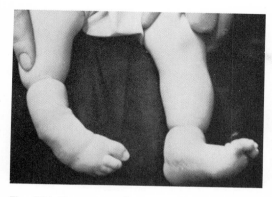

Fig. 258 Constriction bands and bilateral clubfoot. Constricting rings are a developmental defect composed of fibrous bands. The fibrous bands that encircle the limb may restrict circulation as the child grows and, if not excised, will cause a gangrenous condition. Surgery usually consists of a Z-plasty excision of the fibrous scar tissue and is done in two or three stages over a period of several months.

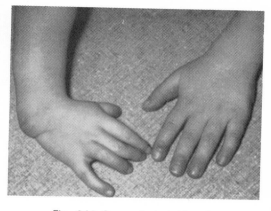

Fig. 260 Congenital clubhand.

The commonest site for circumferential constricting bands is the lower portion of the leg (Fig. 258). However, they may occur at other levels in either the arm or the leg. The severity of these bands varies. They may involve the deep fascia.

Anatomy. The deformity that develops from the absence of a bone is always characterized by loss of the propping or strutting effect of this bone. If a radius is missing, the hand is at a right angle to the forearm in a direction pointing toward the face (clubhand; Fig. 260). It is not unusual to find associated deformities such as absence of the thumb or bifid thumb (Fig. 261), cleft hand (Fig. 262), and presence of a cervical rib (Fig. 263).

When the absence of bones occurs where there is an associated bone, such as in the forearm or the lower part of the leg, the other bone usually becomes enlarged and frequently deformed. When there is absence of the tibia, the leg is usually shorter and the foot tends to turn inward and backward.

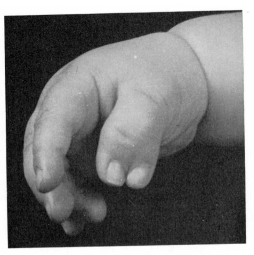

Fig. 261 Bifid thumb. Treatment consists of surgical removal of the accessory thumb.

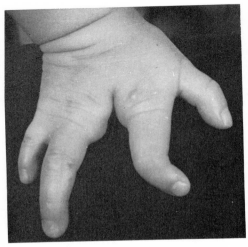

Fig. 262 A cleft hand. Many hands with this deformity are quite functional.

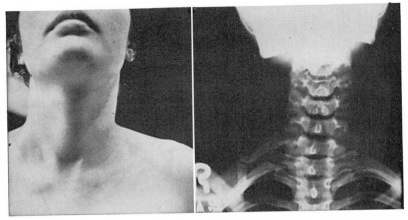

Fig. 263 Cervical rib. The presence of a cervical rib may produce pressure on the brachial plexus and thus cause a radiating pain in the upper extremity. This may be relieved by shoulder exercises and the use of a brace. In some instances, surgical resection of the cervical rib is necessary. (From Kenney, W. C., and Larson, C. B.: Orthopedics for the general practitioner, St. Louis, The C. V. Mosby Co.)

Congenital deformities of this type include limbs that are short and underdeveloped as a result of growth deficiencies. Occasionally, one leg or one arm will be underdeveloped so that it is only about one-half the length of the opposite one.

Syndactyly

Syndactyly is a congenital anomaly characterized by the webbing of two or more fingers or toes (Fig. 264). The web may be formed by skin alone or by skin and subcutaneous tissue, and in severe cases there may be bony fusion between the phalanges.

The treatment consists of surgical separation of the digits and skin grafting of the denuded areas with free full-thickness skin grafts. The commissure or deepest part of the web is fashioned with a flap of skin from the palmar or dorsal aspect of the web. After skin grafting, it is necessary to rigidly immobilize the digits spread apart in a plaster cast or splint for three weeks. The best time for surgery is during the second or third year of life.

Spina bifida

Spina bifida is a common term applied to a group of neurological problems that stem from a developmental defect and consists of incomplete closure of the spinal canal. The defect results in a lack of continuity of the bony ring that normally protects the spinal cord. If the defect is large, it may allow a herniation of the dural sac, which contains the spinal nerves. This herniation or sac is covered only by very thin skin, is present at birth, and is easily detected by inspection. Frequently there will be associated birth defects such as clubbed feet and dislocated hips. The

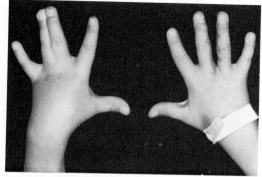
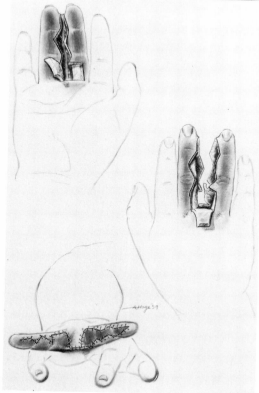

Fig. 264 A, Bilateral syndactyly of the middle and ring fingers, with surgical correction of the right hand. **B,** Schematic drawing of surgical correction of syndactyly of the ring and middle fingers illustrating the dorsal flap (at the base of the fingers) and the zigzag incision utilized to separate the syndactyly. The flap is used to produce a web between the involved fingers. In some instances, split-thickness grafts or full-thickness skin grafts are necessary to secure adequate skin coverage. If syndactyly involves both sides of a finger, only one side is corrected at a given time. This is necessary to prevent interference with the blood supply of the finger and the development of gangrenous tissue. Following surgery, a soft dressing and a plaster cast are applied in a fashion to prevent movement of the fingers. Careful postoperative vascular assessment of each digit is essential. Visualization of each finger may be difficult due to the massive soft dressing but is very necessary. If there is bony fusion of the fingers or discrepancy in finger lengths, the surgery is more difficult and the function and cosmetic results are poorer.

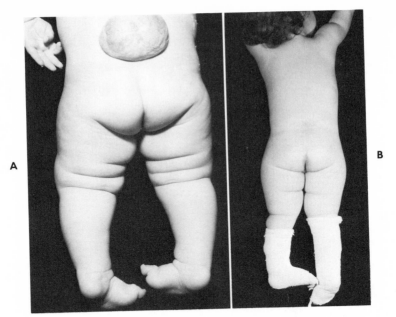

Fig. 265 A, Infant with meylomeningocele and associated clubfoot deformities (talipes equinovarus). **B,** Myelomeningocele has been surgically removed and the feet placed in a cast to correct the clubfoot deformity.

etiology of spina bifida is not understood. The defect develops during the first trimester of pregnancy. Although it usually affects the lumbosacral area, it may occur elsewhere along the spinal column.

Spina bifida occulta is the term applied when the defect is very minor and consists of an incomplete fusion of one or more of the vertebral arches. The patients usually have no residuals such as muscle paralysis, sensory loss, or other complications. A local defect over the involved vertebrae, such as a mild indentation or a localized tuft of hair, may be present. The patient will not recognize any limitations or problems. When the defect in the bony canal is accompanied by an outpouching of the meninges with cerebrospinal fluid, it is referred to as a *meningocele*. If this outpouching contains nerve roots and portions of the spinal cord, it is known as a *myelomeningocele* (meningomyelocele) (Fig. 265, *A*). When the defect is large and the cyst contains neural elements at birth, extensive paralysis and sensory losses usually are found below the level of the defect *(myelodysplasia)*. Frequently, the cyst is covered by only a thin layer of skin and

will become ulcerated easily if contact pressure is not avoided. If incomplete closure includes the vertebrae, the meninges, and the spinal cord, it is referred to as *rachischisis*. Spinal fluid may ooze from this fissure.

The majority of children with spina bifida and myelomeningocele will survive and will have varying degrees of motor paralysis and sensory loss below the level of the defect. This is the group that constitutes a real problem in orthopedic surgery.

Management of myelomeningocele requires the efforts of a team consisting of orthopedic surgeons, neurosurgeons, and pediatricians, as well as urologists, who are needed at a slightly later time.

From an orthopedic standpoint, those children with varying degrees of motor loss will develop distressing deformities such as dislocation of both hips, flexion deformity at the knees, and commonly bilateral clubfeet (Fig. 265, *B*). All of these deformities are difficult to manage, since there is an associated sensory loss in the skin over the same areas, with the skin consequently tolerating little pressure from external supports without the formation of trophic ulcers. In addition, these patients frequently have loss of control of the bowels and bladder.

In the first few months of life, hydrocephalus will occur in a large percentage of the infants with myelomeningocele. Obstruction in the circulatory pathways causes an accumulation of the cerebrospinal fluid and thus expansion of the cranium. For this type of patient, the neurosurgeon frequently provides shunts or artificial conduits from the ventricles of the brain into the subcutaneous tissues of the back or elsewhere to prevent the progression of hydrocephalus. Even though complications can be a problem with this kind of surgery, the procedure has contributed considerably to the survival of the infant with spina bifida. The neurosurgeon also has the choice of removal of the meningocele very early in life, and there is some evidence that this procedure may even prevent an increase of paralysis in the subsequent months.

The urologist is called upon with increasing frequency as techniques are being developed through which the urinary incontinence can be brought under control, either by urinary shunt operations of one kind or another or by continuous bladder drainage. Providing for an unobstructed outflow of urine early in the child's life is necessary to prevent renal damage. This requires very strict vigilance to guard against possible complications.

The orthopedic deformities (paralysis with resultant dislocation of the hips, flexion contracture at the knees, and clubfeet) are treated by various orthopedic means. At present, there is no one standard form of therapy that is applicable in all cases, since there is great variation in the amount of deformity, paralysis, and sensory loss. For the most part, the methods are similar to those discussed under the treatment for each of the individual deformities: clubfeet, dislocated hips, and flexion deformity of the knees. Operative procedures can be utilized if conservative means are unsuccessful. In spite of the sensory loss in the skin, the healing power following operation is quite normal.

The eventual goal of treatment is to provide these severely involved myelomeningocele patients with the ability to walk even though bilateral long leg braces may be required by those with severe paralysis. Even if ambulation is accomplished, the patients must be watched continuously for the advent of pressure sores, especially on the feet. In a few cases, pressure sores and other trophic disturbances develop to such a degree that amputations are demanded. Patients with myelomeningocele with deformities and loss of muscle function constitute a group of patients in whom nursing techniques and vigilance are perhaps more exacting than in any other patient with an orthopedic problem.

Nursing intervention. Infants with spina bifida and myelodysplasia usually are not seen first on the orthopedic service, since in the early stage such conditions are considered to be primarily pediatric and neurologic in nature. However, such individuals frequently spend much time on the orthopedic service. The infant with the milder form of spina bifida (occulta), who displays little outward manifestation of the vertebral cleft, may be admitted to the service because of clubfoot or some other deformity, but on the whole this patient does not present many problems in nursing care. It is the patient with sensory and motor involvement from some degree of cord destruction who will be considered in this discussion.

All of the problems of nursing care encountered in the patient with destruction of the spinal cord through disease, tumor, or trauma, accompanied by the inevitable group of symptoms engendered by this condition, are present in the paralyzed patient with spina bifida. The need to provide nursing care that will prevent or minimize the problems that confront such a patient is apparent. Urinary tract complications, trophic ulcers, and secondary contractures are perhaps the most serious of these problems, and they not only inhibit progress in rehabilitation, but also may be severe enough to pose a threat to the patient's life.

Trophic ulcers are a tremendous problem, complicated as they are by bowel and bladder incontinence. Trophic ulcers have all the menacing features common to pressure areas, and in addition the patient lacks sensation. He is completely unaware of the condition so that there are no warning sig-

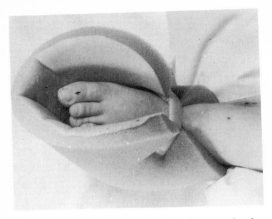

Fig. 266 A heel protector made from polyether urethane foam. Care must be exercised to avoid strapping the protector too tightly and thus restricting circulation. Also, because of body heat and perspiration, the protector should be used only intermittently to prevent maceration of the skin.

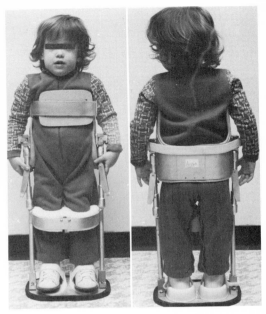

Fig. 267 Stability in the standing position is provided by this standing frame (podium) for the child with spinal bifida with complete paraplegia. The frame provides ankle, knee, hip, and trunk support. Being able to stand provides several benefits for the child. In the upright position, he can participate in more play activities and consequently is a happier child. In addition, the weight-bearing stress helps to prevent osteoporosis and the likelihood of fractures, and maintaining the erect position helps to prevent the development of hip flexion contractures and renal calculi.

nals of pain. Furthermore, lack of nutrition to the area, which is caused by impairment of the sensory nerve supplying the muscles and blood vessels in the part, makes healing difficult or impossible. The nurse should remember that in patients with trophic ulcers the blood vessels surrounding the area have become dilated through failure of the nerve supply that normally regulates blood flow. The blood tends to stagnate, causing the surrounding tissues to become ischemic.

These ulcers develop in the soft tissue over bony prominences. The ischial tuberosities and the sacrum are areas over which the skin and subcutaneous tissue frequently ulcerate. Also, the heels, lateral aspects of the feet, and skin over the malleoli are vulnerable spots. The ulcers develop in a very short period of time, are extremely slow to heal, and can lead to an osteomyelitis, which may necessitate amputation. Prevention depends primarily on relief of pressure on the involved area. This is accomplished by providing for a more even distribution of the body weight and by frequent change of position. The alternating pressure mattress is helpful in changing pressure points, and the use of sponge rubber beneath the hips and heels provides for a more even distribution of the body weight. Heel protectors made of synthetic

sponge rubber may be helpful (Fig. 266), but care must be exercised that they are not strapped too tightly, thus causing restriction of circulation, and that they are not used continuously because body moisture is retained and maceration of the skin may result. Use of the protectors does not eliminate the necessity of changing the patient's position at frequent intervals. The patient with spina bifida who has difficulty ambulating is inclined to spend considerable time in the sitting position. It is desirable that this sitting time be alternated with tilt-table standing, or the prone position, to relieve pressure on the sacral and ischial areas (Fig. 267). When ambulation is started, careful inspection of the skin is necessary to detect beginning signs of pressure caused by the brace or shoe. The care necessary to prevent trophic ulcers is not provided by any one person, but must be the concern of all nursing personnel. In addition, as rehabilitation of the patient progresses, he must assume an ever-increasing amount of responsibility for self-care, which includes skin care.

The tendency toward deformity is very great in these patients. Occasionally a child whose care has been neglected is seen in the orthopedic ward with hips and knees flexed to a right angle, back extremely rounded, and feet inverted to such an extent that the appearance is one of clubfeet found to have developed subsequent to birth. Dislocation of the hips is not uncommon and frequently adds to the dismaying picture. The patient is admitted for some correction of the deformity that will enable him to walk with the aid of crutches and braces. Sometimes the immediate cause of his admission may be the grave nature of the trophic ulcers that have baffled the parents' attempts to heal.

To help prevent the types of deformity mentioned, an exercise program similar to that designed for the paraplegic patient is needed. This exercise program is aimed at strengthening the upper extremities and maintaining joint motion in the lower extremities. In conjunction with the exercise program, training in activities of daily living should be given to encourage self-care and the desire to be self-sufficient.

Since past experiences have shown that these patients are prone to develop contractures and that their hips will dislocate, orthopedic surgeons have devised surgical procedures that help to prevent or minimize these complications. Various types of muscle transplant and tenotomies are done to provide for increased hip stability, to lessen muscle imbalance around the hip joint, and to help prevent or correct flexion contractures. Following any surgical procedure performed on the patient with spina bifida, the nurse should solicit instruction from the surgeon in regard to the patient's care. The surgeon will realize how serious a problem confronts the nurse and will be able to assist in planning safe alterations of position. Frequent changes to the prone position must be such as will maintain the extension of the hips. The back, buttocks, and groin must have attention many times

a day, certainly as often as the child becomes wet. Wrinkled, compressed, and bluish areas must be meticulously cared for. The child's skin will reflect promptly any letup in nursing care, any wrinkles or crumbs in the bed, or any neglect in change of position.

If a cast is used, its care is complicated. It is an extremely difficult task, particularly with female patients, to keep the cast from becoming soggy and foul smelling. Protecting its edges with a durable waterproof material is the first step.

Any apparatus must be considered a menace to the skin of these patients. Astute observation using eyes, fingers, and nose cannot be emphasized too strongly here. Since the patient cannot tell where the pressure is, the nurse must supply this missing sensation by careful frequent inspection of the parts in the apparatus.

The use of soap and water, followed by a dusting powder (borated), and freedom from pressure, moisture, and irritating creases in bed linen are essential in the care of the perineum and buttocks. Frequently, the most resistant areas of ulceration occur in the groin as fissures and beneath the gluteal folds as large deep-seated sores.

Long leg braces with a pelvic band or girdle usually are prescribed when the child is ready for walking (Fig. 268). These, too, must be considered a threat to the integrity of the patient's skin, and the patient's body must be carefully inspected for signs of irritation when they are removed. It usually is not considered advisable for the child to remain in such braces for the entire day. Periods of bed rest without braces but in good body alignment should be alternated with hours of ambulatory exercise. It is not uncommon for the patient with spina bifida to have a weight problem, frequently the result of insufficient activity. When present, obesity becomes a major hindrance to ambulation with crutches and braces.

The parents and patient are most grateful when walking is accomplished, as it frequently is, but often they will not recognize the part each plays in continuing this progress if they are not permitted to watch the meticulous nursing care that accompanies the physical rehabilitation of the child. The complications that may en-

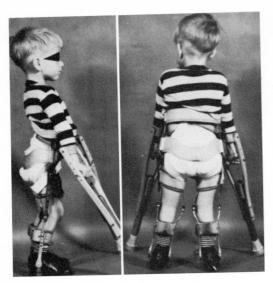

Fig. 268 A small patient with flail lower extremities caused by a lumbosacral spina bifida with myelodysplasia. Long leg braces attached to a body brace plus the use of crutches (Canadian) make ambulation possible. Tightness of the tensor fascia lata has resulted in hip flexion contracture.

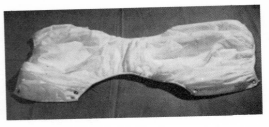

Fig. 269 Side-closing plastic-lined pants with grippers for easy fastening.

sue because of brace pressure on the legs must be pointed out. The necessity for preventing recurrence of deformity by positional correction should be emphasized. The care of the skin, especially around the buttocks and groin, should be demonstrated. The parents must be urged to assist the child to develop as much self-dependence as he is capable of assuming.

In addition to the development of trophic ulcers and contractures, bowel and bladder incontinence is a very real problem for the patient with spina bifida. If intermittent catheterization is not being utilized in the treatment of the urinary dysfunction, it may be desirable to institute a bladder training program. This is started by placing the child on the toilet at frequent specified times throughout the day. Complete emptying of the bladder is encouraged by pressure over the suprapubic area. The mother is instructed in ways in which she may continue the program at home. Adequate fluid intake plus timing of intake are important in preventing urinary tract infection and in promoting a bladder-training program. With the adult patient, the problem of urinary incontinence is prob-

ably one of the most difficult problems he faces. In addition to being a continual source of embarrassment, it is a contributing factor to skin breakdown. Various methods and types of apparatus have been used in an attempt to help the patient with this problem. The male patient may be able to keep himself dry by wearing a rubber urinal that is connected to a drainage bag attached to his leg. Protection for the woman patient may be provided by the use of a perineal pad and plastic-lined pants (Fig. 269). In some instances, the insertion of a Foley catheter is prescribed to help prevent skin breakdown. This is connected to a leg bag during the day and to a drainage bottle at night. When a catheter is in use, the possibility of urinary tract infection is always present. The patient should understand the correct care of the catheter and recognize danger signals that are indicative of need for medical care. To help the patient with incontinence, surgeons are attempting to surgically redirect the urinary flow into the bowel or to the skin surface where aftercare is less troublesome. The nursing care of the patient with a conduit is described in textbooks on urology.

During recent years, clean, intermittent, self-catheterization has become the method of choice of initial therapy for lower urinary tract dysfunction in some patients with myelomeningocele. Studies have shown that patients treated in this manner have had a low incidence of urinary tract complications, and many have shown considerable improvement in renal function and emptying of the bladder. In addition, the mental and emotional outlook of the patient improves greatly. With intermittent catheterization, overdistention of the bladder is prevented, and by preventing undue pressure on the bladder wall, normal blood flow is maintained. Since impairment of the blood supply to the bladder wall diminishes its resistance to bacterial invasion, it is important that the patient and/or the parent realize the necessity of catheterizing frequently enough to prevent undue bladder distention. This necessitates careful instruction of the patient or responsible person plus sufficient practice within the hospital situation to gain proficiency in doing the catheterization procedure.

Fecal incontinence and the regulation of bowel movements constitute another nursing problem encountered in the care of the child with spina bifida. The constipated stools are small and "marblelike," and there may be a constant dribbling of feces. Sphincter control of the anus is not present, and there is no discomfort or special sensation in relation to the need for defecation. Measures to prevent constipation and the development of fecal impaction should be a part of the patient's care. Good bowel hygiene may be promoted by (1) encouraging the child to eat foods with high-residue content, (2) giving bulk-producing medication, (3) maintaining adequate fluid intake, (4) providing exercise as permitted or possible, and (5) establishing a regular time each day for bowel evacuation. It is not sufficient merely to place the child on the toilet each day at a definite time. The child must learn to press on his abdomen, to strain, and to work at having a bowel movement. The insertion of a glycerin suppository is helpful in promoting defecation and in establishing bowel habits.

Control of the urinary and bowel dysfunction and the avoidance of embarrassing accidents, particularly in the young patient with myelomeningocele, will result in significant changes in the individual's sense of self-worth. The development of his personality and abilities will be much more evident. Frequently, no more pathetic individual exists on the orthopedic ward or in the crippled children's school than the patient with this type of problem. The child often feels that he is an outcast because of his inability to take care of his toilet needs. Besides the motor disability that limits him in many ways, he has the social difficulty that becomes harder to bear as he goes into adulthood. Also, those with head enlargement sometimes have the appearance of being subnormal in intelligence which belies their actual mental capacity.

13 Developmental affections

A number of bone and joint affections occur in middle childhood and adolescence with such regularity in age incidence that they are seemingly related to epiphyseal bone growth. Many of these conditions are self-limited within set time intervals and need treatment only to prevent deformity while the condition runs its cycle. Some are capable of inciting pain and therefore demand treatment. The more common of these conditions will be discussed in this chapter.

Coxa plana (Legg's disease; Legg-Perthes disease)

Coxa plana at one time was frequently confused with tuberculosis of the hip because the early symptoms are almost identical. Osteochondritis of the femoral head is caused by a vascular disturbance that produces an ischemic necrosis. The reason for this disturbance is not understood. It is a self-limiting disease, usually occurring in children between 5 and 10 years of age. Boys are more frequently affected than girls, a fact suggesting that trauma may be one of the instigating causes. Muscle spasm is rarely severe, and motions usually are restricted only in abduction and rotation, as contrasted with tuberculosis or arthritis, in which all motions are restricted. In some instances, the child will complain of pain in the knee rather than in the hip.

Pathology. Roentgenograms taken early show small vacuoles on either side or on both sides of the epiphysis. Following this, during the course of a few months to one to two years, the head of the femur undergoes degenerative changes in which segmentation first takes place (Fig. 270). This is combined with liquefaction over the cartilaginous surface of the joint and flat-tening of the upper surface of the head of the femur. In two or three years, when healing finally occurs automatically, the epiphyseal line becomes more nearly horizontal and the head of the femur becomes flattened.

This phenomenon usually does not lead to interference with joint function in early years. It may, however, lead to irritative changes around the hip joint later in life because of the discrepancies in shape between the head of the femur and the acetabulum.

Treatment. During the period of avascular necrosis, the head of the femur is pliable and will heal in a deformed position if weight bearing is permitted. It is apparent that the method of treatment must provide protection for the head of the femur during this process of degeneration.

In the past, treatment consisted of complete bed rest and traction during the developmental stages. If begun early, this type of treatment provides for restoration of the normal shape of the femoral head.

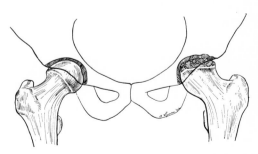

Fig. 270 Coxa plana. The epiphysis of the left hip (at right side in drawing) is in the middle stage, showing extensive segmentation.

However, treatment by bed rest is difficult to accomplish. Because the degenerative changes may continue for one to two years and regeneration of the head of the femur requires approximately a year, the restriction of bed rest to a child who feels well and has boundless energy requires the utmost in cooperation from parents.

Some physicians recommend operation with replacement of the liquefied areas under the femoral head with small bone graft chips from the neck of the femur; some recommend braces to relieve weight bearing, and some recommend the drilling of holes through the neck of the femur into

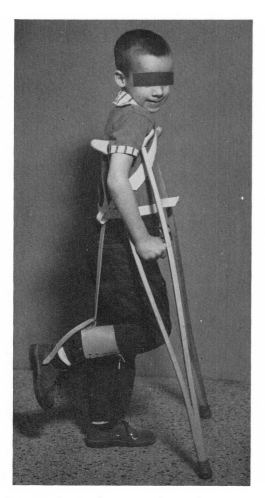

Fig. 271 The Fort harness is designed to prevent weight bearing on the affected extremity. The child wearing this apparatus is taught to walk with crutches, using the three-point gait.

the head of the femur to stimulate bone growth. Some physicians prescribe a leather harness—a Fort harness (Fig. 271)—that prevents bearing weight on the involved limb. The patient is required to walk with crutches. This necessarily places limitations on his activities but does permit his continuing school and living a somewhat normal life.

During recent years, an ambulatory and weight-bearing type of treatment has been instituted. Bilateral long leg casts with an abduction bar or long leg braces are utilized to maintain the limbs in a position of abduction (approximately 45°) and slight internal rotation (20°). With the limbs in this position, the femoral head is held deep in the acetabulum. As the child ambulates and bears weight on the extremities, the acetabulum serves to shape or mold the femoral head during revascularization and new bone formation. To maintain balance while ambulating, it is necessary for the child to use crutches or canes. Active range-of-motion exercise performed routinely will prevent hip contractures, and isometric exercises help to maintain strength in the quadriceps and gluteal muscles (Figs. 272 and 273).

Slipped femoral epiphysis

Slipped femoral epiphysis (Fig. 274) occurs in two types of adolescents: the fat overgrown adolescent (Fröhlich syndrome) and the rapidly growing slender type. The condition is more prevalent in boys than in girls and is frequently bilateral. Trauma may play an important part in the precipitation of displacement and symptoms, but undoubtedly there is some underlying deficiency in calcium metabolism, and perhaps there is a deficiency in the function of the thyroid and the pituitary glands.

Pathology. The three stages to the disease are characterized as follows:

1 In the preslipped stage, the condition manifests itself by the presence of a slight limp to the affected side and a slight limitation of internal rotation of the hip. Roentgenograms in this stage show little or no displacement but light rarefaction of bone on the lower femoral side of the epiphysis.

2 Through trauma or some minor injury during the earlier stages of slipping, the femoral portion of the epiphysis may slide

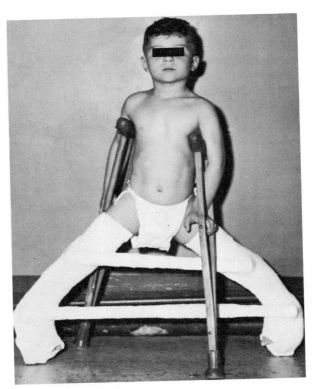

Fig. 272 A type of ambulatory treatment for coxa plana. The long leg casts are designed to hold the hips in abduction and internal rotation so that the major portion of the head of the femur is covered by acetabulum. In this event the acetabulum acts as a guide for shaping of the head as it goes through the repair process. (Courtesy Dr. J. G. Petrie, Montreal, Canada.)

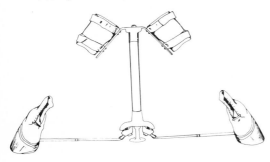

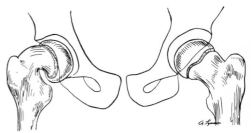

Fig. 274 Slipped femoral epiphysis of the right hip (shown here at the left). Note the horse-neck appearance of the neck of the femur and the erect position of the epiphyseal line.

Fig. 273 A modified Toronto orthosis used in the treatment of coxa plana. The brace serves to maintain the limbs in abduction and internal rotation, holding the femoral head firmly in the acetabulum. Weight bearing and activity are permitted and encouraged. (From Bunch, W. H., and Keagy, R. D.: Principles of orthotic treatment, St. Louis, The C. V. Mosby Co.)

farther upward, and further eversion may occur.

3 More extensive slipping of the epiphysis upward with increased eversion of the limb occurs in the more severe or later stages. The bony changes shown by roentgenograms are accompanied by increased limitation of abduction and internal rotation. When such a degree of displacement exists, there is a rather marked limp, but pain is not a prominent symptom.

The condition usually appears during the rapid growth years—between the ages of 12 and 15.

Diagnosis. If seen in a child 7 to 10 years of age, the symptoms and signs present would be similar to those in Legg-Perthes disease. The age of the patient suggests further investigation. The roentgenographic findings are characteristic. There is an active epiphyseal line, below which the bone seems to flow into its deformity. The neck of the femur assumes a horse-neck appearance.

Treatment. The only treatment during the preslipped stages is immediate internal fixation to prevent possible future slipping.

When definite slipping has occurred within a few weeks before observation, manipulation may be done by the Whitman or Leadbetter method. The leg is brought into forced abduction and internal rotation while the patient is under anesthesia. When reposition of the fragments is established, the foot will no longer evert when the heel is rested on the palm of the hand. A cast may be applied with the leg in abduction and internal rotation, or nailing with a Smith-Petersen nail is frequently recommended. Other operative procedures also are used.

When displacement has existed for months, an operation is necessary to restore alignment and improve joint function. This is accomplished by various types of osteotomy through the neck or trochanteric region of the femur.

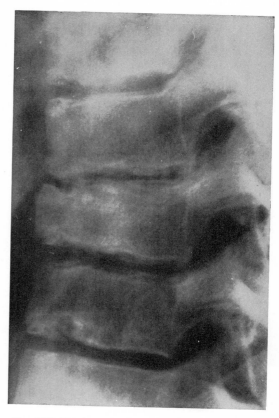

Fig. 275 Epiphysitis of the spine. Note wedging of the vertebral bodies and defects of the anterosuperior and anteroinferior cortical plates. (From Kenney, W. C., and Larson, C. B.: Orthopedics for the general practitioner, St. Louis, The C. V. Mosby Co.)

Epiphysitis of spine (Scheuermann's disease; juvenile kyphosis; osteochondritis deformans juvenilis)

As a result of injury that usually consists in forcible acute flexion in a young individual, there may be trauma to the anterior joint margin of one of the vertebrae. The lumbar vertebrae are the most susceptible (Fig. 275). A small area of bone may be deprived of its normal circulation and undergo degenerative changes. Gradually, it loses its contact with the rest of the vertebral body and becomes encysted.

Symptoms. Symptoms are usually mild and consist of a slight amount of pain on certain motions and possibly an intermittent dull aching sensation in the spine. Roentgenograms show characteristic separation of the vertebral fragment, with the increased density of necrosis and a surrounding area of rarefaction.

Treatment. Immobilization in a position of extension by means of a plaster-of-Paris body cast or a back brace for several months will usually lead either to the healing of the process or to the formation of a bridge of bone between the bodies of the adjoining involved vertebrae. Support provided by the cast or brace will help prevent deformity of the spine (kyphosis; round shoulders).

This patient with juvenile kyphosis should not be permitted to participate in strenuous sports, and bed rest may be necessary if pain is severe. A firm mattress with bed boards is desirable.

Epiphysitis of tibial tubercle
(Osgood-Schlatter disease; osteochondritis of tibial tuberosity)

Epiphysitis of the tibial tubercle (Fig. 276) usually occurs in rapidly growing children, most frequently in boys between 10 and 14 years of age. They complain of pain at the attachment of the patellar tendon on going up and down the stairs and of acute tenderness and swelling in this region. Roentgenograms may show a small beadlike piece of degenerated bone under the epiphysis of the tibial tubercle.

Treatment. Mild cases usually respond to protection by a cast or a reinforced elastic knee support. In severe cases, operative removal of the small piece of degenerated bone may be necessary.

Osteochondritis of knee joint

Although osteochondritis may occur in almost any joint in the body, it is comparatively common in the knee (Fig. 277). It usually appears under the cartilage of the outer surface of the inner condyle of the knee joint.

Cause. The cause is usually injury in which an unusual motion or strain of the joint occurs. Damage and local disturbance of the supply of circulation to a small area of bone and cartilage within the joint may result. The bone becomes separated from its blood supply and undergoes degenerative changes that separate it from the rest of the bone. This piece of dead bone may break through the covering of cartilage and enter the joint. The protective mechanism of the joint attempts to cover this loose bone (commonly referred to as a joint mouse) with cartilage until it finally be-

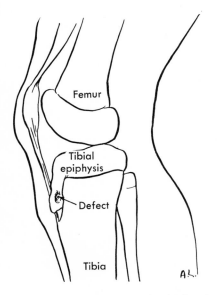

Fig. 276 Epiphysitis of the tibial tubercle.

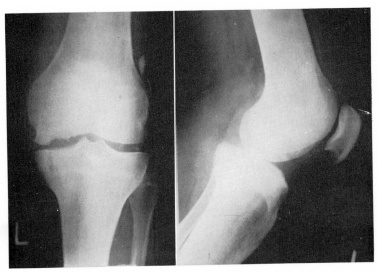

Fig. 277 Anteroposterior and lateral roentgenograms of the knee joint reveal a punched-out margin on the medial condyle of the femur. The "loose body" that arose from the punched-out area is visible in the quadriceps pouch along the lateral aspect of the femoral shaft.

comes smooth and may slip from one point to another within the joint, causing lockage when it is caught between the joint surfaces.

Treatment. When the presence of a joint mouse is definitely established by clinical observation and by roentgenogram, it should be removed. Surgical removal is also recommended if its presence can be determined prior to its becoming dislodged.

Scoliosis

Treatment and nursing intervention. Scoliosis is a lateral curvative of the spine. When there is no abnormality in the shape of the vertebrae and the patient can correct the deformity voluntarily, it is called *functional* or *postural* scoliosis. This type of scoliosis is usually the result of faulty posture, weak musculature, weak ligaments, or compensation for a short leg. Postural types of scoliosis rarely develop into structural types.

If there are changes in the sh vertebrae and thorax that make ble for the individual to correct mity, the condition is referred t *tural* scoliosis. This type may be caused by infantile paralysis (paralytic scoliosis), congenital deformity of the vertebrae (congenital scoliosis), diseases of the lungs, diseases and tumors of the spinal cord and of the ribs, neurofibromatosis, hysteria, etc.

Scoliosis also is described according to the spinal segment involved—e.g., thoracic, lumbar, or thoracolumbar. In severe thoracic scoliosis, the thorax is grossly misshapen. This deformity often consists of a right thoracic curve (referred to as the primary curve) and a left lumbar curve (known as the compensatory or secondary curve). This type of curvature also may be referred to as an S curve (Fig. 278). Curvatures of the thoracic spine are frequently convex to the right, whereas those of the lumbar spine are more often convex to the left. Scoliosis usually is accompanied

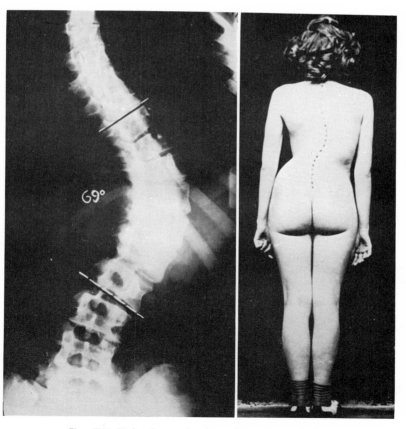

Fig. 278 Right thoracolumbar idiopathic scoliosis.

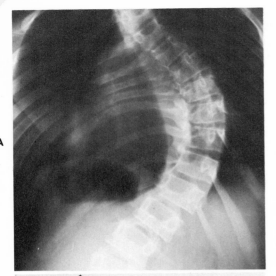

A

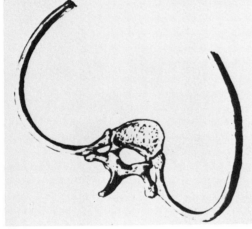

B

Fig. 279 A, Roentgenogram illustrating a right thoracic curve and a left lumbar curve. **B,** Drawing illustrating a cross section of a scoliotic rib cage showing distortion of the ribs, rotation of the vertebral body toward the convex aspect of the thoracic curve, and rotation of the posterior spinous process and pedicles toward the concave side.

by rotation of the vertebral bodies toward the side of the convexity of the curve (Fig. 279). This rotation of the thoracic vertebrae causes the ribs to protrude posteriorly on the convex side of the curve and to be more prominent anteriorly on the side of the concavity. Thus, with a right thoracic curve and a left lumbar curve, one would expect the right scapula and rib cage to protrude posteriorly and the left rib cage to be more prominent anteriorly.

Congenital scoliosis, as the name implies, is caused by a congenital defect, such as a wedge vertebrae, hemivertebrae, fused vertebrae, fused ribs, or other anomaly, and is usually apparent in the small child. *Paralytic* scoliosis develops several months or years after asymmetric paralysis of the trunk muscles and can be caused by a number of neuromuscular conditions; e.g., neuropathic disorders such as poliomyelitis and cerebral palsy and myopathic disorders such as muscular dystrophy. When asymmetric paralysis or weakness occurs, the strong normal muscles on one side of the torso are opposed by weak or flaccid muscles on the opposite side. Consequently, the normal balance of the musculature that supports the spinal column is destroyed. Because of this imbalance, a lateral spinal curvature develops, usually a C-shaped curve. When the cause of an existing scoliosis is not known, it is referred to as an *idiopathic* scoliosis. This is the most frequent type, occurs more frequently in girls than in boys, and usually has its onset at 10 or 12 years of age.

Because scoliosis rarely causes pain until the later stages of the disease, it is frequently unrecognized until the deformity is well established. Sometimes it is not until the child is in the period of rapid growth, between the ages of 12 and 16 years, that the condition becomes so evident it can no longer be overlooked. As with most crippling conditions, early recognition and treatment are vitally important.

It should be remembered that maximal improvement is obtained when the curvature is small and flexible. Routine examinations of school children for the presence of spinal curvature are very desirable. Parents and the general public should recognize the fact that the tendency to wait and see if the child will outgrow the condition is dangerous. This attitude may keep the child from getting treatment during the very time when it would be possible to minimize the effect of the curvature. The belief held by some individuals that scoliosis is a progressive condition and quite hopeless from the standpoint of treatment must be dispelled. The child with even a well-established curvature can be benefited greatly by skillful and continued treatment.

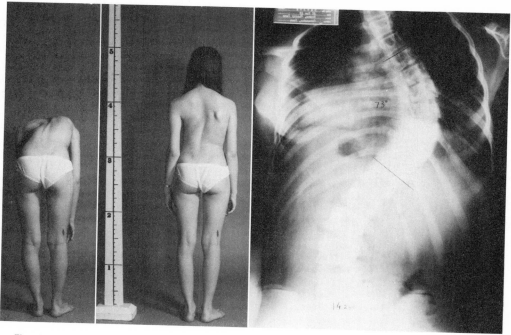

Fig. 280 Clinical photographs and roentgenogram of spine of a 14-year-old girl with a main right thoracic idiopathic soliosis. The thorax is shifted to the right in relation with the pelvis; therefore, the scoliosis is decompensated. Unless treated, these curves tend to increase a few degrees yearly, even after skeletal maturation, causing an increasing thoracic deformity, which may interfere with cardiorespiratory function in later life.

Examination. When examining the scoliotic child, the range of motion of the spine (in all directions) should be noted and limitations recorded. Upon forward flexion, it will be observed that the rotary deformity of the thoracic spine (rib hump) and the thoracic deformity are increased (Fig. 280). An evaluation of the individual's posture may reveal that body alignment is poor. With scoliosis of the thoracic spine, the ribs protrude backward on the side of the convexity of the curve, the thorax is deviated laterally in relation to the pelvis, and the shoulder and scapula on the side of the convexity are higher. The normal contour of the waistline is altered. It is flat on the side of the convexity of the curve and hollow on the side of the concavity. Thus, the arm on the side of the convexity hangs close to the rib cage, and that on the side of the concavity hangs away from the body (Fig. 278).

Scoliosis of the lumbar spine accounts for asymmetry of the hips. The hip on the side of the concavity of the curve is usu-ally more prominent. The level of the iliac crests should be roughly estimated by pressing the hands into the flank areas. Accurate measurements of leg lengths should be made from the anterosuperior spine of the iliac crest to the internal malleolus ("actual" or "true" leg lengths). As this is done, care should be taken that the position of both hips in relation to the pelvis is the same and that they bear the same relationship to an imaginary perpendicular line extending from the cervical spine through the cleft of the buttocks and down between the ankles. Measuring from the umbilicus to the internal malleolus gives the "apparent" leg lengths. A discrepancy in the "true" and "apparent" leg lengths may be present if the normal position of the pelvis is altered.

Discrepancy in shoulder heights should be measured, and to determine the amount of lateral deviation of the spine, a plumb line dropped from the occiput to the floor is helpful. The line normally should pass from the occiput over the posterior spinous

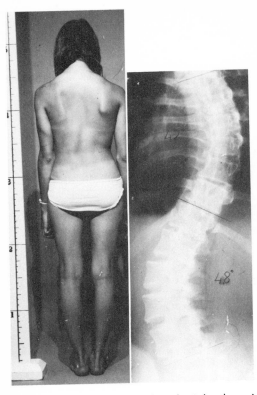

Fig. 281 A 17-year-old girl with right thoracic and left lumbar idiopathic scoliosis. The two curves are well compensated, and the body alignment is good. This is the most common curve pattern in adolescent idiopathic scoliosis. The curves usually do not increase after skeletal maturation and remain well compensated throughout life without causing clinical symptoms.

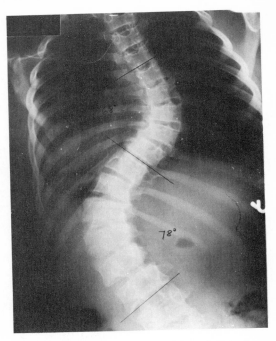

Fig. 282 Curves are measured by placing lines parallel to the first normally shaped vertebral body at the top and bottom of each curve and measuring the angle made where the lines, if extended, come to a common point.

processes of the vertebrae and the gluteal cleft and strike the floor midway between the heels. When there is lateral deviation of the thorax in relation to the pelvis, it means the curvature is decompensated (Fig. 280). However, if body alignment is good, the thorax is over the pelvis, the plumb line is normal, and the curvature is compensated (Fig. 281). Also, when examining the spine for scoliosis, it may be helpful to mark the posterior spinous processes (beginning with the seventh cervical) with a marking pencil.

Roentgenograms of the entire spine taken with the patient in the standing position and in the recumbent position are of value in the diagnosis of the type of curve and shift of the body weight. Measur-

ing and recording the degree of curvature on the initial roentgenogram (Fig. 282) is useful at a subsequent date in determining whether the curve is static or increasing. Roentgenograms taken every three months will show the evolution of the curve. Many curves increase little or not at all, whereas others progress rapidly. Roentgenograms taken with the patient bending to the right and to the left (lateral bending) will give valuable information regarding the flexibility of the curve and its correctability.

Nonsurgical treatment. The scoliotic patient may be treated nonoperatively by use of the *Milwaukee brace* (Fig. 283), which consists of a leather or plastic pelvic girdle that fits snugly and deeply over the iliac crests. This girdle serves as a foundation for a metal pelvic band and three uprights. The single anterior upright is made of aluminum to permit roentgenographic examination. The two posterior uprights are made of steel and are spaced lateral to the spine. These three uprights support

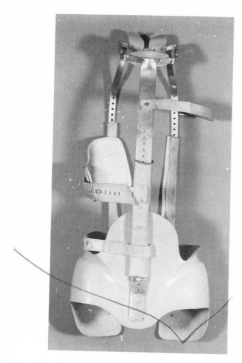

Fig. 283 Anterior view of the Milwaukee brace. Note the plastic pelvic girdle, throat mold, and occiput pads, provisions for adjustment of the brace to increase distraction of the vertebral column, and the adjustable holding pad to provide pressure on the convex aspect of the curve.

the throat mold and occiput pads. The throat mold maintains the head over the occiput pads. In addition to this metal framework, which provides for passive distraction, a holding pad that is attached to the upright bars and placed below the apex of the major curve provides for lateral pressure on the spinal column. The occiput pad and throat mold are adjusted to a position that permits the patient to elevate his head slightly above the head supports. As the child elevates his head above the neck ring and occiput pad, active correction of the spinal deformity is promoted. With relaxation, the neck ring, the thoracic pad, and the pelvic girdle serve as passive holding forces to maintain the spinal correction.

The uprights may be lengthened as correction is obtained or to accommodate the child's growth. Likewise, the holding pad placed over the convex side of the curve may be adjusted as necessary. The brace is designed to correct the spinal curve and to maintain the correction achieved. It should be worn continuously and is removed only for bathing.

Prior to the fitting and wearing of the brace, the child usually is admitted to the hospital. It should be kept in mind, however, that hospitalization over an extended period is not practical and usually not desirable. The child is placed in head and pelvic traction (Cotrel's traction) for ten to fourteen days. The primary purpose of the bed rest and traction is to decrease the spinal deformity by stretching tight ligaments and muscles. It also helps to relieve some of the discomforts caused by poor posture and to make wearing of the brace less difficult. However, it must be remembered that the bed rest and the traction do nothing to hold or maintain the correction—that when the upright position is assumed by the individual, the deformity will be as great as before treatment if some method of holding the correction is not utilized.

The pelvic girdle of the traction apparatus holds the pelvis firmly in position by means of two straps, which are covered with polyethylene foam and which cross on the anterior aspect of the pelvis. These straps fit just above the ilia and are anchored to the foot of the bed (Fig. 284). The pelvic girdle may be removed for bathing but does not need to be removed for toilet needs. The occipital chin strap provides for head traction. Stretching of the spinal column is obtained primarily by the pull placed on the occipital area. The height of the head pulley alters this force. Maintaining a 30° to 40° angle provides for a greater pull on the occipital region. Weight on the headpiece is increased gradually from 2 kg to 4 kg or 6 kg. Removal of the headpiece is permitted for meals and chin care; otherwise it should be worn continuously. A head pillow may be used, and the child may turn from side to side but should not sit up or assume the prone position. These patients often complain of back pain, of being sore and stiff, and of aching jaws. The chin area needs special care to prevent skin irritation. Prism glasses may be used to promote recreational or study activities.

During the hospitalization and fitting of

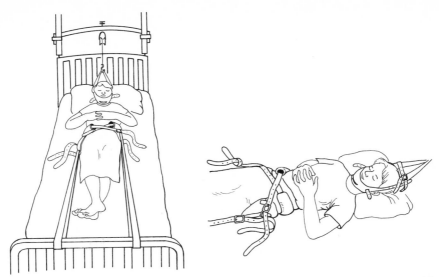

Fig. 284 One type of head and pelvic harness (Cotrel's) that can be used to provide for continuous distraction of the spine. The physician may prescribe that this be worn continuously for several weeks prior to surgery or the application of a brace. By elevation of the head pulley, traction is applied primarily to the occipital bone. The patient is encouraged to actively stretch the trunk insofar as possible by reaching and holding to the head of the bed. The pelvic straps maintain the pelvis in a fixed position. (From the Orthopedic nursing procedure manual, University of Iowa Hospitals and Clinics, The University of Iowa, Iowa City, Iowa.)

the brace, prescribed exercises are taught by the physical therapist. These exercises are of two types. The first type is aimed at maintaining and strengthening the torso muscles (thoracic and abdominal), improving the posture, and maintaining the flexibility of the spinal column. Wearing the body brace restricts normal use of some of the trunk muscles; thus planned exercise to maintain strength of these muscles is necessary. The second type of exercise is aimed at active correction of the major curve and is specific for each individual patient. It is advisable that the parents have a thorough understanding of such exercises as well as of their purpose. Written instructions, illustrated with drawings, would be helpful. It may take considerable ingenuity to keep the child interested in his exercises month after month.

Adjustment to the brace may involve several days. Learning to do things without spinal movement, such as turning the whole body to look sideways, positioning and holding books at eye level, becoming accustomed to sleeping with the brace on, and making needed adjustments in clothing are some of the problems the patient and his parents will encounter. The brace may seem to be too long when the child is sitting, and the upright bars may need adjustment. Also, rest periods in the horizontal position are usually advisable to prevent undue fatigue as the child gets use to the brace. Thus, an opportunity for the patient to adjust to his brace and to gain an understanding of what he must do to attain maximum correction is important. The parents may feel more secure and better prepared to carry out instructions pertaining to the child's exercise, rest, and home activity if they have had an opportunity to observe and participate in the care given in the hospital situation. A better understanding of activities that should be encouraged, those which the patient may safely participate in, is helpful to the parent. Stress or emotional conflicts experienced by the teen-ager due to the condition itself or to the wearing of a cumbersome, seemingly unsightly brace may be detected and dealt with. Sometimes appropriate clothing may make the brace less conspicuous and less of a threat to the teen-ager. Children with scoliosis are at a time of life when appliances are considered a cosmetic encumbrance, particularly by the child with a moderate curvature that has not as yet caused him personal embarrassment. The parents may succumb to pleas to leave the brace off for parties and dances, and ultimately it may be found at checkup that the child is not wearing his brace half the time. Similarly the patient may plead to omit his exercises because he is too busy or too tired. It is important that the scoliotic individual and his parents return for regular checkup visits with the orthopedic surgeon. Roentgenograms are taken, growth charts are maintained, and any increase or decrease in the curvature is carefully evaluated. At this time, brace adjustments can be made and exercise therapy evaluated. Persistence in carrying out the physician's orders, combined with thorough understanding of the long-term nature of treatment and the necessity for checkup at regular intervals, can produce desirable results.

It also should be remembered that for his total welfare the child with scoliosis needs more than supervision of his exercises and the wearing of his brace. Fatigue is to be avoided, and adequate nutrition is particularly important, as is careful supervision of his study, rest, and play habits. Tendencies toward weight loss, excessive weight gain, or periods of rapid growth in height should be observed. In many instances, these may mean that the child should return to the orthopedic clinic earlier than had been planned. Attention to all these details may mean the difference between success and failure in the child's treatment.

It is necessary for the child to wear the brace until bone growth is complete, which may be one to three years, or as long as there is any tendency toward increase of the curve. At maturity, it can be expected that the curvature will cease to progress significantly. Knowing when maturation occurs is not easy, and usually a number of factors are considered, including hereditary factors and development of secondary sex characteristics, plus a careful study of x-ray films of the skeleton. Roentgenograms of the left hand and distal wrist may be used to determine bone age. The chronologic age and the bone age (physiologic age) do not always correspond. Closure of the vertebral epiphyses indicates that growth is complete.

Before permission is given to remove the brace for short periods of time, it is important that stability of correction be demonstrated. This is accomplished by an x-ray film taken with patient in the standing position after the brace has been off for a few hours. If the major curve does not increase, permission usually is given for removal of the brace for several hours twice a week. Roentgenograms are repeated at specified intervals, and if correction is maintained, increased amounts of time without the brace are permitted. Experience has demonstrated that removal of the brace for extended periods should be a slow process and that continued use of the brace at night may be beneficial.

Halo-femoral traction may be used in the treatment of the child with severe and resistant scoliosis. The purpose of the traction is to secure maximum correction of the curvature. The halo consists of a metal head ring held to the outer table of the skull by means of four penetrating pins that are inserted with the patient under anesthesia (Fig. 285). In addition to the head traction, a downward pull or distraction on the vertebral column is necessary and may be secured by applying femoral traction. This means a Steinmann pin is inserted in the distal portion of each femur. Increasing amounts of weights are added to both the head and femoral traction. Approximately three weeks of traction are needed to gain maximum correction of the curves. To maintain the correction gained by the traction, it is necessary for the child to have a surgical fusion of the involved vertebral bodies. Postoperatively, the patient usually is maintained in the traction for several weeks, and then a halo cast is applied. In some instances, femoral traction may be replaced by halo-pelvic distraction (Fig. 362). The hoop portion of the apparatus encircles the pelvis and is held in place by two rods that pierce the ilia. Upright rods connect the hip hoop to the head halo. Correction of the spinal curvature is obtained gradually by manipulating the length of these rods. This type of apparatus immobilizes the spine and enables the patient to be ambulatory prior to surgery and much sooner

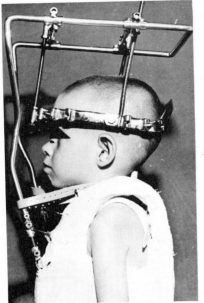

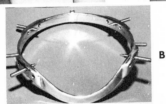

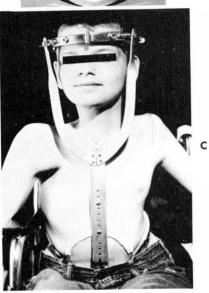

postoperatively than does the femoral traction apparatus. The care of the patient in a halo apparatus is undoubtedly a challenge to the most experienced orthopedic nurse. Care of the apprehensive patient, provision for adequate ventilation of the patient with a respiratory deficit, relief of postoperative pain, prevention of secondary contractures, plus the many aspects of nursing care necessary for a long-term patient are all a part of the care needed by this patient.

Surgical treatment. For some patients, a *spinal fusion* will be necessary to maintain correction of the curvature. In some cases, there is difficulty in obtaining the correction desired and also in holding it by external means. Most of the abnormal curves of the spine are observed carefully over a period of time and measured in degrees. When conservative measures fail to prevent progression of the curvature and increasing deformity cannot be prevented or when the correction gained is not stable, surgical intervention is indicated. Surgery means spinal fusion after correction has been obtained by whatever means may be chosen,

Fig. 285 A, Halo attached to the body cast. B, The metal ring, or halo, that is attached to the skull. C, Halo attached to a Milwaukee brace. (A and B, From Garrett, A. L., Perry, J., and Nickel, V. L.: Stabilization of the collapsing spine, J Bone Joint Surg [Am] 43:474-484, Jun 1961; C, courtesy Dr. Edward Miller, Chicago, Ill.)

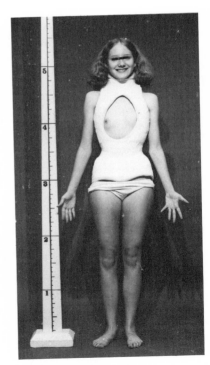

Fig. 286 A plaster body jacket on a patient with idiopathic scoliosis.

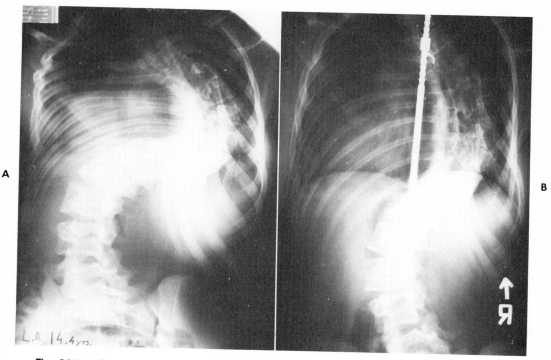

Fig. 287 A, Severe uncompensated dorsal scoliosis. **B,** Dorsal curve considerably corrected and the correction maintained by an implanted Harrington distraction rod.

and most of the fusions are done on patients at about 12 to 14 years of age. In the patients with moderately severe and severely progressive curves who have undergone fusion, it is likely over a period of years that those with idiopathic scoliosis will retain 42% correction of the deformity. This percentage is somewhat lower in those with the congenital scolioses.

There are several techniques for spinal fusion (see Chapter 19). In recent years, the anterior approach has been used for some patients. With this approach, intervertebral discs can be removed as the fusion is done and considerable correction of the curvature obtained. With the posterior approach, the outer cortex of the lamina and spinous processes is removed and raw cancellous bone exposed. The posterior facet joints also are destroyed. The graft (autogenous), which consists of small slivers of bone taken from the iliac crest, are placed along the fusion area. These bone grafts solidify and hold the spine in the corrected position. Usually, fusion done for scoliosis includes one vertebra above the upper end of the curve and two vertebrae below the lower end of the curve.

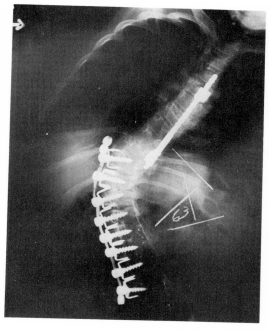

Fig. 288 Roentgenogram taken following the surgical application of the Harrington rod in the dorsal spine and the Dwyer apparatus in the lumbar area for maintenance of correction of the spine in severe scoliosis.

The major problem with the surgical treatment is the failure of fusion—a condition called pseudarthrosis—and this will occur in about one-third of the patients in whom spinal fusion is attempted. When pseudarthrosis is recognized, however, refusion can be obtained by additional bone grafting in most instances. Postoperative care is extremely important. Immobilization of the spine by means of a cast or brace usually is continued for six to twelve months (Fig. 286). It is well to remember that solidification after spinal fusion usually is conceded to be present after about four to six months, although this is subject, of course, to verification by roentgenography.

If the patient is to be immobilized by a brace rather than a cast following a spinal fusion, the nurse should remember that a body brace of any type should be fitted snugly around the pelvis in such a fashion that the lower band grasps the iliac crests. It should be laced or buckled from the bottom as the patient lies in bed. In some instances, the Milwaukee brace is applied and worn continuously for a period of six to eight months or as prescribed. Postoperatively, when bed rest is necessary for an extended period of time, deep-breathing exercises should be encouraged, and exercise of the extremities is desirable to help maintain muscle strength and to prevent the development of secondary contractures. Skin care is an important aspect of the nursing care. Pressure from the pelvic girdle may cause redness and irritation of the skin in the involved areas. If changing the child's position does not relieve the discomfort, an adjustment of the brace may be necessary. Since the patient spends most of his time on one side or the other, the skin over the greater trochanter and the shoulder may show signs of pressure. Bathing the patient must be done with the brace in place.

When the patient is ready for ambulation, the brace is still worn continuously. Later, it is removed at night and then for graduated periods during the day. It is worn for six to twelve months postoperatively, depending on roentgenographic findings. Bone union at the graft site must be strong enough to maintain the correction. Follow-up care will include frequent checks by the orthopedic surgeon to provide for early detection of spinal changes. Pseudarthrosis may occur at a graft site, or the graft may fail to hold the correction.

If a body cast is applied to provide immobilization, the nurse must realize that there is considerable strain on the patient during its application, particularly if he has been bedfast for a long period. The patient will probably be exhausted upon his return from the plaster room. The wet cast should be supported on plastic-covered pillows. Cast edges should be sealed and during the time the patient is confined to bed rest, protection of the buttocks area should be provided to prevent wetting or soiling of the cast. Patients in body casts are helpless, and exacting care is necessary to keep them clean. Skin care around the cast edges and frequent change of position and pressure points are essential aspects of the nursing care.

A form of rod instrumentation introduced by Harrington is another technique. *Harrington rods* are implanted into the spine by clips that hold on the laminae. On the side of the concavity of the curve they can be utilized in a fashion to distract or correct the concavity, and on the convex side they can by compression tend to correct the convexity (Figs. 287 and 288). In experienced hands, the Harrington rods are an effective addition to the surgical treatment of scoliosis but are used in combination with, rather than as a replacement for, the external methods of support.

14 Neuromuscular disorders

Cerebral palsy

Cerebral palsy is the term applied to those conditions characterized by impaired functional muscular control as a result of abnormality in cerebral areas that affect neuromuscular functions. Spasticity is a type of cerebral palsy, although frequently the terms are used erroneously as synonyms.

Predisposing factors. Certain factors that are essentially uncontrollable increase the likelihood of a child's having cerebral palsy during the period immediately surrounding birth.

Being one of firstborn. Being one of the firstborn applies until the mother's fourth or fifth pregnancy occurs. If one of the first births results in cerebral palsy, there is an increased likelihood that later children may suffer the disorder. The incidence in subsequent children, however, is not so great as in the firstborn.

Premature birth. Approximately 40% of all persons with cerebral palsy have a history of prematurity. As might be expected in premature infants, the greater the prematurity, the greater the likelihood of brain damage.

Abnormalities of labor. Infants born following a prolonged period of labor or an unusually rapid labor are more likely to have cerebral palsy.

Abnormalities of delivery. Abnormalities of delivery, such as unusual fetal presentation, major manipulative procedures, and cesarean section, are more likely to produce cerebral palsy.

Multiple births. One of twins, usually the second delivered, has a greater likelihood of being afflicted with cerebral palsy than an infant born singly.

Heavy birth weight. Infants with heavier than average birth weights are more likely to suffer brain damage. This apparently is caused by increased probabilities of cerebral trauma resulting from increased head size.

Race. Cerebral palsy reportedly is somewhat more common in Caucasians than in persons of dark-skinned races.

Sex. Males are slightly more prone to be afflicted with cerebral palsy than females, although a great difference does not exist.

Incidence. Iowa State Services for Crippled Children and the Iowa State Department of Public Instruction report of 1972 indicates the incidence of cerebral palsy to be 1.9 per 1,000 population of those aged 4-21 years. Although 72% of these children showed some degree of mental retardation, well over half were considered educable and the remainder trainable. Many had associated speech and hearing problems, and 20% had sufficient motor dysfunction and mental retardation that their care was more or less custodial.

Cause. Conditions that produce cerebral anoxia and hemorrhage or trauma, either singly or combined, are the most common etiologic agents. These factors, if of sufficient intensity or duration, may operate during the prenatal, natal, or postnatal periods of life and produce an irreversible brain abnormality resulting in cerebral palsy.

Prenatal conditions. The more common of the prenatal conditions include infectious illnesses in the mother early in pregnancy, particularly the mild viral infections; abnormal placental attachments; toxemia; hypotension; anemia; irradiation, particularly if early in gestation and if therapy is directed to the mother's pelvic organs; isoimmunization, such as Rh incompatibility between mother and fetus; and any condition in which the mother suffers intense or prolonged anoxia. The hereditary element per se is a very uncommon cause for cerebral palsy. Investigations have suggested that maternal nutritional deficits preceding and during pregnancy may bear an important relationship to the presence of brain abnormality and cerebral palsy in the offspring.

Natal conditions. The natal period refers to that period of pregnancy from the onset of labor to the birth of a viable child. Incidents that may produce brain damage during this time are primarily anoxia and trauma, either singly or combined. Some of the more common situations producing these damaging cerebral onslaughts are as follows:

1 Depressing maternal anesthesia which, in turn, temporarily enfeebles the vital centers of the infant, thus delaying the onset and effectiveness of natural respirations
2 Placenta praevia or abruptio placentae, which removes a source of oxygen to the infant before his normal respiratory mechanism can operate
3 Delaying birth unduly by force against the presenting part, pending the accomplishment of desired preparations for delivery
4 Prolapsed cord, with delay in delivery of the head
5 Difficult instrumental delivery
6 Acute hypotension in the mother as a result of spinal anesthesia
7 Precipitate birth, resulting in cerebral damage as a result of sudden change in pressure from intrauterine to extrauterine life
8 Breech presentation with delay in delivery of the aftercoming head
9 Vigorous manipulative procedures

Postnatal conditions. Most situations occurring after birth that may lead to brain abnormality are more apparent. The more important of these circumstances include:

1 Kernicterus, often the result of erythroblastosis
2 Brain infections, such as meningitis, encephalitis, and abscesses

3 Cerebral trauma, often resulting from falls or other accidents
4 Intense or prolonged anoxia resulting from any cause
5 Brain tumors
6 Cerebral circulatory anomalies, often leading to rupture

Certain systemic diseases may cause brain damage as a result of secondary effects—e.g., cerebral thrombosis may be a complication of nephritis, nephrosis, or other disease, cerebral embolus may result from subacute bacterial endocarditis occurring as a complication of rheumatic fever, congenital heart disease, or other conditions, and rupture of minute cerebral blood vessels may occur with severe paroxysms of coughing in an infant with pertussis.

The postencephalitic cerebral palsies, which follow some virus-induced disease that has affected the cortex of the brain, are usually severe in nature. Loss of motor function occurs, and varying degrees of impairment in speech and intelligence sometimes are so severe in nature that any

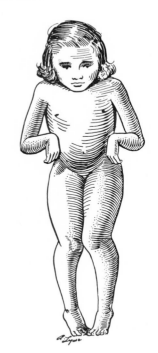

Fig. 289 Cerebral palsy with spastic quadriplegia characterized by flexion at all joints except the ankles, adduction and internal rotation of the thighs, and scissors gait.

return of these functions is despaired of. Until a trial is made, however, pessimistic predictions are hardly justified, for considerable return of function has been possible in a number of the most severely affected patients. These children, struck down suddenly, usually from a healthy and normal childhood, present a most tragic spectacle because of the abruptness and devastation of the disease. Taking a hopeless attitude is all too easy for the nurse and parents in dealing with one of these children, and often the only future they can visualize is to provide complete and conscientious care of the child, with a view to his physical comfort and cleanli-

ness. A more far-sighted attitude would be to utilize the child's unaffected faculties as soon as the acute illness is over. Frequently, more is left than is at first apparent. One very bright boy, 14 years of age, with extremely severe involvement after encephalitis initiated by measles, was distressed immeasurably by not being able to make known his wants. A perplexed but sympathetic student nurse set herself to work out the problem with a piece of white poster paper. She divided her paper into six sections and made a crude drawing in each section: in one a bedpan, in another a urinal, in another a glass of water, etc. When she stood at patient's bedside and

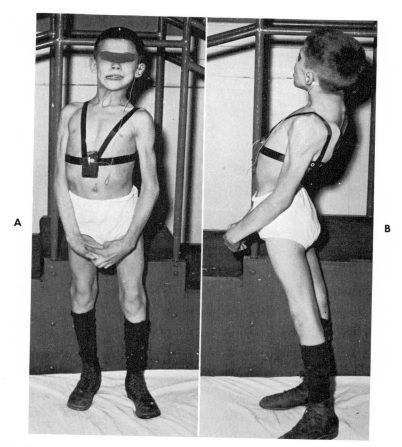

Fig. 290 A, Boy, 12 years of age, with "tension athetosis" and associated hearing loss partially compensated for by a hearing aid. Note generalized hypertrophy of muscles, more involvement of the right shoulder than the left, pronated feet, and voluntary attempt to stabilize purposeless movements of the right upper extremity by clasping with the left hand. **B,** Lateral view of the same boy showing marked lordosis and genu recurvatum as a result of increased tension in an attempt to maintain standing balance as his center of gravity shifts.

Table 1 Basic clinical types of cerebral palsy and their characteristics

Type	Basic clinical characteristics
Spastic	Increased resistance to manipulation; stretch reflex hyperactive deep tendon reflexes; clonus; tendency toward contracture deformities; lower extremities often more involved than upper extremities
Athetoid	Involuntary and uncoordinated motions without conscious control; normal reflexes when in relaxed state; upper extremities often more involved than lower extremities
Ataxic	Disturbance of autonomic balance; nystagmus; adiadochokinesis; difficulty in concentrating vision on a fixed field; normal tendon reflexes
Rigidity	"Lead pipe" resiliency of involved member; tendency to maintain position of extension; absent stretch reflex; near-normal tendon reflexes
Tremor	Intention-tremor contractions occur only with attempted motions; nonintention-tremor contractions present constantly; no hyperactivity of tendon reflexes

pointed to the articles one after another, the boy could move his head sufficiently to let her know what he needed at the moment.

Classification. The most useful classification of cerebral palsy is one based on clinical findings. Autopsy material that is correlated with careful clinical observations in the same person has been insufficient to permit an authentic pathologic categorization according to types.

The basic clinical types of cerebral palsy and their characteristics are listed in Table 1 in decreasing order of frequency of occurrence as recognized by most physicians particularly interested in patients with cerebral palsy (Figs. 289 and 290).

A mixture of types may be present in the same person but probably does not occur in more than approximately 1% of all patients.

The high spinal spastic type of cerebral palsy has been described in addition to the types listed in Table 1. The site of damage in this type is at the level of the juncture between the skull and atlas. The manifestation expected with this lesion is spasticity of the lower extremities.

The extent of involvement is variable from patient to patient. The descriptive terms used to denote extent of involvement are presented in Table 2.

The degree of involvement is perhaps more important than the type of cerebral palsy when possibilities for physical rehabilitation are being considered. A mild degree of involvement suggests that extensive treatment measures are not neces-

Table 2 Terms used to denote extent of involvement

Descriptive term	Extent of involvement
Quadriplegia or tetraplegia	All four limbs
Hemiplegia	One side of body
Triplegia	Hemiplegia plus one limb of opposite side
Diplegia	Like parts of each side of body
Paraplegia	Both legs
Monoplegia	A single limb or part of body

sary and usually can be accomplished by the parents in their home. The patient with a moderate degree of involvement needs special therapy measures that often include the use of braces and sometimes surgical procedures, whereas the one with a severe degree of involvement has only limited possibilities for physical rehabilitation even with the use of all special therapeutic measures available.

Associated defects. The presence of one or more associated disabilities in the person with cerebral palsy occurs more often than not. These disabilities are usually the direct result of the primary brain abnormality. The more common associated defects found in the cerebral palsy population are listed in Table 3.

Social influences. Very few diseases have social factors complicating the condition as extensively as does cerebral palsy. Formerly, all persons with cerebral palsy were considered to be feebleminded; thus institutional placement was the course to

Table 3 Associated defects frequently present in persons with cerebral palsy

Defect	Approximate frequency of occurrence
Mental defectiveness	25% to 40%
Educational retardation	Frequency correlated with degree of severity; very common in patients other than mildly affected
Speech involvement	70% to 80%
Hearing defects	30% to 40%
Oculomotor abnormality	30% to 40%
Convulsive disorder	40%
Perceptual defects	Frequency undetermined; more common in those with athetosis
Symbolic language disability*	Frequency undetermined; probably fairly common
Physical growth retardation	Frequency often related to the degree and extent of involvement; in part due to feeding difficulties
Emotional disturbances	Fairly common, to varying degree

*Includes dysphasia, aphasia, reading disabilities, and allied abnormalities.

follow. Unfortunately, this attitude still exists in a segment of the population, and it has been conducive to the social isolation of afflicted persons in their homes. In addition, many other factors exist—to the detriment of a healthful emotional state in one with cerebral palsy. Some of these are discussed in the following paragraphs.

Parental guilt feelings and martyr complex. Studies have indicated that over two-thirds of all parents of children with cerebral palsy have feelings of personal guilt and consider that the handicapped child is theirs as a cross to bear. One would expect that such attitudes might be conveyed readily by the parents to the child in ways other than verbal expression. Parents who have these feelings to a strong degree are loathe to discuss their problems with others and tend toward voluntary introversion or extroversion and oversolicitousness as a compensatory device.

Family disagreements. Approximately one-half of the parents of children with cerebral palsy in one study admitted serious family disagreements regarding problems presented by their afflicted children.

Parental lack of information. Most parents have little or no accurate knowledge of etiologic factors, possibilities for successful rehabilitation, realistic aims, or even basic understanding of what the term "cerebral palsy" means. Perhaps, as might be expected, the majority of parents exaggerate both the severity of involvement and the mental acuity of their child, either because of lack of knowledge or because of failure to accept the facts. Approximately one-half of the parents of these children make little or no use of literature available on the subject, and most of those who have attempted self-education in this manner have found the reading to be confusing or of no help. It is not unusual to find parents who have no rehabilitation program at home because they are uninformed as to how they should proceed.

Professional help sought. The common response of parents of children with cerebral palsy is (1) a rejection of the initial examiner and the information he gives when it is unfavorable, (2) a search for more favorable information from other sources, and, finally, (3) a realistic acceptance of the child's condition. Thus, in one study of 200 parents of children with cerebral palsy having an average age near 8 years, the average amount of help sought per child was from nine medical physicians, two chiropractors, and one osteopath. Obviously, such shifting parental allegiance is detrimental to the possibility of any helpful approach to the child.

Oversolicitousness. Approximately 40% of parents admit to oversolicitousness toward their child with cerebral palsy. Experience suggests that this is a conservative estimate. Schoolteachers, playmates, and other associates of the child with cerebral palsy are prone to manifest this same attitude and thus enhance the impact of this factor.

Limitations in socialization. Socialization experiences of the handicapped child usually are curtailed proportionately according to the severity of his physical handicap or associated defects. Approximately three-fourths of all children with cerebral palsy who are not in school have few, if any, playmates outside their home. In addition, it is not uncommon to find a child with cerebral palsy of 5 or 6 years of age who has never been inside a supermarket, seen an airport, or had similar experiences that are fairly commonplace for a nonhandicapped child.

Therapy. An effective therapeutic program may require the services of an organized group of professionals in view of (1) the physical handicap itself, (2) the associated defects, some of which are usually present in a person having cerebral palsy, and (3) the social influences encountered by the child with cerebral palsy.

The broad aims of therapy should be to establish locomotion, communication, and self-help, to work toward an appearance of normality in all motor functions, to correct associated defects as effectively as possible, and to provide educational opportunities adapted to the given child's needs.

This plan of therapy may be accomplished in the home or in a hospital, or it may require special and prolonged facilities as provided in a hospital school. In any eventuality, continued home therapy becomes essential for those patients who may have had their therapy initiated in a hospital or hospital school. The needs of the patient and the home facilities available become most important in deciding which approach will be most advantageous for a given patient.

Obviously, to enable one to establish more specific aims in therapy, a thorough evaluation of the entire person becomes a necessity at the beginning of his management and must be repeated as his needs demand. Usually, the scope of this evaluation goes beyond the capabilities of one person, often requiring the services of a physician, a psychologist, a speech pathologist, a social worker, nursing personnel, and other professional persons.

The services of physical therapists, occupational therapists, and speech therapists frequently are necessary to accomplish corrective exercises in a given patient or to instruct and demonstrate to parents sufficiently so that recommended procedures may be accomplished in the home. Parents can accomplish many of the exercises if they are instructed adequately.

Medical help is required in several ways. Of importance is one physician who may act as a coordinator of the rehabilitation program for a given patient because of his particular interest in this condition. He may be a general practitioner or specialist in any one field. It is he to whom the parents may turn for counseling when questions arise. The consultation of other medical specialists frequently is necessary for purposes of correcting associated defects as well as aiding in the basic rehabilitation program.

Appliances such as braces or splints are used frequently for correcting or preventing deformities, reducing incoordinated and purposeless movements of the limbs, or affording increased stability.

Special equipment often becomes necessary as a means of effecting therapy procedures (Figs. 292 to 298). Kneeling benches, stand-up tables, parallel bars, relaxation chairs, and special adaptations of feeding utensils are most commonly used.

Surgical procedures on tendons, nerves, or joints become necessary in some patients with cerebral palsy. Neurosurgery has afforded very limited benefits thus far and is seldom used therapeutically.

Medications have extremely limited usefulness. Certain products have some minor value for their relaxant properties; however, they are only adjuncts to other forms of therapy. Some medications are used to reduce salivary action and drooling. Preparations formerly advocated for improving mental acuity have now been found to have such limited value that they are unimportant. The drugs ordinarily used for control of seizures have similar usefulness in the patient with cerebral palsy.

Parental counseling is of great importance in making a program of therapy effective. The parents must be given basic information regarding cerebral palsy in general and facts pertaining to the condition as it relates to their own child. Realistic planning for rehabilitation (both physical and educational) and eventually for vocational anticipations should be done. The counselor may be the physician who is coordinating the program or some other professional person if he is competent, adequately interested, and sufficiently adept.

A person who has cerebral palsy is likely to have numerous and variable problems related directly or indirectly to his condition. Early recognition and attention to his problems, intelligent planning and accomplishment of a coordinated program of rehabilitation, and wise counseling are measures whereby satisfactory restoration may be effected in the majority of the patients.

Nursing intervention. Cerebral palsy is one of the common causes of crippling in children. Yet it is not unusual for student nurses to complete their entire course of training without caring for such a patient in the hospital. Indeed, nurses often tell their instructors that their most impressive introduction to the patient with cerebral palsy is frequently away from the hospital —on the street or in the home of some friend or neighbor.

Poliomyelitis (infantile paralysis) has received much attention in the past, and much has been done to eliminate this condition. One could hope that a similar amount of public interest might be evinced by this other comparable problem. However, cerebral palsy is a disability that does not strike spectacularly in epidemic form, and its results, although quite disastrous, are sometimes not appealingly dramatic. People are not instinctively drawn toward the unfortunate victim of this condition. They tend to be somewhat appalled and repelled by him, even when their sympathy for him is most manifest. Each nurse, as an individual, may make the lot of the person with cerebral palsy more bearable by interpreting his situation sensibly and realistically to friends or to the community. This service may be a more important one than the relatively small amount of nursing care given these patients in the hospital.

Student nurses discussing this condition frequently reflect the feelings of the public at large when relating their own experience. One student told how, as a child, she would cross the street to avoid passing a certain young boy. He jerked and twisted in all directions, and she was afraid of him. She knows now that the boy suffered from athetosis, and she remembers that he always seemed to try to smile at those who passed him. Another student told of a high school friend whose younger sister "wasn't quite right." She was allowed to play only in a fenced-in backyard. One day the student saw the child in the backyard and noticed that she walked on her toes with her knees crossed and that she drooled and laughed raucously. The student remembers that she shuddered while watching the child and that she felt a great repulsion as though she were looking upon something not quite human. Now, however, she wonders why someone did not tell the parents of that child that perhaps something could be done for her.

Importance of early recognition and treatment. Early recognition is an important factor in the treatment of cerebral palsy. This is not always as easy as it might seem, particularly in the mildly affected child. The more severely affected are not likely to be overlooked. When there is a history of a difficult labor, correlation between certain symptoms in the infant and his obstetric background makes the attending physician and nurse particularly observant. Cyanosis, convulsions, dyspnea, apnea, and twitching indicate an advanced degree of involvement. Increased crying, vomiting, hiccoughs, rigidity, or tenseness may be present in less severely affected babies. All symptoms of this nature should be faithfully recorded on the infant's chart and in considerable detail. Many such babies are also intractably difficult feeders, and this may be a significant factor in diagnosis.

In the infant with very mild involvement, none of the symptoms just mentioned may be present. As the infant grows older, however, certain features make their appearance that should not escape the nurse's attention. The nurse should know at least the elements of normal child development in order to recognize departures from the normal in these children.

It is not at all uncommon for this condition to escape detection until the child begins to walk, although delay in walking may be significant. Sometimes a tendency to walk on the toes (contracture of the

Achilles tendon) accompanied by adduction of the thighs and knees may be the only symptoms noted at this time.

It has been interesting to note that infants 1 year old or less frequently are brought to the physician's office for some slowness in development, such as being unable to sit up or to lift the head, and the story is told that the baby was normal until he had an attack of stomach flu or a cold, or perhaps a fall, when he was about 6 months old. These incidents in the baby's short history could be the cause of the obvious existing cerebral palsy, but in many cases doctors feel that parents have simply not noticed or admitted that symptoms existed until the child reached 6 months of age, when it was no longer possible to ignore certain retardations in development. There is a definite reluctance, even among the well-educated parents, to accept a diagnosis of spastic paralysis. Since there still seems to be a stigma attached to the condition, families tend to be ashamed.

It is very important that treatment be begun early. As far as possible, the training of the child with cerebral palsy should follow the development of the normal child. If the condition is not diagnosed until the child is 3 years of age or older, a great deal of valuable time will have been lost. Nurses will remember that the average child tends to sit at 6 months of age, attempts to creep at about 10 months, and tries to stand alone at 15 months. In the mildly affected child, this sequence might be approximated with only little delay, if training is instituted early enough.

Frequently parents are tempted to follow advice secured from unreliable sources, particularly about taking the child to unqualified practitioners. This tendency is expensive and dangerous, and the nurse must marshal strong (but nonhysterical) arguments against it.

Probably no parents ever need help as badly as those with a child with cerebral palsy. Nurses should know all community resource possibilities for the care and education of such children as well as those available on the state and national levels. Cerebral palsy is an exceedingly complex problem, and the needs of the child for special types of treatment may be very great. Specially trained physical therapists, occupational therapists, speech therapists, and teachers may be required. The local and state chapters of the Easter Seal Society for Crippled Children and Adults usually can give much valuable help on this problem and will be able to refer the nurse to other agencies for additional help. Intelligent, sympathetic information given the family by the nurse sometimes prevents a great outlay of expense and energy in traveling from one place to another in search of a miraculous, quick recovery for the child.

Emotional attitudes toward cerebral palsy. What should be the attitude of the nurse toward these children? As far as possible, it should be the same attitude one has toward a normal child. It has been repeatedly emphasized that workers in this field must remember that the patient is first of all a child and only secondarily a victim of cerebral palsy. Friendliness, interest, affection, and dependability should be manifest in the nurse's actions, for the child needs these things and they add to his feeling of security and personal importance. It should be realized that patients with cerebral palsy are quicker than many other children to detect an unsympathetic presence. They are equally sure to sense a friendly one. It is essential to secure their confidence and friendship, for upon these things much of the success in treatment may depend. Furthermore, the nurse is urged to learn everything possible about the child being cared for, concerning both background and personal history as well as the improvement that the physician believes possible. Has the child come from a home where family life has revolved around him as though he were a pivot? Has he been shoved into the background and treated with great negligence? The nurse's attitude toward the child may need to be altered somewhat by what is learned of his background. We know that the education of the parents is a very important part of the treatment of these children. Treatment must carry on far into the future life of the child; otherwise, its value is questionable from the start. Probably the two features indispensable to successful treatment of the patient with cerebral palsy are (1) the patient's mental capacity to make treatment of permanent value and (2) the understanding and cooperation of the parents.

Too often the afflicted child has been utterly spoiled by the time he comes to the hospital. It may be because of a parent who has decided, with almost a religious fervor, to devote her whole life to the child to compensate for his being crippled. No responsibility of any kind has ever been given him, and he has never had to suffer the consequences for any misdeeds. Hospital experience will not be easy for such a child, but if the situation is directed by an intelligent and understanding nurse, it can be of great benefit. The child's moments of rebellion and temper will occur less frequently as he sees his unbecoming behavior duplicated in others like himself on the clinical unit. The nurse's manner (quiet, firm, and understanding but unwavering where principle is concerned) will play a great part in the child's emotional development. This is so important that nurses should never underestimate their share in the treatment of these children. Too often the nurse believes that the physical therapist, occupational therapist, and teacher are the ones who really contribute toward the rehabilitation of these children—that nurses have little to do with it. This attitude is quite false. The child spends more time with the nursing group than with any other while he is in the hospital. The nurse's attitude and teaching, by precept, example, and practice, can do much toward the emotional development of the child. This service to him is not to be minimized.

Intelligence in cerebral palsy is not measurable by appearance. Facial contortions, a raucous voice, emotional instability, gutteral speech, apparent inability to understand what is being said, laziness, and lack of desire to do things for himself do not always signify low mentality. Opinions concerning the mental capacity of persons afflicted with cerebral palsy vary considerably. Estimations of mentality based on mental tests that require some type of motor response are not considered reliable. As better instruments for measurement are devised, however, and as knowledge of the various types of cerebral palsy increases, a more adequate estimation of the child's educability is becoming possible.

Whereas too much optimism is always to be avoided until the child has been given the benefit of an examination by a specialist, to recommend custodial care for a badly affected child without such an examination is exceedingly unwise.

Defects of speech, hearing, sight, and sensation may be present. It can easily be seen that any of these defects might make the child seem less alert than he actually is. The athetotic child is particularly likely to be slow to differentiate between sounds, and his ability to distinguish words may be greatly impaired. Defects of sight vary from lack of control of eye muscles and squinting to strabismus and nystagmus.

Clinical types of cerebral palsy are classified as spastic, athetoid, ataxic, rigidity, tremor, etc. The list grows as the knowledge of the disease progresses. The most frequent in occurrence are the spastic and the athetoid, and discussion of nursing care will be confined largely to patients with these types.

There is considerable variation in the treatment of spastic and athetoid cerebral palsy. The child who presents the uncomplicated cortical involvement, the true spastic child, has a set of symptoms that make efforts toward muscle reeducation the most important consideration. This child, confronted by a blocking of his voluntary efforts to perform an action, frequently tends to show signs of gradually developing frustration and apathy. There is reason enough to explain this, for each time the rigid spastic child attempts a movement, a sort of tug-of-war goes on between opposing muscles. Normal activity demands relaxation of one set of muscles while the other set contracts, but in the spastic child this does not happen. Constantly repeated blocking of his efforts may finally convince him that the trial is not worth the effort, and he becomes harder to motivate than the patient not so afflicted. Reeducation of muscles forms the basis of treatment, and muscle checking to ascertain which muscles are strong, which are weak, and which are normal is essential to the program. In addition, the emotional manifestations that characterize these children need some concurrent attention. They are not, as a rule, gregarious or outgoing. They tend to be fearful of new situations and of unknown experiences. They dread sharp, unexpected noises and are very much afraid of falling. Their fear of falling is based on experience, for a fall in an unrelaxed position is indeed an unpleasant occurrence.

The athetoid patient, on the other hand, can make normal movements without the block in the antagonist muscle that confronts the spastic patient, but he is deluged by a flood of involuntary, purposeless movements that are beyond his control. He develops muscle tensions very early in life in an attempt to overcome this. Relaxation is the basis of treatment with the athetoid patient. Surgery and braces are seldom used because permanent fixed deformity does not occur in uncomplicated cases. These children are subject to spells of emotional instability approaching rages, but they are, on the whole, more outgoing and affectionate and less self-conscious than the rigid, spastic patient.

In ataxic cerebral palsy, the chief difficulty may be maintenance of equilibrium. Because it is hard for the ataxic patients to balance themselves, walking may be exceedingly difficult. Otherwise, they seem to have less severe involvement than those with spastic and athetoid cerebral palsy.

Certain principles apply to all types of cerebral palsy, and to avoid repetition these will be set down together. Such treatment as applies to one type or the other is usually ordered by the physician who makes the diagnosis.

Relaxation, although paramount in athetosis, is important to all types of cerebral palsy. Too much stimulation of any nature is inadvisable. Surgical units, clinical units used as centers of play for a noisy group of children, and loud music are not good for these patients. The environment should be particularly quiet before meals, before the physical therapy treatments, and before retiring. The need for a controlled environment in the home also is to be emphasized. The atmosphere on the clinical unit should be one of fairly even tenor at all times. Fatigue comes quickly, even with small effort. It must be watched for and its symptoms recognized. The child tends to want to go on beyond his fatigue level. Rest periods need to be a little longer for these children, because they go

to sleep only after a considerable period of lying in a quiet room. In observing them after they have relaxed and gone to sleep, one will note that their exhaustion is sometimes out of all proportion to the activity in which they have engaged. One of the chief lessons the patient with cerebral palsy must learn is how to relax voluntarily. In order to help the child do this, nurses should be familiar with the methods used by physical therapists in teaching relaxation. Sometimes it is possible to help the child by reference to some familiar relaxing incident, experience, or sensation; e.g., he might be asked to think about a soft and cuddly kitten, or a handful of sand, or a feather or leaf floating in the wind.

Nurse's responsibilities in speech training. It is now generally conceded that the ability to talk is a primary need in patients with cerebral palsy and that it is much more important than, for instance, learning to walk. Speech is bound up closely with every other type of learning, and every experience might be said to have its speech component. Nurses should attempt to supplement the child's speech therapy with conversation appropriate to each experience the child has during the day—i.e., talk about clothes as the child dresses and about food as he eats.

Speech training for the patient with cerebral palsy should be given by qualified speech therapists. To be most effective, it should be begun early, preferably between 2 and 5 years of age. If this training is begun early, it will not be necessary for the child to unlearn the poor habits of communication that children with speech difficulties usually have. Parents may help prepare the child for speech training by having regular periods each day devoted to talking to the child. If the child is very young, talking should be accompanied by looking at pictures or handling the objects about which the adult is talking (Fig. 291). This simple beginning in speech training will aid considerably in the child's development. It is natural for the child to try to imitate and echo the sounds he hears, and the child with cerebral palsy should not be deprived of this experience.

A factor that must be remembered by both nurses and parents is that the child

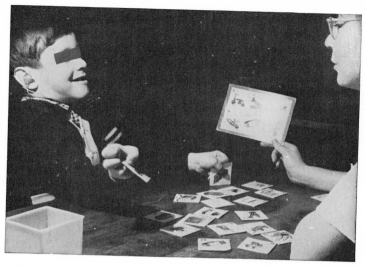

Fig. 291 Speech therapist using a combination of pictures and lipreading to aid speech in a deaf athetoid child. The patient's eyes are blocked in the photograph to conceal identity. (From Kenney, W. C., and Larson, C. B.: Orthopedics for the general practitioner, St. Louis, The C. V. Mosby Co.)

must be urged to ask for the things he wants. If he can get what he wants without asking for it, he will not have to try. Speech therapists emphasize the fact that it is not wise to interpret the child's speech by satisfying his wants too easily. Much of the motivation to speak more accurately may thereby be lost.

Although poor habits of speech should, of course, be discouraged in the hospital when the nurse knows the patient is capable of doing better, it is unwise to constantly call attention to the child's speech, particularly in a nagging manner. An emotional block toward the whole speech problem may be induced by nagging. Encouragement and assistance rather than correction should characterize the nurse's approach to this matter.

Teaching child to feed himself. The ability to feed himself is an important accomplishment for the child with cerebral palsy. Equipment for eating therefore should be optimal. Consultation with the occupational therapist frequently will reveal to the nurse ways of adapting existing hospital equipment to fit the needs of the child for handling his own food. Spoons can be built up with sponge rubber that can be wound around the handle to make a bulky object easy for the child to grasp (Fig. 292). If this is covered with plastic ma-

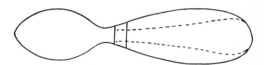

Fig. 292 Spoon built up with sponge rubber and covered with plastic material to make a good grasping handle for the child with cerebral palsy.

terial and secured at the base with waterproof tape, it can be washed and dried with the other hospital silver. A specially constructed chair with a slight backward tilt and a table with a space hollowed out for the child's body are especially useful (Fig. 293). If the table can be constructed with depressions to receive a bowl, a glass, or cup so that things will not slide away from the child as he reaches for them, it will be particularly suitable for his use. On a table that lacks this feature, however, it has been found that small rubber mats, frequently used under tumblers, and bowls equipped with suction cups will help to keep the dishes from slipping. It is advisable to have the child's elbows supported by the table while he eats, since much greater relaxation will be obtained in that way. The feet should rest on a solid surface and not dangle in midair. A large waterproof bib will relieve the

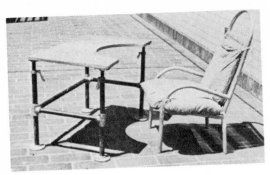

Fig. 293 Adjustable table and chair made by hospital carpenter for patient with cerebral palsy.

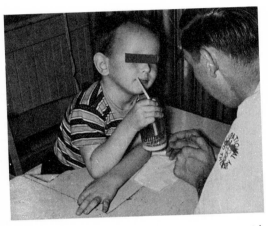

Fig. 294 Therapist teaching a patient with cerebral palsy to drink through a straw. (From Kenney, W. C., and Larson, C. B.: Orthopedics for the general practitioner, St. Louis, The C. V. Mobsy Co.)

child from fear of spilling food on his clothes. Many other details for making mealtime a more comfortable experience for the child can be worked out so that the period is less an ordeal for both the nurse and the patient than it sometimes is when no special equipment is provided.

Because much of the muscle coordination needed for chewing and swallowing also is necessary in speech, it is advisable that as soon as possible the child be given food that requires chewing. Chewing will aid considerably in developing control of the jaw and throat muscles. Some speech therapists advise that the child's training in swallowing can be aided materially by a lollipop. In sucking a lollipop, the child

will learn many of the tongue motions that are necessary in swallowing. A drinking straw is useful in teaching the child to narrow his mouth motion (Fig. 294).

Most of those who work with cerebral palsy patients advise that training for eating should not be done at mealtime. To avoid an emotional block, it is better for the child to learn at a time when his nutrition is not involved. Training in many of the details that concern eating often are incorporated in the physical and occupational therapy program. Such skills are accomplished very gradually, and the child learns to master one motion thoroughly before he is advanced to another. If he can learn to raise an empty glass to his mouth, first by being guided by the therapist's hand and then by his own effort, he has advanced considerably toward being able to feed himself. After he has mastered the empty glass, a very small amount of liquid is added to it, and this is continued until he can lift a glass containing the usual portion of liquid.

Drooling is almost always a matter of great concern to the parents of the child with cerebral palsy. Training to overcome this habit usually is begun concurrently with speech therapy because it is considered to be the result, at least in part, of an inactive tongue. Speech clinicians tell us that something can be done for drooling in almost every instance. As the child learns to chew, suck, and swallow, he will automatically develop these reflexes that will aid in the control of drooling. It is also possible to aid the child in learning to swallow by having certain periods of the day when he practices swallowing rhythmically. For instance, in one exercise the mother or nurse counts to five and the child is instructed to swallow on the fifth count. Repeated faithful efforts in this will show results in the child's gradual ability to control drooling.

The child should have the benefit of quiet surroundings and suitable equipment when he is eating. In the hospital, where distractions are numerous, this is sometimes hard to provide without depriving the child of the companionship of those his own age. Consultation between nurse, physical therapist, and occupational therapist frequently will result in a flexible plan for the child that can be altered as his ability to feed himself and cope with distraction develops.

It must always be remembered that the child may need help, particularly with the last part of his meal. The severely affected patient cannot be deserted and expected to accomplish even minor tasks for himself. He may need help in adjusting his equipment. When he shows obvious symptoms of fatigue, he needs assistance. If he becomes disheartened by being given too much to do or too difficult tasks to perform, he tends to lose interest and courage. The nurse should keep this in mind even when leaving him to perform a simple function of dressing or eating. Encouragement and assistance will do much to promote in the child a feeling of accomplishment without tiring or discouraging him. There is a delicate difference in the matter of creating in the child's mind the ability and desire to do things for himself and confusing him by the assignment of tasks that are beyond his capacity.

It is essential to teach the child to watch what he is doing. Once his concentration span is exceeded, he learns little by his fumbling efforts. The nurse must not be fooled, however, by the child's little tricks of feigning fatigue with a long-drawn-out sigh or a look of helplessness. He is likely to make tentative trials in this direction for the benefit of new nurses. (This is human nature and not peculiar to the patient with cerebral palsy.) Patience, understanding of the child's personality, and considerable firmness are necessary in combating these episodes, but such attitudes must be motivated by continued interest in the child's welfare, for he quickly detects when this is absent.

Nursing care for child in hospital. Sometimes the child with cerebral palsy is kept in the nursery unit of the orthopedic division long after his age would permit him to be moved. This is done so that he may remain in a crib. A child 8 years of age with fairly normal intelligence does not respond well to this kind of treatment. He resents it, and it does something to his spirit. If the child can be moved into a unit with children of his own age group, some provision for this must be made.

A great effort should be put forth to speak to these children very distinctly. It is not considered wise to repeat oneself because it seems that the child has not understood. If there is some type of hearing defect, it may take him several seconds or more to understand and carry out the order or answer the question asked him. Consideration must be given the problem he has with the mere task of motor response. If words are repeated, his ability to respond is interrupted by deluging him with more stimuli. Facial expression should be carefully controlled, or he will detect impatience and be discouraged at the outset. He must be spoken to clearly, simply, and directly, and sufficient time must be allowed for him to comprehend and organize his response. Repetition is in order only when he has asked for it.

It should be recognized from the outset that it is an injustice for the nurse to rush through the care of the patient with cerebral palsy. These children do not make progress under the care of a hurried, overwrought nurse. Their response to this haste is unmistakable—a tightening of all muscles, rigidity, and increased tenseness—the very things for which they were brought to the hospital to overcome. If it is at all possible, the nurse should postpone care of these patients until last in order to be able to give them more time to attempt to do things for themselves. This is sometimes impossible because of early morning assignments to physical or occupational therapy, but the opportunity should not be neglected when it can be managed. Allowing the child to wash and dry his own face and hands or to brush his teeth may take what seems an unjustifiable amount of the nurse's time, but the reward attendant upon these efforts seems so great that no nurse should overlook it.

Toilet habits are not usually difficult to establish in the mentally unaffected patient with cerebral palsy and should be begun as early as with normal children. Specially constructed low toilet seats with armrests are desirable so that the child may be left alone. Continued use of the bedpan long after the child is progressing toward a considerable degree of independence is not wise. For the child who spends most of his time in bed, some arrangement should be made to place him securely and comfortably on the pan and leave him alone rather than to stand at his side holding him—a practice not conducive to good toilet training.

Very early in his training should come

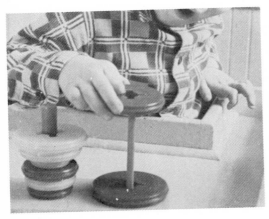

Fig. 295 Patient with cerebral palsy learning to grasp and release the hand by use of a large toy. Later, smaller objects will be used. Note also that the patient is in a standing table to help develop his ability to stand erect. (From Kenney, W. C., and Larson, C. B.: Orthopedics for the general practitioner, St. Louis, The C. V. Mosby Co.)

an appeal to the child to develop proper habits of cleanliness, such as clean hands, brushed teeth, and neatly combed hair. This may seem a small matter, but it will go far toward giving him a feeling of personal worth—without which no other training is of much avail.

Nurse's responsibility in teaching patient. While the patient with cerebral palsy is in the hospital, all the services affecting him must be coordinated. Methods of relaxation followed by careful muscle reeducation in physical therapy and hours of urging toward self-help in occupational therapy and in the schoolroom can be undone by the solicitous nurse who does not realize that the ultimate aim of treatment is to enable the patient to care for himself to the limits of his ability. It is far easier at mealtime to feed the child than to sit beside him guiding, urging, and, if need be, assisting him to eat. But if he is allowed to feed himself only on those days when the nurse is not busy, he will lose the desire to do it at all; it has been observed over and over again that the child loses the will to feed himself if there are days when the nurse does it for him. He likes the presence of another person, and it is not necessary

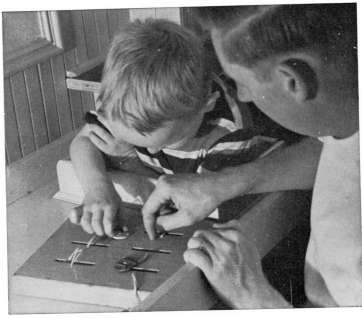

Fig. 296 Patient with cerebral palsy using a large model requiring, in general, the same type of movements needed to lace the shoes. (From Kenney, W. C., and Larson, C. B.: Orthopedics for the general practitioner, St. Louis, The C. V. Mosby Co.)

for him to put forth any effort. Another factor that leads directly to his caring less about doing things for himself is frequently his realization that it is a nuisance to the nurse to wait for him. These children are observant. They soon recognize signs of irritation or bother on the nurse's face. It is not uncommon for a child with athetosis to break into fits of uncontrolled weeping in the middle of a meal for no greater reason than that he feels himself a nuisance. Possibly because of this necessity to hurry, hurry, hurry on the part of busy nurses on orthopedic surgical units, the spastic child feels that he has no business being there.

The child's own wants in the matter of attempting new activities deserve consideration. The motive is strong at this time, and attention will be directed with greater success at something he really wants to do. Guidance is necessary to prevent frustrating disappointments.

Because one of the great aims of all treatment is to give the child as great a degree of independence as is compatible with his condition, considerable attention must be given toward assisting him to care for his own physical necessities. Teaching him to manage his own clothes is a point of great importance. This may be a very slow process in the badly affected child and may start with nothing more spectacular than an attempt to fold his garments as they are taken off. The less skilled movements naturally come first, but some attempt can be made to prepare him to assume more of the task by allowing him to practice with certain toys (Figs. 295 and 296) or a good-sized doll with clothes containing hooks and eyes, buttons, and zippers, as well as drawstrings and snaps.

When the child begins to walk in the hospital, the nurses should know exactly how he has been taught in the physical therapy department so that consistency in instruction may be carried out. It is particularly important to note the child's walking posture and to discourage slumping attitudes. It will help very little for the child to have fifteen to twenty minutes of careful instruction in the physical therapy department once a day if he is allowed to form careless habits of walking the rest of the time on the unit.

Nurses may learn from physical therapists how mirrors can be used in the physical training of the child with cerebral palsy. It is a remarkable fact that often such a child, learning to walk by the aid of lines drawn in front of a mirror, will straighten his body almost as though by reflex when he comes within the range of vision of the mirror. He does not like the look of the stoop-shouldered youngster he sees ahead of him, and he will do his best to alter that appearance. Physical therapists frequently advise parents to use a weighted doll carriage in assisting the child to walk. Walkers are thought by some authorities to be inadvisable because the child, unless closely supervised, tends to push himself along without lifting his feet from the ground

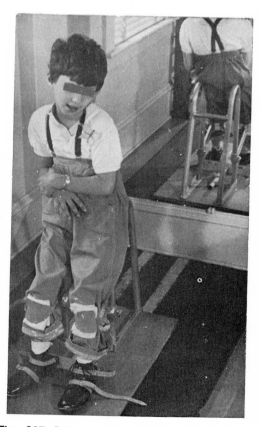

Fig. 297 Patient with cerebral palsy in stabilizer to achieve standing balance. (From Kenney, W. C., and Larson, C. B.: Orthopedics for the general practitioner, St. Louis, The C. V. Mosby Co.)

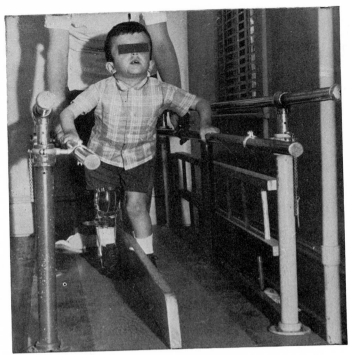

Fig. 298 Patient with cerebral palsy learning reciprocal gait in the parallel bars. Note the center piece to prevent scissoring. (From Kenney, W. C., and Larson, C. B.: Orthopedics for the general practitioner, St. Louis, The C. V. Mosby Co.)

and thereby develops undesirable habits of progression. Parallel bars (Fig. 298), which furnish a sort of stabilized canelike support for the child, are considered more useful. Frequently, some type of support for the child's feet can be constructed to give a wider base for standing and walking. "Duck shoes" or "ski shoes" have been used for this purpose, and these are firmly fastened to the child's everyday shoes during his walking exercises. They are dispensed with as soon as possible, and the child is urged to attempt walking in the normal fashion.

The nurse caring for the patient with cerebral palsy over a considerable period of time will soon learn that there are certain occasions and conditions under which the child relaxes best. Soothing music, gentle rhythmic movements of the limbs, warmth, light massage, and immersion in warm pools frequently are efficacious in assisting the child to relax. Knowing that a great deal of the patient's progress depends directly upon his ability to meet new situations and environments successfully, the nurse will seek to increase the

child's ability to relax in other, less favorable circumstances. This will require time and thought and will be accompanied by many setbacks, but carry-over is possible if the child has normal intelligence.

Nursing care after surgical treatment. Student nurses frequently see patients with cerebral palsy only when they are admitted to orthopedic units for surgery. This is by no means the best time to make the child's acquaintance because he is likely to be more tense and emotional than at any other time. For this reason, it would be desirable to have him admitted long enough before surgery for the nurses to establish some measure of rapport with him and to reassure him of their friendliness, interest, and desire to help him. Only in this way can his great burden of apprehension and insecurity be alleviated. Fortunately, most surgeons feel that it is very unwise to operate on such children until they have become adjusted to their surroundings. Furthermore, operations on rigid spastic patients are usually performed after a period of muscle training. If this interval devoted to muscle reeducation is spent in the hospital, the nurse can help the patient make his adjustment to the hospital situation more satisfactorily than is possible if he enters immediately preceding surgery.

Many operations have been made necessary in these patients because of failure to prevent secondary contractures that come about from constant positions of creeping, crawling, and sitting. These positions are the ones maintained by the child a great portion of the time if he is unable to walk. Parents should be instructed to have the child alternate these positions with some periods in the prone position, which tends to stretch the contracted flexors of the hip and to overcome the forward position of the shoulders. Another variation can be obtained in the back-lying position with a small pillow beneath the dorsal spine. At such times, elevation of the bed or crib on boxes at the head will permit the child to see what goes on around him and not leave him with a feeling of isolation from hospital or home activities.

Postoperatively, these children sometimes display great apathy and prostration—greater than the mild surgical procedure they have been subjected to would seem to warrant. The nurse is urged to respect the child's desire to be let alone as much as is compatible with good care. If he is in casts (long leg or hip spica) after surgery on nerves or tendons, every alteration of his position tends to cause agonizing muscle spasm in the extremities. Even without such movement, his face will be contorted with expressions of pain at very frequent intervals as a result of spasm in the muscles at the site of surgery. Often, these spasms make him very resistant to any type of nursing care, and only the most skillful handling on the part of the nurse will be tolerated willingly. The patient must be turned very gently. No portion of the trunk must be allowed to change position during the turning process. Steady support along the body and cast are essential during any change of position.

Postoperative nausea seems to be unduly prolonged in the spastic child. The intake of such children must be checked carefully.

The skin of these children tends to break down easily when subjected to constant pressure. Attention to their every complaint regarding a sensation of pressure is extremely important. Loss of some degree of sensation, however, is not uncommon in these children, and pressure areas may form beneath casts without any complaint from the child. Scrupulous care of the skin, accompanied by frequent inspection of the cast for odor, rough edges, and the like, is indispensable.

If an adductor tenotomy has been performed, the site of incision in the groin is a frequent cause of concern to the nurse, particularly if the child is very young or is one who cannot be depended upon to call for the bedpan. Waterproof adhesive tape may be used to cover and seal the dressing. Usually the nurse is given permission to change these dressings when the necessity arises. Although careful aseptic technique must be carried out, it is a recognized fact that these tissues seem to be resistant to urine-induced infections.

When the physician has ordered the casts to be bivalved and the patient removed from them for certain periods during the day, it often has been observed that the child will cry bitterly when the splints are put on again. Acute muscle spasm and tenseness sometimes make it almost impossible to reapply these splints, and, if force is used, the child frequently has a miserable night. It is advisable to try to bring about relaxation of the child's muscles rather than to use force in this circumstance. A prolonged bath in warm water sometimes helps to relax muscles and makes application of the splints less painful for the child. The nurse's humane urge to leave off the splints after an unsuccessful attempt to apply them must be tempered by the realization that the tendency toward recurrence of deformity in these patients is very great, and much of the improvement gained by the operation may be sacrificed if splinting is not carried out faithfully.

This difficulty is not so pronounced in the application of the braces that may be ordered later for the postoperative spastic patient. By the time braces are ready, any postoperative tenderness has subsided. It has been found convenient to have the shoes that are attached to such braces cut open to the toes and have eyelets made over the dorsum of the foot, since much easier manipulation of the foot is possible in this way. Grasping the sock over the child's instep and thereby guiding the foot into the shoe serves to overcome the tendency of the foot to go into plantar flexion as the shoe is applied.

Teaching parents home care of child. Instruction for follow-up home care is so vital that the success of all hospital treatment may be said to depend upon it. Demonstrations and information are far from sufficient. If possible, the parents should spend several days in preparation for taking the child home. The mother should be allowed to watch the treatments and nursing care on several occasions and to observe certain emergencies that arise in connection with the child's daily routine so that she will see how these are dealt with in the hospital. It is particularly important for the parents to realize how serious an error it is to break down or interfere with the patient's nascent sense of his own independence and worth. On the other hand, although parents should be urged to encourage the child in his activities, some warning may be needed if they seem to be overly ambitious for the child's progress. Sometimes the parents' enthusiasm and desire for the child constantly to do better serve only to increase his tension, and he may be totally unable to relax in their presence. Furthermore, they should understand that the child occasionally will go through a period when there seems to be no improvement whatever. Since these plateaus are part of the natural cycle for the patient with cerebral palsy, too much concern should not be attached to them.

In giving instructions for home care to the parents, the nurse may help them see the advantages of enlarging the child's horizon by means of friendships with other handicapped children as well as with normal children. The orthopedic public health nurse may be of considerable help to the parents in finding these friends. Assisting the child to forget himself is believed by some to be the major objective of treatment, since loss of agonizing self-consciousness is one of the surest ways to improve motor skill.

Some attempt to educate the child's friends and associates in their approach and relationship with him may be advisable. Only friends who are by nature considerate of others should be encouraged. Outright rudeness or thoughtless remarks made to the handicapped person often discourage him from further attempts at socialization. To help the child in meeting the inescapable crises, some explanation needs to be given to him about human nature and its variable response to the handicapped person. He should be helped to realize very early that both children and grown-ups frequently will display unintelligent, ignorant attitudes toward him, which are unthinkingly cruel on some occasions and foolishly sentimental on others. Perhaps the child old enough to comprehend these attitudes can be made to realize that he himself must develop attitudes of tolerance and forbearance toward persons of limited abilities.

There are many crafts adaptable for the home use of the child with cerebral palsy. Finger painting is excellent for the child whose hand grasp is poor. Work with clay and embroidery or burlap with yarn and large blunt needles provide training toward muscle coordination. Looms and basketry are also excellent. Occupational therapists advise us that whatever craft the cerebral palsied child undertakes should be within his mental and physical capacity. The materials chosen for work should not be difficult to handle. In addition, the work should be the child's own, not that of the parents, nurses, or therapists. Motivation can too easily be destroyed if many alien hands interfere with the child's progress in making something that he would like to think of as entirely his own.

Community projects for the assistance of patients with cerebral palsy are numerous, and the alert public health nurse can help to interest local groups in the subject. One particularly good idea that has been worked out in one community is a so-called lending "library" of equipment for these patients; e.g., reclining chairs, specially constructed tables with adjustable legs, dishes, etc. Another example of community cooperation is a manual training class that has taken as a special project the construction of equipment recommended by a local orthopedist for use by persons with cerebral palsy.

Public health nurses can be of inestimable help to the parents in many ways. They should know definitely what instructions were given the parents before the child was taken home, as well as the treatment and success of treatment that the child had in the hospital. It is essential that they have this information before the child goes home so that there will be no interruption in care or backsliding. Even a week without continued treatment can undo much of what was accomplished in the hospital.

Muscular dystrophy

Types. A number of neuromuscular disorders are included under the term "progressive muscular dystrophy." The most common type is pseudohypertrophic muscular dystrophy. This type affects boys much more frequently than girls, and symptoms (Fig. 299) may be noted by the time the patient is 2 or 3 years of age. The mother becomes aware that the child stumbles and falls more readily than do other children. He may not be able to run and tends to walk on his toes with a slightly waddling gait. The calf muscles become enlarged. As the disease advances, intermittently, the waddling nature of the gait increases and an exaggerated hollow develops in the back (Fig. 300). The muscles around

the thighs, hips, and shoulders atrophy. The fibers of the enlarged calf muscles become displaced by fat and fibrous tissue. It is characteristic that when these children are placed in a sitting position on the floor they arise first to their knees and hands, awkwardly bring each leg up separately to a flexed, weight-bearing position, and then, with their hands against the knees and thighs, gradually force themselves up into an erect position (Gowers' sign; Fig. 301). Even then, they have great instability, and a small blow against the knees or other parts of the body may throw them off balance and cause them to fall to the floor.

In later stages, extensive wasting of the muscles occurs, and the limbs and spine may assume grotesque deformities. Respiratory infections become more difficult to control and frequently are the cause of death. A second cause of death is involvement of the heart muscle. In recent years the use of antibiotics has helped to prolong the life of the child with muscular dystrophy.

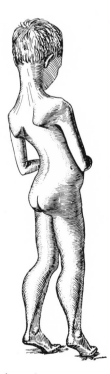

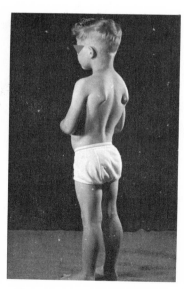

Fig. 299 Child in early stage of pseudohypertrophic progressive muscular dystrophy. Note winging of scapulae, lumbar lordosis, and enlarged calf muscles.

Fig. 300 Moderately advanced pseudohypertrophic progressive muscular dystrophy. Note enlarged calves, contracted heel cords, swayback, and winged shoulders.

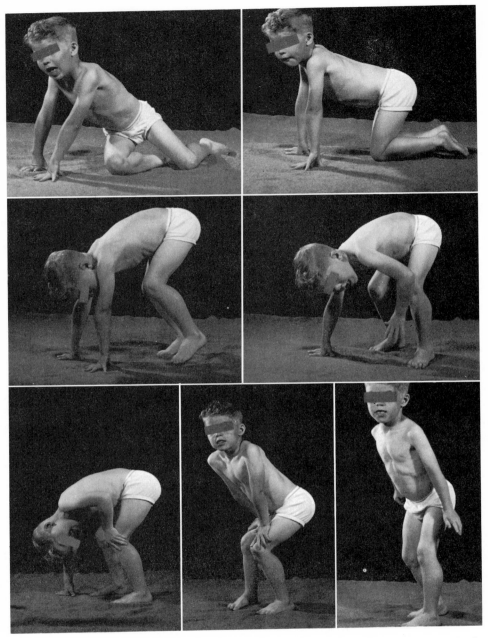

Fig. 301 Child with pseudohypertrophic progressive muscular dystrophy arising from the floor in a typical fashion. After getting on his hands and knees, he braces his hands against his thighs and pushes himself to an upright position (Gowers' sign).

The cause of pseudohypertrophic muscular dystrophy is unknown. There is a definite hereditary factor, and it is transmitted in the same manner as hemophilia —through an unaffected mother to the male children. A test that determines the blood level of creatine phosphokinase (CPK), an enzyme, may be used as an aid in the identification of muscular dystrophy carriers as well as in early detection of the disease. At the present time no cure is known, and the prognosis is poor. Much research has been and is being done, however, in an attempt to find the cause and thus a method of treatment.

Facioscapulohumeral muscular dystrophy is a second progressive type that affects both sexes. Symptoms of this type may appear during the early teens or sometimes later in life. It is not so incapacitating as pseudohypertrophic muscular dystrophy, and most of the patients live a relatively long and useful life.

Limb-girdle muscular dystrophy, a third progressive type, affects males and females equally and has its onset usually in the second or third decade of life. It develops more rapidly than the other types and may incapacitate the individual within a few years.

Nursing intervention. Even though the prognosis is poor, much can be done to help patients with muscular dystrophy to live useful and happy lives. Education for the child should not be neglected. Attendance at a regular school is desirable as long as his physical condition permits. When this is no longer possible, his education should be continued in a school for handicapped children. As the disease progresses and the physical activities that he can participate in lessen, reading may become his chief means of entertainment.

Children with muscular dystrophy should be encouraged and taught to help themselves as much as possible and for as long as possible. They may be slow and clumsy, but active use of their muscles helps maintain strength, which, when lost, is never regained. Parents need help in understanding this, and because muscular dystrophy is a slowly progressive disease, the parents or other family members must assume most of the responsibility for the child's care. Preventing joint contractures is of the utmost importance. It is necessary that the family be taught the value of a foot support, to prevent development of drop foot, and proper bed positions to prevent knee-flexion and hip-flexion contractures or other deformities.

Excessive weight frequently becomes a problem as the child grows older and is less active. Overeating is to be guarded against.

The nurse should remember that the family of a child with muscular dystrophy needs guidance and assistance in securing equipment that facilitates care and at the same time lessens the demands on the mother's physical strength. Rehabilitation aids, such as a trapeze for the bed or a lift for moving the patient from bed to wheelchair, should be made available.

Many patients with muscular dystrophy have received assistance through the Muscular Dystrophy Association, an organization founded in 1950 by the parents and families of muscular dystrophy victims. Through its local and state chapters, it assists the muscular dystrophy patient by providing school facilities, physical therapy, braces, wheelchairs, and other items needed for his care. It also administers grants to finance research.

Poliomyelitis

The very fortunate trend toward the disappearance of poliomyelitis has resulted from the widespread use of poliovirus vaccines (Salk and Sabin) in the United States. The vaccine has been used extensively since 1955.

IPV (inactivated poliomyelitis virus) contains vaccines for types 1, 2, and 3 and is administered by subcutaneous or intramuscular injections. It is given in three doses, the second dose from two to six weeks after the first and the third dose seven months later. OPV (attenuated oral live poliovirus) contains vaccines for strains 1, 2, and 3 and represents the three monovalent vaccines. The vaccine is liquid and may be given by dropper or teaspoon. The dosage varies depending on the potency of the pharmaceutical preparation. The trivalent oral poliovirus (TOPV) is used almost exclusively in the United States because it is easier to administer and produces an immune response which, without regular booster doses, appears to be similar to immunity induced by natural poliomyelitis infection.

The three-dose immunization (TOPV) should be started at 6 to 12 weeks of age, with the second dose given no less than six to eight weeks later and the third dose administered eight to twelve months after the second one. The schedule, recommended by the Public Health Service Advisory Committee, will produce an immune response to all poliovirus types in well

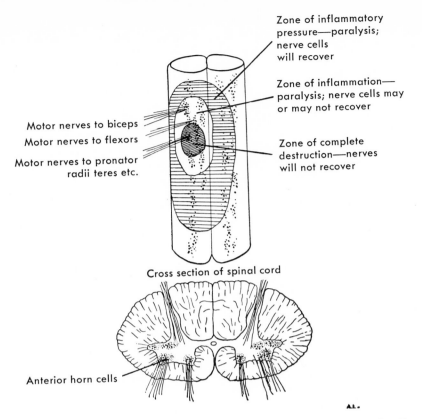

Zone of inflammatory pressure—paralysis; nerve cells will recover

Zone of inflammation—paralysis; nerve cells may or may not recover

Zone of complete destruction—nerves will not recover

Motor nerves to biceps
Motor nerves to flexors
Motor nerves to pronator radii teres etc.

Cross section of spinal cord

Anterior horn cells

Fig. 302 Schematic drawing of spinal cord showing the method of attack of poliomyelitis.

over 90% of the recipients. Upon entering elementary school, all children who have completed the primary oral poliovirus series should be given a single follow-up dose of trivalent oral poliovirus. All others should complete the primary series.

In spite of the decreased incidence of poliomyelitis, this discussion is included for the benefit of the student who may encounter poliomyelitis in other countries or need to care for patients with residual deformities and paralyses from previous epidemics in the United States.

The causative organism is known definitely to be a virus, three strains of which have been isolated. An attack of poliomyelitis does not develop immunity to more than one strain of the virus.

Pathology. The destructive lesions in poliomyelitis are in the anterior horn cells of the spinal cord. The motor system of the body consists of three groups of cells: (1) those in the brain that initiate the mo-

tions, (2) those in the medulla and ganglia that coordinate the motions, and (3) those in the spinal cord (the anterior horn cells) that transmit the impulses to the muscle cells.

The anterior horn cells are distributed in groups throughout the entire spinal cord but are concentrated in the groups that supply nerve impulses to the upper and lower extremities. These groups of cells are arranged more or less in small groups supplying nerve impulses to the upper and lower extremities. These groups of cells are arranged more or less in small groups supplying individual muscles, such as the deltoid, the biceps, the gluteus maximus, the quadriceps.

During an attack of poliomyelitis, the following may occur: (1) There may be several areas where complete destruction of cells, either by local activity of the disease itself or by destructive effects of the toxins formed, may cause an actual degenerative process of varying size and degree. (2) Waste products and edema may endanger the vitality of a major group of cells around the destroyed area. (3) Beyond this are large inflammatory changes that temporarily incapacitate a much larger group of cells (Fig. 302). Return of functional power in the muscles supplied by these cells is fairly rapid.

In the completely destroyed areas, there will never be any return of muscle power. In the intermediate zone, the cells may recover or may disintegrate, according to the demands placed upon them. Rest is the important factor. Only the cells damaged by relatively mild inflammatory change will recover under almost any condition.

The rapid recovery that takes place, within one to three weeks after an attack of poliomyelitis, occurs because the muscles are innervated by the cells that have been impaired temporarily by the inflammatory process.

The recovery that may or may not take place in the following weeks or months is directly related to the number of cells destroyed by the edema and waste products of the disease activity.

The permanent paralysis is directly related to the number of cells destroyed by the local activity of the disease.

Improvement continues in patients with poliomyelitis for at least several years. Any improvement after a few months, however, is not the result of any further recovery of the nerves but rather an improved functioning of the muscle fibers whose nerves of stimulation have already recovered.

There are two other types of involvement with poliomyelitis. The *bulbar* type consists of an involvement of the nerve cells high up in the spinal cord. If the inflammatory condition reaches the vital centers, the condition is fatal. If the damage is not sufficient to cause death, a relatively complete recovery usually occurs within a few weeks or months. These patients may require use of the respirator during the more active stage of the disease because of the paralysis of the intercostal muscles and the diaphragm. *Poliomeningitis* manifests symptoms that are frequently very similar to those found in other forms of meningitis, including delirium, stiff neck, strabismus,

and incontinence. Actual paralysis of the muscles is not usually present. There may be flaccidity or spasticity of the extremities.

Symptoms and signs. Poliomyelitis usually begins rather abruptly with a headache and an intestinal disturbance. There may be an elevation of temperature from 99° to 102° F. There is usually some evidence of spinal cord irritation that is recognized by stiffness of the neck with some resistance and pain in the back when attempts are made to raise the head from the bed. Paralysis, when it develops, usually occurs somewhere between the third and seventh day after the onset of the illness. In some cases, however, the initial symptoms are so mild that the disease is not recognized until paralysis has set in. The patient may then fall because of weakness of a limb.

In those persons in whom paralysis does not develop, all symptoms may disappear within two or three days. It is unwise, however, to make any statement regarding the severity of the disease earlier than forty-eight hours after the disappearance of all fever, since apparently mild cases may subsequently become severe. When paralysis develops, there may be pain on movement of the limbs and joints or on pressure upon the muscles involved. After the acute symptoms, the patient is usually quite comfortable except for this.

Diagnosis. Diagnosis is confirmed by the spinal tap and identification of the virus (one of three strains now known). Many recently identified viruses such as the ECHO group can cause symptoms, exclusive of paralysis, that simulate the acute stage of poliomyelitis. A spinal fluid examination that reveals a slight increase in pressure, a clear appearance, and a cell count of from 10 to 300 or slightly higher is considered very significant. The cell count, if performed early enough, shows a predominance of polymorphonuclear leukocytes, but these are succeeded within twenty-four to forty-eight hours by lymphocytes. Spinal sugar is normal; nurses will remember that it should be about one-half the amount of the blood sugar. Chlorides are normal, and the Pandy test for spinal globulin may be positive, 1+ to 4+. The total protein is usually increased, and an elevation of 45 mg/mm^3 or above is thought to be significant.

If laboratory facilities are available, the poliomyelitis virus should be looked for, by the use of suitable culture techniques, in the stool of the patient or in throat washings.

Because it has been established that the virus may leave the body of the patient (or healthy carrier) in the discharges from the bowel or the nose and throat, it seems safe to assume that person-to-person contact must play a large part in the spread of the disease. Although the upper respiratory passages are no longer considered the primary routes of infection, nevertheless, the exact manner in which the virus enters the body is not completely understood, and care should be used in handling the discharges from the bowel and the nose and throat of any patient suspected of having poliomyelitis.

It is now an accepted fact that the virus of poliomyelitis remains in the gastrointestinal tract sometimes over a period of weeks, and, therefore, considerable attention must be given to the matter of disinfecting stools.

Health teaching and prevention of poliomyelitis. At the present time, the nurse's most important responsibility pertaining to poliomyelitis lies in the area of prevention. Helping parents understand the necessity of having members of the family receive the poliomyelitis vaccine and providing them with information on immunization programs available in their community are vital if this disease is to be prevented. The oral vaccine is available at a minimal cost, and every child and adult should receive this protection against poliomyelitis. Additional teaching done by the nurse is based on a few rules of hygiene dictated by current concepts of the disease. Because in many cases it seems unquestionable that the virus is ingested, all foods should be protected from filth, flies, dirty hands, and animals. If food is to be eaten raw, it should be washed well. Hands should be carefully washed not only before meals but before eating food. Milk should be certified or pasteurized, and the water supply should be from approved sources.

Treatment and nursing intervention. During the acute and febrile stage of poliomyelitis, rest is all-important. The treatment of choice consists of the use of a firm bed and relaxation of the affected extremities in a position of physiologic rest. In the upper extremities, the shoulders are maintained in slight abduction, the elbows flexed or extended, and the wrists at slight dorsiflexion. In the lower extremities, the knee and hip are flexed a few degrees, and the foot is held in a position at right angles to the leg.

Warm moist packs may be applied to the involved parts and passive exercises done to help maintain a normal range of motion. This treatment seems to have the advantage of eliminating stasis in the muscles, thereby preventing spasm and contractures, maintaining flexibility, and making the patient comfortable. Nothing, however, can effect the recovery of the nerve cells in the anterior horn of the spinal cord.

Deformity should be prevented during the convalescent stage. However, if it does occur or if weaknesses persist, the limbs must be protected by braces or the deformities corrected.

Passive joint movement is usually done several times during the day. Every effort is put forth to maintain complete range of joint motion in all joints from the earliest days of the disease. Warm pool treatments or hot tub baths are sometimes given several times during the week as part of the treatment. Intensive packing of tight or contracted muscles, followed by forcible stretching, may be done after the acute period of pain and spasm is over.

Bulbar involvement. Both medical treatment and nursing care in bulbar poliomyelitis are based on four considerations: preventing asphyxia, averting exhaustion, maintaining adequate nutrition, and checking secondary infections. Restlessness, wakefulness, an increase of mucus in the throat, difficulty in swallowing, drawing the head back, rigidity, and an expression of apprehension are significant and should be reported without delay.

Involvement of muscles of respiration. In the spinal type of poliomyelitis or in the combined spinal and bulbar type, weakness of shoulders and arms is sometimes an early sign that impairment of some muscles of the chest (pectorals) and those of respiration (intercostals and diaphragm) may take place. The nurse must be alert for signs of approaching respiratory embarrassment when caring for a patient with obvious involvement of the upper extremities.

Poliomyelitis has become a rare illness during the past two decades. The dreaded epidemics have disappeared. However, the occasional sporadic case still occurs, and there are those individuals affected with the disease prior to the use of the vaccine who may have residual paralysis and need corrective surgery and special orthotic equipment to help them ambulate and maintain independence.

Brachial palsy in newborn infants

Cause. Brachial palsy consists in a paralysis of the arm caused by damage to the brachial plexus during the birth process. It may occur spontaneously during a relatively difficult labor, or it may result from the use of instruments or traction on the arm in abnormal labor.

Difficult, prolonged labor seems to play a definite part in its etiology, since anesthesia is employed in these cases, and considerable muscle relaxation is present during birth.

Types. There are three types (all becoming less frequent with improved obstetric methods). (1) Erb's palsy (upper-arm type) is caused by injury to the fifth and sixth cervical nerve roots and results in paralysis of the muscles around the shoulder. The arm remains adducted and internally rotated, and the forearm is held in a pronated position. (2) Klumpke's palsy (lower-arm type) results in a more severe form of paralysis, caused by injury to the eighth cervical and first thoracic nerve roots. The function of the intrinsic muscles of the hand and the wrist and finger flexors is lost. A clawlike hand may develop. (3) The whole-arm type may involve all the nerve roots of the brachial plexus, resulting in a flail arm and the loss of sensation in the extremity. The arm is rotated inwardly by the unparalyzed pectoral and scapular muscles. These muscles become contracted if the condition remains untreated for any great length of time, and the deformity becomes fixed.

The prognosis in Erb's palsy is good. It is poor in paralysis of the whole arm or of the lower arm (Klumpke's).

Treatment and nursing intervention. Early recognition of brachial paralysis is not difficult. It is frequently suspected by the obstetrician when he delivers the child. The causative factor is a forcible separation of head and shoulder during delivery. This produces a tearing injury of the nerves of the brachial plexus. The nurse giving the initial bath will note the characteristic position of the arm as it hangs flaccidly with the elbow in extension, the shoulder adducted and rotated inward (often accompanied by a cupping appearance of the shoulder), and the hand pronated, palm facing the back (Fig. 303). The infant does not use the arm and will object to its being moved for him during the first days of life. This reaction gradually subsides, and the arm can be moved without pain to the child.

In the milder form of brachial palsy, the nerves are injured and the paralysis is usually caused by stretching of the brachial nerve trunks. As recovery takes place, treatment is directed at the prevention of contractures. This is accomplished by providing for active or passive motion of the

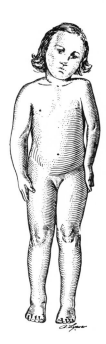

Fig. 303 Brachial palsy of the left arm in a 6-year-old child. Inward rotation and adduction of the shoulder, pronation of the forearm, and atrophy of the arm are shown.

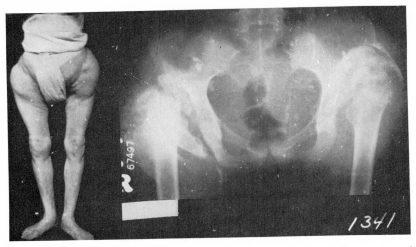

Fig. 304 Charcot joints. The roentgenogram illustrates the extensive destruction of bone. The patient experiences little or no pain, but such joints are quite unstable, and weight bearing is difficult.

joints involved. Sometimes a "Statue of Liberty" position, which consists of abduction and external rotation of the shoulder, flexion of the elbow, and supination of the forearm, is prescribed for short periods several times daily. This position may be maintained by means of a splint or by careful positioning of the infant's body and arm. Freedom of the arm is permitted at other times. This is important, since no one position should be maintained continuously.

In the most severe lower or whole arm paralysis, there is usually formidable damage or complete severance of some of the roots of the brachial plexus. Inspection by operation and suturing of these nerve roots is seldom justified. Again, early care and management must provide for passive range of motion and changes of position for the involved extremity. This treatment is directed at the prevention of contractures. Later, tendon transplants or other surgical procedures may be performed to correct any existing deformity and to improve function.

Charcot joints and other neuropathies

Charcot joints are not truly neuromuscular disorders but are allied enough to be included in this chapter.

It has been established—clinically and roentgenographically—that bone, cartilage, and ligaments can, at times, literally melt away, leaving a very misshapen, unstable, unserviceable, and yet quite painless joint. This is known as a neuropathy and occurs particularly in association with certain nerve tissue disorders such as neurosyphilis, diabetic neuritis, syringomyelia, and occasionally paraplegia. The name Charcot has been applied to such joints (Fig. 304).

The only treatment is treatment of the underlying cause: penicillin for neurosyphilis, diet and insulin for the control of diabetes, and radiation therapy for syringomyelia. The unstable joint does not heal, but occasionally the progression of the process can be checked. Joint fusion or application of braces will provide stability for the affected joints.

15 Arthritis

Rheumatism is a general term that includes disorders in which pain and stiffness of the muscles or skeleton are prominent features.

Arthritis is a form of rheumatism in which the joints primarily are affected. It is estimated that roughly 1% of the people in the United States have arthritis. With the associated social, economic, and emotional burdens on the families of patients with arthritis, the importance of the nursing care of the patient becomes obvious.

Arthritis is a chronic disease causing varying degrees of disability, frequently quite severe. Unfortunately there is no cure for most of the forms of arthritis. The desired goal in the care of the patient must be to help him function efficiently as a human being and as a member of society. It follows, then, that the treatment program must consider the patient's physical and emotional health and any social problems that may be present, especially as they relate to family members and economic situation. If the treatment program does not include all these, it is inadequate and will fail to achieve the goal that common sense tells us is the only logical objective. Indeed, this should be the kind of attention and desired goal in the care of any patient, no matter what his ailment.

The described objective in the care of the patient with arthritis cannot be adequately achieved by any one person. The combined efforts of a number of specially trained persons—the patient's personal physician, consulting physicians, nurses, physical therapist, occupational therapist, social worker, and vocational counselor—will be needed at various times. The overall program is directed by the physician who has the responsibility for the patient's long-term care and who must know all the facets of the patient's problems.

The physician who has the primary responsibility for the patient's care must not only attend to his medical needs, but must also assist him in other areas. The role of the nurse, as will be shown, is very important in the total treatment program. The physical therapist has close contact with the patient and similarly contributes a great deal. Many patients have disabilities that make it difficult or impossible for them to perform everyday tasks that we take for granted, such as putting on shoes or socks. The occupational therapist can help the patient by showing him ways of adapting to his disabilities, by demonstrating techniques for simplifying everyday tasks, and by providing devices to aid him in performing these activities. The social worker can help in working out family problems, in providing contact with special service agencies, and frequently giving moral support to the patient who has emotional problems contributing to his disability. The vocational counselor contributes a real service when he helps the patient find a new occupation when he can no longer continue at his previous work because of his disability.

There are numerous types of arthritis. The three discussed below (rheumatoid, degenerative, and gouty arthritis) are relatively common. Other, less common types usually resemble one of these three clinically, and the principles of nursing care can be applied accordingly.

Rheumatoid arthritis

Rheumatoid arthritis is a chronic systemic disease of unknown cause. Anemia, low-grade fever, weight loss, and other disturbances of the patient's general health may occur, but joint pain and swelling are the symptoms that usually cause the patient to seek medical care. Varying degrees of deformity and destruction of joints commonly occur, causing different kinds and amounts of disability. The joint damage may be so severe in some instances as to result in complete invalidism. Rheumatoid arthritis occurs more commonly in women than in men, in a ratio of 2 or 3 to 1. It may occur at any age, from infancy to advanced old age, but most often appears between 20 and 50 years of age.

The prominent symptoms are stiffness, especially upon arising in the morning, and joint pain and swelling involving multiple joints. The swelling is caused by inflammation of the synovium, the tissue lining the joint capsule, and by accumula-

tion of fluid within the joints. The inflammatory process results in hypertrophy of the joint synovium and the formation of granulation tissue that is referred to as pannus. Growth of the granulation pannus spreads to the articular cartilage, causing destruction of the cartilage and eventually erosion of the subchondral bone (Fig. 305). Palpation of a joint with an inflamed synovial membrane usually reveals tenderness, swelling, and a sponginess or bogginess. The outward appearance is that of a swollen joint, which is warm to touch and painful when moved. There is a definite tendency for involvement of the same joints on both sides of the body, and the arthritis usually affects more joints as time goes on. Although any joint in the body may be involved, there is a predilection for the small joints of the hands and feet. The wrists, elbows, ankles, and knees also are commonly involved. The swelling that appears in the hands usually is present in the proximal interphalangeal joints (middle knuckle). The intrinsic muscles of the hand are considerably atrophied, and for this reason the thickened edematous middle knuckles seem particularly enlarged. This deformity is spoken of as a spindle deformity and is quite characteristic (Fig. 306).

As a result of the chronic joint inflammation, important anatomic changes may occur, with consequent limitation of joint function. Involvement of the joint capsule and supporting ligaments may cause weakness, stretching, or rupture of these struc-

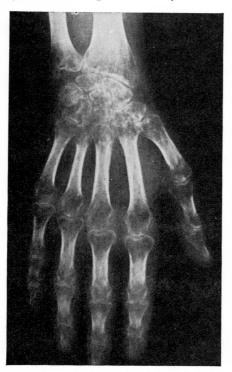

Fig. 305 Roentgenogram of the hand in rheumatoid arthritis showing localized demineralization and narrowing of the joint space. (From Kenney, W. C., and Larson, C. B.: Orthopedics for the general practitioner, St. Louis, The C. V. Mosby Co.)

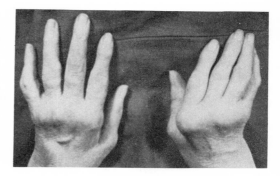

Fig. 306 The hands in rheumatoid arthritis. Note the enlarged metacarpophalangeal joints and the spindle-shaped fingers that are seen with swelling of the proximal interphalangeal joints. The ulnar deviation of the fingers on the right hand is a common deformity.

tures, resulting in instability. When the instability is severe, partial dislocation of the joint, referred to as subluxation, may occur. In other instances there is scarring of these supporting tissues, causing limitation of motion. This is termed contracture of the joint capsule or ligament. When scarring occurs within a joint, limitation of motion (called ankylosis; Fig. 308) also occurs. It may be so severe as to result in a completely motionless joint. Actual destruction of cartilage and bone within the joint often is found in rheumatoid arthritis. When severe, it may result in greatly impaired joint function. Muscle weakness is common and may contribute to the patient's disability.

The diagnosis of rheumatoid arthritis is determined by a number of factors. The patient's history is important and usually reveals the presence of sporadic aches and pains, and then pain that is more pronounced, and finally attacks that occur more frequently with swelling of the small joints of the hands or feet. The presence and duration of early morning stiffness are significant. Laboratory reports may reveal slight elevations of the erythrocyte sedimentation rate and the leukocyte count. The latex agglutination test is a helpful diagnostic procedure but is not specific for arthritis. It may be positive in several connective tissue diseases. The procedure is based on the fact that the presence of abnormal macroglobulins (referred to as rheumatoid factor) in the serum will cause the clumping together of small biologically inert particles (latex-bentonite) that have been coated with human gamma globulin. Early in the course of the disease, roentgenograms show little change in the joint structure. However, in chronic arthritis, narrowing of the joint space (loss of cartilage), changes in the joint contour, the presence of bony spurs, and erosive changes of the bone are evident in varying degrees.

The course of rheumatoid arthritis usually is one of periods of increased disease activity alternating with intervals of decreased disease activity (exacerbations and remissions). There may be great variation in the intensity and duration of the periods of increased activity from time to time. It is very difficult, therefore, to predict the course of the disease in an individual patient. A small percentage of patients with

rheumatoid arthritis will have a mild course with little disability. Most patients will have varying degrees of disability that increase with the duration of the disease. These patients remain largely independent of others for self-care and are usually able to pursue occupations not requiring vigorous physical activity. Severe incapacitation will occur in relatively few patients.

Ankylosing spondylitis, also known as rheumatoid spondylitis and Marie-Strümpell arthritis, is a chronic form of arthritis affecting primarily the sacroiliac joints and spine (Fig. 307). Frequently it leads to severe ankylosis or limitation of motion of the back. It affects men approximately four times more frequently than women and usually occurs between 16 and 40 years of age. Pain and stiffness of the back are the common symptoms of this disorder. In-

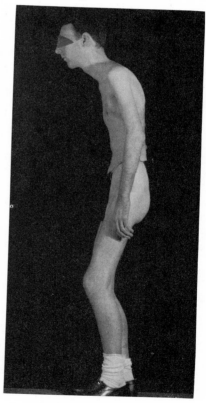

Fig. 307 Typical posture in ankylosing spondylitis (Marie-Strümpell arthritis) of the spine. The hip and shoulder joints also may be involved. (From Smith-Petersen, M. N., Larson, C. B., and Aufranc, O. E.: Osteotomy of the spine for correction of flexion deformity in rheumatoid arthritis, J Bone Joint Surg [Am] **27**:1-11, Jan. 1945.)

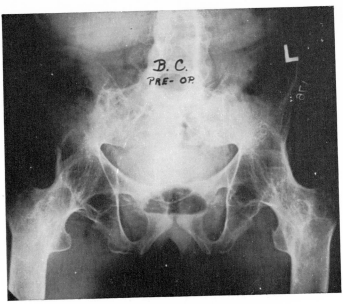

Fig. 308 Roentgenogram in Marie-Strümpell arthritis. Both hip joints, both sacroiliac joints, and the zygapophyseal joints have been destroyed and have undergone bony ankylosis. Note the calcification of the vertebral ligaments. No motion in this portion of the back and in the hips is possible. (From Kenney, W. C., and Larson, C. B.: Orthopedics for the general practitioner, St. Louis, The C. V. Mosby Co.)

volvement of the extremity joints occurs in some patients and is usually less severe than in typical rheumatoid arthritis. The course of ankylosing spondylitis is variable, just as is rheumatoid arthritis. It is usually a progressive disease involving more of the spine with the passage of time.

Rheumatoid disease occurring before the age of 16 years is referred to as juvenile rheumatoid arthritis (Still's disease; Figs. 311 and 312). It is very similar to adult rheumatoid arthritis in that joint deformity, loss of joint motion, and subluxation of the joint may occur. Control of pain, proper splinting, positioning, and exercise are important. The child with a severe rheumatoid arthritic condition that is present throughout the growing years may have premature closure of the epiphyses. When this occurs, growth is abnormal.

Treatment and nursing intervention. Because rheumatoid arthritis is a chronic systemic disease, consideration must be given to the care of each patient's general health as well as to the treatment of the joint problems and to daily nursing care.

General considerations. Adequate rest, relief of pain, prevention of deformity, proper nutrition, treatment of any other diseases present, and assisting the patient to understand his disease and develop a proper attitude toward it are the important general features of treatment. There is no cure for rheumatoid arthritis, and it must be clearly understood that all treatment is directed at maintaining good general health and helping the patient to function at his best possible level.

Years of experience have shown that a successful basic treatment program for rheumatoid arthritis must include adequate rest, relief of pain, and a regular exercise program. The patient with rheumatoid arthritis requires eight to twelve hours of sleep each night and, when the disease is in an active period, frequent rest periods during the day. In the event of an acute flare-up of the arthritis, several days of bed rest are helpful in reducing joint inflammation and systemic symptoms. However, remaining in bed for prolonged periods of time is undesirable because it leads to increased muscle weakness and limitation of joint motion.

No drug has been found to be more desirable than aspirin for relief of pain, and this is the basic ingredient of the drug therapy portion of the treatment program. Aspirin often controls pain satisfactorily when given in adequate dosages—eight to sixteen or more 0.3 Gm tablets daily. Many patients will not require any other medication. In other patients, additional drugs are needed, but the aspirin is continued as the basic drug.

Physical therapy is a basic part of the treatment program for most patients with rheumatoid arthritis. It should consist primarily of therapeutic exercises having one or both of the following objectives: improvement or maintenance of muscle strength and/or improvement or maintenance of range of motion of joints. Efforts directed at the first objective, especially, should be the major concern of the physical therapist. Therapists often apply heat to painful joints for temporary relief of pain and stiffness. Since the duration of beneficial effect of such treatment is quite brief and since rheumatoid arthritis is a protracted disease, this method of pain relief has limited practicality in the long-term management of these patients. More appropriate pain relief can usually be obtained by adjustment of the drug regimen. When combined with other intensive physical therapy techniques (e.g., just before a patient begins a therapeutic exercise period), heat therapy may offer justifiable benefit to the patient.

Other factors must be considered in the basic treatment program for a patient with rheumatoid arthritis. Adequate nutrition is accomplished by a balanced diet having sufficient caloric intake to maintain normal weight. Overweight, even of moderate degree, is deleterious and should be corrected by diet. The adverse effect of obesity must be clearly explained to the patient, and the importance of weight reduction, when needed, should be strongly emphasized. Special diets, supplements, or vitamins have no value in the treatment of rheumatoid arthritis. Treatment of other diseases that are present should be done to improve the patient's general health.

Because rheumatoid arthritis is a chronic disease and the patient often has pain and is limited in the performance of daily activities, it is common for him to become discouraged and to develop a poor outlook for the future. Thus moral support is a very important aspect of treatment and can mean the difference between success and failure of the overall program. It is important that the patient develop the proper attitude toward his disease. Obviously, a give-up or hopeless reaction is undesirable and, when severe, may be a major factor in causing disability. On the other hand, failure to acknowledge any limitations can cause the patient much difficulty, too. The person who adopts a realistic attitude toward his disease, lives within the limitations imposed by it, and follows advice for treatment definitely does better than the one who does not. Physicians, nurses, and others concerned with a patient's care have a great deal of responsibility in this regard because it is from them that he derives many of his ideas and attitudes concerning his illness. Those who care for the arthritic patient must have a realistic but hopeful approach to the patient and his disease. Frequent contact with the patient provides the nurse with ample opportunity to benefit him in this area. Attitudes of pity or unconcern will certainly have an undesirable effect.

Prevention of deformity is of the utmost importance. When deformity is severe, it may be the major cause of disability in an arthritic patient. Many components of the treatment program contribute to this aspect of therapy, such as rest of an inflamed joint, medication to relieve pain, and physical therapy treatments to maintain joint motion and muscle strength. Braces or splints to support the joints may be indicated. Some are used only when the patient is resting or sleeping and others only when the patient is up and about. Specially designed or modified shoes may be very helpful in relieving foot pain caused by deformity.

An often neglected but very significant area for the prevention of deformity is the bed in which the arthritic patient spends one-third to one-half of his time. The mattress must be firm with a bed board between it and the spring. The pillow should be thin so as to cause minimal flexion of the neck (Fig. 309). Pillows should never be placed beneath the knees because this will very likely lead to the development of flexion contractures of the hips and knees

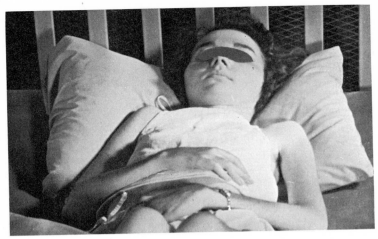

Fig. 309 Position frequently assumed by arthritic patients: shoulders adducted and elbows and wrists flexed.

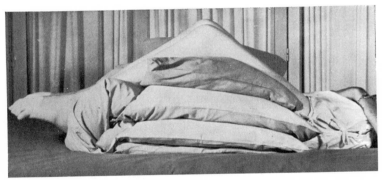

Fig. 310 Permanent flexion contractures of the knees and hips (common deformities in arthritis) caused by the continuous use of pillows to support the knees in a flexed position.

(Fig. 310), which is a serious deformity. A pillow placed between the knees to separate the legs slightly, however, is definitely helpful in preventing adduction deformity of the hips. The bed should be relatively high because often the patient has weak leg and hip muscles. The use of a footboard on the bed to prevent contracture of the heel cord (drop-foot deformity) and to keep the bed covers off the feet is important. Maintaining proper body alignment when resting is helpful in preventing deformity (see Chapter 3). The arthritic patient should lie with the joints extended as far as is comfortable a good portion of the time. A sandbag or a trochanter roll placed along the lateral aspect of the lower extremity helps to maintain a neutral position of the hip joint. This prevents external

rotation of the limb, an undesirable position for the patient with acute hip involvement.

Daily nursing care. Many aspects of daily care that the nurse learns to do routinely needs to be modified or individualized for the arthritic patient. Simple things that are ordinarily done without thinking, such as going to the bathroom, turning in bed, or even moving an extremity, may be ordeals for an arthritic patient because of pain or disability. He frequently requires a great deal of time. To hurry him or become impatient will only cause him unnecessary pain or dissatisfaction with the nurse. The latter will retard or prevent the development of satisfactory rapport with the patient. In the morning especially, or after a period of rest, the arthritic patient moves slowly because of the stiffness so charac-

teristic of the disease. Pain also is frequently increased at these times. It is worthwhile for the nurse to listen to the patient,
for often he has learned special ways of
taking care of his needs that make it easier
for him. Because there is an almost infinite
variety in the types and degrees of disability in arthritic patients, care must be
individualized according to each patient's
needs. It is important to determine what
the patient can and cannot do by himself.
He should be expected to do those things
of which he is capable, but he will require assistance in others. There is a distinct tendency of some patients to grow
increasingly dependent on others, even for
those things that they can do for themselves. This, of course, is to be discouraged,
and the patient should be led to do more
and more for himself as his therapy progresses.

Standard nursing care activities such as
bathing, shaving, brushing teeth, and making up beds are necessary parts of the
patient's care and are not to be ignored.
Because of disability, assistance may be
required but should be given only if
needed. The patient should be encouraged
to establish a daily routine for performing
self-care. Because arthritic patients may
spend considerable time in bed, special attention to skin care is important. Cleanliness and the use of skin lotion when necessary are most helpful. Careful attention
must be given to pressure points located
over bony prominences, such as the elbows,
spinous processes of the vertebrae, sacrum,
trochanters, ankles, and heels, to prevent
decubitus ulcers. Soft foam-rubber pads
will offer some protection for these areas,
but the most important preventive measure
is frequent change of position. Observation
of the patient performing his daily activities
will give clues for making his efforts easier
or less uncomfortable. A trapeze can be
placed over the patient's bed to aid him
in turning and in getting in and out of
bed. The patient with troublesome weakness or pain in the legs will benefit from
the use of a chair with a relatively high
seat. It is much easier for him to get in
and out of such a chair than from a low
one. Armrests provide additional assistance
in getting in and out of a chair. If troublesome hand deformities are present, eating

utensils with modified handles may be
beneficial. Likewise, a chair in the shower
to enable the patient to sit down while
bathing, a bath sponge on a long handle,
a long-handled shoehorn, and a rod with
a hook at one end to help in putting on
socks may be very helpful to the patient.

Many routine daily activities present potential injury hazards for the arthritic patient because of his weakness or instability.
The bathtub and shower should be provided with handrails and nonslip floor
mats. Wheelchairs, when the brakes are
not applied, can be treacherous; all patients
should be firmly warned of this. The rubber
tips of crutches and canes are essential for
safe use. When they are missing or worn,
the danger of a serious fall is always
present. Therefore, they should be checked
frequently. Stairways must have handrails.
Some of these precautions may seem unnecessary or obvious, but for the arthritic
patient they are very important.

Special forms of treatment. Special forms
of treatment include medication, braces,
splints, and traction, and surgery.

Drugs. No matter what medications are
used in the treatment of rheumatoid arthritis, it must be remembered that none is
curative. They are useful only to aid in
the relief of pain and stiffness, and probably
none has an effect on the disease itself.
Therefore, these medications are never a
substitute for the basic treatment program;
they are additions to it and are of less
importance than the basic program itself.
Because pain in active arthritis is caused
by inflammation, it follows that most of
the drugs are used to suppress inflammation. Medications that have this effect include aspirin, phenylbutazone, indomethacin, the antimalarial drugs chloroquine
and hydroxychloroquine, gold, and the various cortisone-like drugs that are frequently
called corticosteroids or steroids.

Aspirin is the basic drug in treatment
of rheumatoid arthritis. It is definitely helpful in the large majority of patients, quite
safe for long-term use, and well tolerated
by most patients. Plain aspirin is the desirable form for most patients and the least
expensive. Most patients require relatively
large doses, 0.6 to 1.5 Gm four times daily
on a regular schedule. In many patients,
the maximum tolerated dose is necessary,

just short of that dose which causes symptoms of aspirin excess. Greater effectiveness is achieved by the patient's taking aspirin regularly, four doses daily, than when it is used sporadically. A convenient schedule for most patients, and one that minimizes abdominal distress, is a dose with each meal and at bedtime, the latter with a snack or milk. The difference in effectiveness between small and large doses of aspirin is often significant and warrants careful adjustment to determine the maximum dose tolerated by the patient in order to gain the greatest benefit.

The common symptoms of salicylism (aspirin toxicity) are tinnitus (noises in the ears), decreased hearing acuity, vertigo, headache, lassitude, drowsiness, dimness of vision, nausea, vomiting, hyperventilation, and depressed mental function. Of these, tinnitus and hearing loss are the most common and are usually the first to appear. Chronic aspirin therapy causes gastritis in a significant number of patients and gastric ulcer in a lesser but still important number. Both of these problems most commonly occur with epigastric pain. Not all patients taking aspirin who have such pain necessarily have gastritis or ulcer, however. Minor epigastric distress may be eliminated by the use of buffered aspirin. Those patients known to have previous gastritis or gastric ulcer and those who cannot tolerate buffered aspirin should be given enteric-coated aspirin.

Some arthritic patients have found ibuprofen (Motrin), a relatively new drug, to be beneficial in reducing joint pain and lessening the duration of morning stiffness. It is a nonsteroidal anti-inflammatory agent that has analgesic and antipyretic activities. Its mode of action is not understood. Gastrointestinal disturbances may occur with this drug. Some additional adverse reactions that have been reported include tinnitis, dizziness, edema, and headache.

For many patients with rheumatoid arthritis, aspirin is not adequate for control of pain and stiffness resulting from joint inflammation. In these cases, additional drugs are necessary. It is strongly emphasized that aspirin be continued in the maximum tolerated dose and that other drugs be added. Of the several drugs listed previously, one or more may be used in combination with aspirin. All are compatible, one with any other. The particular drug chosen will depend on several factors: previous attempts at therapy, severity of disease, cost to the patient, and others.

Phenylbutazone is an anti-inflammatory drug of relatively low potency and may be helpful in some patients. A one-week trial of therapy is adequate for assessment of efficacy. If no benefit has occurred, it should be discontinued. If helpful, it may be continued. The initial dose is 100 mg four times daily for one week, followed by the smallest effective amount. Adverse effects include salt and water retention, which occurs in all patients. This may lead to edema formation, worsening of hypertension, or congestive heart failure in patients with serious heart disease. Abdominal distress similar to that described for aspirin is common. Less frequently, dermatitis or stomatitis occurs. The serious forms of toxicity, although uncommon, involve the bone marrow, causing agranulocytosis or aplastic anemia; the latter is especially serious because approximately 50% of cases end fatally. Long-term therapy with this drug is not recommended if at all avoidable. If used on a long-term basis, monthly blood counts must be obtained. Even then, severe toxicity may occur unpredictably.

Indomethacin is an anti-inflammatory drug helpful in some patients with rheumatoid arthritis. The usual initial dose is 25 mg twice daily, increasing by 25 mg every four days to 25 mg four times daily. Maintenance doses are 75 to 150 mg daily. A three-week trial of therapy at 100 mg daily is adequate to determine effectivnesss in most patients. If beneficial, it may be given for a prolonged period of time relatively safely. Serious adverse reactions are rare, although gastritis and gastric ulcer similar to distress from aspirin may occur. Less serious but distressing side effects frequently requiring discontinuance of the drug include headache, dizziness, vague but unpleasant mental symptoms, abdominal distress, and diarrhea.

Two antimalarial drugs, *chloroquine* and *hydroxychloroquine*, have been found to be beneficial in the treatment of some patients with rheumatoid arthritis. Their efficacy is approximately equal. Hydroxychloroquine is thought by most to be less toxic.

The usual dose of this drug is 400 mg daily for six weeks; then 200 mg daily, given at bedtime to minimize nausea. A three-month trial period is required to determine whether it is effective. If so, treatment may be continued. Nausea, flatulence, blurring of vision, and diplopia may occur initially. Usually these require only temporary reduction of the dose and are transient. Deposition of the drug on the cornea causes a gritty sensation in the eye. This clears if the drug is stopped for several weeks. Treatment may then be resumed at a lower dose. Dermatitis and leukopenia occasionally occur, requiring discontinuance of the drug. The most serious and least frequent adverse effect is retinal toxicity. It is insidious, unnoticed by the patient until serious visual loss has occurred, and irreversible. This toxic effect requires that, prior to starting treatment and every six months while the drug is given, the patient's eyes and visual function be examined by an ophthalmologist. Only with this precaution is the use of the drug safe.

Gold compounds have been used for approximately thirty-five years in the treatment of rheumatoid arthritis. Like most of the drugs mentioned, gold is not beneficial in all cases. An adequate trial requires treatment for twenty to twenty-five weeks. The common adverse effects of gold therapy are dermatitis, stomatitis, and proteinuria. Less frequently, leukopenia, thrombocytopenia, or anemia occur. Precautions to detect adverse reactions should be taken promptly. In most instances, stopping gold therapy is the only treatment needed, but serious reactions require vigorous treatment.

Corticosteroids have been used in the treatment of rheumatoid arthritis for nearly twenty-five years. They are potent drugs with respect to their capacity to control joint pain and stiffness and also in their capacity to cause adverse effects. The large majority of patients with active arthritis have a favorable response to these drugs with prompt reduction of pain and stiffness.

A large variety of preparations is available, but none has been shown to be more effective or to cause fewer adverse effects than prednisone. It also is less expensive than most of the other forms. The recommended initial dose is 2 mg three or four times daily. After one month, if there has been good control of pain, reduction of the daily dose by 1 mg at three-week intervals is begun, reducing to the smallest dose that gives good control of pain. In patients with more severe arthritis larger doses may be necessary.

The numerous adverse effects of corticosteroid therapy are related to the dose and duration of treatment. The most frequent effect is obesity with redistribution of body fat to the trunk and face, resulting in cushingoid facies. With some preparations, salt, and water retention lead to edema, hypertension, heart failure in some patients with heart disease, or electrolyte disturbances. Increased susceptibility to infection is a common problem. Glaucoma and cataracts may occur, as may serious emotional disturbances, diabetes mellitus, and osteoporosis. Peptic ulcer disease has long been held to be caused by corticosteroid therapy, but there is little sound evidence to support this impression. Interference with healing of an ulcer, however, is likely, as is delayed healing of any wound. With the small doses often effective in treatment of rheumatoid arthritis, the risk of many of these complications is minimal.

Corticosteroids are also often effective when injected into an inflamed joint. This form of treatment has none of the risks associated with systemic therapy, but the beneficial effect is confined to the treated joint, and the effect is temporary, averaging two to three weeks. A more recently available preparation, triamcinolone hexacetonide, gives significantly longer duration of beneficial effect. The doses of the various preparations vary greatly, and the information supplied by the manufacturer should be followed.

Braces, splints, and traction. As a result of the weakening and stretching of the joint capsule or supporting ligaments, or because of severe destruction of cartilage and bone within the joint, troublesome instability of the joint may be present. This may cause severe pain or result in a joint that is too unstable to function properly. The use of a movable brace to give added support to the joint can be quite helpful at times. Such a brace is most often used for support of the knees and ankles.

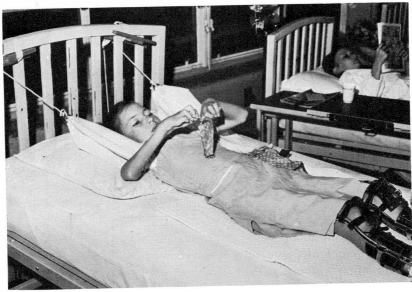

Fig. 311 Method of maintaining abduction of the arms in patient with juvenile rheumatoid arthritis without interfering with activity of the hands.

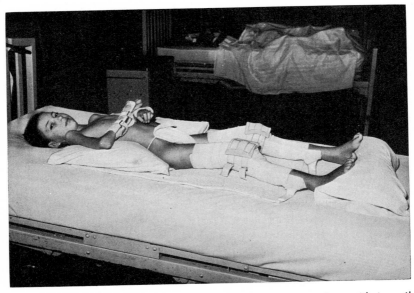

Fig. 312 Rest position with a pillow under the dorsal spine in patient with juvenile rheumatoid arthritis. An adducted position of the arms is undesirable for long periods and should be alternated with positions of abduction and external rotation. Note the night splints applied with Ace bandages to prevent flexion contractures of the knees. Bars attached at the ankle area prevent rotation of the limbs.

During treatment for relief of joint contractures, the use of a rigid support that places a mild, steady, stretching force on the contracture is of definite benefit. Such a support is referred to as a splint. Splints are used most frequently on the knees but can be used for contractures of other joints (Figs. 311 and 312). Splints also are of benefit when used to support an acutely inflamed and painful joint. In this instance, the support gives relief of pain and aids in the prevention of a contracture. Recent development of effective rigid splints for support of unstable wrists and knuckle joints of the hands offers promise for effective relief of this difficult problem. Such splints can be worn when working.

Proper application of braces and splints to the extremities is important for proper function and for the prevention of pain and pressure sores. In this respect, the nurse has an important responsibility to the patient using these devices. Early recognition of these problems will prevent unnecessary discomfort or a troublesome complication for the patient. The nurse should become thoroughly familiar with the proper use of braces and splints.

Occasionally, traction is used in an attempt to relieve severe contractures. This may be applied either to the skin or to the skeleton. A patient in traction requires meticulous nursing care in order to prevent complications, one of the most common being pressure sores resulting from contact with either the bed or the traction apparatus. Because of pain and stiffness resulting in a reluctance to move, the arthritic patient is quite vulnerable to decubitus ulcers. Therefore, his care requires strict attention to details on the part of the nurse. Important are such simple things as frequent changes in position, clean bed linens kept smoothly in place, minor adjustments in the position of the traction apparatus, and protective sponge rubber padding over pressure points when necessary.

Surgery. Surgical treatment of rheumatoid arthritis is indicated in many patients. Operations are performed for removal of swollen synovial tissue (synovectomy) in joints around tendons, repair of severely weakened or ruptured ligaments and tendons, and release of severe contractures. Joints that have severe destructive changes may require the insertion of a prosthesis (an artificial joint or joint portion), a repair procedure (arthroplasty) or, at times, bony fusion (see Chapter 20). The principles and details of nursing care pertaining to both arthritic and orthopedic surgical patients must be applied simultaneously in these patients—sometimes a challenging task.

Degenerative arthritis (osteoarthritis; degenerative joint disease)

Degenerative arthritis, as the name implies, is the result of joint deterioration, specifically of the joint cartilage and underlying bone. This process results in varying degrees of joint destruction but usually is not of great severity. The weight-bearing joints of the lower extremities are most often affected, and as a rule only one or a few joints are involved. The cause of degenerative arthritis is not known, although there is clearly an association with the aging process of joint cartilage. Osteoarthritis of the hip joint may be referred to as malum coxae senilis. It is not a systemic disease but is confined to the joint. The onset of this disease is usually during middle or old age.

The major complaint of patients with degenerative arthritis is joint pain upon weight bearing or motion, which is relieved by rest. Frequently there is also stiffness of the involved joint that is relieved by a few minutes or less of activity. The joint may appear to be normal on examination. Frequently, however, there is grating during motion (crepitus), and there may be bony enlargement. Accumulation of fluid is not uncommon, but the amount is usually not large.

When degenerative arthritis with significant pain has been present for a relatively long period of time, mild to moderate contracture of the joint capsule, along with muscle weakness, often occurs. This results in limitation of joint motion. Although relatively uncommon, severe joint destruction may result in marked limitation of motion and more severe pain.

One of the most common sites of occurrence of degenerative arthritis is in the distal finger joints, those nearest the fingertips. The bony enlargement of these joints has been given the name of Heberden's nodes (Fig. 313). The cause for involvement of these small nonweight-bearing joints is unknown. Women are affected approximately twenty times oftener than men, and there is a definite hereditary factor in this form of arthritis. Frequently there are no symptoms. It is not uncommon, however, for the patients to have mild aching pain. Hand function is seldom significantly affected.

The course of degenerative arthritis usually progresses very slowly. The severity of symptoms parallels fairly closely the amount of use of the involved joint. Most patients have mild to moderate restriction of activity, largely because of pain; relatively few patients have severe limitation of

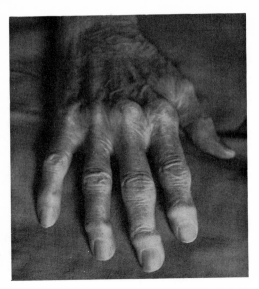

Fig. 313 Heberden's nodes. In degenerative arthritis, the distal interphalangeal joints may become painful and deformed. (In rheumatoid arthritis, the metacarpophalangeal joints and the proximal interphalangeal joints are involved.)

physical activity. Rarely will a patient be severely incapacitated because of degenerative arthritis.

Traumatic arthritis is degenerative arthritis occurring in a joint that has been previously injured. The injury may have been in the nature of infection, repeated dislocation, fracture, or another type of arthritis. There is an interval of time, months or even years after the injury, before the degenerative arthritis appears. It may be mild or severe, depending upon the severity of the previous injury and other factors.

Treatment and nursing intervention. Because degenerative arthritis involves only a few joints, patients with this form of arthritis usually are more easily cared for than those with rheumatoid arthritis. Occasionally patients with severe involvement (e.g., of both knees or both hips) will have considerable disability. The presence of other diseases affecting their general health may cause, in conjunction with their arthritis, disability more severe than would result from the arthritis alone. In patients with heart disease that limits physical endurance, the presence of moderately severe degenerative arthritis in a hip or knee may cause walking to be much more laborious with the result that endurance is further re-

duced. Very often patients with this form of arthritis are elderly and may require modification of care and treatment routines.

The basic principles of treatment for degenerative arthritis are the same as those for rheumatoid arthritis, including rest, relief of pain, and physical therapy. Because degenerative arthritis is not a systemic disease, the patients require no more bed rest or sleep than if they did not have arthritis. Rest of the involved joints, however, is very desirable because it provides for relief of pain. Usually this can be accomplished by resting in a chair. Some patients, however, must lie down for relief of pain, especially when the hips are involved. Frequent interruption of activity with short rest periods is much more effective than occasional long periods of rest.

The need for medication to relieve pain is usually not great. Two or three aspirin tablets three or four times daily usually is sufficient. At times, when aspirin alone is not adequate, the addition of phenylbutazone or indomethacin for a five-day to ten-day period is often helpful. The other drugs used in the treatment of rheumatoid arthritis have no value in this disease. Specifically, steroids, the cortisone-like drugs, should never be given orally. Injection of a steroid into a joint with troublesome pain, however, is frequently helpful in relieving symptoms. The same doses are used as in rheumatoid arthritis.

A large proportion of patients with degenerative arthritis are cared for in the home. Mild degrees of the condition are very common among the population beyond middle age. These persons usually will be hospitalized only when reconstructive surgery is necessary, although they may enter the hospital briefly for corset or brace fittings or for periods of physical therapy.

The health supervision the nurse can give in the home may be an important detail. Health supervision will include attention to details for improvement of the patient's posture and general habits of working, sitting, and standing. Constant sitting for a patient with degenerative arthritis of hip or spine is a bad practice. It often leads to flexion contractures of the hips, adduction of the hips, and a tendency toward dorsal kyphosis. Within the limits of the patient's tolerance, activity is to be encouraged. A person with this kind of arthritis is not one who should be encouraged to assume a life of idleness or a sedentary occupation when other activity is possible.

If shoe corrections have been prescribed, nurses should check frequently to see that they do not become worn down and useless. Shoe corrections provide support and comfort to pronated feet, which are common in this condition, and they may have a great deal to do with improvement in posture. If a brace or corset has been ordered, frequent inspection of the apparatus and supervision of its application are important. If postural exercises have been prescribed, the nurse should have a full understanding of these in order to assist and encourage the patient in their performance.

Another point of importance in which the nurse may play an important role is that of giving reassurance. Worry is not an uncommon feature encountered in patients having this condition. They should be brought to understand that degenerative arthritis does not tend to cause rigid joints and that it does not go from one joint to the other as does rheumatoid arthritis. When the patient understands this, he is relieved of a great burden, particularly if he has a secret fear of becoming a helpless cripple.

Physical therapy plays an important role in the treatment of degenerative arthritis. The objectives are the same as in rheumatoid arthritis. This aspect of the treatment program is a major factor in preventing increasing disability by maintaining muscle strength.

Local treatment may consist of heat, best given in the form of hot packs applied to the affected joints and adjacent painful muscles. Therapeutic exercise to strengthen muscles and improve joint motion should be done in most cases following the application of heat.

The use of a cane or crutches is often helpful in relieving pain by decreasing the amount of weight borne by the joint. Contractures causing limitations of joint motion are not uncommon. Frequently contractures can be greatly improved with exercises and, at times, night splints. Occasionally surgery will be required. Marked joint destruction associated with severe pain or limited motion, or both, may require surgical treatment. This is usually in the form of an arthroplasty, a repair of the joint or a total joint replacement.

Gouty arthritis

Gout is a disease resulting from the abnormal metabolism of uric acid. There is an increase in the amount of uric acid in the body that is reflected in an increase in its concentration in the blood. The clinical picture of gout is characterized by this elevation of blood uric acid concentration along with recurrent attacks of acute, severely painful arthritis. In some patients,

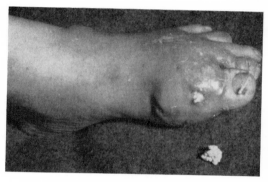

Fig. 314 Gouty arthritis with involvement of the first metatarsophalangeal joint, urate crystals, and a draining sinus from a large tophus.

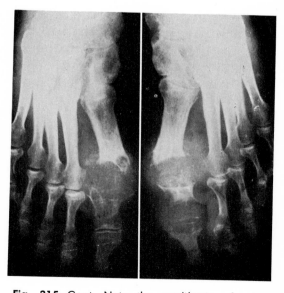

Fig. 315 Gout. Note the predilection for involvement of the first metatarsophalangeal joint. (From Kenney, W. C., and Larson, C. B.: Orthopedics for the general practitioner, St. Louis, The C. V. Mosby Co.)

deposits of uric acid known as tophi occur in various places in the body (Figs. 314 and 315). Approximately 95% of the patients with gout are men. There is no doubt of an hereditary factor in this disease. In approximately one-half of the patients, a history of gout in family members can be obtained. The age of onset, determined by the first attack of acute gouty arthritis, is usually between 20 and 60 years.

The typical acute attack of gout begins rather abruptly. There is severe constant pain, and the joint becomes swollen and red. The usual attack lasts for three to ten days when untreated.

For unknown reasons, the large joint of the great toe is involved much more commonly than any other joint. Other joints in the foot, the ankle, and the knee are also commonly affected. Any joint in the body, however, may be involved.

The course of gout is quite variable, ranging from one or a few attacks during a lifetime to a progressively severe disease with marked crippling, when untreated, in some patients. In most patients, however, the course falls between these two extremes. With proper treatment, attacks of acute gout are infrequent and crippling deformities do not occur.

Treatment and nursing intervention. Few patients with gout require hospitalization for orthopedic treatment. Medications are available that are very effective in controlling the disease. *Colchicine* is the traditional drug of choice for treatment of the acute attack. It is given in the dose of one tablet (either 0.5 or 0.65 mg) every hour until the attack improves, until nausea, vomiting, or diarrhea occurs, or until a total dose of twelve tablets has been taken. Relief of the attack is almost always striking. *Phenylbutazone* is equally effective for relief of the acute attack, or it may be combined with colchicine in a stubborn attack.

Colchicine is also important for prevention of recurrent attacks, and the dose is usually two or three tablets daily. *Probenecid (Benemid)* is an equally important drug used in the treatment of gout. Its function is to increase excretion of uric acid by the kidney, reducing the total amount of this substance in the body. It has no effect on the acute attack of gout. For it to be effective, probenecid must be taken regularly, every day.

Allopurinol is another drug that is effective in reducing the concentration of uric acid in the body. Its mechanism of action is that of decreasing the production of uric acid in the body, a mechanism quite different from that of probenecid. Allopurinol, too, must be taken regularly in three or four daily doses for maximum effectiveness.

Severe dietary restriction, once a standard part of the treatment program, is no longer advocated because it does not contribute greatly to reducing the amount of uric acid in the body. Avoidance of foods high in purine content (such as liver, kidney sweetbreads, sardines, anchovies, and meat gravies) is a reasonable measure.

When properly treated, gout rarely causes deforming arthritis. The untreated or inadequately treated patient, however, may develop a variety of deformities and contractures of joints. In addition, there may be severe destruction of multiple joints in the late stages of chronic gouty arthritis. These problems require the same principles of treatment and nursing care as those in other forms of arthritis.

16 Infection

Osteomyelitis

Osteomyelitis is of three types: acute infectious, acute localized, and chronic.

Cause. Acute infectious osteomyelitis usually is caused by pyogenic bacteria that reach the bone through the bloodstream. The most common organism is the *Staphylococcus*, and the next most common is the *Streptococcus*. Other organisms that may cause the disease are the *Pneumococcus*, typhoid, colon, gas, and tubercle bacilli, *Gonococcus, Actinomyces, Coccidioides, Echinococcus,* and *Spirochaeta pallida*.

The virulence of the organism frequently determines the severity of the disease. In some instances, especially when the infective agent is the *Staphylococcus* or *Streptococcus*, the disease may be of the violent fulminating type, and death may occur within twenty-four or forty-eight hours after onset of the infection. Young children are most often affected with the systemic type, and those areas of the body most subject to trauma are the ones most frequently involved.

In acute localized osteomyelitis the infection often results from compound fractures or penetrating wounds into the bone. Such infections are rarely virulent and usually are not accompanied by a general reaction in the entire affected bone, as is seen in metastatic infections.

Chronic osteomyelitis occurs in the person whose body has built up considerable resistance to the particular type of organism causing the infection. It is characterized by intermittent exacerbations of pain and inflammation—usually brought on by an attempt to throw off sequestra.

The etiology of osteomyelitis presents some factors important to nurses in their health teaching. It is, of course, a well-recognized fact that compound injuries of bone may lead to osteomyelitis, but what is not always so well understood is that any lowering of the resistance or integrity of the tissue may predispose toward the disease. The body's resistance being lowered by exposure, fatigue, malnutrition, or infected tonsils and teeth seems to be a definite factor in the etiology. Bruises, blisters, deep slivers or splinters, impetigo, sties of the eyelids—all are given consideration as possible etiologic agents by writers on this subject. Any type of skin lesion deserves careful attention. When teaching the patients, the nurse should seek to make it understood that a child with extensive skin abrasions should not be allowed to resume normal athletic activities until the lesions are healed. Blisters on the heel—very common in young people—should be carefully disinfected and protected from irritation from the shoe by felt pads. This cannot be overemphasized. A history of boils is a common feature in osteomyelitis, and these deserve medical attention. Remember that the *Staphylococcus*, chief organism in the common boil, is the same *Staphylococcus* that is a cause of the more serious osteomyelitis. It also must be remembered that persons with extensive boils carry the same phage type of *Staphylococcus* in their nose in 80% to 90% of the cases.

Pathology. Acute osteomyelitis usually begins at the end of the long bones, where there is the greatest number of blood vessels. The disease usually is caused by the combination of two factors: (1) local selectivity resulting from trauma and (2) metastatic infection from some remote source of focal infection in the body.

After the bacteria are implanted in the bone, they grow and cause pressure and

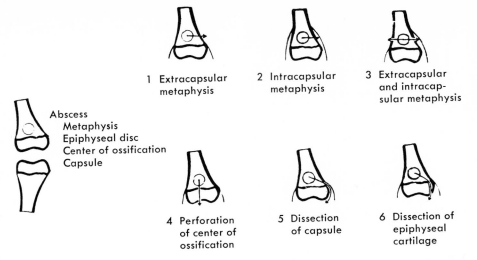

Fig. 316 The pathways for pus to decompress itself from the focal point in bone in acute osteomyelitis in the lower femur. **1,** The circle or central nidus of infection near the metaphyseal side of the epiphyseal plate can decompress into the surrounding soft tissues, producing a soft tissue abscess. **2,** The pus may burrow near the epiphyseal plate and discharge into the joint, producing a septic joint. **3,** Simultaneously, the infection may erode bone and discharge into soft tissues at one point and into the joint at another. **4,** Rarely the infection can erode the epiphyseal plate cartilage and enter the epiphysis. **5** and **6,** Variations of dissection by the pus as it destroys the capsule and enters the joint.

destruction of bone. The pressure serves to spread the infection (Fig. 316), which finally breaks through the bone surface and produces elevation of the periosteum. Most of the circulation to the bone enters through the periosteum, and the stripping effect of pus under pressure cuts off circulation to the bone. Death of the bone occurs. The periosteum maintains its circulation and under this stimulation tends to grow and lay down new bone, forming the characteristic involucrum (Fig. 317). This involucrum may extend part of the way along the shaft or along the entire distance of the shaft. Within this involucrum of newly formed bone, the dead bone (sequestrum) becomes completely detached and must either be removed by surgery or gradually work its own way out by abscess and sinus formation.

Course. The symptoms of acute osteomyelitis begin with a feeling of illness, possibly headache, nausea, and a rather rapid increase in temperature. The earliest local symptom is likely to be severe sudden pain, boring in nature, near the region of a joint. Systemically, a chill followed by high temperature may introduce the condition.

Abruptness and severity of pain are emphasized as the two most notable features of this condition.

In the acute stages, it is difficult at times to tell whether the involvement is in the joint or in the neighboring bone. The differentiation usually can be made by the fact that a certain range of painless motion is present when osteomyelitis is near a joint, but when joint involvement is present, any degree of motion is painful. The bloodstream may become infected so that positive cultures of the organism can be obtained, and the leukocyte count may rise to a very high level. Unfortunately, roentgenography is of no value in the early stage of osteomyelitis. Positive roentgenographic evidence of infection may not be found before two or three weeks. Even then the findings may be misleading when the progress of the disease has been altered by the administration of antibiotics. Localized swelling and tenderness of the involved area occur within twenty-four to forty-eight hours.

Treatment. Surgery and the use of antibiotics offer the best means of treatment of osteomyelitis. The proper antibiotic is selected on the basis of organism sensitivity,

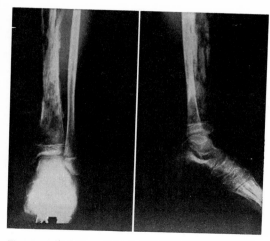

Fig. 317 Chronic osteomyelitis of the tibia. Note destruction of the bone, the sequestrum, and the proliferation of new bone (involucrum). (From Kenney, W. C., and Larson, C. B.: Orthopedics for the general practitioner, St. Louis, The C. V. Mosby Co.)

which can be determined by blood culture or aspiration from the local site. Transfusions, infusions, and supportive care also must be given.

In children under 2 or 3 years of age, when the bone and periosteal tissues are flexible, it may be questionable whether surgical decompression offers any advantage. Incisions and drainage of localized abscesses may be beneficial.

In the average case of acute osteomyelitis the disease usually develops less abruptly. Some patients have been treated successfully by the use of antibiotic drugs alone. With other patients, relief of pressure within the bone and periosteum by incision and drainage is necessary. Much depends on the local and general reaction of the patient within the immediate hours and days following onset of the disease. Immobilization in casts or in splints seems decidedly helpful in most cases, particularly because of the effect of muscle relaxation.

The treatment of chronic osteomyelitis depends largely on the complete removal of all dead bone (sequestra) and the prolonged use of antibiotics. The use of antibiotic drugs at the first sign of bacterial activity will frequently avert the attack.

Nursing responsibilities in various methods of treatment. Perhaps it is significant

that methods for treating osteomyelitis developed during wartime. The first method was the Carrel-Dakin treatment used during World War I.

A second method that most nurses have read about is the Orr treatment, the closed plaster method of treating osteomyelitis. This treatment had its inception in World War I but was not used on a large scale until the Spanish Civil War. Because of the results from its use in World War II, it was generally accepted as the treatment of choice for osteomyelitis.

The Orr method has been somewhat modified by chemotherapy and the antibiotic drugs, but the principles that Orr laid down are still considered sound and form the basis of modern treatment. Briefly stated, the Orr treatment consists of immediate adequate surgical drainage (saucerization), the establishment of complete rest for the involved area by the use of a plaster-of-Paris cast that includes the joint above and the joint below the infected area, the use of petrolatum packing to maintain drainage of the affected area, and postoperative care in which rest and freedom from the interference of dressings are paramount features.

Odor from the closed plaster cast, however, may often present a real problem. Fortunately, the effect of the odor on the patient is not nearly so troublesome as it is on members of the hospital staff and visitors. The nurse can give effective reassurance to the family only if she herself understands the principles underlying the closed plaster method of treating infected bone wounds and the amazing results that have been obtained by use of this method.

Although the use of penicillin and other antibiotics has changed the treatment of osteomyelitis in some respects, provision for adequate rest of the involved area is still considered very important. In the acute stage of the disease, the tendency is to institute drug therapy before resorting to surgery. However, the administration of antibiotics does not always ensure recovery and must often be accompanied by adequate drainage. There always has been controversy over surgery in the acute stage, particularly when bacteremia and general prostration are present. It is recognized that the systemic features of the disease may often be of more immediate importance than the relief of local symptoms. If surgery is performed in the acute stage, it is usually swift and conservative, consisting of a series of drill holes made through the metaphyseal portion of the bone to evacuate pus and relieve tension. More adequate drainage may need to be supplied later. Penicillin may be a lifesaving treatment in patients with the more severe forms of osteomyelitis accompanied by septicemia, provided the laboratory tests indicate that the organism isolated is sensitive to this antibiotic. In certain other cases, proper choice of another antibiotic may be indicated. The patient usually is given the drug parenterally every three hours and, if localized abscesses occur, the drug may be used in the wound as well.

In some instances, the organism causing osteomyelitis is found to be resistant to one or more of the anti-infective drugs, but penicillin will be used because it is a powerful bacteriostatic agent. It is particularly fitted to the treatment of osteomyelitis because it is not inhibited by the presence of pus or large numbers of bacteria.

General nursing care. The patient's general condition should be of as much concern as the local condition. Fluids should be given abundantly by mouth if the patient is able to retain them and intravenously if he is unable to do so. Blood transfusions are often part of the early treatment of this disease. The presence of sufficient protein and vitamin C in the diet of these patients is important because both of these substances are vitally necessary for wound healing.

A highly important fact to remember in caring for the patient with osteomyelitis is that deformity is a common sequela of the disease. The patient tends to hold the limb in a position that causes the least possible strain on the inflamed bone. Nearby joints are likely to be held in a position of flexion in order to relax muscles. In a patient with osteomyelitis of the lower end of the femur, flexion in the hip, flexion in the knee, and a tendency toward outward rotation of the whole leg may be observed. Drop foot is another feature that develops early. It is customary that as soon as drainage has been established, the physician in charge will have a splint applied to the patient's extremity to hold it in an optimal position.

However, if a period of days goes by, during which wet dressings are being used and no splint is in readiness, the nurse must improvise equipment to keep the foot in a normal position. Many writers describe patients in whom a single focus of osteomyelitis is satisfactorily healed but the patient is nonetheless permanently crippled by flexion deformities of the knee and hip and an equinus position of the foot. Contractures of muscles alone may cause the deformity. Although edema is common in the early stages of osteomyelitis and splinting may be difficult, some attempt at maintaining optimal joint positions should be made.

Wet dressings alternated with dry dressings are sometimes ordered to be applied several times each day for the patient with an infected wound. During application of these dressings, unnecessary manipulation must be avoided, and extreme gentleness is necessary when positioning the extremity. If heat is ordered to the area, this is usually accomplished by wrapping the extremity with an electric heating pad. This assures constant and continuous application of heat to the desired area. Controlling and checking the amount of heat being applied is important, since the patient's pain may be so severe that he cannot determine when there is too great a degree.

Laboratory findings play an important part in helping the physician prescribe treatment for the patient with osteomyelitis. Frequent blood cultures and determination of the blood level of antibiotics may be done. Urinary findings, hemoglobin studies, and white blood cell counts are also necessary.

Handling of affected area. The patient with osteomyelitis or septic arthritis is usually extremely apprehensive, and part of this apprehension is caused by his fear of being moved. He may even cry out if the bed is touched. Because it will be necessary for the nurse to move these patients to a certain extent, the manner of handling an acute inflamed joint or extremity will be discussed.

Persons who have had osteomyelitis or a septic joint tell us that the pain caused by being moved is almost intolerable. The moving of an acutely inflamed joint should not be undertaken without help. All the help in the world, however, will do no good if the principles of joint immobolization are not understood and faithfully carried out. It is not enough that the joint or the part infected is carefully immobilized; the joint above and the joint below also must be immobilized to prevent movement in the infected area. This will be readily understood when the mechanism of muscle action on joints is recalled. The muscles that act to move one joint also may serve as flexor or extensor of the one above or below it. Because this is true, moving a knee in which (or near which) a septic condition exists can be accomplished painlessly only by immobilizing the hip and ankle as well as the knee. This will require three hands: one under the hip, one under the knee, and another to support the ankle and foot steadily. Every movement of the hands in lifting must be smooth, unhurried, and infinitely careful. If the patient is turned to the side, the limb must stay on the same level as his body and not be allowed to sag when he is turned. His body should be supported by firm pillows. Gentleness in handling is imperative for another reason. Pathologic fractures have been known to occur as early as ten days after the onset of osteomyelitis. Such fractures frequently are overlooked because the accompanying pain is often wrongly attributed to the concurrent disease.

Complications. Besides the drug reactions that may possibly occur from the use of the antibiotics or the sulfonamides, nurses should be alert to any signs that might indicate the progression of the disease to other parts of the skeleton. Any swelling, redness, or pain near a bone must be reported at once.

Amyloidosis, a waxy degeneration of the liver, spleen, and other organs, is a late and often terminal symptom. It may be manifested by the presence of blood, pus, or albumin in the urine.

As a result of loss of bone substance, there is considerable danger of pathologic fracture during and after osteomyelitis. The extremity that has been involved must be handled with great care even after the period of tenderness and pain has passed. When the patient is allowed to be out of bed, he must be guarded against falls, jerky movements, or any mishap that might

threaten the integrity of the weakened bone. Sudden pain, crepitus, or deformity must be reported immediately. A sudden malposition of the limb may be the first indication that fracture has occurred in that area. Pain is sometimes disguised by the general discomfort of trying to walk after many weeks in bed.

Aftercare. In some patients with osteomyelitis, long hospitalization is necessary, and careful follow-up after discharge is indispensable. The duties of the public health nurse in educating the family concerning the need for close observation and supervision of the activities of the patient are manifest. The dangers of neglect and the possibility of deformity, fracture, and stiffness of joints must be carefully pointed out, as must the possibility of recurrence. The chronicity of the condition also must be explained to avoid discouragement. Frequent return to the clinic for checkup must be stressed.

Dressings. Another important factor in the care of a patient with osteomyelitis is that of protecting other patients and medical personnel from the organism causing the infection. The hospital personnel must know and understand the importance of aseptic technique. The value of and the need for proper hand washing cannot be overstressed.

Negligent technique often accompanies the dressing of draining bone wounds. The monotony of changing these dressings over a period of weeks or months may account for this lowering of standards. Nurses should remember that open wounds such as those encountered in patients with chronic osteomyelitis provide almost perfect culture media for bacteria. Cross infection is an ever-present danger in such wounds, and cross infection may sometimes mean the difference between recovery and chronic invalidism to the patient. Cross infection may be brought about by many agents, such as dust and lint particles in the air, soaked dressings that come in contact with contaminated bed linen or casts, upper respiratory passages, the fingers of nurses and physicians during dressing periods, and, of course, unsterile instruments and dressing equipment.

Carelessness in sterilizing instruments and in using unwashed hands to apply dressings has been the rule rather than the exception in changing septic dressings. In some instances, it has been the custom to remove all dressings before patient rounds, so that the attending physician may see the wounds without unnecessary delay. This is a dangerous procedure because contamination and cross infection can take place so readily in a unit where dressings on many wounds are removed at the same time. The time a wound is exposed to the air should always be kept at a minimum.

In removing dressings from contaminated wounds, it is advisable to cut the bandage and remove it in one piece. If the bandage is unwrapped, it tends to lose lint and dust into the air, and this lint may very easily hold bacteria that will infect wounds of other patients in the area.

It is extremely important that all patients with infected wounds be housed in a separate unit. Protection against cross infection is necessary. Cross infection with a new staphylococcal strain may not be evident unless the antibiotic sensitivities are tested or unless phage typing of the *Staphylococcus* is done.

Acute pyogenic arthritis (septic or purulent arthritis)

Acute pyogenic arthritis is most frequently a disease of childhood and is caused by pyogenic organisms such as the *Staphylococcus* and *Streptococcus*. According to the virulence of the organism and the susceptibility of the host, the onset and reaction may be mild, medium, or severe. Any joint may be involved, but those most commonly involved are the joints most susceptible to trauma, such as the knee, hip, ankle, elbow, shoulder, and wrist.

Infection commonly results from the combination of trauma and focal infection and enters the joint through the bloodstream or by means of a penetrating wound into the joint.

Symptoms and signs. When the infection is mild, the joint reaction may consist of only the stimulation of synovial fluid production. This is called an effusion.

If the virulence is greater, local reaction is further stimulated and fibrinous material (coagulated white blood cells) may cover the surfaces of the joint.

If the reaction is violent, the joint may be filled with pus under considerable pressure and the symptoms are much exaggerated. The temperature may rise to 103° or 104° F, the joint may become reddened, and a fusiform swelling may occur. Joint irritation is notoriously painful on any attempt at motion. Therefore, violent muscle spasm of a protective nature usually accompanies joint irritation and exaggerates the tension and pain. There is usually a marked increase in the number of white blood cells.

Treatment. Early recognition and early treatment with appropriate antibiotics is the best means to prevent destruction of the joint. If response to antibiotics is not dramatic within forty-eight hours, surgical drainage must be considered as an emergency measure in the treatment.

Before the advent of antibiotics, this type of joint infection was an extremely serious condition. An antibiotic or a chemotherapeutic agent is now usually administered immediately to such patients, and surgical treatment is used only when necessary. The joint affected is immobilized by means of simple traction or a bivalved cast. Warm moist dressings often will be ordered for the joint. Fluids and blood transfusions will be given, and aspiration of the joint under aseptic conditions may be done. If the patient can be brought through the acute phase of this disease, his chances for recovery are good.

In the more severely affected patient, in whom fibrin is deposited on the joint surfaces, more extensive treatment is indicated. Joint washings may be done by using two syringes inserted on opposite sides of the joint. Quantities of physiologic saline solution are flushed through the joint until the return is clear. Then penicillin solution may be injected into the joint. Immobilization should be accomplished by splints or by Buck's extension.

If the joint reaction is severe and there is pus formation, incision and drainage are usually necessary. Drainage can be accomplished by a single or double incision adequate to allow complete exposure of the joint. All fibrinous material is picked out with forceps, and the joint is washed clean with physiologic saline solution. Penicillin solution can then be infiltrated throughout the joint, and the incision can be closed. The joint is immobilized in a splint or a plaster-of-Paris cast, and the temperature and symptoms are watched closely.

If there should be continued elevation of temperature or continued pain, it may be necessary to bivalve the cast and inspect the joint. In a severely affected patient, it may be necessary to open the wound and institute free drainage. Such technique exposes joints to secondary infection and should be avoided if possible.

General treatment should consist in the administration of proper chemotherapy combined with transfusions, infusions, and physical therapy treatments.

As noted previously, great care must be exercised in moving the patient with acute pyogenic arthritis.

Tuberculosis of bones and joints

Prior to the late 1930's, tuberculosis was a dreaded disease affecting any part of the body but more particularly the lungs, bones, joints, and kidneys. It was looked upon as a lingering malady from which only a few recovered. The incidence was higher where crowded living conditions, squalor, and poor nutrition were present. The causative organism, the tubercle bacillus, was borne from person to person, through the air and by ingestion. Dairy herds infected with the bovine-type organism transmitted the disease directly in the milk.

Public health measures, such as segregation of persons with active disease, disposal of infected cattle, pasteurization of milk, improved living conditions and nutrition, plus the discovery of appropriate antibiotics, have nearly eradicated the disease. Sanatariums throughout the country, built and operated solely for the care of tuberculous patients, have now been put to other uses. However, in other parts of the world in which public health measures are less efficient, tuberculosis remains a formidable problem.

In the United States and in those countries of the world with strict enforcement of public health measures, an occasional sporadic case of tuberculosis does occur. The major concern is the early diagnosis of these cases since therapy can offer an excellent opportunity for cure. Tuberculosis must be kept in mind as a possible diagnosis in the presence of slowly developing pain, swelling, or limp involving the knee or hip joints, slow, progressive, more or less painless swellings in tendon sheaths, or vaguely localized unrelenting backaches.

Whenever tuberculosis is suspected, there are tests that can fairly accurately establish the diagnosis. The tuberculin skin sensitivity test is available. However, a more accurate test is the actual microscopic demonstration of the tubercle bacillus in tissue biopsy or by culture of the bacillus in material (pus) aspirated from the involved area.

Therapy. Tuberculosis of bones and joints may be treated by antituberculous drugs and/or surgery.

Drugs. A number of drugs have been shown to be effective in the arrest of the tubercle bacillus. These drugs are used in various combinations in different centers. Commonly used antituberculous drugs are as follows.

Isoniazid (INH) in doses of 5 mg/kg of body weight up to 300 mg daily may be continued for two years if tolerated. Numbness or paresthesias may occur and should be used as a guide to reduction or even discontinuance of the drug.

Ethambutol hydrochloride in doses of 15 mg/kg of body weight is frequently combined with isoniazid. Optic neuritis has been reported with the use of this drug, so it is necessary to test the visual fields frequently and also to check for color discrimination ability. Any alterations in visual perception by these tests should be used as a guide to alteration in the dosage of this drug.

Streptomycin is a helpful adjuvant in those patients in whom the tubercle bacillus is thought to be more virulent or in whom the isoniazid and ethambutol are slow to control the systemic symptoms of the disease. It is given in doses up to 1 Gm per day and ordinarily used only in patients over 35 years of age and then not to exceed 90 Gm in the overall treatment. The restrictions are occasioned by the possibility of damage to the eighth cranial nerve, which affects hearing. Frequent checks for early hearing losses should indicate reduction or discontinuance of the drug.

Rifampin is very effective against the tubercle bacillus. However, it is more effective in pulmonary tuberculosis than in tuberculosis of bones or joints and also is much more expensive than the other drugs.

Surgery. There is a place for surgical therapy in the management of tuberculosis of bones and joints. The indication for surgical intervention is based on a knowledge of the pathology created by the tubercle bacillus.

As with other infecting organisms such as staphylococcus, the tubercle bacillus is carried by the bloodstream to any part of the body. It may lodge in the smaller vessels near the ends of bones or in periosteum and set up a local inflammatory reaction. A part of the reaction is a good deal of local tissue death that results in caseous material (tuberculous pus) which differs from the usual abscess formed by staphylococcus. The caseous material is less liquid than staphylococcus pus contains unabsorbed dead tissue debris. The body reaction to this caseous material is less acute than body reaction to staphylococcus pus—thus the term "cold abscess" has been used to describe it. It is also less painful than an abscess from staphylococcus and may remain unresolved for weeks or months.

In some cases of tuberculosis of bones or joints, the amount of tissue death in the bone and the associated cold abscess remain even though drugs have controlled the tubercle bacillus and prevented further tissue destruction.

Surgical drainage of these persistent abscesses may be the only way to eradicate the tuberculous pus. When such abscesses are evacuated surgically, the surgical wound should be closed to prevent contamination by other organisms from the skin surface. Should such a cavity become secondarily infected, there may be persistent drainage from a chronic sinus for months. The most common tuberculous abscesses to require surgical drainage are those in the spine where the primary destruction has occurred in one or more vertebral bodies and intervening discs. Drainage of these vertebral abscesses is accomplished by a surgical procedure designated as costotransversectomy to describe the posterolateral approach to the spine by removal of a transverse process at its articulation with a rib if the abscess, as it commonly is, is located in the dorsal spine.

Following such surgical therapy on the spine, it is customary to immobilize the spine until the bone and soft tissue defects have repaired. If the defects are large and a later collapse of the remains of one or more vertebral bodies is considered likely, there is further surgical treatment that can prevent the possible collapse of the spine. Dr. A. R. Hodgson of Hong Kong has advocated surgical removal of diseased vertebral bodies and replacement by bone grafts to prevent collapse of the spine (Fig. 359).

Tuberculous abscesses in a bone near a joint can be debrided surgically to promote ingrowth of new bone to repair the defect. At times, this may salvage a joint that would otherwise become deformed or totally destroyed and nonfunctional. If total

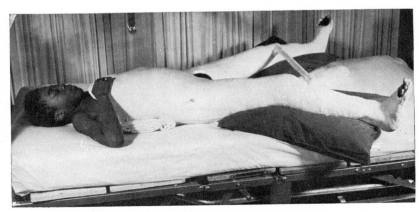

Fig. 318 A complete body cast has been applied to maintain immobilization and good position for this patient with tuberculosis of the spine. Note the placement of pillows to support the extremities.

destruction of a joint has occurred and deformity supervened, such a deformity can be corrected for alignment surgically and a solid fusion of the joint accomplished that will maintain correction and aid in the control of the tuberculous infection.

Surgery is the only means of removal of tuberculous foci such as that causing chronic tenosynovitis of the flexor tendons at the wrist.

Nursing aspects of skeletal tuberculosis. Tuberculosis of the joint usually develops

as an insidious disease and is secondary to foci located elsewhere in the body. At the onset there is only occasional pain, with muscle spasm around the joint, and there may be slight elevation of the temperature without leukocytosis. Symptoms may include weight loss, fatigue, and anorexia. Skeletal tuberculosis is acquired from persons who have active or quiescent tuberculous lesions in the lungs and is rarely transmitted to other persons except through careless handling of dressings

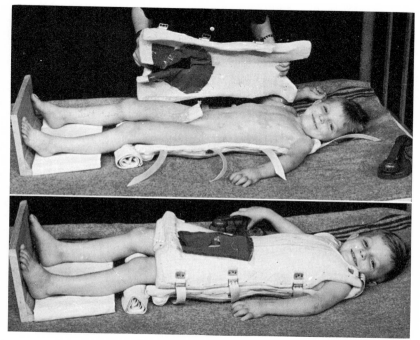

Fig. 319 The plaster shell or plaster bed is frequently used to immobilize the spine after fusion. Each half is lined with stockinet. The straps and buckles make it possible to remove either half for bathing and skin care. Before the patient is turned, the straps are buckled tightly. (Courtesy Iowa State Services for Crippled Children.)

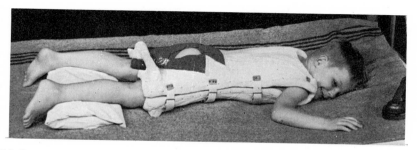

Fig. 320 Prone position. The anterior and posterior halves may be buckled in place to prevent the child from rising up and turning. Note the waterproof material placed about the perineum and buttocks. (Courtesy Iowa State Services for Crippled Children.)

from draining sinuses. It must be remembered that the disease is progressive when untreated. Also, roentgenograms of the chest are necessary to rule out the presence of concomitant pulmonary tuberculosis. Unnecessary exposure of family members, other patients, or health personnel must be avoided. Prophylaxis is of prime concern and, briefly stated, consists of early diagnosis and adequate treatment of discovered cases. Treatment of the disease includes the use of antituberculous drugs, good nutrition, and rest. Provision for general as well as local rest is important. Casts, body jackets, braces, or splints are utilized to provide immobilization of an involved joint (Figs. 318 to 320). With the early use of drugs, it is hoped that the progress of the infection can be controlled and joint function maintained.

The first symptoms of spinal tuberculosis (sometimes referred to as Pott's disease after Sir Percival Pott who first described the syndrome nearly 200 years ago) are usually stiffness, muscle spasm, and a tendency to reach things on the floor by bending the knees rather than the back. Pain may be referred to the limbs. These symptoms may be intermittent and be relieved by comparatively short periods of rest. The intermittent characteristic may cloud the early diagnosis. The characteristic deformity in tuberculosis of the spine is the development of a gibbus (Fig. 321), an angulation or pronounced anteroposterior curve of the spine such as is seen in the hunchback. This deformity results from destructive lesions in the spine causing collapse of one or more vertebral bodies.

Paralysis in tuberculosis of the spine occurs occasionally. Strangely, it is rarely the result of the mechanical disturbance in the alignment of the spine but rather the effect of abscesses, granulation tissue, and other accompanying factors in the tuberculous disease.

Abscess formation in the cervical region may develop in the pharynx, causing difficulty in breathing. In the dorsal region, it may occur in the mediastinum and may rupture into the lung. In the lumbar spine, an abscess may develop between the lumbar muscles or in the gluteal region, or it may follow the course of the iliopsoas muscle and joint in the groin. This is the most common form (psoas abscess). Spasm of the muscles of the thigh and a tendency toward flexion and lateral rotation of a limb that is accompanied by great pain on motion may suggest to the physician that a psoas abscess is in the process of formation long before a fluctuating mass may be seen in the groin. Drainage of an abscess is common when the abscess is progressive and not controlled by antituberculous drugs. Approach to an abscess in the dorsal spine usually is made through costotransversectomy. If there is a great deficiency of bone at the conclusion of the operation, bone grafts (spinal fusion) can be added to bridge the gap between the vertebral bodies.

Care of the patient after spinal fusion has been described in Chapter 17. Joints that have undergone arthodesis usually are well immobilized in plaster of Paris before the patient is returned from the operating room, and nursing care is the same as that for any other surgical patient wearing a plaster cast.

When ambulation is permitted following spinal fusion, the support may be an am-

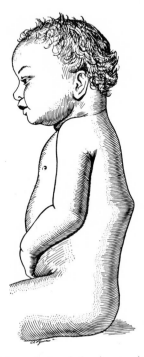

Fig. 321 Tuberculosis of the lower dorsal spine with angulation, or gibbus.

bulatory cast, jacket, or brace. The Taylor body brace or some modification of it is commonly used. It consists of two thin flexible steel bars that form a support for the vertebral column, one lying on either side of it, and which fit the curves of the back perfectly. A pelvic band made of steel and leather is fastened at the bottom of these supports. The nurse applying these braces should always remember that the pelvic band must closely encircle the pelvis slightly below the iliac crests. With the band in the position, the brace will be properly placed with regard to the rest of the body.

Tuberculosis of the hip usually begins with a limp of gradually increasing severity. The hip becomes slightly flexed, abducted, and externally rotated, and the individual has a tendency to walk on the toes of the affected side. In advanced cases, atrophy of muscles about the joint may be apparent. Night cries are frequently present. These are caused by a definite mechanism. The muscles relax in sleep and the joint is unprotected. In the subconscious state, body movements may occur and the joint may become irritated. There is an immediate violent spasm of the muscles that causes severe pain by bringing the irritated joint surfaces together, and the individual cries out as he awakens.

As the disease progresses, the destruction of the head of the femur and possibly of the acetabulum increases. The characteristic destruction that occurs in the hip joint in a more advanced case is shown in Fig. 322.

During the early stages, recumbent treatment is combined with the use of drugs. It is hoped that with rest (local and general), good nutrition, and hygienic surroundings, combined with drug therapy, joint motion may be saved. Immobilization of the joint may be maintained by plaster splinting or by traction.

In patients with more severe disease, fusion of the hip may be necessary. There are several methods of accomplishing fusion, but all successful methods consist of some form of bone graft between the femur and pelvis, and growth of this graft leads to solid bone formation between these two structures and the elimination of joint function. Tuberculosis seems to lose its affinity for a joint when motion and fric-

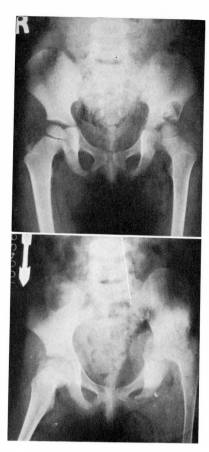

Fig. 322 Roentgenograms of a tuberculous hip. In the upper film, the head of the left femur and the joint space are still well defined. As the infectious process continues (lower film), the joint cartilage is destroyed, calcium is deposited, and eventually motion in the joint is destroyed.

tion are eliminated. After fusion operations, a plaster-of-Paris cast is applied from the chest to the toes of the affected side. The position of the hip joint is of considerable importance. There should be a 10° to 20° flexion and, if there has been some destruction, about a 5° adduction to give the best weight-bearing line. Approximately six to eight months are required for bone healing after hip fusion. This must be determined by roentgenography.

To help the family in home care of the patient with skeletal tuberculosis, the nurse must have enough imagination to understand how the home situation will vary from the hospital situation. Ability to compute a diet for the patient with tuberculosis that provides adequate protein, minerals, and vitamins and that takes into consideration the family income is an important feature. Many little details that seem almost too small to be mentioned must be dealt with thoroughly. In addition, the hospital nurse will make a referral to the local visiting or public health nurse.

Since patients must continue with antituberculous drugs at home, it is desirable that a visiting nurse make home visits and evaluate symptoms and progress. The cost of drugs must not be forgotten. Prior to discharge, appropriate arrangements should be made for supplying the needed medicine.

17 Painful orthopedic problems in adults

Spinal affections

Back pain is a common complaint and can occur at any age and from many causes. In childhood, the most likely cause would be infection; in adolescence, a developmental defect such as epiphysitis (Scheuermann's disease) or spondylolisthesis; in young and middle-aged adults, some type of mechanical strain on ligaments or discs; and in elderly persons, some form of osteoporosis or metastatic disease. The spine, being a series of bones and joints, is subject to the same pathologic conditions that affect bones and joints elsewhere in the body, such as congenital defects, infections, arthritis, metabolic disorders, and malignant processes, either primary or metastatic.

The functions of the spine are to provide the spinal cord a bony protection against direct injury, to support the head, trunk, and vital organs in an upright position, and, most importantly, to provide a flexible pole to continually adjust the balance of the body to its own center of gravity, no matter what the task—be it tightrope walking or moving furniture.

Countless times each day the spine is called upon to flex, extend, or rotate to adjust body balance as we walk, run, sit, stand, stoop, or twist, often accompanied by extra weight as we lift or carry loads. The supporting structures of the spine (viz., the discs and ligaments) have limits of tolerance to these mechanical demands beyond which they deteriorate and become painful. Aging affects the tolerance of these tissues to mechanical stresses. Use of the spine in the proper position will lessen the mechanical stresses.

Knowledge of the anatomy of the spine will help the nurse understand the cause and effect of various pathologic states—how they produce backache and how they should be managed.

The spine is composed of a series of bony vertebral units separated one from the other by an intervening intervertebral disc and made continuous one with the other by strong ligaments. Motion occurs through the intervertebral disc guided by the arrangement of the facets and limited by arrangement and position of the ligaments (Fig. 18).

The disc is composed of a center, the nucleus pulposus, which is surrounded by dense collagen fibers, the annulus fibrosus. The nucleus pulposus contains complex proteins and mucopolysaccharides that hold water under pressure. The pressure permits the disc to function as a shock absorber and responds to sudden compression loads by bulging against the annulus fibrosus with a return to normal shape when unloaded. With advancing age, the water content of the nucleus pulposus diminishes and collagen tissue gradually replaces the nucleus (Fig. 323), with the result that the motion between two vertebrae is diminished. This accounts for restricted painless spine motion that is common in advanced age.

Rapid degeneration of the disc with loss of intradiscal pressure allows the disc to become unstable (Fig. 324). Instability is painful whenever the disc is suddenly or repetitively loaded by lifting or stooping and twisting. The nucleus pulposus or a part thereof may be extruded through de-

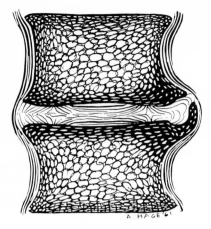

Fig. 323 Drawing of tissues in advanced age illustrating narrowing of the intervertebral disc and replacement of the nucleus pulposus by collagen.

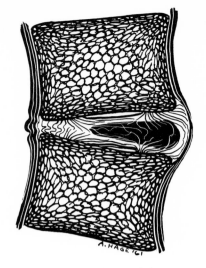

Fig. 324 Disc instability.

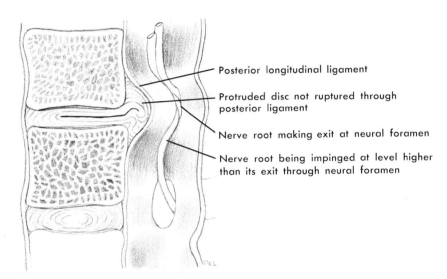

Posterior longitudinal ligament

Protruded disc not ruptured through posterior ligament

Nerve root making exit at neural foramen

Nerve root being impinged at level higher than its exit through neural foramen

Fig. 325 Diagram of a ruptured intervertebral disc.

generated cracks in the annulus fibrosus and encroach on nerve roots within the spinal canal (Fig. 325). This constitutes a ruptured disc and produces not only a painful back, but also radiating pain down the leg known as sciatica. The distribution of sensory loss will help to identify the precise nerve root affected (Fig. 326). Nature tends to repair degenerated discs over a period of time, including those that have ruptured. Operative removal of ruptured disc fragments must be done immediately if there are signs that nerve deficits are increasing.

The nerve deficits will be paralysis of muscle groups, sensory losses to touch, reflex losses, and loss of bladder control. The straight leg–raising test will be markedly restricted.

Where the pain is confined to the low back associated with instability, the natural repair will be enhanced if the healing degenerated disc can be held in neutral position and motions avoided. The patient can be instructed in postural control of the back, provided with back support to aid in the control, and given exercises at the

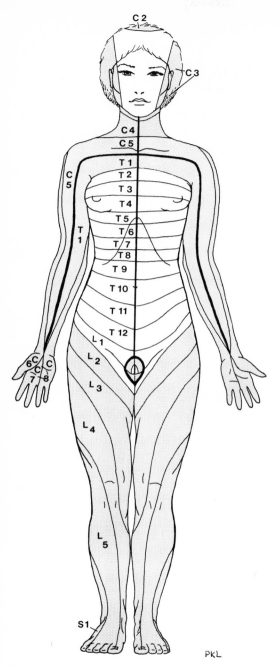

Fig. 326 Anterior view of the body illustrating the sensory dermatone levels.

gliding joints, are placed at each disc level to guide the motion of the disc. There is a capsule and synovium around each facet, and each is susceptible to the same pathologic conditions as any other joint in the body. Anatomic variations in the symmetric arrangement of the facets are common. The pedicles and laminae that extend from each side of the vertebral body and meet in the midline posteriorly form a bony ring that surrounds and protects the spinal cord at each vertebral segment throughout the entire spine. Incomplete development of the pedicles occurs in 5% of the population. This is serious, since the bony ring is then incomplete and the posterior elements will be unattached to the body of the vertebra. This permits a sliding forward of one vertebra on the other, a condition known as spondylolisthesis (Fig. 328). The presence of this defect can be detected in early childhood. However, there is a 50/50 chance that it may never cause a backache. When backache is present, it is likely that the disc at the abnormal level has degenerated (Fig. 329) and become unstable.

When properly developed, the posterior arch of the vertebral unit will have an outrigger or bony process protruding backward from its center called the spinous process. This is the base for the attachment of many of the posterior muscles that control the spine. There is a very strong ligament from one spinous tip to the next (interspinous ligament), and this serves the useful purpose of limiting forward bending of the spine. Should the spine be forcefully bent forward, this ligament could tear and would be called a "sprung back."

Nursing intervention. With acute low back strain, spasm of the lumbosacral muscles occurs, and in some instances spasm of the hamstring muscles also may be present. The muscle spasm, which is a protective mechanism, greatly limits spinal motion and makes moving about or changing position difficult, as well as painful and fatiguing. As the examiner palpates the lumbar area, the muscles are firm, and localized tender or painful spots may be present. If the muscle spasm is asymmetric, a slight lateral curvature of the spine may be present and the individual will walk with a "list" to one side. Severe spasm of the lumbar muscles tends to flatten the lumbar

proper time to strengthen the muscles that control the spine motions.

There are other anatomic structures that are important to a properly functioning spine (Fig. 327). The facets, two small

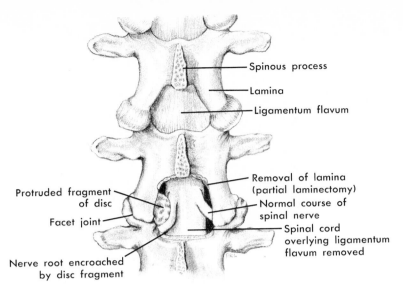

Spinous process

Lamina

Ligamentum flavum

Removal of lamina
(partial laminectomy)

Normal course of
spinal nerve

Spinal cord
overlying ligamentum
flavum removed

Protruded fragment
of disc

Facet joint

Nerve root encroached
by disc fragment

Fig. 327 Posterior view of the vertebral column showing a ruptured nucleus pulposus causing pressure of a nerve root.

spine, and as this curve is obliterated, the spinal column assumes a C shape.

The patient with low back pain also may complain of sciatic pain that radiates down the leg. This type of pain can be caused by irritation of the nerve or by pressure on the lumbosacral nerve roots. The examiner will check for this pain by gently raising the relaxed leg (with the patient in the supine position with the knee extended and the hip flexed). This will cause increased back and leg pain. If the limb is elevated until back pain is felt and then lowered slightly, the sciatica can be reproduced by passively dorsiflexing the foot (Lasègue's sign). Complaint of pain or discomfort in the popliteal space usually is due to tight hamstring muscles.

Early mild back strain is usually treated by recumbency and heat. Heat in the form of a heating pad or hot moist packs may provide considerable relief for the patient with back strain. Back-strapping with adhesive tape also may provide temporary relief in mild cases. Adhesive strips 3-4 in wide and long enough to extend from the anterior iliac spine on one side across the back and beyond the anterior iliac spine on the other side are used. Considerable traction is exerted on each strip as it is applied, and a lumbar pad of felt to supply pressure

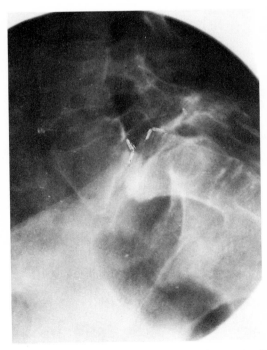

Fig. 328 Roentgenographic appearance of spondylolisthesis. Note the fifth lumbar vertebra displaced forward on the sacrum a distance of half its width.

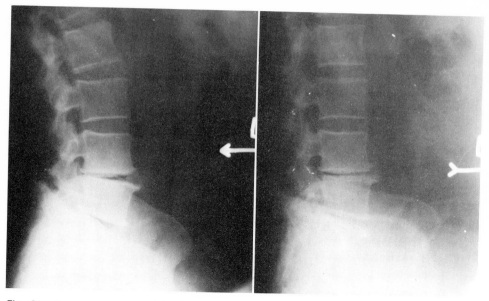

Fig. 329 Roentgenograms of the lumbar spine in the lateral view showing a degenerated disc that is narrowed and also bony spurs at the anterior margins of the vertebral bodies adjacent to the disc. The posterior annulus fibrosus is pinched between the vertebral bodies when the spine is extended.

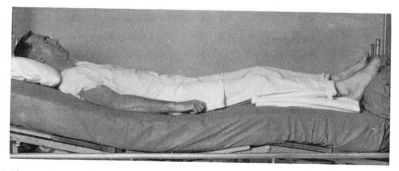

Fig. 330 The patient with acute back pain is usually more comfortable with the backrest elevated 20° to 45° and the knees flexed slightly (semi-Fowler position).

over the sacral region may be used under the tape. Three or four strips of adhesive tape are necessary, and these should extend from the trochanter level to above the iliac crests. The patient may be either standing or lying in bed while these are applied. It has been found that in the former position he can provide assistance if he stands in a corner and braces himself against the walls with his hands. Strapping gives only temporary relief, but occasionally symptoms may subside and the patient will be able to return to his work.

When bed rest is ordered for severe pain in the lower portion of the back, a firm mattress with a bed board between the mattress and the springs is essential. The patient is most comfortable in a semi-Fowler position. In this position, with the backrest elevated approximately 20° to 45° and the knees flexed slightly (Fig. 330), there is less tension of the back muscles and of the hamstrings. At times, the attending physician may wish to apply traction to relieve spasm of the thigh and back muscles, and Buck's extension or pelvic traction is used intermittently. During the acute stage, the patient may be uncomfortable in any position and for this reason is allowed to assume whatever attitude he can find that gives relief. An analgesic and a muscle relaxant usually are prescribed, and morphine may be necessary to control pain. Nurses tend to minimize low back pain as one of the minor afflictions until they have cared for a patient with an acute condition and watched the intense suffering that he endures.

After a period of bed rest, and when the acute pain has subsided, exercises are ordered for the purpose of improving the patient's body mechanics and thereby building up a resistance against further back strains as the result of postural deviations. Nurses should make an attempt to observe these exercises as they are taught in the physical therapy department. Usually, such exercises are begun by having the patient (first in the lying position and then while standing) flatten the lumbar spine by active contraction of the abdominal and gluteal muscles. Diaphragmatic breathing also is emphasized. Sometimes the exercises are done by the patient in bed as often as every hour during the day. He may be taught to contract the gluteal muscles five or ten times, using a steady, slow rhythmic contraction. A second important bed exercise for this condition is one in which the patient lies on his back and raises his head and shoulders a short distance from the bed without using his elbows to brace himself. This strengthens the abdominal muscles and may be done five to ten times an hour until the exercise is being performed a hundred times daily.

Therapeutic corset. Practically all physical therapy treatment for patients with back pain is designed to create a set of corset muscles sufficiently strong to serve as an internal splint for the low back. Until this can be accomplished, some kind of corset or brace is customarily prescribed. Nurses should understand that a corset for this condition should be prescribed by the physician. Patients who attempt to purchase corsets for low back pain without the advice of an orthopedist frequently spend a great deal of money on garments that are absolutely inefficient and may even exacerbate their condition. Corsets for low back pain have a dual purpose: provide a type of immobilization for the painful back and

assist in maintaining the trunk in good posture. Use of the therapeutic corset is often a somewhat perplexing problem to the student who has relatively little chance to obtain experience in its application (Fig. 331). Students should be given the opportunity to watch the prescription corsetiere doing the final fitting and to observe points of special importance in the construction and application of the garment.

The corset is made to fit the curves of the back so that no loose or gapping spaces occur anywhere. Its length must be sufficient to assist in the control of buttock muscles, and it should be high enough to approximate the lower portion of the shoulder blades. The front of the corset must be long enough to support the abdomen adequately, and a careful fitting over the iliac crests is necessary to prevent the garment from sliding up.

Perineal straps are sometimes used to prevent the corset from rolling up, but these are not considered essential if the fit of the garment is adequate (sacroiliac belts frequently have these straps attached). Pads made of flannelette sewed into place over the sacrolumbar region of the corset are not uncommon, but again these are considered superfluous if the corset is carefully constructed to fit the curves of the back. Back-lacing is considered desirable for proper fitting in therapeutic corsets.

The patient should be observed while sitting after the corset is applied to see that it does not slip from its original position. A garment that fits loosely or that rolls up is of no value. The front stays should not press down on the pubic bone because this will cause the patient considerable discomfort.

Preventing recurrence of back strain. Teaching and helping the patient understand how he may avoid recurrence of back strain is an important aspect of his care. This not only involves his wearing the prescribed support and continuing with the exercise program started in the hospital, but also involves an understanding of the principles related to correct body mechanics. Using correct methods of stooping, lifting, and carrying objects, sitting in a straight-back chair as opposed to a soft, low, deep-seated chair, sleeping on a firm mattress, and avoiding sudden twisting

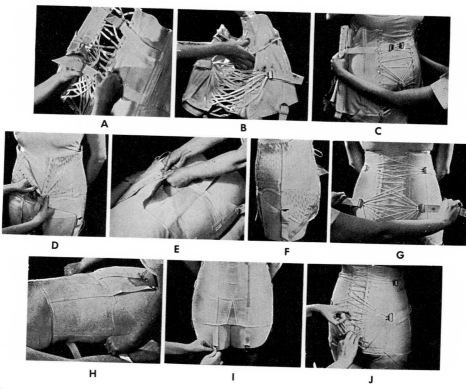

Fig. 331 Application of a corset for conditions of the low back. **A,** Release the buckles by turning them backward on the straps, holding the buckle between the first finger and thumb, and slide toward the end of the strap to within two inches of the end. **B,** After releasing the buckles, it is advisable to bend the corset bones in the top and bottom in the back in order to conform to the curves of the body. **C,** Standing position. Place the support on the body with the center back well down under the gluteus muscles (as shown). The bottom of the front should curve down to the pubic bone; the bones of the support, if any, should not press on the pubic bone. **D,** Hooking the support in the standing position. If the top hook of the support is fastened first, it will hold the support on the body while the fitter hooks the rest of the support from the bottom upward. **E,** Reclining position. Same procedure as in standing position. **F,** Fastening side stocking supporters. In both standing and reclining positions, fasten side stocking supporters in such a manner that the front portion will draw straight down on the side as shown. **G,** Pulling the adjustment straps in the standing position. Draw, slightly, the top strap or lacer sufficiently to settle the support at the waistline. Then hold the lower straps, one in each hand, and give a steady pull, thus laying a foundation around the pelvis. **H,** Reclining position. The patient must raise her body to enable the fitter to obtain a proper grip on the straps and to give a firm, steady, outward pull. Procedure is the same as for standing position. Caution: always tighten the opposite straps at the same time, one in each hand, and not first one and then the other. **I,** Fasten front stocking supporters straight down without tension. **J,** Inspection of fitting. See that there is no slack in any of the lacers; if slack is present, retrace lacers with the fingers. Tuck ends of the adjustment strap backward through the loops designed to receive them. When correctly adjusted, the back opening should not be more than two or three inches wide; if it is, a garment of larger size should be chosen. Have the patient sit down to make sure that the support is comfortable and that it does not slip from its proper position on the body. (Courtesy S. H. Camp & Co.)

movements of the spinal column are important factors in preventing recurrence of back strain (Chapter 3). The prevention of sudden twisting movements of the spine necessitates care in or the avoidance of walking on icy walks, a rough terrain, or a steep incline where maintaining body balance is more difficult. Also, the lifting of heavy objects may have to be avoided indefinitely.

Herniated disc. Rupture of an intervertebral disc is a well-recognized cause of pain in the lower back. Initial treatment of the patient is usually conservative, and providing for recumbency on a firm mattress is an important aspect of his care. A semisitting position is sometimes found to be efficacious for the comfort of the patient.

Maintaining comfort and relief of pain are concerns of the nurse. Information from the patient pertaining to the location of the pain, whether it is continuous or intermittent, and factors that tend to lessen or to intensify it are helpful. Patients with back pain experience different kinds of pain and may describe it as "sharp and shooting" or as a "deep aching" pain. When pain is present, a disc usually is suspected, and the precise location of the radiating pain is helpful in determining the location of the disc involved. If the pain is radiating to the anterior thigh, involvement of the third lumbar root is indicated; if to the lower thigh and the medial upper tibia, the fourth lumbar root; if to the lateral calf and the great toe, the fifth lumbar root; and if the back of the calf and the lateral heel, the first sacral root.[16] Irritation or injury of the nerve roots (in the lumbar spine), in addition to causing pain, may cause other abnormal changes in the lower extremity, including sensory and motor disturbances, reflex changes, and atrophy and weakness of muscles. Sensory changes may lessen the patient's perception of light touch and the ability to discriminate between sharp and dull.

As stated previously, muscle spasms frequently cause the patient great discomfort. The application of heat by means of hot moist packs or, in some instances, a heating pad may give relief. Pelvic traction or Buck's extension also may be applied to help lessen the muscle spasm. In addition, a muscle relaxant such as Valium frequently is prescribed, and analgesics also are made available. However, the administration of narcotics may be necessary to provide relief for the patient. Careful assessment to determine whether the patient is getting pain relief is essential and should be accurately recorded by the nurse.

Care in positioning and turning the patient can help minimize pain. When turning, it is important that the shoulders and hips be moved in one plane (logrolling). Twisting of the spine is avoided by teaching the patient to turn in a logrolling fashion. A wide drawsheet that extends from the shoulders to below the hips may be used. A pillow is placed between the patient's thighs. The nurse, reaching across the patient, grasps the rolled drawsheet and gently turns him toward her onto his side. The patient's hips should then be pulled back toward the center of the bed and the uppermost limb adjusted on the pillow previously placed between the thighs. The patient with a herniated disc also may be turned by the method described for the patient with a spinal fusion (p. 338). A child's bedpan or a bedpan with a tapered back will cause the patient with back pain less discomfort than the ordinary adult bedpan. To place the patient on the pan, he is rolled onto his side, the pan and a small pillow to support the lumbar region are placed in position, and he is then rolled back, onto the pan. Having him use the trapeze should be avoided. Support to hold the covers off the feet and to prevent drop foot is a necessity if there have been motor or sensory changes in the limbs.

Since conservative treatment usually consists of several weeks of bed rest, the patient with this problem may become quite discouraged and feel that little progress is being made. He may fear being operated upon or question whether he will be able to return to his usual activities without recurrence of the condition.

Treatment following relief of the acute symptoms usually includes an exercise program aimed at strengthening the abdominal and gluteal muscles. Strengthening of these muscles tends to lessen the anterior tilt of the pelvis and the amount of lumbar lordosis.

Prior to ambulation, the patient is fitted with a corset or brace that provides support and immobilization of the back. The purpose of the support is to prevent recurrence of the condition, and it should be worn when the patient is not in bed. Also, a pair of good walking shoes should be worn when the patient is permitted to begin activity. Another important aspect in preventing recurrence of this condition is instruction of the patient in correct body mechanics. Proper methods of lifting and stooping must be practiced and strenuous activity avoided if recurrence is to be prevented. The practice of correct body mechanics also includes use of good sitting posture. The use of a straight-back chair as opposed to the upholstered chair is recommended for the person with a back problem. Strain on involved nerves may be caused by sitting with the knees crossed or by sitting with the knees in extension, such as elevating the feet on a footstool or driving a car with a low seat. In addition, any sudden twisting movement of the spine should be avoided.

Laminectomy. Laminectomy may be necessary for the patient with a lesion of an intervertebral disc. This is particularly true if it is a recurrence of a disc problem. The surgical procedure provides for removal of the portion of the nucleus pulposus that is protruding or ruptured from the intervertebral disc. To do this, a portion of the lamina of one or more vertebrae is removed. The nursing care of a patient after laminectomy without fusion is a relatively simple problem—quite different from the nursing problem encountered following laminectomy for the person having a fractured spine or tumor of the spinal cord. When spinal fusion is not done simultaneously with the laminectomy, the patient usually is permitted to move about in bed at liberty and is encouraged to exercise his feet and legs at frequent intervals. Nurses are instructed to observe his ability to do this after the operation and to record this carefully during the early postoperative period. The patient should be placed on a firm mattress. Maintenance of the supine position may be ordered for the first twenty-four hours postoperatively. Pressure on the operative area helps prevent formation of a hematoma. The usual precautions in turning patients with conditions of the spine should be observed in the care of each of these patients. The body is turned in one plane, and twisting of the spine is carefully avoided. Side-lying positions are often permitted and a pillow placed between the legs will help to relax the back muscles. Likewise, a pillow to support the upper arm will prevent sagging of the shoulder. Early ambulation is frequently prescribed for the patient who has had a laminectomy. This, in itself, helps to prevent many postoperative complications, such as urinary retention, distention, phlebitis, and hypostatic pneumonia.

Spinal fusion. The nursing care of the patient who has had a spinal fusion is similar to that needed by most patients following major surgical procedures. Frequent monitoring of the vital signs is essential. Measures to control pain and to prevent lung congestion, dehydration, and phlebitis are instituted, and attention to urinary output is important. There may be a mild and temporary decrease in the tone of the urinary and gastrointestinal tracts as a result of the inevitable shock to the sympathetic nervous system. Abdominal distention caused by a paralytic ileus and urinary retention may occasionally be postsurgical problems. Oral fluids are started slowly, and the diet is increased as the patient tolerates it. In addition, attention to positioning and turning and providing for immobilization of the spine are necessary aspects of the patient's care.

The patient immobilized in a plaster bed or anterior and posterior shells (Fig. 332) is usually most comfortable if pillows are used to support the legs along their entire length. Some relaxation of the back muscles is obtained by this slight elevation. Furthermore, it is thought by many surgeons to be a means of overcoming a threat of thrombophlebitis in the femoral vessels. The pillows should not be placed in such a fashion that flexion of the knee is exaggerated.

Prior to surgery, the shells used for immobilizing the patient must be well prepared. Wrinkles and ridges should be eliminated. The stockinet or lining must be pulled out to cover all the raw edges and be fastened securely. Velcro straps are added, and the final finishing is done by a brace maker. The area around the buttocks usually needs to be protected

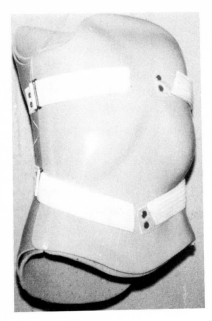

Fig. 332 Polyethylene anterior and posterior body shells fastened together with Velcro straps and lined with thin foam rubber. These splints are light in weight, easily cleaned, and durable but are nonabsorbent. Patients may complain of perspiring and of being warm.

with a waterproof material. All this should be done before surgery because the patient can seldom spare either section of the shell long enough for repair afterward. The advisability of having the patient lie in the plaster bed for a time before surgery is great. Any points of discomfort incidental to the shell can then be discovered before he is immobolized in it.

Turning may be done the first evening if the patient's condition permits. If the patient lies on his back, careful check of the pulse and blood pressure will be necessary to detect hemorrhage, since the dressings are not visible.

It is advisable to have sufficient help so that the initial turning may be accomplished with as little discomfort to the patient as possible. He is naturally apprehensive at this time, and everything should be done to give him a sense of security. Later turnings will be accomplished much more easily if this is done. The patient in a well-fitting plaster bed can be turned with relatively little pain to his back. If the graft (cortical bone) has been taken from the

tibia, slight changes of position in the knee joint will cause muscle pull on the tibia. This necessitates careful handling of the involved limb. If cancellous bone is used, the graft is taken from the iliac crest. This incision also is a tender area and may cause considerable discomfort.

In preparation for turning, the patient is moved in one plane to the side of the bed. The undersheet is then changed by a nurse on the opposite side of the bed. Pillows are arranged to receive the leg from which the graft has been taken, and a support is made ready for the feet. The plaster shell (Figs. 320 and 321) should be securely fastened at the axillary level and around the hips.

If possible, the arm toward which the patients is to be turned should be placed above his head. However, after operations on the dorsal spine, it is sometimes better to have the arm on the side toward which the patient is to be turned stretched downward along the side of the cast. The nurse standing at the side of the bed toward which the patient has been pulled must take responsibility for seeing that this arm is freed immediately after turning is completed. Otherwise, the pressure of the plaster shell on the arm may cause considerable bruising. The patient is turned toward the clean side of the bed in one plane. One nurse places her hands on the patient's shoulders and hips, and the other nurse assumes responsibility for the leg from which the graft was taken.

Once turned, the patient should be made as comfortable as possible. The feet should be supported on a pillow placed under the ankles so that the toes do not dig into the bed. The posterior shell of the cast is removed, the dressings are carefully inspected for signs of hemorrhage or drainage, and the surrounding skin is washed and then rubbed gently with alcohol. The circulation of the back, head, neck, and thighs is important for the well-being of patients who have had spinal surgery and should be given frequent attention. Consequently, gentle back rubs, including the scalp, neck, and thighs, should be given. The patient should be urged to lie prone for as long as he can do so in order to reestablish circulation in the dependent areas of the back and thighs. He may ask to be turned back almost immediately, but a little explanation

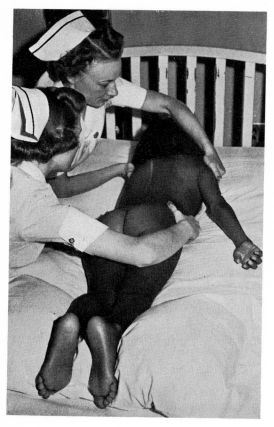

Fig. 333 One method of turning a patient (from prone to supine position) after a spinal operation when no supportive apparatus is used. The patient is rolled toward the nurses and, to avoid twisting movements of the spine, the shoulders and pelvis are turned simultaneously. The same method of supporting the shoulders and pelvis may be employed when the patient is turned from the supine to the prone position.

of the purpose of the position often will help in prolonging the period.

Frequently, patients with spinal fusions are not immobolized in plaster. Extreme care and gentleness are essential in turning such patients to avoid motion of the spine, which will be accompanied by excruciating pain. To maintain good alignment, some physicians request that these patients be kept flat, either on the abdomen or on the back. In other instances, the patients are permitted to move and turn as they wish.

When the patient not in a cast or brace after spinal fusion is being turned from his back to his abdomen, the same technique

is applied as that used with the patient in a plaster shell. First, the patient is moved to one side of the bed. If the bed is made with a wide drawsheet, the sheet can be used as a slide for the patient. This helps to avoid twisting movements of the spine. Clean linen is placed on the opposite half of the bed. Two nurses stand at the side of the bed toward which the patient is to be turned. The patient's arms are kept close to his side, and he is instructed to make his body rigid. The first nurse places her hands on the patient's far shoulder and arm, and the second nurse grasps the patient's hip and thigh (Fig. 333). To avoid twisting of the spine, the shoulders and pelvis must be maintained in the same plane and turned simultaneously. Slowly and gently, the two nurses turn the patient onto his abdomen toward themselves. Following this, it is necessary to move the patient back to the center of the bed. This again can be accomplished with the drawsheet. When the patient lies in the prone position, the dorsum of his feet need to be supported by a pillow. His arms may be placed in any comfortable position.

If the patient is turned on his side, the nurse will remember what constitutes a good side-lying position. The pillow between the legs to prevent adduction of the uppermost limb will avoid added strain on sore back muscles.

During the early days after surgery, carelessness in turning rarely takes place. The patient is so apprehensive that it is necessary to guard one's every movement lest unnecessary pain be caused. After ten days or two weeks, however, when the patient's general condition is on the upgrade and the acute pain in the leg and back is much diminished, haste and carelessness sometimes do occur, for nurses on busy units tend to try to turn such patients with insufficient help. Healing in spinal grafts takes place slowly, as does all bone healing, and gentle handling must continue for many weeks. The so-called critical time after spinal operations is considered to be four to five weeks. Particular care in handling the patient during this time should be observed. Spinal pseudarthrosis can occur because of careless postoperative handling of the patient with spinal fusion.

Edema of the face sometimes occurs in

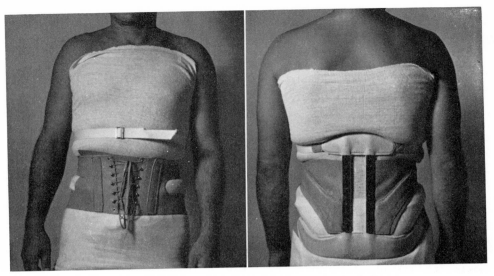

Fig. 334 Anterior and posterior views of a low back brace.

the patient with cervical fusion. A temporary impairment of bowel function often occurs after the spinal fusion, and the use of a suppository is usually ordered between the fourth and sixth days. Rectal impaction should be avoided. The establishment of regular habits of elimination will soon help to overcome the need for bowel care and should be part of the patient's routine. The back and legs of the patient must be supported while he is on the bedpan so that all sections of the body are in the same plane. Also, these patients will have less discomfort if a bedpan with a tapering back is used instead of the regular bedpan. Attention to such details will sometimes pay surprising dividends in helping the patient to resume normal habits of elimination.

Patients who must lie prone are in danger from pressure over the iliac crests. This is particularly true of the thin patient in a bivalved cast. Reddened or bluish areas around the bony crests should receive immediate attention because skin breakdown there is extremely rapid.

The patient's progress and his resumption of normal activities, such as sitting, standing, and walking, will depend upon the condition that made the spinal fusion necessary. Progress usually is more rapid following fusion for disabilities of the low back than for tuberculosis or similar infec

tions of the vertebrae. It is urgent that patients who are to remain inactive for a prolonged period have constant intelligent nursing care to parts of the musculoskeletal system that are not primarily affected but which must be kept functional for when they become ambulatory. The physician may prescribe deep-breathing exercises, exercises for maintaining muscle tone in the feet, quadriceps setting, and, later, flexion and extension of the knees. Outward rotation of the hip, if not controlled by a cast or plaster bed, should be prevented by sandbags or a trochanter roll. Unless contraindicated, the patient should be provided with occupations that will ensure normal varied use of the arms and shoulders.

The patient usually will be provided with a brace or a body cast before he is allowed out of bed. It is essential that the nurse know how to apply the brace correctly and that she recognize its importance to the patient's ultimate recovery. The brace is worn continuously until permission for its removal for short periods is given by the physician.

Applying back braces. Nurses should remember that low back braces (Fig. 334) and spring back braces may ride up considerably, particularly on heavy women. Perineal straps to prevent this are sometimes used but are never very comfortable. If the brace has a well-fitting pelvic band, it will often overcome the tendency of the brace to ride up. The pelvic band should fit low enough to hold the upper part of the buttocks adequately. When the brace is applied, the abdominal leather apron must be laced very snugly at the lower portion, with diminishing snugness as the lacing ascends. It is important in applying back braces to observe that the spinal uprights are far enough apart not to press on the vertebral prominences but close enough together to fit well between the scapulae.

Another important point to remember is that it is essential that a back brace allow the patient to sit with the hips at right angles, with no impingement of the metal or the leather on the groin. The patient must be able to sit without having the brace pushed up by the chair.

Spinal braces, such as the Taylor back brace, are not infrequently used for postoperative immobilization after fusions in the low back (sacroiliac fusion, sacrolumbar fusion, or combinations of the two). These supports often are applied in the operating room, and the patient wears them continuously for a period of several months. For back care, he is carefully turned in the brace. The metal and leather part of the apparatus is then lifted off the back, but the canvas apron that supports the abdomen is left under the patient as he lies prone, making it easy to reapply the brace after the back has been cared for. A thin cotton vest of some knitted material usually is worn beneath the brace.

Foot disabilities

Anatomy of foot. The feet bear the weight of the body when walking or standing and serve as levers in raising and propelling the body forward. Each foot consists of seven tarsal bones, five metatarsal bones, and fourteen phalanges. At birth, much of this structure is soft tissue (cartilage), and for this reason the foot of the newborn infant (when deformity exists) lends itself to corrective measures much better than the foot of an older child. There are two main arches, the longitudinal and the transverse (metatarsal). These arches are present at birth. The baby's foot, however, may appear quite flat because of a fat pad that fills the longitudinal arch space.

The medial aspect of the longitudinal arch extends from the os calcis to the head of the first metatarsal. The lateral aspect extends from the os calcis to the head of the fourth and fifth metatarsals. This arch is supported by two groups of muscles: those of the inner and those on the outer side of the ankle. The inner group of muscles consists of the anterior tibial, normally attached below the internal cuneiform, the posterior tibial muscle, normally attached to the scaphoid, and the flexors of the toes, whose tendons act by leverage under the astragalus (sustentaculum tali) to support the arch. All these muscles work in coordination and are assisted, to some extent, by the intrinsic muscles of the foot. The outer side of the foot is supported by the peroneal muscles—longus, brevis, and tertius. These muscles tend to balance the arch-elevating effect of the muscles of the inner side of the foot and at the same time work in unison to support the arches of the foot.

The metatarsal arch extends medially from the base of the fifth metatarsal to the base of the first metatarsal. This arch is supported by the balanced action between the flexors and the extensors of the toes combined with the intrinsic muscles of the foot.

When muscle action fails, from disuse or disease, the strain is transmitted to ligamentous structures, such as the plantar fascia, and to other ligaments around the joints. Strain is often accompanied by inflammatory change. Thus, it can be readily understood that the patient who has been at bed rest needs adequate support for his arches when ambulation is permitted. This patient needs a well-fitted shoe—not soft slippers.

Movements of foot. When caring for the bed patient, it is essential to know the normal movements of the foot and ankle. If these motions are not contraindicated and are performed passively or actively, joint contractures can be prevented. Plantar flexion (equinus position) and dorsiflexion of the foot take place at the ankle joint. Inversion (supination) and eversion (pronation) movements of the foot are made possible by the subastragalar joint. Adduction and abduction motions take place in the midtarsal joints. Flexion and extension of the toes take place at the metatarsophalangeal and the interphalangeal joints.

Shoes. Today, walking is being encouraged as one of the best forms of exercise. This is especially true for the older person. Painful feet provide little incentive for the young or old person to be active. If ambulation is to be done with comfort, well-cared-for feet and well-fitted shoes are of prime importance.

Characteristics of well-fitted shoe. Properly fitted shoes are an important factor in the prevention of foot deformities. If pain and foot discomfort are to be prevented, the shoe size and shape should conform to the foot. The foot must not be forced into an ill-fitted shoe. The shoe length, with weight-bearing, should extend approximately one-fourth to one-half inch beyond the end of the great toe. A shoe that is too short will cause crowding of the toes, and the great toe will be forced into a hallux valgus position. A straight inner last is desirable. Continuous wearing of pointed shoes will result in a hallux valgus deformity and the formation of a bunion (Fig. 335). In a properly fitted shoe, the sole at the ball of the foot must be wide enough to permit free movement of foot muscles. The length should be proportioned so that the ball of the foot is accommodated at the widest part of the shoe. This part of the shoe needs to be flexible to permit bending of the toes. The shank should give fairly good support. The heavy person or the person who stands for long hours may need

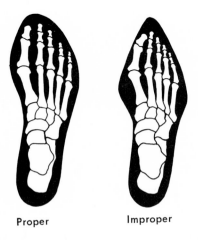

Proper   Improper

Fig. 335 Note that the shoe with a pointed toe forces the great toe into a hallux valgus position.

a stronger shoe and a more rigid shank than the person who sits for long periods. The shank of a child's shoe, unless ordered otherwise by his phyiscian, should be flexible. The heel should fit the heel of the foot. Sling-back shoes give little or no support, do not hold the heel in position, and tend to cause blisters and calluses. The height of the heel depends upon the purpose of the shoe. A shoe that is to be worn when working or walking should have a heel of reasonable height. It is difficult for the person who walks or stands in high heels to attain good posture and to practice good body mechanics. The weight of the body is thrown forward on the ball of the foot. This results in calluses and strain on the metatarsal arch.

Children's shoes. The infant who has not started to walk needs covering for his feet only to keep them warm. The shoes need to have soft soles that permit motion of the feet and use of foot muscles. When the child learns to walk, his shoe should have a thin leather sole sufficient to protect his foot but flexible enough to permit normal motion and use of the muscles, particularly at the ball of the foot. The best shoe for a growing infant, especially if there is any abnormality, is of the high-topped variety with a firm sole, narrow heel, and broad toe.

Care of feet. Good hygienic care of the feet, daily bathing, and massage will help to relieve tired, aching feet. Contrast baths improve circulation and the tone of foot muscles. The person who spends many hours on his feet may secure relief from aching feet by changing shoes during the working hours. Wearing the right-sized stockings and care in trimming the nails will help to prevent painful ingrown toenails and dangerous infection. The nails should be trimmed straight across. Irritation and pressure caused by ill-fitted shoes will result in corns and calluses. A corn is an overgrowth of the outer layer of skin and is nature's way of protecting the soft tissue. Pads may be used to relieve the pressure. To secure permanent relief, however, it is necessary that the shoe fit properly and that pressure on the area be relieved. Maintaining clean healthy skin will help greatly in preventing athlete's foot (dermatophytosis). Wearing clean stockings and permitting shoes to air and sun are of considerable value. Blisters and abrasions of the skin should have proper care. This is particularly important for the older person who has poor circulation or the person with diabetes whose tissues heal slowly.

Foot strain

Foot strain caused by inherently weak muscles can begin with the first steps that a child takes. This weakness may persist and cause foot strain throughout life.

A second common cause of foot strain is ill-fitted shoes. There has been a tendency in the past for style to take precedence over comfort—high heels, narrow toes, a narrow sole, etc. Although this is being partly overcome with the availability of shoes that conform to the shape of the average foot, such correct shoes are still none too popular. Although ample width is essential in the metatarsal region, a shoe should not be loose or ill fitted at the instep and heel. One of the common causes of foot trouble, particularly in women, results from wearing shoes made sufficiently large in circular dimension but with the sole narrower than the ball of the foot. This is likely to cause strain on the metatarsal arch, because pressure is exerted upward along the lateral borders of the foot (Fig. 336), and, in spite of the fact that the person has ample room within the confines of the shoe itself, there is no freedom of muscle action.

A third cause of foot strain is inadequate muscle and ligamentous support. (The arches of the foot are supported by ligaments, tendons, and muscles.) The child who is growing very rapidly may complain of some foot discomfort. Muscle strength is not keeping up with the growth of the body. Prolonged inactivity will result in weakness and atrophy of the soft tissues supporting the arches of the foot. If weight bearing is permitted in soft bedroom slip-

pers, the patient may develop painful feet. Excessive body weight puts an additional strain on the foot. The muscle and ligamentous support of the arches may become inadequate, and the inevitable result is painful, flattened arches. Excessive exercise in soft rubber-soled shoes, when the individual is not accustomed to such activity, may result in foot strain and pain.

Bunions

There are two types of bunions: acquired and hereditary. Acquired bunions are definitely caused by wearing shoes that are too pointed and too narrow or too short.

Hereditary bunions are caused at least in part by a congenital abnormality. The space between the first and second metatarsals is increased (Fig. 337) so that bunion development is unavoidable when almost any type of shoe is worn.

Hallux valgus is an abnormal position of the big toe. Bunion is an overgrowth of bone. The two are commonly associated (Fig. 338).

The pain and discomfort from bunions can, in most instances, be relieved by properly fitted shoes and by support of the metatarsal arch. Arch supports, metatarsal bars, and sufficiently wide shoes are essential. Persons who suffer from these deformities are not always willing to accept the type of shoe necessary for relief. Sometimes bunions may be so severe that bony correction is required.

Operative procedures are directed at correction of the abnormal position by various techniques, the commonest of which is re-

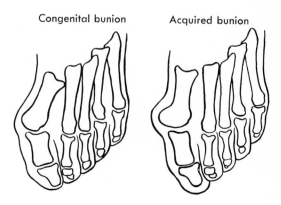

Congenital bunion   Acquired bunion

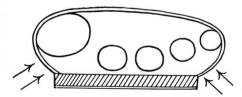

Fig. 336 Pressure exerted to cause metatarsal arch strain when shoe is improperly built. Such a shoe may have plenty of room.

Fig. 337 Note difference in angle between first and second metatarsals.

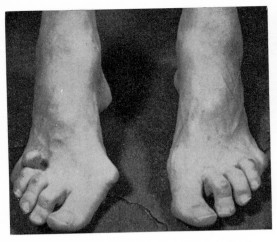

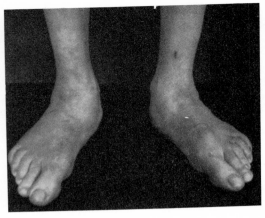

Fig. 338 Hallux valgus deformity with bunion, overlapping fifth toe (right), hammer toes, and corns.

Fig. 339 Pronation of the foot, a common postural disturbance. Note the flattened or depressed position of the longitudinal arch. If the foot is observed from the back, the Achilles tendon curves toward the midline. Frequently, the patient with pronated feet will complain of backache and of pain in the calves of the legs.

moval of the proximal portion of the first phalanx (Keller operation), and the bunion is corrected by removal of bony overgrowth.

In the congenital type, osteotomy at the base of the first metatarsal may be combined with tendon transplantation according to the method of McBride. An osteotomy at the distal end of the metatarsal also may be necessary to restore the alignment.

Arch strain

Longitudinal arch strain. The pain in longitudinal arch strain in both children and adults usually is felt in the arch and in the leg muscles. As a rule, the pain caused by arch strain is present only after exertion and fatigue. If there is an inflammatory condition accompanying such a strain, it is usually characterized by aggravation of the pain upon arising in the morning or upon sudden activity after short periods of rest. Pain present only after activity usually is the result of muscle and ligamentous strain rather than inflammation of the joints and ligaments.

Treatment is designed to relieve the strain on the anterior and posterior tibial muscles by means of temporary arch supports made of felt and leather and designed to the individual requirement. Felt is used instead of steel because the latter is rigid and tends to decrease the muscle development for correction. Particularly if knock-ankle deformity (Fig. 339) is present, a

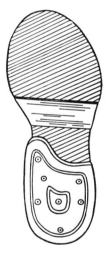

Fig. 340 Thomas (or orthopedic) heel often used in combination with a metatarsal bar.

Thomas or orthopedic heel (Fig. 340) with an inner elevation also may be added.

A distinction should be made between acute arch strain and permanent or chronic flatfoot. In the latter, the use of rigid arch supports of stainless steel or Monel metal is justifiable. In acute arch strain, exercises with temporary lifts and supports may be of distinct value in restoring muscle power after the strain has been relieved. In chronic flatfoot, however, exercises are of

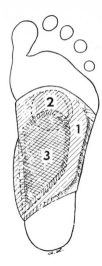

Fig. 341 Design for arch support based on the normal weight-bearing surface. The pads are felt or rubber covered with leather. Pad **3** fills the normal arch space. Pad **1** distributes pressure evenly over a larger area. Pad **2** increases pressure under the metatarsal arch at any desired point.

little value. At times, high-topped shoes may be necessary to offset the demands on the muscles that also control the ankle.

Metatarsal arch strain—metatarsalgia. The metatarsal arch is supported primarily by muscles, and, when the muscle action fails because of abuse or disuse, strain is placed upon the ligamentous structure and upon the arch. If strain is severe enough, there is a flattening of the arch and weight is taken on the heads of the second, third, and fourth metatarsals. The person with this condition will develop a callus over the ball of the foot, and walking will become quite painful. To relieve this pain, felt or rubber pads covered with leather may be placed just posterior to the heads of the second, third, and fourth metatarsals. The padding gives support to the arch and relieves pressure. The physician may also request that a metatarsal bar (anterior heel) be attached to the shoe. This, again, gives the arch support and relieves pressure on the metatarsal heads.

In strains of either longitudinal or metatarsal arches, a support of felt or rubber covered with leather may be designed from the pedograph or outline of the weight-bearing surface of the foot (Fig. 341). It is the object of supports not only to relieve pressure in the area of the foot that does not come in contact during weight bearing, but also to distribute the pressure evenly throughout the area not bearing weight and a small portion of the weight-bearing area.

One of the main requirements in strain of the metatarsal arch is to provide sufficient room for action of the muscles that support the metatarsal arch. Therefore, adequate width of the shoe in the metatarsal region is necessary. Many persons with broad short feet need shoes that are EE or EEE in width, which are difficult yet possible to obtain.

Exercises. The treatment described is aimed at relieving the symptoms and enabling the person to get about without discomfort. If the condition is to be corrected, however, the strength of the muscles that normally support the arch must be restored. This may be accomplished by active exercises. The following exercises for the metatarsal and the longitudinal arches and for contracted heel cords are frequently prescribed.

For metatarsal arch. One exercise prescribed to strengthen the metatarsal arch is the towel exercise. A towel is placed on the floor, and the feet are placed parallel to each other about an inch apart with the heels just over the posterior border. The toes are then contracted alternately one foot with the other so that the towel is gradually accumulated under the arch. Another exercise for the metatarsal arch is the marble exercise. Ten to twelve marbles are placed on the floor and, by action of the flexor tendon are picked up, moved, and released rhythmically. A pencil also may be used. The toes also may be contracted rhythmically over the edge of a step (Fig. 342) or a large book upon which the subject is standing.

For longitudinal arch. In the standing position, the feet and toes are inverted so that the weight is borne on the outer border of the feet. This exercise should be repeated thirty times. Another exercise for the longitudinal arch is performed by rising on the balls of the feet, raising the heels, and everting the ankles. This is to be repeated twenty to thirty times.

For contracted heel cords. Two exercises for contracted heel cords are performed as

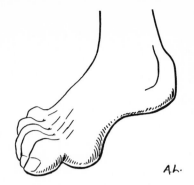

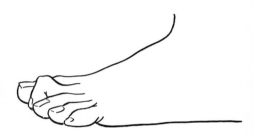

Fig. 343 Clawfoot deformity with retraction of the toes and high arch (cavus).

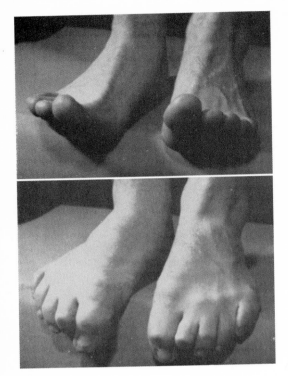

Fig. 342 Contracting the toes rhythmically over the edge of a stairstep to strengthen foot muscles.

Fig. 344 Hammer toe. A corn usually forms on the top and the end of the toe.

follows: (1) stand on the heel, raising and inverting the forefoot, and (2) stand with the ball of the foot on the edge of a stairstep and drop the weight downward, stretching the heel cords. These exercises should be done at least twice daily and should be repeated, starting at about twenty times for each and increasing to about fifty.

Other foot disabilities

There are other causes for disabilities in the foot as a result of disease, trauma, and disturbances in circulation.

Apophysitis. Apophysitis is a disease of the heels of growing children as a result of traumatic and metabolic disturbance. There is an irritation of the posterior epiphysis of the os calcis. Pain and tenderness are characteristic. Treatment consists of removing the counter of the shoe and temporarily raising the heel one-half to three-fourth of an inch.

Koehler's disease. Koehler's disease is characterized by pain, tenderness, and slight swelling about the tarsal scaphoid. It is caused by trauma, direct or indirect, and by circulatory disturbances in the bone, causing degenerative changes and compression within the scaphoid. It is relieved by casts or by arch supports and a lift or wedge along the inner side of an elongated heel.

Freiberg's disease. Freiberg's disease is a condensation or infraction in the distal end of the second metatarsal, usually resulting from trauma and aseptic necrosis and characterized by shortening of the metatarsal, tenderness about the metatasal head, and some strain of the metatarsal arch. It is treated by support of the metatarsal arch.

Clawfoot and hollow foot. Clawfoot (Fig. 343) and hollow foot consist of a contracture of the muscles and ligaments of the plantar arch as a result of relative overactivity of the extensors of the toe as compared to the flexor action. This may be influenced or instigated by continued metatarsal arch strain, arthritis, or spastic or infantile paralysis. The condition is frequently accompanied by calluses under the metatarsal heads and by corns on the dorsal surface of the interphalangeal joints of the toes. The treatment may require proper support of the metatarsal arch with arch supports and metatarsal bars, tenotomy of the extensor tendons to the toes, tendon transplantation of the extensor tendons to the metatarsal necks, or, in severe cases, resection of the metatarsal heads or proximal portions of the phalanges.

Hammer toes. Hammer toes (Fig. 344) may be either congenital or acquired as a result of contracture of the extensors of the toes. The first interphalangeal joint is usually prominent and flexed. A corn usually develops on top and on the end of the toe. Correction can be obtained easily by resection of a portion of the proximal phalanx so that the toe is shortened and the muscle contracture released.

Knock-ankle and flatfoot deformities. Knock-ankle and flatfoot deformities in children are common and frequently are accompanied by bowlegs or knock-knees and internal rotation of the tibiae so that the child walks with a pigeon-toe and knock-ankle gait. It is difficult to tell whether or not there is a true flatfoot deformity in young children when they are beginning to walk because of the frequent existence of a fat pad under the arch. Arch supports are not often indicated, and the correction usually can be accomplished by lifts and elongated heels. When the internal rotation and pigeon-toe deformity is not severe and the principal deformity is knock-ankle, an elongated heel with an inner lift of one-eighth to one-fourth of an inch will usually correct the deformity within a few months.

When the pigeon-toe deformity is severe with marked internal rotation of the ankle on the knee, it is best to use cable rotators attached to the outside or the inner side of the shoe. They spiral the leg and are fastened to a belt at the waist (Fig. 139). The adjustment of these rotators may exert the necessary tension to maintain correct alignment. In six to eighteen months the alignment becomes fixed and the deformity disappears.

Bowlegs in children are not uncommon up to the second year of age and probably compensate for foot deformity, or vice versa. After the bowleg deformity has sub-

sided, a reversion to the knock-knee status may take place and persist to the seventh or eighth year. During this time, frequent changes in shoe elevations may be necessary to meet the current requirements of balance.

Bursitis

Location of bursae. Throughout the body there are a number of places where bony prominences are exposed to irritation, either from outward pressure or from the friction effect of tendons, ligaments, and even the skin over these prominences. Such prominences are protected by small sacs (bursae) or compartments filled with a lubricating synovial fluid produced from the walls of the sac. This allows the gliding of the various structures over the bony prominences without friction. A bursa may develop in an area where none normally exists if persistent irritation continues. The ordinary location of these bursae (Fig. 345) is as follows:

1 Shoulder
  a Subacromial
  b Subcoracoid
2 Elbow
  a Olecranon
3 Hip
  a Gluteal (under attachment of glueteus maximus)
  b Trochanteric (greater trochanter and lesser trochanter)
  c Ischial (weaver's bottom)
4 Knee
  a Prepatellar (housemaid's knee)
  b Pretibial (under patella tendon)
  c Superficial pretibial (over tibial tubercle)
  d Popliteal
  e Bicipital
5 Foot
  a Achilles (under the attachment of the Achilles tendon)
  b Retrocalcaneal (anterior to the Achilles tendon)
  c Inferior calcaneal (under the attachment of the plantar fascia to the heel—policeman's heel)
  d Bunion (may develop on either the inner or the outer side of the foot when there is bony prominence of the metatarsal head as seen in hallux valgus)

Symptoms. Inflammation of a bursa may develop gradually as the result of a repeated strain or injury or acutely as the result of more severe damage. Pain, swelling, and marked tenderness are present. When active motions involve the function of the

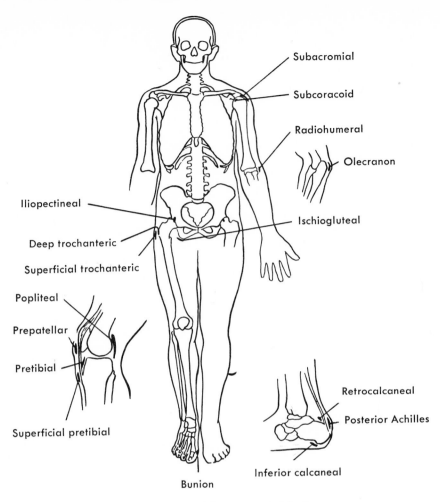

Subacromial

Subcoracoid

Radiohumeral

Olecranon

Iliopectineal

Ischiogluteal

Deep trochanteric

Superficial trochanteric

Popliteal

Prepatellar

Pretibial

Retrocalcaneal

Posterior Achilles

Superficial pretibial

Inferior calcaneal

Bunion

Fig. 345 Locations of the most common bursae.

bursa, pain is greatly aggravated. Passive motions, however, usually are not so painful as they would be if there were joint involvement.

Acute inflammation of a bursa may develop when bacteria or toxins from remote focal infection settle there.

Treatment. The cause of bursitis, such as irritation and infection, should be removed.

In the noninfectious types of bursitis, complete rest and the application of heat are important. A sling or a flannel spica applied to the extremities often is effective in giving relief.

Subdeltoid bursitis is one of the commonest forms and may need special treatment. The subdeltoid bursa is situated between the deltoid muscle and the rotator

cuff of the shoulder. The inflammation arises in this bursa secondary to degeneration in one of the tendons of the rotator cuff, usually the supraspinatus. Calcium is deposited into the degenerated area, and it is often possible to see a calcific deposit in a roentgenogram of the shoulder that is painful as a result of bursitis. Pain is the outstanding symptom and frequently radiates down the arm. Restriction of motion in the shoulder may be so severe that this condition has been referred to as frozen shoulder.

Treatment of subdeltoid bursitis will depend on whether it is in the acute or the chronic stage. In acute bursitis, the treatment is aimed at relief of pain. The simplest way to release the calcium that is under tension and is responsible for the active pain is to insert a needle and wash it out. This can be done with procaine HCl (Novocain). At times, the calcium is inspissated (dried out to form a hard pebble) and may require surgical excision. Many times the acute attack will cure itself by absorption of the calcium; however, this may require a period of a few days, during which time the patient must be well medicated for pain and the shoulder must be immobilized in a sling.

Chronic bursitis does not demand immediate treatment to relieve pain, although pain is present. The main consideration is to stop irritation of the degenerated rotator cuff so that it may heal. Avoidance of extreme motion and lifting, plus use of local heat, may control the symptoms and allow the process to subside. Many physicians prescribe radiation therapy, but the beneficial effect is variable. Pendulum exercises to regain lost motion are perhaps the most important treatment. Local injection of hydrocortisone into tender areas often helps to relieve pain.

18 Bone tumors

Three types of tumors occur in bone: (1) benign (nonmalignant), (2) malignant, and (3) metastatic from other tissues or organs. Benign tumors grow slowly and do not tend to destroy surrounding tissues or spread to other parts of the body through the bloodstream or lymphatic system. These include osteocartilaginous exostosis, enchondroma, chondroblastoma, chondromyxoid fibroma hemangioma, osteoid osteoma osteoblastoma, and giant cell tumor (Fig. 346).

Malignant tumors (sarcomas) usually grow rapidly and may be of considerable size before they are recognized by the pa-

tient. They often have spread to other parts of the body through the bloodstream before being brought to the attention of a surgeon.

Tumors metastatic from cancer of other tissues, such as the breast, prostate, lung, kidney, or thyroid gland, are quite common because bone marrow has a rich blood supply and cancer cells are easily spread through the bloodstream.

Benign tumors

Generally, the cause is not known for all types of benign tumors. Some of the benign tumors are thought to be aberrations of the growth and development of tissues. The

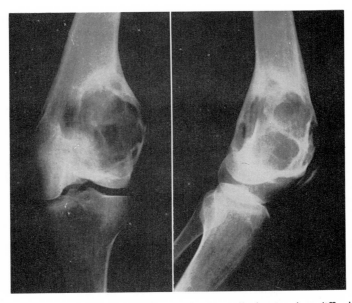

Fig. 346 Giant cell tumor (osteoclastoma), which is usually benign but difficult to differentiate from certain malignant osteogenic sarcomas even after biopsy. Characteristically, these tumors expand the shaft, show little bone reaction, involve the epiphyses of the long bones, and seldom break into a joint cavity. (From Kenney, W. C., and Larson, C. B.: Orthopedics for the general practitioner, St. Louis, The C. V. Mosby Co.)

osteocartilaginous exostosis (Fig. 347) is considered to be caused by displacement of cartilage cells at the epiphyseal plate. As bone growth takes place, the displaced cells cause enlargement near the ends of long bones that may be bumped easily because of their prominence. Some patients may have exostoses of many bones (Fig. 348). At times, malignant change takes place in one of these tumors. All of the other benign tumors have little or no visible external manifestations because they are confined within bone.

The symptoms in patients with benign tumors are generally mild pain in the affected bone or prominence, as in the patient with an exostosis. The diagnosis is made with the aid of roentgenograms and surgical biopsy.

Treatment is simple removal, excision, or curettage. Therefore, the nursing care involves routine postoperative management of a patient in a plaster dressing or soft bandages.

Malignant tumors

Most bone sarcomas are classified according to the type of tissue formed by the malignant cells; examples are osteogenic sarcoma (Fig. 349), fibrosarcoma, chondrosarcoma, hemangiosarcoma, and round cell sarcomas: Ewing's sarcoma, reticulum cell sarcoma, and multiple myeloma (Fig. 350). As is true for benign tumors, the cause is generally not known. Certain preexisting conditions, such as Paget's disease of bone, may cause bone sarcoma to develop. At

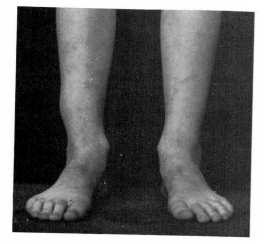

Fig. 347 Osteocartilaginous exostosis of the fibula. Note enlargement of the lower end of the right leg. This tumor is painless unless bumped.

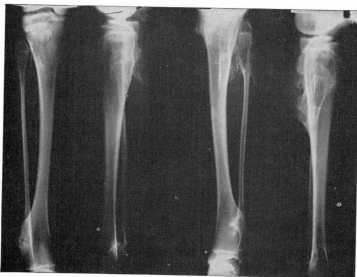

Fig. 348 Multiple osteocartilaginous exostoses. These exostoses are capped by cartilage that tends to mature when normal epiphyses close. The tumors are familial and benign but can produce symptoms if mechanically injured. Rarely (after incomplete surgical removal or with repeated trauma) they may become malignant. (From Kenney, W. C., and Larson, C. B.: Orthopedics for the general practitioner, St. Louis, The C. V. Mosby Co.)

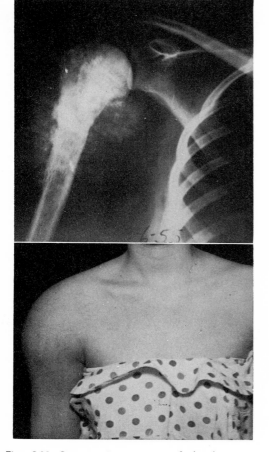

Fig. 349 Osteogenic sarcoma of the humerus. This is a primary malignant tumor of bone. It occurs in late childhood or young adulthood and usually is located in a long bone near the end of the diaphysis. Early symptoms are severe pain and swelling. This type of bone lesion metastasizes early, and the prognosis is poor. Treatment consists of amputation or extensive local resection, and in some instances roentgentherapy is advised.

times, irradiation therapy given for nonmalignant lesions may induce malignant tumors after a latent period of several years or more.

Diagnosis. A history of intermittent pain that is particularly troublesome at night, tiredness, a limp, and swelling of a part of an extremity without previous trauma or obvious infection may lead one to suspect a tumor (Fig. 351). Such a combination of symptoms requires immediate medical attention. Sometimes the parent will belittle the symptoms as being the result of some

recent fall or trauma. The patient frequently looks healthy when admitted to the hospital for the first time. The night pain may increase in severity. Roentgenograms, including tomograms, are a helpful adjunct to proper diagnosis. In certain of the bone sarcomas, laboratory work is of value. For instance, osteogenic sarcomas tend to produce a high alkaline phosphatase in the blood serum. Because the treatment and prognosis of bone sarcoma vary with the type of tumor, a surgical biopsy is the surest way to establish an accurate diagnosis. Roentgenograms of the chest will help to determine whether or not obvious metastases are present in the lungs. Metastases, however, may not be visible at the time of the initial examination but may be manifested after treatment has been instituted.

Treatment. The treatment of malignant bone tumors is surgical removal either by wide local resection (when it is both technically feasible and consistent with conservation of function) or by amputation. In most medical centers, multidrug chemotherapy is used as an adjunct to surgical removal.

Local resection is more frequently possible in the upper extremity than in the lower extremity. When tumors are present near the knee joint, function is usually better after amputation and the use of an artificial limb. At the midshaft of the femur and the upper end of the femur, resection and replacement either with a metallic prosthesis or an intramedullary rod with supplementary bone transplants may provide function without sacrificing the extremity. When metastasis can be demonstrated, as in the chest, surgical removal of the original tumor obviously will not cure the patient, but it may be necessary to control pain and to prevent the local tumor from becoming an ulcerated, fungating, foul-smelling mass.

Radiotherapy or radioactive cobalt in combination with chemotherapy will be used in patients in whom the tumor is radiosensitive. Some tumors, such as Ewing's sarcoma (Fig. 352), can be controlled for months to years by this treatment. Reticulum cell sarcoma may be cured by this method. Irradiation is often helpful in relieving pain even though it may not be curative.

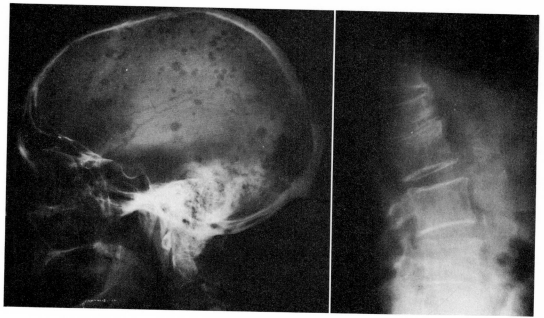

Fig. 350 Multiple myeloma involvement of the skull and vertebral column. This condition occurs in an older age group (40 to 60 years) and most commonly involves the axial skeleton (skull, vertebrae, sternum, and ribs). Roentgenograms of involved bone reveal punched-out areas. Multiple myeloma begins in the medullary cavity, is malignant, and can progress rapidly. Pain from pathologic fracture may be the first symptom, or pain in the back region may cause the individual to seek medical care. Due to the excessive bone destruction, hypercalciuria can occur. Increased fluid intake and the use of diuretics help maintain body hydration and promote excretion of the calcium. A sufficient increase in the serum level of calcium (hypercalcemia) produces a number of symptoms, including gastrointestinal disturbances, increased cardiac muscle irritability, and confusion. Steroids may be administered to help lower the calcium blood level. Corsets, splints, or other forms of support frequently are prescribed to facilitate activity and mobilization. This is important in preventing disuse osteoporosis and further loss of calcium. The presence of Bence Jones protein in the urine is diagnostic of multiple myeloma. Anemia, decreased resistance to infection, and renal impairment are frequent complications. Antineoplastic drugs used in the treatment of multiple myeloma include phenylalanine mustard and cyclophosphamide (Cytoxan). The prognosis is not favorable.

Metastatic tumors

Tumor that is metastatic to bone from cancer of other tissues is the most common tumor found in bone. It usually occurs in patients over 40 years of age, when cancers of the breast, prostate, intestinal tract, lungs, and other tissues are most common. The cancer deposit is most frequently found in those bones rich in red marrow, such as the spine, pelvis, and ribs (Fig. 353). As a rule, pain occurs at this site of deposit, but occasionally the first indication of bone involvement is a fracture resulting from some trivial accident. Compression fractures of the spine are common when cancer cells have weakened the struc-

ture of the bones of the vertebrae, or there may be pathologic fractures of the hip, shoulder, or pelvis. Proper diagnosis of the type of cancer is essential to proper treatment. Therefore, one needs information afforded by the roentgenogram and, if it is possible to obtain tissue from the metastasis, the histologic diagnosis. In certain locations, needle biopsy may be necessary rather than an open surgical biopsy. Metastases from the breast or prostate may be controlled for variable periods of time by the use of hormones and chemotherapy. In most instances, radiotherapy and analgesic drugs are necessary for the control of pain. Bone scans have facilitated the early detection and treatment of metastatic lesions. Increased uptake of the radioactive strontium in the affected area identifies the lesion before sufficient bone change has taken place to be visualized on a roentgenogram. The early treatment helps to alleviate pain and to decrease bone destruction (Fig. 354).

Nursing intervention

Mention of the word cancer to the patient and family provokes an immediate image of painful lingering death. Not all cancer means imminent predictable death, however. Therefore someone knowledgeable in the physiologic behavior of each variety of cancer, be it primary tumor or secondary metastases in bone, should inform the patient and family of the expectations pertinent to treatment, restrictions in life style, and ultimate likely outcome. The attending physician is primarily responsible to inform, counsel, dictate therapy, and pro-

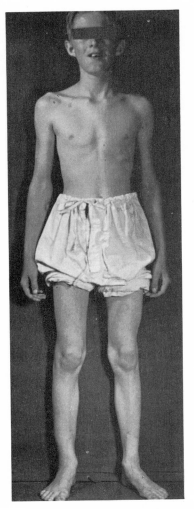

Fig. 351 Ewing's sarcoma of the lower end of the right fibula. This type of tumor usually occurs during the early teen-age years, is of medullary origin, and develops in the shaft portion of the long bones. Many times the patient has a history of trauma to the area. Symptoms usually consist of pain and tenderness, fever may be present, and laboratory studies reveal a leukocytosis. Response to irradiation and chemotherapy is usually favorable for a period of time; then metastasis occurs. The prognosis for life with this type of tumor is now improved.

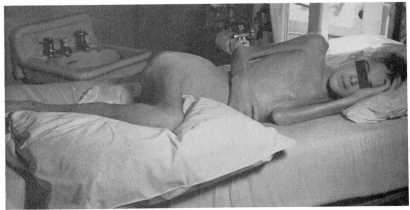

Fig. 352 Ewing's sarcoma, terminal stage.

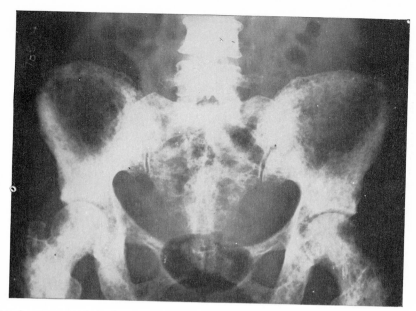

Fig. 353 Carcinoma of the breast metastatic to bone. Solitary metastases usually are to the vertebrae or femur. The more common type of lesion is osteolytic, but occasional cases show bone formation and resemble metastatic carcinoma of the prostate. (From Kenney, W. C., and Larson, C. B.: Orthopedics for the general practitioner, St. Louis, The C. V. Mosby Co.)

vide the psychologic as well as physical support to the patient and family as is required throughout the ordeal. The physician also should instruct all members of the medical team—nurses, therapists, technicians—as to their role in supporting the patient and family.

Specific explanations given in a meaningful and kindly way and reassurance in relation to the treatment and care will help promote peace of mind for the cancer patient. The needed treatment and possible side effects should be discussed. The patient needs to understand what is expected of him, and if he can be helped to express his anxieties and to ask questions, it will be a less frightening experience for him. Care and treatment of the cancer patient necessitates that the health worker be a concerned listener, one who has time for the patient, and one who has insight into his own attitudes about cancer and death, as well as the many facets of the disease and its treatment.

Nursing care of patients with malignant bone tumors does not differ greatly from the care given to a patient with malignancy of any part of the body. The postoperative

care of patients who have had amputations or disarticulations will correspond to that of patients with amputations for any cause. If a local resection has been performed, the patient undoubtedly will be in a plaster dressing and the care is the same as that for one in a plaster cast.

Splinting of the extremity may be done to prevent pain or injury to the affected part. The chance of pathologic fracture occurring at or near the site of the tumor is to be kept in mind, for very little trauma or manipulation is necessary to bring about such fractures. This should be remembered during the bed-making process or when the patient is being turned, and especially if he is allowed out of bed. In the latter case, he should be carefully protected against bumps or falls. Fracture may occur from a relatively trivial mishap, and complaints of pain in the area may be considered to be due to the lesion unless the nurse is vigilant in observation. Also, gentleness and proper support are necessary when the patient is being transferred from cart to bed and vice versa.

The prognosis for the patient who has a local recurrence or a metastatic lesion is

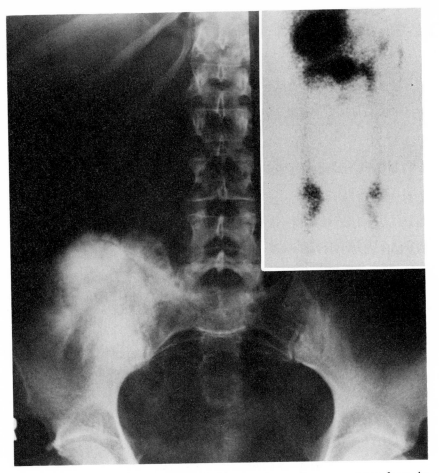

Fig. 354 Dense abnormal bone formation (white area) may be seen arising from the right iliac bone. The appearance is that of an osteogenic carcoma. **Inset,** Bone scan. The patient is injected with a radioactive tracer compound that localizes in the body where there is bone formation. The picture is obtained by "scanning" the patient with a special "gamma camera" that detects the gamma rays emitted by the radioactive tracer after it has localized in the areas of the body with bone formation or "turnover." Areas that have accumulated the tracer show as dark or "hot" areas in the picture. This scan shows normal tracer "uptake" in the legs and left pelvis but an abnormal increased uptake in the area of the right iliac bone corresponding to the area of the osteogenic sarcoma. Some of the compound is excreted in the urine, so there is "activity" in the urinary bladder also. This patient's cancer is obvious on the plain x-ray film, but the bone scan can help detect metastases in other areas that are not so obvious. Also, some cancers and other abnormalities can be detected by bone scanning before they become visible on regular x-ray films. The bone scan is not specific for cancer; areas of arthritis, fractures, osteomyelitis, etc. where increased bone turnover is occurring will show "hot." Therefore, clinical and x-ray correlation is needed.

usually poor. False hope must not be given the cancer patient. The patient should be told the facts as simply and gently as possible. He should be helped through the stages of initial denial, anger, and depression to reach acceptance and hope.[220] Providing for comfort measures and helping the patient realize that pain can be controlled may relieve some of his concern about the future. In some instances, assistance in planning for home care may lessen anxieties and provide for a happier situation. The nurse who is able to help the patient cope with problems day by day as they arise is offering the cancer patient a reassuring and helpful relationship.

Radiotherapy. Although not curative, radiotherapy is helpful in the treatment of some types of bone malignancy. Cancer cells are destroyed, and relief of pain may be apparent early in the course of treatment. When radiation therapy is prescribed, instructions should be sought from the radiologist regarding the patient's care. Marks on the skin made with an indelible pen indicate the area to be treated, and these should not be washed off. It is important that the skin area involved be protected from trauma such as friction caused by harsh linens or tight garments. The use of soap or lotion on the area is omitted. Adhesive tape applied to hold a dressing in place is very traumatizing to the sensitive skin and should be avoided. Sunbathing is not permitted, since the patient's skin at this time is particularly sensitive to light. The application of either heat or cold is also contraindicated. In some instances, the patient receiving radiation therapy can be made more comfortable and his skin protected by placing him on a square of sheepskin. This is particularly true if he is emaciated and unable to be out of bed. If breaks in the skin do occur, the physician should be informed of the problem, and any ointment prescribed should be applied to a surgical dressing that is placed on the involved area. Rubbing of the skin is avoided. As treatment progresses, changes in the skin become apparent. Helping the patient understand that the redness (erythema), the scaling (desquamation), and the crusting are expected may help to lessen his concern about the treatments he is receiving.

Maintaining adequate nutrition for the patient with a malignancy can be a very real nursing problem. It is important that his food intake include vitamins, proteins, and other blood-building foods to counteract the advancing anemia. The patient's appetite is frequently poor, and there is the added fact that radiation treatment may cause nausea and vomiting. An anorexia diet may help, and sometimes frequent small meals are tolerated better than the usual three. Oral hygiene and time to rest prior to eating may be helpful. Assistance with meals will lessen fatigue. Drugs (antiemetics) that help to combat nausea may relieve some of the discomfort and thus help the patient maintain an adequate intake of food and fluid.

Complete blood counts at fairly frequent intervals are ordered for the patient receiving radiation therapy. The weakness and fatigue experienced by the patient receiving such therapy will be more tolerable if he understands that it is caused by the effect of the radiation on the bone marrow, and not necessarily symptoms of the disease, and that following completion of the therapy new erythrocyte cells will begin to form again. The need for frequent rest periods and the need to conserve energy will be understandable. A white blood count may be taken daily. A decrease in the white blood count (leukopenia) increases the individual's susceptibility to infection, and contact with a person who has an infection should be avoided. Good body hygiene and prompt care of a beginning infection are essential. If the white blood count falls sufficiently, reverse isolation may be utilized.

Antineoplastic drugs. Drugs used in the treatment of bone lesions include antimetabolites, alkylating agents, hormones, antibiotics, and other miscellaneous agents. Specific drugs include adriamycin, methotrexate with citrovorum rescue factor, vincristine, actinomycin D, and cyclophosphamide (Cytoxan). These drugs are used in rigidly controlled protocols with appropriate surgery or radiation therapy. Disease-free intervals in patients with Ewing's sarcoma are most encouraging. Clinical trials in patients with osteosarcoma show promise.

The antimetabolites are chemical compounds that interfere with the utilization of essential metabolites, thus interrupting cell growth. One example of this type of drug is 5-fluorouracil (5-FU). The alkylating agents slow the growth of cells by reacting with molecules within the malignant cell. These drugs are toxic to healthy cells as well as to cancerous cells. Mechlorethamine (nitrogen mustard) is an example of this kind of drug. The route of administration varies with the agent. Some may be given by mouth, others by infusion, and some by arterial perfusion.

Since toxic manifestations do occur with the use of antineoplastic drugs, the nurse must seek specific information about the drug being administered. Nausea, vomiting, and diarrhea are frequent side effects and can lead to dehydration and an electrolyte imbalance. Dryness of the mouth and inflammation of the oral mucosa require good oral hygiene, a bland diet, and, in some instances, antibiotics. Leukopenia, thrombocytopenia, and anemia are due to bone marrow depression. The lowered white blood count increases the individual's susceptibility to infection, and the lowered platelet count may cause bleeding due to impairment of the normal blood-clotting mechanism. Alopecia (loss of hair, eyebrows, eyelashes) may occur due to damage to the hair follicles. The hair loss is temporary, with regrowth usually taking place in several months. If steroids are being administered, toxic effects include fluid retention and hypertension. A low-salt diet may be necessary to lessen fluid retention, and this usually necessitates the administration of potassium to prevent hypokalemia. Also, the possibility of the cancer drug interacting with routine drugs being administered the patient must be kept in mind.

The toxic manifestations caused by the antineoplastic drugs necessitate exacting care in their administration and careful assessment of the patient to determine his ability to tolerate the drug. Blood counts, blood chemistries, and urinalyses are completed prior to and at frequent intervals throughout the treatment to detect significant changes, and the patient's general well-being, nutritional status, evidence of fatigue, presence of infection, and skin condition must be carefully monitored.

Unit IV STUDY QUESTIONS

CONGENITAL DEFORMITIES/DEVELOPMENTAL AFFECTIONS

1 How will a sound knowledge and understanding of the normal infant assist the nurse in providing better care for children with congenital deformities?

2 What should be included in a routine assessment for musculoskeletal anomalies of the newborn infant?

3 Explain the difference between subluxation of the hip and a dislocated hip in the newborn infant.

4 a What nursing problems will confront the mother caring for her child in a hip spica cast?
  b What can the nurse do to help the mother give good nursing care to the child?

5 Why is it important that the following conditions be diagnosed and treated early?
  a Congenital dislocation of the hip
  b Torticollis
  c Clubfoot

6 What symptoms may be observed that would indicate a congenital dislocation of the hip
  a Before weight bearing?
  b After weight bearing?

7 Discuss overcorrection as a means of treatment in congenital deformities.

8 List two types of spina bifida and describe each.

9 Be prepared to discuss the nursing care of the patient with spina bifida as related to the following:
  a Prevention and healing of trophic ulcers
  b Prevention of deformities and secondary contractures
  c Care of incontinence
  d Problems of the patient with spina bifida with braces
  e Problems encountered following surgery
  f Psychologic, social, and economic factors
  g Provision of adequate home instruction and follow-up care

10 What should be included in a posture evaluation or assessment to detect early signs of idiopathic scoliosis?

11 The patient with severe scoliosis frequently is placed in some type of corrective apparatus. Review briefly the treatment and nursing care of the patient who is wearing a Milwaukee brace or a halo-body cast.

12 Procedures to stabilize the spine may be done for the scoliotic patient. Explain what is meant by a spinal fusion and discuss the nursing care of patient who has undergone such a procedure.

13 Pseudarthrosis may occur following a spinal fusion. Explain.

14 When the condition known as coxa plana occurs, there is avascular necrosis of the head of the femur. To prevent deformity during the period of necrosis, it is necessary to protect the head of the femur. Discuss methods used to accomplish this, and review nursing implications.

15 a What is meant by slipped femoral epiphysis?
   b It is desirable that treatment for slipped femoral epiphysis be started early. Explain.

16 In what age group do the following conditions occur?
   a Coxa plana
   b Slipped epiphysis

17 Distinguish between the following terms:
   a Kyphos
   b Gibbus
   c Scoliosis
   d Lordosis

NEUROMUSCULAR DISORDERS
Cerebral palsy

1 Study and list the possible causes of cerebral palsy.

2 What early symptoms might indicate the presence of cerebral palsy?

3 Discuss briefly the differences in treatment of the two main types of cerebral palsy.

4 Discuss the nurse's part in habit training of patients with cerebral palsy.

5 What are some of the problems that might be encountered in the postoperative care of the patient with cerebral palsy?

6 Does the physical disability in cerebral palsy influence the patient's mental and emotional development? Explain.

7 a Can you visualize the problems with which parents and family are confronted when a child is born with cerebral palsy?
   b What assistance can the nurse give the parents?

Muscular dystrophy

1 Briefly review the types of muscular dystrophy and the symptoms and treatment of each.

2 As a rule, the youngster with muscular dystrophy is cared for in the home. What can the nurse do to help the family provide proper care for this type of patient?

Poliomyelitis

1 Discuss the nurse's duties pertaining to prevention of poliomyelitis.

2 Explain the sequence of giving the Sabin oral vaccine (OPV).

ARTHRITIS

1 Review the anatomy and structure of:
  a Knee joint
  b Hip joint

2 a What is the basic objective in the care and treatment of a patient with arthritis?
   b What are the roles of the various people who may be involved in the patient's care?

3 What are the principles that guide the nurse in her care of a patient with arthritis?

4 Differentiate between the following rheumatic conditions:
   a Rheumatoid arthritis
   b Osteoarthritis
   c Septic arthritis
   d Gouty arthritis
   e Traumatic arthritis
   f Marie-Strümpell arthritis
   g Juvenile rheumatoid arthritis

5 What is meant by the term "rheumatoid factor"?

6 Review the drugs commonly used in the treatment of rheumatoid arthritis, including dosage, expected effect, and possible toxic reactions.

7 What are the basic ingredients of a treatment program for a patient with arthritis?

8 a To what details of care and arrangement of the patient's bed must the nurse give attention?
   b What is the objective?

9 Contractures, to a large degree, are preventable. What important contributions can be made by the nurse in this regard?

10 The patient with arthritis who lives within the limitations imposed by his disease does better than those who do not. How may the nurse help the patient to adopt this attitude?

INFECTION

1 Case finding is an important factor in the prevention of tuberculosis.
   a Why is this important in the prevention of skeletal tuberculosis?
   b Review the nurse's responsibility pertaining to this aspect of patient care.

2 Review the drugs commonly used in the treatment of skeletal tuberculosis, including possible toxic reactions.

3 Review symptoms, treatment, and nursing care of a child with acute pyogenic arthritis of the hip joint.

4 When dressing a draining wound, the nurse should use precautions to protect herself and other patients from the organism involved. Precautions also are needed to prevent cross infection. Review technique necessary to obtain these objectives.

5 Define the following terms:
   a Brodie's abscess
   b Cold abscess
   c Ankylosis
   d Arthrodesis
   e Fusion
   f Gibbus
   g Involucrum
   h Kyphos
   i Night cries
   j Saucerization
   k Sequestrum

6 An inflamed joint is quite painful. Describe method(s) of supporting and moving an extremity that will cause the patient a minimum of discomfort.

PAINFUL ORTHOPEDIC PROBLEMS IN ADULTS

1 Conservative treatment of low back pain may include bed rest and intermittent traction. Explain recommended bed position(s) and type(s) of traction used.

2 Frequently, a patient with low back pain is fitted with a brace or corset for support and immobilization. Explain why this is helpful, and describe correct application of the back brace or corset.

3 The patient with low back pain caused by muscle strain is instructed in correct body mechanics. Why is this an important aspect of his care?

4 A herniated disc may be the cause of back pain. Review anatomy of the spine and explain the meaning of a herniated nucleus pulposus.

5 Explain how care following a laminectomy differs from care following a spinal fusion.

6 After an extended period of bed rest, it is desirable for the patient to wear shoes that provide support for the feet. Explain why this is recommended.

7 Exercises may be prescribed in addition to arch supports for the treatment of fallen arches. Explain.

8 Review criteria that may be used in evaluating a properly fitted shoe.

BONE TUMORS

1 a Differentiate between malignant and benign bone tumors.
   b List several benign tumors.

2 Review symptoms, diagnostic procedures, and treatment as they relate to Ewing's sarcoma, osteosarcoma, multiple myeloma, and metastatic bone lesions.

3 Discuss nursing care of the patient receiving radiotherapy to a metastatic lesion of the spine.

4 Review complications that may occur in the patient with a metastatic bone lesion.

5 List several primary cancerous lesions that frequently metastasize to bone.

6 Review drugs used in the treatment of bone malignancy, including possible toxic reactions.

Unit IV REFERENCES

CONGENITAL DEFORMITIES

1 Altshuler, A., Meyer, J., and Butz, M. K.: Even children can learn to do clean self-catheterization, Am J Nurs 77:97-101, Jan 1977.

2 Banks, H. H., editor: Musculoskeletal disorders I, Pediatr Clin North Am 14:299-532, May 1967.

3 Banks, H. H., editor: Symposium on musculoskeletal disorders II, Pediatr Clin North Am 14:533-722, Aug 1967.

4 Banks, H. H., editor: Symposium on birth defects and the orthopedic surgeon, Orthop Clin North Am 7:261-524, Apr 1976.

5 Beare, J. I.: Osteogenesia imperfecta, Nurs Times 66:453-455, 9 Apr 1970.

6 Bonine, G. N.: The myelodysplastic child; hospital and home care, Am J Nurs 69:541-544, Mar 1969.

7 Braney, M. L.: The child with hydrocephalus, Am J Nurs 73:828-831, May 1973.

8 Bull, M. J., Shucart, W., Haller, J. S., Zimbler, S., Granger, C. V., Labib, K. B., Rodrigues, K., Retik, A. B., and Marks, A.: The pediatrician and myelodysplasia, Orthop Clin North Am 7:475-479, Apr 1976.

9 Childs, V.: Physiotherapy for spina bifida, Physiotherapy 63:218-221, Jul 1977.

9a Chuinard, E. G.: Femoral osteotomy in the treatment of congenital dysplasia of the hip, Orthop Clin North Am 3:157-174, Mar 1972.

10 Cowell, H. R.: Genetic aspects of orthopedic diseases, Am J Nurs 70:763-767, Apr 1970.

11 Curtis, B. H.: The hip in the myelomeningocele child, Clin Orthop 90:11-21, Jan-Feb 1973.

12 D'Arcy, E.: Congenital defects. 1. Some finding concerning the impact on the family, Nurs Times 65:1421-1422, Nov 1969.

13 Dubowski, F. M.: Children with osteogenesis imperfecta, Nurs Clin North Am. 11:709-715, Dec 1976.

14 Ferguson, A. B., Jr.: Orthopedic surgery in infancy and childhood, ed. 4, Baltimore, 1975, The Williams & Wilkins Co.

15 Ford, H. A.: Nursing a spina bifida child in a general hospital, Nurs Times 66:293-295, 5 Mar 1970.

16 Gill, G. G., and White, H. L.: Mechanisms of nerve root compression and irritation in backache, Clin Orthop 5:66-81, 1955.

17 Hasham, A. I., Meyer, J., Altshuler, A., Butz, M., Norderhaug, K., and Uehling, D. T.: Clean intermittent catheterization for meningomyelocele, Wis Med J 74:S117-118, Oct 1975.

18 Hill, M. L., Shurtleff, D. B., Chapman, W. H., and Ansell, J. S.: The myelodysplastic child; bowel and bladder control, Am J Nurs 69:545-550, Mar 1969.

19 Hilt, N. E., and Schmitt, E. W., Jr.: Pediatric orthopedic nursing, St. Louis, 1975, The C. V. Mosby Co.

19a Howorth, B.: Development of present knowledge of congenital displacement of the hip, Clin Orthop 125:68-87, Jun 1977.

20 Kapke, K. A.: Spina bifida: mother-child relationship, Nurs Forum 9(3):310-320, 1970.

21 King, J. D., and Bobechko, W. P.: Osteogenesis imperfecta; an orthopaedic description and surgical review, J Bone Joint Surg [Br] 53:72-89, Feb 1971.

22 Knapp, M. E.: Physical medicine and rehabilitation in pediatrics. Part I. Postgrad Med 46:173-176, Dec 1969.

23 Knapp, M. E.: Physical medicine and rehabilitation in pediatrics. Part II. Postgrad Med 47:219-224, Jan 1970.

24 Knight, K.: Congenital dysplasia of the hip, ONA J 4:165-167, Jun 1977.

25 Lavoie, D., Liermann, C. J., Fletcher, A. B., and Corbett, D.: Spina bifida: immediate concerns—long-term goals, Nursing (Jenkintown) 3:42-47, Oct 1973.

26 Littlewood, J. M.: Spina bifida, Nurs Times 66:5-8, 1 Jan 1970.

27 Lloyd-Roberts, G. C.: Orthopaedics in infancy and childhood, London, 1971, Butterworth & Co. (Publishers), Ltd.

28 Lowry, M. F.: Congenital dislocation of the hip, Nurs Times 66:72-74, 15 Jan 1970.

29 Madden, B.: Orthopaedic aspects of spina bifida, Physiotherapy 63:186-190, Jun 1977.

29a Marlow, D. R.: Textbook of pediatric nursing, ed. 4, Philadelphia, 1973, W. B. Saunders Co.

30 Menelaus, M. B.: The orthopaedic management of spina bifida cystica, Edinburgh, 1971, E. & S. Livingstone, Ltd.

31 Murray, B. S., Elmore, J., and Sawyer, J. R.: The patient has an ileal conduit, Am J Nurs 71:1560-1565, Aug 1971.

32 Passo, S. D.: Positioning infants with myelomeningocele, Am J Nurs 74:1658-1660, Sep 1974.

33 Ponseti, I. V., and Campos, J.: Observations on pathogenesis and treatment of congenital clubfoot, Clin Orthop 84:50-60, May 1972.

34 Ponseti, I. V.: Diagnosis and treatment of congenital dislocation of the hip in the infant, J Lancet 81:298-301, Jul 1961.

35 Ramsey, P. L.: Congenital hip dislocation, Postgrad Med J 60:114-120, Oct 1976.

36 Salter, R. B.: Role of innominate osteotomy in the treatment of congenital dislocation and subluxation of the hip in the older child, J Bone Joint Surg [Am] 48:1413-1439, Oct 1966.

37 Smith, C.: Talipes. 1. Anatomy of the foot, Nurs Times 71:138-139, 23 Jan 1975.

38 Smith, C.: Talipes. 2. Clinical features of talipes equinovarus, Nurs Times 71:176-177, 30 Jan 1975.

39 Smith, C.: Talipes. 3. Nursing care of a
    child wearing a splint, Nurs Times **71**:222-
    223, 6 Feb 1975.
40 Smith, C.: Talipes. 4. Further types of talipes
    deformity, Nurs Times **71**:270, 13 Feb 1975.
41 Spickler, L.: Osteogenesis imperfecta, ONA
    J **3**:163-165, May 1976.
42 Steele, S.: Nursing care of the child with
    long-term illness, New York, 1971, Appleton-
    Century-Crofts.
43 Tachdjian, M. O.: Diagnosis and treatment
    of congenital deformities of the musculo-
    skeletal system in the newborn and the in-
    fant, Pediatr Clin North Am **14**:307-357,
    May 1967.
44 Tachdjian, M. O.: Pediatric orthopedics,
    Philadephia, 1972, W. B. Saunders Co.
45 Taylor, J. F., Oyemade, G. A., Shaw, E.,
    Ankers, P., Davies, C., and Jenkins, A.: Pri-
    mary treatment of rigid congenital talipes
    equino-varus, Physiotherapy **62**:89-93, Mar
    1976.
46 Twomey, M. R.: Arthrogryposis multiplex
    congenita, Nurs Times **72**:1117-1119, 22 Jul
    1976.
47 Twomey, M. R.: Nursing care study: osteo-
    genesis imperfecta, Nurs Times **73**:123-126,
    27 Jan 1977.
48 Wiley, L., editor: Spina bifida: immediate
    concerns—long-term goals, Nursing (Jenkin-
    town) **3**:42-47, Oct. 1973.
49 Zachary, R. B.: The improving prognosis in
    spina bifida, Clin Pediatr **11**:11-14, Jan
    1972.
50 Zimbler, S.: Orthopedic evaluation and treat-
    ment of the myelodysplasia patient, Orthop
    Clin North Am **7**:483-487, Apr 1976.
51 Zimbler, S.: Practical considerations in the
    early treatment of congenital talipes equino-
    varus, Orthop Clin North Am **3**:251-259,
    Mar 1972.

DEVELOPMENTAL AFFECTIONS

52 Anderson, B. and D'Ambra, B.: The ado-
    lescent patient with scoliosis: a nursing care
    standard, Nurs Clin North Am **11**:699-708,
    Dec 1976.
53 Andriacchi, T. P., Schultz, A. B., Belytschko,
    Belytschko, T. B., and DeWald, R. L.: Mil-
    waukee brace correction of idiopathic scolio-
    sis, J Bone Joint Surg [Am] **58**:806-815,
    Sep 1976.
54 Baker, E. A., and Zangger, B.: School screen-
    ing for idiopathic scoliosis, Am J Nurs **70**:
    766-767, Apr 1970.
55 Bame, K. B.: Halo traction, Am J Nurs **69**:
    1933-1937, Sep 1969.
56 Blount, W. P.: The nonoperative manage-
    ment of scoliosis, ONA J **3**:19-21, Jan 1976.
57 Blount, W. P.: Use of the Milwaukee brace,
    Orthop Clin North Am **3**:3-16, Mar 1972.
58 Blount, W. P., and Bolinske, J.: Physical
    therapy in the nonoperative treatment of
    scoliosis, Phys Ther **47**:919-925, Oct 1967.
59 Blount, W. P., and Moe, J. H.: The Mil-
    waukee brace, Baltimore 1973, The Williams
    & Wilkins Co.

60 Brooks, H.: Cortel or red rope traction, ONA
    J **2**:173-174, Jul 1975.
61 Cantrell, D.: Scoliosis, RN **39**:55-56, Nov
    1976.
62 Cocchiarella, A., Challenor, Y., and Katz,
    J. F.: Orthosis for use in Legg-Calve-Perthes'
    disease, Arch Phys Med Rehabil **53**:286-288,
    Jun 1972.
63 Cordell, L. D.: Slipped capital femoral
    epiphysis: long-term results, Postgrad Med
    60:135-141, Oct 1976.
64 Dunn, B. H.: Scoliosis detection, ONA J
    2:282-283, Nov 1975.
65 Edmonson, A. S.: Postural deformities, In
    Crenshaw, A. H., editor: Campbell's Opera-
    tive orthopaedics, ed. 5, St. Louis, 1971,
    The C. V. Mosby Co.
66 Erwin, W. D., Dickson, J. H., and Harring-
    ton, P. R.: The postoperative management
    of scoliosis patients treated with Harrington
    instrumentation and fusion, J Bone Joint
    Surg [Am] **58**:479-482, Jun 1976.
67 Ferguson, A. B., Jr.: Orthopaedic surgery
    in infancy and childhood, ed. 4, Baltimore,
    1975, The Williams & Wilkins Co.
68 Goldstein, L. A.: The surgical management
    of scoliosis, Clin Orthop **77**:32-56, Jun 1971.
69 Harrington, P. R.: Technical details in rela-
    tion to the successful use of instrumenta-
    tion in scoliosis, Orthop Clin North Am **3**:49-
    67, Mar 1972.
70 Harrington, P. R.: The etiology of idiopathic
    scoliosis, Clin Orthop **126**:17-25, Jul-Aug
    1977.
71 James, J. I.: Infantile idiopathic scoliosis,
    Clin Orthop **77**:57-72, Jun 1971.
72 Kamhi, E.: Legg-Calvé-Perthes disease, Post-
    grad Med **60**:125-130, Oct 1976.
73 Keim, H.: Scoliosis, Clin Symp **24**:2-32,
    Feb 1972.
74 Keiser, R. P.: Treatment of scoliosis, Nurs
    Clin North Am **2**:409-418, Sep 1967.
75 Kelly, P. J.: Osteomyelitis in the adult,
    Orthop Clin North Am **6**:983-989, Oct 1975.
76 Killian, M.: Halo apparatus, ONA J **3**:246-
    249, Aug 1976.
77 La Breche, B. G., Levangie, P. K., and
    Sharby, N. H.: Cotrel traction: a new ap-
    proach to the preoperative management of
    idiopathic scoliosis, Phys Ther **54**:837-842,
    Aug 1974.
78 Lonstein, J.: Screening for spinal deformities
    in Minnesota schools, Clin Orthop **126**:33-
    42, Jul-Aug 1977.
78a Love-Migmogna, S.: Scoliosis, Nursing
    (Jenkintown) **7**:50-55, May 1977.
79 Maczak, S.: Harrington rod insertion: the
    immediate postoperative period, ONA J **4**:
    229-230, Sep 1977.
79a Matzka, L.: Nursing care—scoliosis surgery,
    ONA J **2**:251-255, Oct 1975.
80 Mir, S. R., Cole, J. R., Lardone, J., and
    Levine, D. B.: Early ambulation following
    spinal fusion and Harrington instrumentation
    in idiopathic scoliosis, Clin Orthop **110**:54-
    62, Jul-Aug 1975.
81 Moe, J. H.: Methods of correction and sur-

gical techniques in scoliosis, Orthop Clin North Am **3**:17-48, Mar 1972.

82 Moe, J. H.: The Milwaukee brace in the treatment of scoliosis, Clin Orthop **77**:18-31, Jun 1971.

83 Morton, J., and Malins, P.: The correction of spinal deformities by halo-pelvic traction, Physiotherapy **57**:576-581, Dec 1971.

84 Nichol, C.: Legg-Perthes disease, Can Nurse **72**:31, 34-36, Jun 76.

85 O'Connor, B. J.: Scoliosis: classification and diagnosis, ONA J **3**:84-88, Mar 1976.

86 Pappas, A. M.: The osteochondroses, Pediatr Clin North Am **14**:549-570, Aug 1967.

87 Patterson, T. D.: Scoliosis, RN **39**:58-60, 65-69, 74, 76, 80, Nov 1976.

88 Perry, J.: The halo in spinal abnormalities: practical factors and avoidance of complications, Orthop Clin North Am **3**:69-80, Mar 1972.

89 Petrie, J. G., and Bitenc, I.: The abduction weight-bearing treatment in Legg-Perthes' disease, J Bone Joint Surg [Br] **53**:54-62, Feb 1971.

89a Ponseti, I., Pedrini, V., Wynne-Davies, R., and Beaupere-Duval, G.: Pathogenesis of scoliosis, Clin Orthop **120**:268-280, Oct 1976.

90 Raney, R. B., Sr., and Brashear, R. H., Jr.: Shands' Handbook of orthopaedic surgery, ed. 9, St. Louis, 1978, The C. V. Mosby Co.

91 Raynolds, N.: Teaching parents home care after surgery for scoliosis, Am J Nurs **74**:1090-1092, Jun 1974.

92 Risser, J. C.: Scoliois: past and present, J Bone Joint Surg [Am] **46**:167-199, Jan 1964.

93 Roberts, J. M.: New developments in orthopedic surgery, Nurs Clin North Am **2**:383-390, Sep 1967.

94 Roberts, J. M.: Scoliosis, the clinical overview, RN **39**:57-58, Nov 1976.

95 Segil, C.: Current concepts in the management of scoliosis, Nurs Clin North Am **11**:691-698, Dec 1976.

96 Sells, C. J., and May, E. A.: Scoliosis screening in public schols, Am J Nurs **74**:60-62, Jan 1974.

97 Trott, A. W.: Orthopedic problems of the adolescent, Postgrad Med **49**:83-87, Mar 1971.

98 Twomey, M. R.: Halo pelvic traction; a new method of correcting deformities of the spine, Nurs Times **66**:1225-1228, Sep 1970.

99 Wiley, L., editor: Scoliosis: affectionate yet firm postoperative nursing care, Nursing (Jenkintown) **4**:49-55, Aug 1974.

100 Winter, R. .: How to find a spinal deformity —look for it, Mod Med **43**:38-43, 1 May 1975.

NEUROMUSCULAR DISORDERS
Cerebral palsy

101 Banks, H. H., and Panagakos, P.: The role of the orthopedic surgeon in cerebral palsy, Pediatr Clin North Am **14**:495-515, May 1967.

102 Blockley, J., and Miller, G.: Feeding techniques with cerebral-palsied children, Physiotherapy **57**:300-308, Jul 1971.

103 Bobath, B.: Motor development, its effect on general development, and application to the treatment of cerebral palsy, Physiotherapy **57**:526-532, 10 Nov 1971.

104 Bobath, K.: The normal postural reflex mechanism and its deviation in children with cerebral palsy, Physiotherapy **57**:515-525, 10 Nov 1971.

105 Cailliet, R.: Bracing for spasticity. In Licht, S. H., and Kamenetz, H. L., editors: Orthotics etcetera, New Haven, 1966, Elizabeth Licht, Publisher.

106 Cotton, E.: Integration of treatment and education in cerebral palsy, Physiotherapy **56**:143-147, Apr 1970.

106a Dubowitz, U.: Analysis of neuromuscular disease, Physiotherapy **63**:38-45, Feb 1977.

107 Ferguson, A., Jr.: Orthopaedic surgery in infancy and childhood, ed. 4, Baltimore, 1975, The Williams & Wilkins Co.

108 Haynes, U. H.: Nursing approaches in cerebral dysfunction, Am J Nurs **68**:2170-2176, Oct 1968.

109 Keats, S.: Cerebral palsy, Springfield, Ill., 1970, Charles C Thomas, Publisher.

110 Keats, S.: Operative orthopedics in cerebral palsy, Springfield, Ill., 1970, Charles C Thomas, Publisher.

111 Knapp, M. E.: Cerebral palsy I, Postgrad Med **47**:229-232, Feb 1970.

112 Knapp, M. E.: Cerebral palsy II, Postgrad Med **47**:247-252, Mar 1970.

113 Kolderie, M. L.: Behavior modification in the treatment of children with cerebral palsy, Phys Ther **51**:1083-1090, Oct 1971.

114 Pothier, P. C.: Therapeutic handling of the severely handicapped child, Am J Nurs **71**:321-324, Feb 1971.

115 Raney, R. B., Sr., and Brashear, H. R., Jr.: Shand's Handbook of orthopaedic surgery, ed. 9, St. Louis, 1978, The C. V. Mosby Co.

Muscular dystrophy

116 Carini, E., and Owens, G.: Neurological and neurosurgical nursing, ed. 6, St. Louis, 1974, The C. V. Mosby Co.

117 Cohen, J.: Laboratory diagnostic measures in generalized muscular disease, Pediatr Clin North Am **14**:461-477, May 1967.

118 Gardner-Medwin, D.: Management of muscular dystrophy, Physiotherapy **63**:46-51, Feb 1977.

119 Johnson, E. W., and Kennedy, J. H.: Comprehensive management of Duchenne muscular dystrophy, Arch Phys Med Rehabil **52**:110-114, Mar 1971.

120 McKeran, R. O.: The muscular dystrophies, Nurs Times **72**:1515-1518, 30 Sept 1976.

121 Miller, J.: Management of muscular dystrophy, J Bone Joint Surg [Am] **49**:1205-1211, Sep 1967.

122 Muscular Dystrophy Associations of America, Inc.: Patient and community services program, New York, 1971.

123 Ogg, E.: Milestones in muscle disease re-

search, New York, 1971, Muscular Dystrophy Associations of America, Inc.

124 Siegel, I. M.: Pathomechanics of stance in Duchenne muscular dystrophy, Arch Phys Med Rehabil 53:403-406, Sep 1972.

125 Spencer, G. E., Jr.: Orthopaedic care of progressive muscular dystrophy, J Bone Joint Surg [Am] 49:1201-1204, Sep 1967.

126 Wershow, H. J.: Muscular dystrophy: a positive approach to care, Nurs Outlook 14:49-53, Jan 1966.

127 Zundell, W. S., and Tyler, F. H.: The muscular dystrophies, New Eng J Med 273:537-543, 596-601, 2 Sep, 9 Sep 1965.

Poliomyelitis

128 Gunn, A. D. G.: Poliomyelitis protection, Nurs Times 73:58, 13 Jan 1977.

129 Huckstep, R. L.: Poliomyelitis in Uganda, Physiotherapy 56:347-353, Aug 1970.

130 Peach, A. M.: Poliomyelitis—a conquered fear? Nurs Times 66:107-109, 22 Jan 1970.

131 Raney, R. B., Sr., and Brashear, H. R., Jr.: Shand's Handbook of orthopaedic surgery, ed. 9, St. Louis, 1978, The C. V. Mosby Co.

132 Top, F. H., Sr., and Wehrle, P. F., editor: Communicable and infectious diseases, ed. 7, St. Louis, 1972, The C. V. Mosby Co.

Brachial palsy in newborn infants

133 Adler, J. B., and Patterson, R. L., Jr.: Erb's palsy, J Bone Joint Surg [Am] 49:1052-1064, Sep 1967.

134 Bresnan, M. J.: Neurologic birth injuries. 1, Postgrad Med 49:199-205, Mar 1971.

135 Bresnan, M. J.: Neurologic birth injuries. 2, Postgrad Med 49:202-206, Apr 1971.

ARTHRITIS

136 Abruzzo, J. L.: Rheumatoid arthritis: reflections on etiology and pathogenesis, Arch Phys Med Rehabil 52:30-38, Jan 1971.

137 Baden, A. M.: Ambulatory nursing: children with arthritis: some everyday help, Nursing (Jenkintown) 3:22-24, Dec 1973.

138 Ball, B., moderator: Helping patients adjust to rheumatoid arthritis, Nursing (Jenkintown) 2:11-17, Oct 1972.

139 Beeson, P. B., and McDermott, W., editors: Cecil-Loeb Textbook of medicine, ed. 13, Philadelphia, 1971, W. B. Saunders Co.

140 Bergersen, B. S.: Pharmacology in nursing, ed. 13, St. Louis, 1976, The C. V. Mosby Co.

141 Bowden, S. A.: New surgery for arthritic hands, Nursing (Jenkintown) 6:46-48, Aug 1976.

142 Brassell, M. P., Schaal, F. M., Rossky, E. G., and Spergel, P.: Helping patients adjust to rheumatoid arthritis, Nursing (Jenkintown) 2:11-17, Oct 1972.

143 Bryan, R. S., guest editor: Symposium on rheumatoid arthritis, Orthop Clin North Am 2:600-771, Oct 1971.

144 Calabro, J. J., Katz, R. M., and Maltz, B. A.: A critical reappraisal of juvenile rheumatoid arthritis, Clin Orthop 74:101-119, Jan-Feb 1971.

145 Clark, H.: Osteoarthritis: an interesting case?, Nurs Clin North Am 11:199-206, Mar 1976.

146 Driscoll, P. W.: Rheumatoid arthritis: understanding it more fully, Nursing (Jenkintown) 5:26-32, Dec 1975.

147 Ehrlich, G. E.: Arthritis management, Nurs Digest 4:24-26, Winter 1976.

148 Grahame, R.: Rheumatoid disease. 1. Clinical aspects, Nurs Times 67:664-667, 3 Jun 1971.

149 Grahame, R.: Rheumatoid disease. 2. Caring for patients, Nurs Times 67:701-704, 10 Jun 1971.

150 Harris, R.: Plaster splints for rheumatoid arthritis. In Licht, S. H., and Kamenetz, H. L., editors: Orthotics etcetera, New Haven, 1966, Elizabeth Licht, Publisher.

151 Henry, J. B., and Pinals, R. S.: Evaluation of tests for rheumatoid factor, Postgrad Med 48:49-52, Dec 1970.

152 Hoaglund, F. T.: Osteoarthritis, Orthop Clin North Am 2:3-18, Mar 1971.

153 Lockie, L. M.: Current evaluation of drugs for treating arthritis, Postgrad Med 49:100-104, Apr 1971.

154 Loxley, A. K.: The emotional toll of crippling deformity, Am J Nurs 72:1839-1840, Oct 1972.

155 McEwen, C.: Synovectomy and the rehabilitation of the patient with rheumatoid arthritis (editorial), J Bone Joint Surg [Am] 53:621-623, Jun 1971.

156 Management of arthritis, Postgrad Med 51: 20-114, May 1972.

156a Marmor, L.: Arthritis surgery, Philadelphia, 1976, Lea & Febiger.

157 Millender, L. H., and Sledge, C. B., editors: Symposium on rheumatoid arthritis, Orthop Clin North Am 6:603-912, Jul 1975.

158 O'Dell, A. J.: Hot packs for morning joint stiffness, Am J Nurs 75:986-987, Jun 1975.

159 Pendleton, T., and Grossman, B. J.: Rehabilitating children with inflammatory joint disease, Am J Nurs 74:2223-2226, Dec 1974.

160 Pigg, J.: Ambulatory nursing: 50 helpful hints for active arthritis patients, Nursing (Jenkintown) 4:39-41, Jul 1974.

161 Pitorak, E. F.: Rheumatoid arthritis: living with it more comfortably, Nursing (Jenkintown) 5:33-35, Dec 1975.

162 Potter, T. A., and Nalebuff, E. A., editors: Symposium on the surgical management of rheumatoid arthritis, Surg Clin North Am 49:731-952, Aug 1969.

163 Rheumatoid arthritis. Part I, Physiotherapy 56:382-408, Sep 1970.

164 Rheumatoid arthritis. Part II, Physiotherapy 56:430-458, Oct 1970.

165 Roaf, R., and Hodkinson, L. J.: Textbook of orthopaedic nursing, ed. 2, Oxford, 1975, Blackwell Scientific Publications, Ltd.

166 Robinson, W. D.: Rheumatoid arthritis. In Beeson, P. D., and McDermott, W., editors: Cecil-Loeb Textbook of medicine, ed. 13, Philadelphia, 1971, W. B. Saunders Co.

167 Rodman, G.: Gout and other crystalline

forms of arthritis, Postgrad Med **58**:6-14, Oct 1975.

168 Salter, R. B.: Textbook of disorders and injuries of the musculoskeletal system: an introduction to orthopaedics, rheumatology, metabolic bone disease, rehabilitation and fracture, Baltimore, 1970, The Williams & Wilkins Co.

169 Shafer, K. N., Sawyer, J. R., McCluskey, A. M., Beck, E. L., and Phipps, W. J.: Medical-surgical nursing, ed. 6, St. Louis, 1975, The C. V. Mosby Co.

170 Simmons, E. H., and Brown, M. E.: Surgery for kyphosis in ankylosing spondylitis, Can Nurse **68**:24-29, May 1972.

171 Smiley, D.: Rheumatoid arthritis, Postgrad Med **58**:17-24, Oct 1975.

172 Stillman, J. S.: Osteoarthritis, Postgrad Med **58**:37-43, Oct 1975.

173 Suppes, F. T., Moskowitz, R. W., Lockie, L. M., and Hoolander, J. L.: Arthritis, Postgrad Med **47**:160-167, Mar 1970.

INFECTION

Osteomyelitis/Tuberculosis of bone and joints

174 Bergersen, B. S.: Pharmacology in nursing, ed. 13, St. Louis, 1976, The C. V. Mosby Co.

175 Boland, A. L., Jr.: Acute hematogenous osteomyelitis, Orthop Clin North Am **3**:225-239, Mar 1972.

176 Ferguson, A.: Orthopedic surgery in infancy and childhood, ed. 4, Baltimore, 1975, The Williams & Wilkins Co.

176a Hodgson, A., and Stock, F.: Anterior spine fusion for the treatment of tuberculosis of the spine, J Bone Joint Surg [Am] **42**:295-309, Mar 1960.

177 Lawyer, R. B., Jr., and Eyring, E. J.: Intermittent closed suction-irrigation treatment of osteomyelitis, Clin Orthop **88**:80-85, Oct 1972.

178 Medoff, G.: Current concepts in the treatment of osteomyelitis, Postgrad Med **58**:157-161, Sep 1975.

179 Miller, J. E., editor: Symposium: bone infections, Clin Orthop **96**:2-344, Oct 1973.

180 Raney, R. B., Sr., and Brashear, H. R., Jr.: Shand's Handbook of orthopaedic surgery, ed. 9, St. Louis, 1978, The C. V. Mosby Co.

181 Rhodes, K. H.: Antibiotic management of acute osteomyelitis and septic arthritis in children, Orthop Clin North Am **6**:915-921, Oct 1975.

182 Stetson, J. W., DePonte, R. J., and Southwick, W. O.: Acute septic arthritis of the hip in children, Clin Orthop **56**:105-116, Jan-Feb 1968.

183 Smith, C.: Osteomyelitis, Nurs Times **70**:862-865, 6 Jun 1974.

184 Taylor, J. F.: Osteomyelitis. 1. The acute form, Nurs Times **72**:486-488, 1 Apr 1976.

185 Taylor, J. F.: Osteomyelitis. 2. The chronic form, Nurs Times **72**:535-537, 8 Apr 1976.

186 Top, F. H., Sr., and Wehrle, P. F., editors: Communicable and infectious diseases, ed. 7, St. Louis, 1972, The C. V. Mosby Co.

187 Williams, S. R.: Nutrition and diet therapy, ed. 3, St. Louis, 1977, The C. V. Mosby Co.

PAINFUL ORTHOPEDIC PROBLEMS IN ADULTS

188 Adams, J. P.: Foot problems in adults, Postgrad Med **42**:1-6, Jul 1967.

189 Bateman, J. E., editor: Symposium on pitfalls in foot surgery, Orthop Clin North Am **7**:751-1048, Oct 1976.

190 Cooper, S.: Low back pain caused by rupturing of the nucleus pulposus, ONA J **2**:224-230, Sep 1975.

191 Cooper, S.: A patient teaching plan for conservative treatment of low back pain. Part I. Development, ONA J **3**:301-306, Oct 1976.

192 Gill, G. G., Jr., and White, H. L.: Mechanisms of nerve root compression and irritation in backache, Clin Orthop **5**:66-81, 1955.

193 Harrold, A. J.: Laminectomy for disc disorders, Nurs Times **67**:406-408, 8 Apr 1971.

194 Harmon, V.: Taking the pain out of back procedures, Nursing (Jenkintown) **4**:91-92, Sep 1974.

195 Hickling, J.: Spinal traction technique, Physiotherapy **58**:58-63, 10 Feb 1972.

196 Hogan, L., and Beland, I.: Cervical spine syndrome, Am J Nurs **76**:1104-1107, Jul 1976.

197 Lucas, D.: Spinal bracing. In Licht, S., and Kamenetz, H. L., editors: Orthotics etcetera, New Haven, 1966, Elizabeth Licht, Publisher.

198 Matthews, J. A.: The effects of spinal traction, Physiotherapy **58**:64-66, Feb 1972.

199 Mitchell, W. J.: Orthopedics. In Conn, H., et al., editors: Family practice, Philadelphia, 1973, W. B. Saunders Co.

200 Mooney, V., Cairns, D., and Robertson, J.: The psychological evaluation and treatment of the chronic back pain patient—a new approach, Part I, ONA J **2**:163-165, Jul 1975.

201 Musick, D. T., and MacKenzie, M.: Nursing care of the patient with a laminectomy, Nurs Clin North Am **2**:437-445, Sep 1967.

202 Parry, W., and Yates, D. A. H.: Minor back injuries, Nurs Times **72**:1468-1471, 23 Sep 1976.

203 Piercey M. L.: Assessment of low back pain, Nurse Pract **1**:18-21, Mar-Apr 1976.

204 Raney, R. B., Sr., and Brashear, H. R., Jr.: Shand's Handbook of orthopaedic surgery, ed. 9, St. Louis, 1978, The C. V. Mosby Co.

205 Robb, S., Bunion surgery, Am J Nurs **74**:2181-2184, Dec 1974.

206 Rothman, R. H., guest editor: Symposium on disease of the intervertebral disc. Orthop Clin North Am **2**:307-592, 1971.

207 Stauffer, R. N., Ivins, J. C., and Miller, R. H.: The lumbar disk syndrome and its operative treatment, Postgrad Med **49**:87-93, Feb 1971.

208 Wells, R.: Lumbar laminectomy and/or fusions, ONA J **1**:33-36, Sep 1974.

209 Wiley, L., editor: Rupture of the cervical disk, Nursing (Jenkintown) **3**:33-39, Apr 1973.

210 Williams, P. C.: Low back and neck pain, Springfield, Ill., 1974, Charles C Thomas, Publisher.

211 Yates, D. A.: Indications and contra-indica-

      tions for spinal traction, Physiotherapy **58:** 55-57, 10 Feb 1972.
212 Zamosky, I., and Licht, S.: Shoes and their modifications. In Licht, S., and Kamenetz, H. L., editors: Orthotics etcetera, New Haven, 1966, Elizabeth Licht, Publisher.

BONE TUMORS

213 Bergersen, B. S.: Pharmacology in nursing, ed. 13, St. Louis, 1976, The C. V. Mosby Co.
214 Bochow, A. J.: Cancer immunotherapy: what promise does it hold? Nursing (Jenkintown) **6:**50-56, Oct 1976.
215 Bouchard, R., and Owens, N. F.: Nursing care of the cancer patient, ed. 3, St. Louis, 1976, The C. V. Mosby Co.
216 Elliott, C.: Radiation therapy: how can you help?, Nursing (Jenkintown) **6:**34-41, Sep 1976.
217 Ferguson, A.: Orthopaedic surgery in infancy and childhood, ed. 4, Baltimore, 1975, The Williams & Wilkins Co.
218 Hoffman, E.: "Don't give up on me," Am J Nurs **71:**60-62, Jan 1971.
219 Jacobs, P.: Tumours of bone, Nurs Times **68:**1572-1575, 14 Dec 1972.
220 Kübler-Ross, E.: On death and dying, New York, 1969, Macmillan Publishing Co., Inc.
221 Lichtensten, L.: Bone tumors, ed. 5, St. Louis, 1977, The C. V. Mosby Co.
222 Livingston, B. M., and Krakoff, I. H.: L-asparaginase; a new type of anticancer drug, Am J Nurs **70:**1910-1915, Sep 1970.
223 McCorkle, R.: The advanced cancer patient: how he will live and die, Nursing (Jenkintown) **6:**46-49, Oct 1976.

224 Marino, L. B.: Cancer patients: your special role, Nursing (Jenkintown) **6:**26-29, Sep 1976.
225 Marino, E. B., and LeBlanc, D. H.: Cancer chemotherapy, Nursing (Jenkintown) **5:**22-33, Nov 1975.
226 Peterson, B. H., and Kellogg, C. J., editors: Current practice in oncologic nursing, St. Louis, 1976, The C. V. Mosby Co.
227 Raney, R. B., Sr., and Brashear, H. R., Jr.: Shand's Handbook of orthopaedic surgery, ed. 9, St. Louis, 1978, The C. V. Mosby Co.
228 Rickel, L.: Emotional support for the multiple myeloma patients, Nursing (Jenkintown) **6:**76-80, Apr 1976.
229 Ross, E. K.: What is it like to be dying? Am J Nurs **71:**54-60, Jan 1971.
230 Schulz, R., and Aderman, D.: Clinical research and the stages of dying, Nurs Digest **4:**47-48, Jan-Feb 1976.
231 Schumann, D., and Patterson, P.: Multiple myeloma, Am J Nurs **75:**78-81, Jan 1975.
232 Shafer, K. N., Sawyer, J. R., McCluskey, A. M., Beck, E. L., and Phipps, W. J.: Medical-surgical nursing, ed. 6, St. Louis, 1975, The C. V. Mosby Co.
233 Sklaroff, D. M., and Charkes, N. D.: Diagnosis of bone metastasis by photoscanning with strontium 85, JAMA **188:**1-4, 6 Apr 1964.
234 Staudt, A. R.: Femur replacement, Am J Nurs **75:**1346-1348, Aug 1975.
235 Stuart, E.: Amputation for osteogenic sarcoma, Nurs Times **68:**1453-1454, 16 Nov 1972.

19 The orthopedic surgical patient

Nurses will remember from their surgical nursing experience that hemorrhage, wound infection, and pain are the three great obstacles to success in surgery. In orthopedic surgery, impairment to circulation caused by mechanical obstruction must be added to these. Nurses should be alert for symptoms that indicate the presence of any of these conditions.

General considerations

A great number of reconstructive operations on bones are performed on people past middle age. Steindler stated that when the constitutional background of the patient is abnormal, it will have a definite primary influence upon the surgical risk. It is for this reason that laboratory tests are done on a large scale. In addition to the routine laboratory tests done on all surgical patients, such as blood count, hemoglobin estimation, bleeding and clotting time, and urinalysis, the orthopedic surgeon often requests determinations of serum calcium, phosphorus, and phosphatase, as well as of the blood sedimentation rate. Renal function tests also may be ordered.

Nurses should be able to read laboratory sheets with some degree of facility in order to understand the condition of their patients more satisfactorily. The nurse's understanding preoperatively of the risk facing the individual patient will enable her to assist in his recovery more confidently. A high sedimentation rate is not a good prognostic sign. Excessively high or low blood pressure may lower the patient's vital capacity. Specific gravity of less than normal in the urine adds to the gravity of the outcome. Blood urea nitrogen of over 35 mg/100 ml of blood indicates a considerable degree of kidney damage. It is a well-known fact that postoperative mortality in patients with nephritis complicated by hypertension is high. Any patient who has been confined to bed over an extended period is not considered a good surgical risk.

Dehydration, present or threatened, is an outstanding danger that should be recognized. During and after surgery, parenteral fluids and, in some instances, solutions containing electrolytes are given to replace fluid loss and to provide for normal intake needs. Blood loss is carefully estimated and, if sufficient, is replaced with whole blood, plasma, or one of the plasma volume expanders. Careful checking by the nurse to make certain that the patient receives the correct type and amount of fluid is essential. Disastrous results can occur if fluids are given too rapidly or if too much of an electrolyte substance is given. This necessitates accurate recording of intake and output.

The mental condition of the patient is a critical factor. This is particularly true with the spastic child. When possible, the patient with cerebral palsy should be allowed to obtain some mental equilibrium before surgery is performed. Some surgeons scoff at preoperative psychic depression. Others feel quite definitely that such depression adds to the gravity of a postoperative prognosis, particularly when premonition of death exists. Such mental states should be reported to the physician by the nurse as accurately as a definite physical symptom.

Excessive obesity causes the surgeon concern because of the impairment in respiration that sometimes accompanies it. Wound infection and fat embolism are possibilities to be feared, especially in obese patients. A marked degree of weight loss is not considered a good indication, because a loss of glycogen reserve is likely to exist. After surgery, persistence of nausea and vomiting will increase the gravity of such a patient's condition extremely because acidosis may occur very quickly.

Inhalation anesthesia usually is preferred by orthopedists, largely because it is a controllable anesthesia; i.e., it can be discontinued at once if the patient's condition seems to warrant it. Spinal anesthesia is sometimes used in older persons or in those with hypertension. Danger signals in this type of anesthesia are rapid fall of blood pressure and diminution of the respiratory rate.

Preoperative preparation of patient

Preoperatively, a general physical examination will be performed by the physician. Base line information pertaining to the health status of the patient makes it possible to compare preoperative and postoperative physical findings and laboratory reports. This is helpful in determining the patient's postoperative needs.

All oral intake is omitted after midnight for patients receiving a general anesthesia. The use of cathartics prior to surgery is seldom recommended, and enemas may or may not be given the evening before surgery. Sedatives are especially advisable for the nervous individual and may be ordered to ensure the patient a restful night. Preoperative medications usually are given two or three hours prior to the time of surgery. The nurse also must keep in mind that special medication orders may be necessary for the surgical patient who is diabetic, the individual who routinely takes an anticonvulsive drug or a cardiovascular medication, and for the individual receiving steroid therapy. In most instances, it is essential that these drugs not be omitted the morning of surgery.

Attention to the physical, laboratory, and preoperative routine should not deter the nurse from offering the psychologic support that must accompany much of the preparation of any patient for surgery. Most orthopedic conditions are not acute. The patient has perhaps anticipated the operation for some time. Probably, if he is an adult, he has debated over a long period of time the advisability of having the procedure performed. The emotions he feels are a mixture of hope and fear—hope, perhaps, that he will regain the use of a long-paralyzed limb and fear that the surgery and long convalescence may be of no avail. It is an important moment in his life. The nurse should recognize this and realize that the difference between the operative procedure for the orthopedic patient and that done for the ordinary surgical patient lies in his hope that some lost function of his body will be restored. This hope often overrides the natural fear. Preoperatively, the nurse needs to establish rapport with the patient and to listen to him in order to gain some knowledge of his background and his hopes for improvement and recovery. Preoperative teaching may be done at this time. The patient should have knowledge of what to expect following surgery—the type of apparatus to be used (e.g., cast, traction, etc.), activity limitations, the significance of position changes, deep-breathing exercises, etc., and, perhaps most important of all, the assurance that the care necessary to minimize pain will be provided. Also, this is a good time to explain to the patient his own part in his recovery and the necessity for patience and cooperation to ensure a successful outcome.

Preparation of operative site

Because the consequences of infection in bone surgery are so grave and may lead to crippling through stiffness of the joints or chronically infected bone, the preparation of the operative site must be carefully and conscientiously executed. The exact procedure used will vary from clinic to clinic. However, there has been a tendency to omit the long forty-eight-hour or seventy-two-hour sterile orthopedic preparation. Instead, the orthopedic patient may be given a preparation similar to that given the general surgical patient.

The antiseptic solutions used vary in different clinics. The method of preparation, however, is much the same. It is now well recognized that mild soap and water are probably the best agents available not only

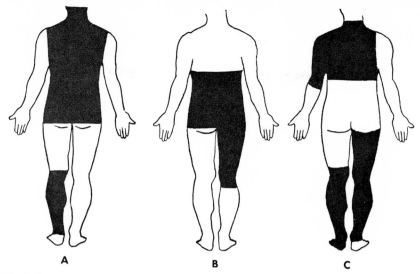

Fig. 355 A, Sites commonly prepared for surgery of the spine with autogenous graft from the left tibia. **B,** Site prepared for bone operation on the hip. **C,** Sites prepared for operations on the shoulder, ankle, and knee.

for removing dirt and grease from the skin, but also for eliminating bacteria safely and effectively. Some surgeons believe that no other antiseptic is necessary for cleansing the skin.

After the preliminary cleansing of the skin, shaving is the next step in the preparation of the operative site. The area to be shaved is usually designated by the physician in the preoperative orders, but the nurse should know what constitutes the area of preparation for all types of orthopedic surgery. Surgery performed on the toes will usually require a surgical preparation to the knee; surgery on the ankle, to the midthigh. In spinal surgery, the area will depend on the site of injury or disease. If the operation is to be performed in the high cervical area, the shaving will no doubt include the back of the neck and occiput and will continue to the buttocks. Preparation for lower spinal fusions will include the back of the buttocks and the upper parts of the thighs and will extend upward to the shoulders. If a graft is to be taken, the leg will be prepared from ankle to midthigh or groin. Knee operations usually indicate preparation of the leg from the toes to the groin. For operations on the hips, the preparation usually extends to well below the knee and to the lower

border of the ribs, the umbilicus being the limit anteriorly and the spine posteriorly. The pubic area is always included. The nurse must remember that a preparation for surgery on one joint should include preparation of the joint above. This is not always a rule, but it provides a generous enough area that little dissatisfaction will be found (Fig. 355).

Nurses should develop a deep respect for the importance of the skin, recognizing the fact that the intact skin serves as a mechanical barrier to keep bacteria out of the body. Indeed, some investigators feel that a clean, healthy, and intact skin may actually have a self-disinfecting power. Nothing that is done during the sterile preparation should lessen in any way the defensive powers of the skin.

The shaving must be done most carefully. It is not a procedure to be hurried. The blade should be new and of good quality. Two things can happen with a hurried shave: denuding of the skin area and/or omitting a small field of fine hair. Hair is not easy to disinfect and may be a source of infection. A denuded area is a grave threat and may mean postoperative infection. The surgeon may refuse to operate because of it. Abrasions of the skin of any sort should be reported.

After the area is shaved, the extremity for operation must have special attention. It must be thoroughly washed and absolutely clean. The persistence of grime on the feet or hands after this washing should be reported to the surgeon. The toenails or fingernails must be clipped and thoroughly cleaned. Frequently, it is necessary to soak the foot or hand in warm sudsy water for thirty minutes prior to scrubbing.

After these preliminary but important details have been attended to, the procedure that follows will vary somewhat according to the wishes of the surgeon. In general, however, the area that has been shaved is well scrubbed with mild soap and water for three to five minutes. Mechanical cleansing of the skin prior to the preparation in the operating room is of the utmost importance and must be done conscientiously.

A tray or cart containing the supplies needed for the preparation of the operative site should be on every orthopedic service (Fig. 356). It should contain an extension light, a razor with fresh blades, unsterile towels for protecting the bed from moisture, bottles containing mild liquid soap,

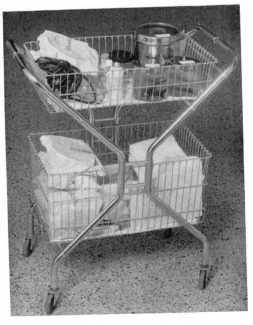

Fig. 356 Equipment necessary for cleansing and preparing the skin for a surgical procedure can be taken to the bedside in this lightweight cart.

and the preferred antiseptic. A small cup or basin for the water needed for the shaving, paper sacks, cotton balls or sponges, gloves if they are used, and brushes will complete the tray.

Blood transfusions

The transfusion of blood has become a common procedure and is done frequently on a busy hospital service. Yet a blood transfusion carries a death risk as great as that from an uncomplicated appendectomy. The observations made by the nurse during this procedure are a vital part of the patient's care. The alert well-informed nurse can prevent some dangerous reactions, and her prompt recognition and treatment of others can be lifesaving.

When the blood is delivered to the patient area prior to the time that it is to be given, it should be placed in a refrigerator and kept at a temperature above freezing until it is to be transfused. Blood should not be permitted to stand at room temperature for several hours.

Before the transfusion is started, both the physician and the nurse should compare the patient's name and registration number on the label of the blood container with that on the patient's identification wrist band. In addition to the patient's name, the type of blood and the Rh factor appearing on the bottle label should be checked against the accompanying slip. Dangerous reactions and deaths have occurred because blood has been given to a patient for whom it was not intended.

During the entire transfusion, the recipient should be watched carefully. It is essential that the drop indicator on the transfusion set be checked frequently and adjustments in the rate of flow be made as necessary. The soft tissues around the needle should be checked for swelling. A hematoma caused by blood going into the subcutaneous tissues can be very painful and may result in serious slough of tissue. The complaints of a patient receiving blood must not go unheeded. Any complaint of respiratory difficulty, such as pain or tightness in the chest, fast breathing, wheezing, coughing, pain in the abdomen or lumbar region, or the appearance of chills or hives, is an indication for the nurse to stop the transfusion and to notify the attending physician. The appearance of respiratory difficulties may necessitate the prompt application of tourniquets on all four extremities, the upper arms and the thighs. The purpose of the tourniquets is to prevent pulmonary edema by pooling the blood in the extremities away from the heart. The tourniquets should be pulled tight enough to hold back venous blood but not tight enough to occlude arterial pulses. The tourniquets should be released one at a time for two minutes, then replaced and another one released. No tourniquet should be in place more than ten minutes without a respite.

Do not permit the tubing to empty completely before discontinuing the transfusion. Near the end of the transfusion, watch the apparatus carefully so that the blood flow may be stopped when there is still 20 ml or so in the container or tubing. If the transfusion has been discontinued because of a reaction, place the used equipment containing the residual blood in the refrigerator. The labels and unused blood should be available for posttransfusion tests in the investigation of transfusion reactions.

After a transfusion, take the patient's temperature at two-hour, four-hour, and six-hour intervals. An elevation in the temperature should be reported to the physician.

A twenty-four–hour collection of urine may be ordered for patients receiving transfusions. Note the volume and color of each specimen as it is collected. Oliguria is the output of a dangerously small amount of urine, usually less than 600 ml in a twenty-four-hour period. If a single specimen, collected over a known period of time, has a volume of less than 25 ml/hr, or if a red color is present in a urine specimen after transfusion (probable hemoglobinuria), save the specimen and notify the physician.

Immediate transfusion reactions

Transient fevers. Transient fevers are often initiated by a chill. The fever may occur during or soon after transfusion. One cause may be the presence of polysaccharides called pyrogens in the blood mixture. These pyrogens are produced by the growth of nonpathogenic bacteria in the fluids or equipment used in the transfusion. These substances are not destroyed by sterilization. A second cause may be the presence of small amounts of heated plasma protein left in reused equipment. A third cause may be the onset of a hemolytic reaction in which the donor's or recipient's erythrocytes are destroyed. Early hemolysis may be excluded by drawing a fresh specimen of the patient's blood, centrifugating it, and demonstrating the lack of pink coloration in the plasma or serum.

Urticaria. Hives occur in about 1% of the patients receiving blood transfusions. During or soon after the transfusion, patches of hives or angioneurotic edema appear on the skin. This can be promptly dealt with by an intramuscular injection of 0.3 ml of a 1:1000 solution of epinephrine. The transfusion can then be continued.

Hemolysis. Destruction of the red blood cells may result from one of the following:

1 Damage to the donor's blood by improper storage, overheating, or freezing, or the mixing of the blood with distilled water, glucose solutions, or solutions other than isotonic sodium chloride

2 The transfusion of blood containing red blood cells that are destroyed by the recipient's antibodies

3 The administration of blood whose plasma contains strong antibodies against the recipient's blood cells

Some of these incompatibilities cannot be detected by the usual laboratory tests. However, some may occur from errors in blood grouping or crossmatching, errors in labeling blood containers, or errors in reading the labels by the nurse or physician. Hemolytic reactions often start with a chill and fever, accompanied by pain or a constrictive sensation in the chest and pain in the lumbar regions or thighs. These symptoms should indicate the immediate discontinuance of the transfusion, notification of the physician, examination of a fresh urine specimen for hemoglobinuria, and the collection of a fresh blood specimen from the patient for examination of plasma hemoglobin. Between six and twenty-four hours after transfusion hemolysis has occurred, the patient may develop painless jaundice that lasts a day or two. Two dangerous complications may result from hemolysis. A state of immediate shock may occur in which the patient has few symptoms except lethargy and low blood pressure. Death may occur in a few hours. More insidiously, the kidneys may be damaged so that the urinary output is less than 600 ml in a twenty-four-hour period. Complete cessation of urinary excretion is called transfusion anuria; when some urine, but an insufficient amount, is produced, it is termed oliguria.

The prognosis is the same for both complications—normal urinary excretion may resume any time up to three or four weeks, or death may occur from renal failure.

Circulatory overload. Circulatory overload occurs when the increase in blood volume from transfusion causes acute cardiac failure and pulmonary edema. The patient suddenly becomes extremely short of breath, with wheezing respirations and cyanosis of the lips. When these signs occur, the transfusion should be discontinued at once and tourniquets (as described previously) placed on all four extremities. Preparation should also be made for a phlebotomy, which the physician may wish to perform.

Air embolism. Air embolism occurs rarely, but it is possible whenever a leak is present in certain parts of the transfusion apparatus, or when all the blood has run out and air follows it into the vein. The patient has pain in the chest with severe dyspnea and cyanosis. The nurse can hear thumping in the heart at a distance. Prompt action may be lifesaving. If air embolism occurs, the transfusion should be discontinued and the physician notified. The patient should be placed on his left side so that the air bubbles float upward in the right ventricle away from the outlet to the lungs, and oxygen should be administered.

Delayed transfusion reactions

Delayed transfusion reactions need not concern the nurse directly but are mentioned for general information.

Transmission of disease. In the United States, infectious hepatitis (serum type), or homologous serum jaundice, is the most common disease transmitted by transfusion. The donor is a carrier of the causative virus but usually has no clinical signs or symptoms of the disease; thus there is no method of excluding him from giving blood. The incubation period in the recipient is roughly from 60 to 120 days. The patient may become jaundiced with signs of severe liver damage, and there is considerable mortality.

In some parts of the world, transfusion malaria is a serious problem. With ordinary storage of blood, the malarial parasites outlive the erythrocytes. The only method of preventing the disease is to reject all donors who have had untreated malaria within five years.

Transfusion syphilis is usually not possible to contract from blood that has been refrigerated for more than two days, because the causative treponemas are readily killed at low temperatures. Syphilis may be transmitted by transfusion of fresh blood when the donor has a chancre and enough time has not elapsed to confirm the diagnosis of syphilis by a positive Wassermann reaction. The disease differs from that acquired by physical contact in that when the blood of a syphilitic person is given to another person, the recipient will acquire the disease but without the chancre. The incubation period of syphilis acquired in this manner is from one to four months.

Isosensitization of recipient. If a patient does not possess a particular blood antigen, he or she may be sensitized when cells containing this antigen are received in transfusion. Antibodies gradually develop in the recipient over weeks and months, so that a succeeding transfusion with the same antigen results in destruction of the red blood cells. Women who are Rh-negative also may be sensitized from a fetus that received Rh-positive antigens from the father's genes. In this case, the mother's antibodies may hemolyze the red blood cells of her infant to produce a disease called erythroblastosis fetalis. The red blood cells of a woman sensitized in this fashion also will hemolyze blood containing the antigen when it is received in transfusion.

Postoperative nursing care

A recovery room where intensive nursing care can be provided for the postoperative patient is almost a must in the modern hospital. Here the recovery room nurse can give undivided attention to the postanesthetic patient. Constant observation for signs of shock and hemorrhage or for an obstructed airway is a vital part of the nurse's concern. Positioning the patient to maintain a patent airway, allowing for free drainage of vomitus or mucus and preventing the relaxed tongue from falling back against the pharynx, is more difficult if traction or a body cast has been applied postoperatively. This type of apparatus often makes use of the side-lying position impossible. If the supine position is used, leaving the oropharyngeal or nasopharyngeal airway in place until the pharyngeal reflexes have returned is helpful in maintaining an unobstructed airway. The tongue is held forward, and suctioning of secretions can be done more easily.

The administration of blood or intravenous fluids started in the operating room usually continues in the immediate postoperative period. Emergency equipment and drugs are readily available, and the timely use of suction and oxygen have greatly reduced postoperative hazards. In addition to a recovery room, many hospitals provide postoperative units or intensive care units where the patient who has had major surgery may receive care for several days. By grouping these patients together in small units, superior and constant nursing care can be provided. Many postoperative complications can be prevented when good nursing care is provided the first few days after surgery. Encouraging and helping the patient to cough and to breathe deeply at frequent intervals are almost routine postoperative orders. Use of a breathing tube to build up carbon dioxide is helpful when deep breathing and coughing are vital to the patient's welfare. Intermittent positive pressure breathing apparatus also may be used to facilitate air exchange and to prevent lung congestion. Antiembolic stockings, an aid in the prevention of phlebitis, are routinely worn postoperatively. If oozing of blood into the wound is expected following surgery, a drainage tube may be inserted prior to closure. With mild suction, blood is removed and formation of a hematoma prevented. Preventing dehydration and maintaining electrolyte balance for the postsurgical patient are also concerns of the nurse.

After any type of orthopedic operation, it is important that the nurse know the lim-itations of activity for the patient. This is essential for intelligent care, and it is as unwise to restrict the patient unnecessarily over a long period as it is to allow him more activity than the physician wishes. Every orthopedic nurse should ascertain the limits for each patient. When and how often may he be turned? Will he be allowed to lie on his side with proper support, or is the prone position more advisable? May he have his backrest elevated at intervals? It is also advisable for the nurse to inspect the cast early. Are all the toes visible? Is the cast cut out enough around the buttocks for good care? (It is almost never necessary for the cast to come down over the gluteal crease, and if it is left in this fashion, it is usually the result of oversight.)

As said many times in this book, close observation of circulation in extremities in plaster is one of the nurse's chief responsibilities. To quote directly from Jones and Lovett, "Every plaster cast where there is any definite slowing of the return of blood in the fingers or toes or any considerable swelling of fingers or toes should be immediately bivalved, the lid removed, and all constricting soft bandages cut through. The latter point is more important."*

It must be remembered, too, that apparatus or casts applied for the remedy of acute conditions, such as fractures, osteomyelitis, or septic joints, may be followed, or rather are likely to be followed, by constriction and circulatory embarrassment as late as three or four days afterward. The cardinal symptoms the orthopedic nurse should watch for are (1) pain, (2) color— cyanosis, anemia, or blanching, (3) swelling, (4) depressed local temperature, (5) diminished sensation, (6) loss of motion, and (7) sudden elevation of temperature that cannot be accounted for (see Chapter 6).

Postoperative complications

Nurses caring for patients who have had bone surgery should be familiar with the symptoms of fat embolism. This condition will usually occur within the first twenty-four hours but can be distinguished

---

*From Jones, R., and Lovett, R. W.: Orthopedic surgery, Baltimore, 1929, The Williams & Wilkins Co.

from symptoms of shock by the fact that it usually does not occur until twelve hours after surgery (see Chapter 5). The condition is severe and frequently fatal. The patient must be kept absolutely quiet. If he is in a cast, no attempt should be made to remove it in trying to save his life.

Thrombophlebitis may occur as the result of immobolization or enforced bed rest (see Chapter 5).

Pulmonary embolism is another grave complication that sometimes follows surgery. It comes on much later than fat embolism, usually in from ten to twenty days, although it may occur much later. If the embolus is large, death may occur instantly. If there is a partial block, the patient will complain of sudden severe chest pain. (See Chapter 5.)

Gradual stretching of nerves may bring about epileptiform convulsions. These are not so grave as the convulsions that accompany fat embolism and occur later, usually from two to six days after operation. The dyspnea is slight, the pulse does not become increased, the respiratory rate is approximately normal, and recovery may be expected after two to four days. Treatment is removal of plaster and sedation.

The presence of backache after operation as a result of the complete relaxation of the muscles of the back during anesthesia is so commonly known that it seems hardly necessary to mention it. It is almost axiomatic that the lumbar spine be supported with a firm pad during anesthesia and after return to bed to prevent this disturbing postoperative complication.

Urine retention may occur in patients who have had orthopedic surgery. It is frequently necessary to catheterize patients who have had operations on the back or hip. This may continue to be a problem for several days postoperatively, and the utmost care must be taken to prevent cystitis or kidney infection.

It is not uncommon for the patient who has had a major orthopedic operation to have abdominal distention. Rectal tubes, enemas, and neostigmine methylsulfate may be ordered to relieve discomfort. In some instances, relief is not obtained until gastric suction has been started.

The alert orthopedic nurse will provide measures to prevent postoperative pneumonia. This applies to any surgical patient but is of special importance for older persons.

The risk of operative intervention on spinal deformities of great extent (severe scoliosis or kyphosis) is increased by the effect these deformities have upon the rib cage, lungs, and heart. The large vessels of the thorax also may be affected. Patients with severe scoliosis should be observed postoperatively for dyspnea, cyanosis, and edema of the lower extremities.

Prevention of wound infection

In surgery of bones and joints, the greatest possible care is exercised to prevent infection. The outcome of most orthopedic operations depends largely on bone union, and bone will not unite in the presence of infection. Furthermore, the presence of postoperative infection of bones and joints often leads to lifelong crippling. For these reasons, techniques used by nurses in preoperative skin preparation and in postoperative dressings should be as nearly faultless as possible.

The prevention of wound infection will depend to a large extent on attention to the following details:

1 Careful preoperative skin preparation
2 Meticulous operating room techniques
3 Observation of wound site to keep dressings and cast intact and free from contamination
4 Careful wound dressing technique— masks, use of forceps rather than fingers, segregated space for dressings, and individual dressing trays
5 A clean ward for clean patients where no patients with infected bone conditions are housed simultaneously
6 Careful removal of any foreign bodies or dead tissue from wounds, since such foreign objects will increase the susceptibility to infection five-hundred-fold

Postoperative drainage from clean surgical wounds should be reported by the nurse as soon as it is observed. Staining of the cast or dressing either by serum or by purulent drainage must be watched for. Immediate reenforcement of saturated dressings with a sterile pad so that capillary action will not bring about further contamination is important.

Children who have been walking barefoot are often predisposed to tetanus infection. When dirt is grimed into the soles of the feet before surgery, it is sometimes difficult to attain the surgical cleanliness desired. The physician should be informed of this circumstance. Occasionally, prophylactic antitoxin may be given to these patients before surgery is performed.

Dressing of orthopedic surgical wounds should be done by the most scupulous technique. Patients with infected wounds should be segregated from those with clean ones. Clean wounds are always dressed before infected ones, and there should be a separate dressing tray for each patient. Greater control of environment is, of course, possible if a special room is set aside for dressings. Wartime experiments showed conclusively that many hazards exist in wound dressings that were not formerly recognized as being important. For example, if patients with clean wounds and patients with infected bone are housed in the same open clinical unit, the bedclothing may be a source of contamination. Bedclothes contain great quantities of lint and dust, and if they are exposed to purulent discharges from wounds and dressings, these particles may be loaded with bacteria. The gradual spread of certain strains of bacteria through an entire ward by this method was demonstrated forcefully during World War II.

For this reason, it is advisable not to dress wounds until at least an hour after all the beds have been made so that dust and lint may have a chance to settle. Sweeping or dusting is never done during dressing periods. Even turning a patient in bed may be hazardous in that it will release quantities of lint and dust. Blankets and soiled linen should be carefully handled and never shaken on the unit as the beds are made. They should not be thrown on chairs or on the floor where dust and lint may be deposited. It is preferable to have containers for soiled linen on the unit so that the linen can be placed in them immediately upon removal from the bed. In some institutions, nobody is admitted to the unit during the dressing period and windows and doors are kept closed. Doctors, nurses, and the patient wear masks while the dressing is being done.

Bandage scissors are sometimes a source of infection in surgical dressings. It is inexcusable to cut the outer dressings of both infected and clean wounds without disinfecting the scissors. In removing dressings, it is wise to cut the bandage and remove it in one piece. Unwrapping soiled bandages may fill the surrounding air with bacteria-loaded lint that may infect other wounds. It is considered safer not to touch anything with the hands until the outer bandage is applied unless the hands have been washed in the meantime. All saturated dressings should be reenforced immediately after they are observed, and when the wound is a clean one, the reenforcement must be sterile to avoid contamination by capillary action. This means, of course, that the dressing should be applied with a sterile forceps. The practice of placing sterile dressings on a wound by hand is uniformly condemned by surgeons.

Early ambulation after orthopedic surgery

Although bed rest is being scaled down to very short periods following surgery for conditions other than skeletal, a certain amount of recumbency is still indispensable for some orthopedic patients. Even on orthopedic units the tendency is to promote as early ambulation as is compatible with the healing time of bone.

New sets of skills are necessary for the nurse who wishes to help the patient toward an early and uncomplicated convalescence. There is nothing helter-skelter about the procedure. It requires wisdom, understanding, and knowledge of new techniques. It is not merely a matter of saying "arise and walk." Equipment for preparing the patient for ambulation is seen in most hospitals today. One sees trapezes on many beds and portable overhead frames that make it possible for patients to exercise the arms and shoulders preparatory for using crutches. Sawed-off crutches are often provided the badly affected patient for learning to manage crutches while he is still in bed. Pulleys and ropes for resistive exercises are not uncommon. Printed lists of simple instructions for bed conditioning exercises prescribed by the physician are seen.

Present-day nurses know that standing is preferred to sitting for the patient's first out-of-bed periods, and they understand the relationship of the cough and the elimination of mucus to his welfare. There are certain dangers that attend the patient who is allowed out of bed early only to sit for many hours in a chair. For patients who must sit, it is important to see that the seat is not too long, because a long seat causes pressure on the popliteal vessels, with the inevitable danger of thrombosis. A backward tilt to the seat is preferable because it serves to keep the hips from slipping forward toward the edge of the chair—a posture that encourages sagging shoulders and rounded back. The elderly thin patient must not sit with his legs crossed because of the danger of peroneal palsy from pressure on the very superficial peroneal nerve on the outer aspect of the knee.

Wheelchair restraints should provide a good sitting position for the patient. The hips should be maintained in contact with the back of the chair, and the shoulders should be persuaded to an upright position so that stooping forward does not occur as the patient operates the chair.

No restraint is foolproof, and all of them need constant adjusting.

The procedure for getting a patient out of bed by having him turn to his side, flex his hips and knees as though sitting, and then swiveling him gently to the sitting position is entirely acceptable in orthopedic nursing. Unfortunately, most orthopedic patients are encumbered with apparatus that makes getting up a much more complicated procedure. Nevertheless, adaptations may be made to fit the needs of each patient without too much difficulty.

20 Special operative procedures

A surgical operation is often the most effective means of relieving a deformed extremity or painful joint. The nurse must be aware of the operations available and have some knowledge of the indications, the techniques, and the likely results. With this information, she will be able to reassure the patient preoperatively and give meaningful management postoperatively and be watchful for complications relevant to each operation.

Operative techniques vary considerably from one surgeon to another and from one time to another. However, the basic principles for which certain operations were designed remain the same; i.e., a crooked leg from any cause requires realignment that can be accomplished by osteotomy. The type of osteotomy, whether opening wedge, closing wedge, or dome, is a technical consideration dependent on the individual surgeon's judgment.

In the following discussion of operative procedures, broad categories will be pointed out and advantages of specific techniques indicated.

Arthrodeses

Any operation designed to stiffen (fuse) a joint is an arthrodesis. The most common reason for stiffening a joint is to relieve pain by eliminating motion, to provide stability where normal ligamentous stability has been destroyed, and/or to correct deformity by realignment at the level of fusion. The disadvantage is that function will be altered; e.g., a stiff knee prevents the bend required in ascending stairs or in putting on socks.

Triple arthrodesis. Triple arthrodesis is a surgical procedure to correct deformity of

the foot secondary to birth defects (e.g., residuals of clubfoot) or to stabilize the foot where muscle imbalance from neuromuscular disease exists. Three joints are excised (subtalar, astragaloscaphoid, and calcaneocuboid), and the foot is held in corrected position in a cast until bony fusion occurs (Fig. 357). The major postoperative complication is swelling, which obstructs circulation to the distal foot. This can be relieved by cutting and spreading the cast.

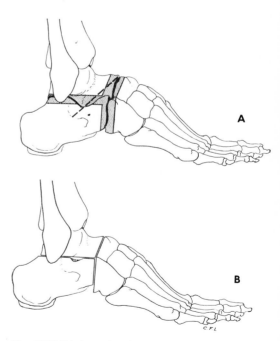

Fig. 357 Triple arthrodesis. **A,** *Broken line,* position of skin incision; *shaded area,* amount of bone resected. **B,** Position of bones after surgery. (From Crenshaw, A. H., editor: Campbell's Operative orthopaedics, ed. 5, St. Louis, The C. V. Mosby Co.)

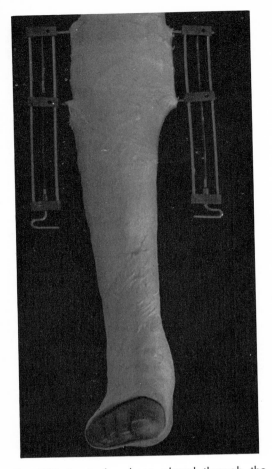

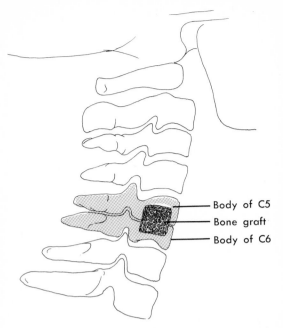

Body of C5
Bone graft
Body of C6

Fig. 359 Anterior fusion of the fifth and sixth cervical vertebrae. Note that the intervening disc has been removed. A bone graft, usually taken from the iliac wing, has been slotted into the vertebral bodies to provide immobilization as well as to serve as a scaffold to be replaced by living bone.

Fig. 358 A pin has been placed through the lower end of the femur and the upper end of the tibia to maintain compression apposition during the healing stage after an arthrodesis of the knee. The two hand screws allow for daily adjustment to bring the two bone wires closer together to maintain compression at the site of the fusion.

Knee fusion. Knee fusion is reserved for those patients in whom instability of the knee is so great that total joint replacement surgery will not resolve the problem. When knee fusion is indicated, the desired position can be maintained by skeletal compression fixation (Fig. 358).

Spinal fusion. Surgery for fusion of the lower lumbar spine was one of the early orthopedic procedures performed to aid the healing of tuberculosis of the spine. Although still a common orthopedic operation, it is no longer done for tuberculosis but rather to relieve back pain or to pre-

vent increasing deformities as in congenital defects of the spine and progressive forms of scoliosis.

There are many techniques to achieve fusion, and the surgical approach to the bony vertebral column may be either the front (anterior fusion) or the back (posterior fusion). Fusion is accomplished by bone grafts slotted into vertebral bodies across the disc space (anterior fusion; Fig. 359) or placed on the lamina from one segment to the next (posterior fusion; Fig. 360).

Immobilization of the spine after anterior fusion requires a minimum of external support since the graft is placed in such a way as to lock two vertebrae together. Posterior fusions however, require external support, and if the fusion involves many vertebral segments, as in scoliosis, internal fixation is added. Internal fixation in posterior fusions is provided by Harrington rods (Fig. 361) and in anterior fusions by Dwyer apparatus (Fig. 288).

External support is accomplished in lum-

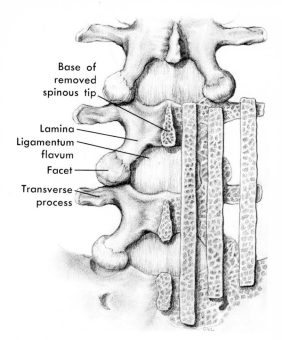

Fig. 360 Posterior fusion. The diagram has combined three varieties of spinal fusion using bone grafts from the tibia to bridge and to fuse between laminae, to fuse facets, and to provide lateral fusion from transverse process to transverse process. The placement of the grafts is the operator's choice, and the graft material may be bone chips taken from the iliac wing.

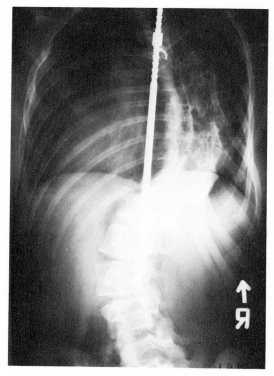

Fig. 361 Scoliosis with Harrington rod distracting the dorsal spine to correct the dorsal curve.

bar and low dorsal fusions by either plaster casts or special braces. In high dorsal fusions, better support can be provided by halo-pelvic traction (Fig. 362). Complications will depend on which technique was followed, and it would be well to communicate with the surgeon in charge to be informed of any special postoperative management.

Abdominal distention with ileus can occur, particularly after anterior abdominal approaches to the spinal column. In extensive, long posterior fusions for scoliosis, transient paresthesia or paraplegia (pseudoparalysis) can occur. Painful pressure points from external immobilization apparatus should be relieved promptly to prevent pressure sores.

Spinal fusion is done to provide stability within the spine. Fusion of painful unstable discs will relieve pain; fusion in scoliosis will stabilize the spine in the corrected position and prevent recurrence of deformity.

Arthrotomy

Arthrotomy is a surgical incision into a joint. Incision into a joint provides an exposure for direct visualization of intraarticular structures. Direct visualization (exploratory arthrotomy) may be the only way to verify an anatomic or pathologic diagnosis. Also, drainage of joint infection is accomplished through arthrotomy.

Arthrotomy for internal derangement of knee

The knee, the elbow, and the phalangeal joints are the only true hinge joints in the body. The knee, being a weight-bearing joint, is the most susceptible to strain and ligamentous injury. Such injuries commonly occur in athletes and industrial workers and usually are the result of twisting motions or lateral strain. When the knee is in complete extension, stabilization is accomplished by the internal and external lateral ligaments.

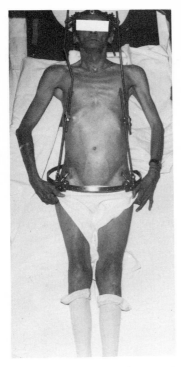

Fig. 362 Patient with cervical spine instability in halo-pelvic apparatus. The hoop portion of the traction encircles the pelvis and is held in place by two pins inserted in the iliac portion of the pelvis.

These become taut in the extended position but relax somewhat in flexion (Fig. 363). The anterior cruciate ligament also is tightened in extension and tends to stabilize the joint in complete extension.

The posterior cruciate ligament prevents forward displacement of the tibia on the femur when the knee is in flexion.

Types of injury. Rupture of the anterior cruciate ligament may occur when the knee is forced into a backknee position. Rupture of the posterior cruciate ligament may occur when the force is exerted on the lower leg from behind with the knee in flexion.

The most common athletic injury is tearing of the internal lateral ligament. It is caused by exerting pressure against the other side of the knee when the foot is anchored against the ground. This is often called football knee and requires a period of three to six weeks to heal. The first three to four weeks are spent in a walking cast that extends from the groin to above the ankle. After this, a knee support is frequently used for a period of several weeks. The reinforced, laced, elastic type seems to be the most efficient. The knee-cage brace with a steel reinforcement and joint may be preferable in some cases.

Rupture of the cruciate ligaments usually is caused by rather severe knee injuries. Fortunately, most of these ruptures will heal if cast immobilization is used for sufficient periods of time. If not, operations for the replacement of the ligaments with tendons or strips of fascia become necessary.

Rupture of the internal and external semilunar cartilages occur frequently. Rupture of the internal cartilages is the most common. It occurs as a result of a twisting motion. The foot is anchored on the ground, and the body and thigh twist when

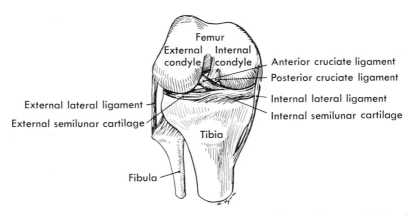

Fig. 363 Ligaments of the knee joint and semilunar cartilages shown with the knee in flexion.

the knee is flexed, in a way that causes rotation of the condyles of the tibia on the condyles of the femur. Rupture of the external semilunar cartilage occurs as a result of a reversal of this motion.

The rupture may occur as a detachment of the anterior attachment of the cartilage or the posterior attachment of the cartilage, or it may be the bucket handle type in which the cartilage is split, part of it entering the central comparment of the knee joint and part of it remaining in the normal position along the outer margin of the joint. Repeated locking is indicative of this type.

Treatment. Immediate operation is not always necessary in semilunar cartilage injury. Many patients will recover if closed reduction is accomplished with or without anesthesia and a walking leg cast is applied for a period of three to four weeks. If there is recurrence, then removal of the cartilage usually is indicated. Removal produces a mild rotatory instability of the knee that usually can be overcome by maintaining strong stabilizing muscles to the knee and usually does not lead to any interference with the function of the joint. There are many active athletes who have had a cartilage removed.

After surgery no cast is used, but a compression bandage helps prevent postoperative hemorrhage. Quadriceps setting and straight leg–raising exercises as well as protected weight bearing, are begun after twenty-four to thirty-six hours. About three months are required for full recovery.

Arthrography and arthroscopy

An **arthrogram** is a roentgenogram of a joint that contains an injected radiopaque dye. The dye (Fig. 364) fills the intracapsular space, and any outline distortions from the normal as seen in the radiograph may provide helpful information in the diagnosis of intra-articular pathology. The injection of the dye demands sterile technique, and the dyes commonly used are absorbed so removal is unnecessary. Arthrograms have a limited usefulness because of the difficulty in interpretation of the radiographs.

Arthroscopy is a special diagnostic surgical procedure for visualization of intra-articular structures through an arthroscope. An arthroscope is a telescopic instrument with a light source and a viewing lens whose pointed aperture can be inserted into a joint in a fashion similar to a large needle. Since the instrument does penetrate the body, sterile precautions pertain as for any operative procedure. The advantage over arthrotomy is that there is minimal morbidity and the patient can resume normal activity within twenty-four hours. The

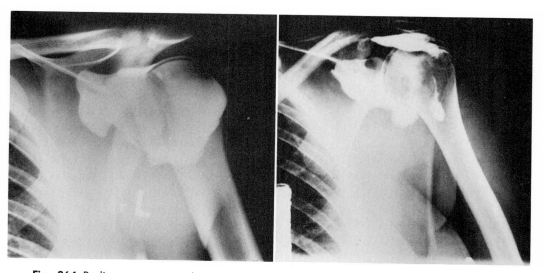

Fig. 364 Radiopaque material injected into the joint demonstrating the confines of the synovial cavity. Any material seen outside of these boundaries would indicate a rent or tear in the lining; e.g., a tear in the rotator cuff.

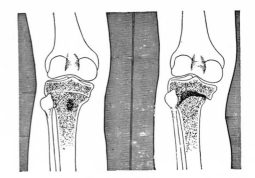

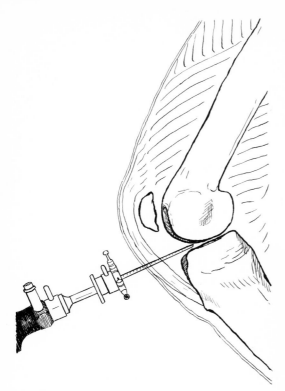

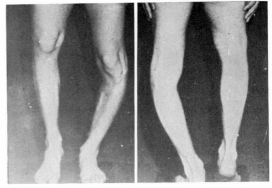

Fig. 366 Line drawing illustrating osteotomy of the tibia used in the correction of genu valgum deformity.

Fig. 367 Anterior and posterior views illustrating extreme bowing of left tibia.

Fig. 365 Diagram indicating the location of the seeing eye of the arthroscope. A fiberoptic flexible-stem scope is also available. Direct visualization of the interior of the joint is possible. However, some areas remain anatomically inaccessible. At present, the knee joint is the only joint in which the arthroscope is used.

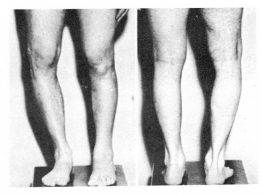

Fig. 368 Postoperative photographs of patient shown in Fig. 367 showing correction gained by osteotomy of the proximal end of the tibia.

use of the arthroscope is exclusively for the knee joint (Fig. 365).

Osteotomy

Osteotomy is an operation wherein a bone is cut in such a way as to permit any desired realignment of its shape or direction. Osteotomy was designed originally to correct a rachitic bowleg deformity. The upper tibia was cut transversely with an osteotome and the two resultant bone fragments placed in an alignment that matched the normal leg. The tibia was hinged, as it were, at the osteotomy site, and the deformity was corrected by bending the hinge to the desired new angle. The tibia was then immobilized until the osteotomy site healed in the corrected position (Figs. 366 to 368).

The techniques available to accomplish osteotomy vary, depending upon the anatomy of the soft tissues and the bone at the site elected. In general, osteotomies are described as transverse, oblique, or dome in

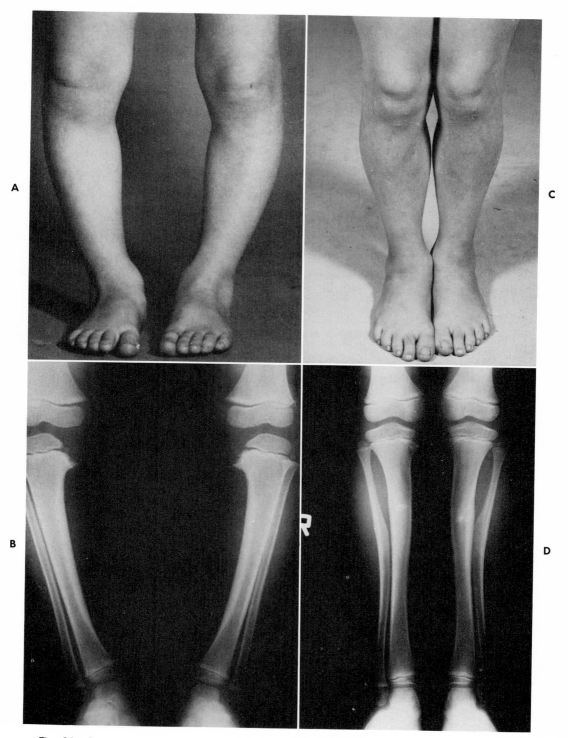

Fig. 369 Congenital bowlegs (genu varum). **A** and **B**, Clinical photograph and roentgeno-gram of the bowlegs in stance. **C**, Clinical photograph after correction. **D**, Roentgeno-gram showing healed osteotomy where operative correction occurred at junction of upper one-half with lower two-thirds of the tibia.

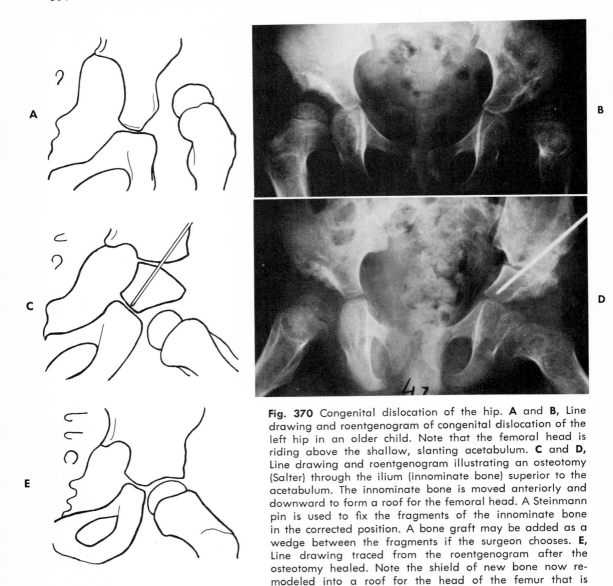

Fig. 370 Congenital dislocation of the hip. **A** and **B,** Line drawing and roentgenogram of congenital dislocation of the left hip in an older child. Note that the femoral head is riding above the shallow, slanting acetabulum. **C** and **D,** Line drawing and roentgenogram illustrating an osteotomy (Salter) through the ilium (innominate bone) superior to the acetabulum. The innominate bone is moved anteriorly and downward to form a roof for the femoral head. A Steinmann pin is used to fix the fragments of the innominate bone in the corrected position. A bone graft may be added as a wedge between the fragments if the surgeon chooses. **E,** Line drawing traced from the roentgenogram after the osteotomy healed. Note the shield of new bone now remodeled into a roof for the head of the femur that is near normal.

shape and direction, and by removal of a wedge of bone at the osteotomy site, a deformity may be corrected by closing the wedge.

The direction of correction to be attained can be specifically described; i.e., transverse, closing wedge valgus osteotomy of the tibia. To maintain the newly corrected position, some form of internal fixation is commonly used, such as threaded pins, plate and screws, or nail and plate, whichever is suitable.

The more common conditions in which osteotomy is indicated are illustrated in Figs. 369 to 373.

Epiphyseal arrest

Unequal growth of the legs may be an aftermath of injury to the epiphyseal plate that occurred in early childhood. Correction of this condition by equalizing the length of the legs is an important consideration in orthopedic surgery.

Phemister and others a number of years

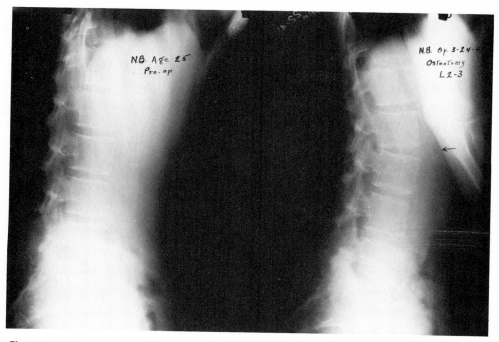

Fig. 371 Osteotomy of the spine, showing the application of the principle of osteotomy to the spine to correct the forward-bent position in spondylitis.

ago showed that arrest of epiphyseal growth could be effected by forms of localized epiphyseal destruction or disturbance. Their plan was based on the fact that equalization of leg lengths could be obtained by such disturbance and that retardation of growth at the epiphyseal line could be accomplished by a block osteotomy over the line with a 90° rotation of fragment (a square plug). When this is rotated, it causes a fusion or elimination of the growth line, resulting in the stoppage of growth of the limb. The state of the epiphysis as shown by roentgenography and a family history of height statistics give clues as to the time that epiphyseal growth should be stopped.

Blount has shown clinically that the principle of epiphyseal arrest can be applied to

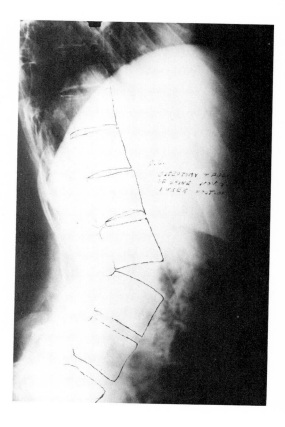

Fig. 372 Osteotomy of the spine showing the amount of correction that can be attained by an opening through the disc space after surgical removal of the posterior ring of the vertebral unit. After correction, a posterior spinal fusion is done to provide stability and maintain correction.

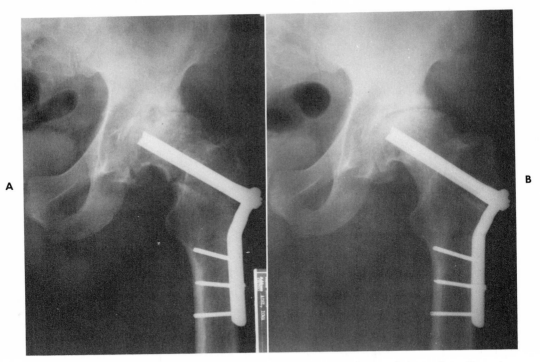

Fig. 373 A, Roentgenogram of degenerative arthritis of the hip with loss of cartilage in the joint space and early subchondral cyst formation. The osteotomy at the base of the neck of the femur has been fixed with a nail and side plate. **B,** Roentgenogram of the osteotomy one year later. Note that the osteotomy is well healed, and a new joint space has regenerated. The patient is pain-free.

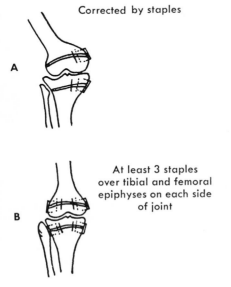

Fig. 374 Drawings showing epiphyseal arrest used in the correction of knock-knee, **A,** and for leg shortening, **B.**

many more problems. By the use of stainless steel staples, it can be applied not only to the equalization of leg length, but also to the calculated control of knock-knees and bowlegs. Moreover, this process may be stopped and controlled by the timely removal of the staples. Blount has found that one staple on each side may break as a result of epiphyseal growth strain. About three staples are necessary to stop the growth. Strangely enough, however, if the staples are removed before complete closure of the epiphyses, growth is restored. These findings open up a new field of leg equalization as well as the correction of bowleg and knock-knee deformities at a calculated time before puberty or the closure of the eiphyseal lines.

In addition, deformities such as a flexed knee or a hyperextended knee can be corrected by staple fixation. Use of the staples can be discontinued at the proper time (Fig. 374).

Total joint replacement

When the Federal Drug Administration in 1969 permitted the use of methyl methacrylate (referred to as bone glue or bone cement, polyethyl plastic) in the human body, a new era of joint replacement began.

Physicians and engineers have designed mechanical joints to replace injured, worn out, congenitally deformed, or diseased joints in the human body. Bone cement provided the method for fixation of these joint implants to the living bony skeleton. Whereas these new joints are mechanical implants into the human body and, as in the hip (the first total joint developed), have already shown remarkable capacity to relieve pain and allow function, the whole field of total joint implants must be considered to be in a state of trial. The long-term (lifetime) effectiveness of bone cement is unknown, and there is no final acceptance of the present materials or designs of joint replacement implants. Research will continue for discovery of the most suitable mechanical design and material to simulate normal joint function and provide a lifetime service. It is clear that mechanical total joint replacement, even though on trial, has been publicly accepted to the near exclusion of previous methods of joint reconstruction such as fascial or cup arthroplasty. The research in joint mechanics and materials testing has added greatly to our knowledge of normal joint function and will no doubt improve future implant designs. Perhaps more importantly, continued research into causes of crippling will open the way to better prevention of functional losses and less need in the future for operative joint replacement.

Hip joint

The procedure for total joint replacement of the hip is implantation of two component parts: one for replacement of the acetabulum and the other for replacement of the head and neck of the femur (Fig. 375). Each component is fixed in position with bone glue, and the position of each must relate as in a normal joint. The normal joint has stability, flexibility, and directional action dependent on muscle force. These properties, when combined, must permit the person with an implant to sit, stand, walk, run, and perform independent self-care activities all in near-normal fashion. Also, the joint must be painless and require no external support such as cane, crutches, or braces. Any individual with a diseased or injured hip joint with irreversible pathology and in whom functional losses or contractures are present is a candidate for total hip joint replacement (Fig. 376). Any age group is acceptable, although there is some caution in persons who anticipate longevity beyond twenty years, since the natural tolerance time for implant materials in the body is unknown. Even the young (under 40 years of age) who are informed and willing to accept the unknown are candidates. The only contraindications to total hip replacement are the presence of active infection and/or inadequate bone to support one or the other of the component parts, and such circumstances are rare.

The main complication in the immediate postoperative period is that of dislocation where the femoral head component loses its proper relationship with the acetabular component. This comes about when there is laxity of the muscles about the hip or when a certain leg position exceeds the stable relationship of the femoral head component to the acetabular roof. Ordinarily, the surgeon is aware of the possibility of dislocation from testing during the operation and should leave written orders for proper postoperative positioning of the hip. In case of a sudden pain, followed by continued pain and protective muscle spasms attendant to any attempted motion at the hip, dislocation should be suspected and reported to the surgeon.

The postoperative management will be ordered by the surgeon. However, it is fairly routine that crutch walking is begun in the uncomplicated case within five to seven days and the patient ready for discharge within ten to fourteen days to a self-care program at home.

Nursing intervention. The fracture patient with aseptic necrosis of the femoral head or the patient with arthritic changes (rheumatoid arthritis or osteoarthritis) in the hip joint not only has a painful joint, but his ability to ambulate is markedly decreased. For months, and perhaps years, the arthritic patient has been experiencing limited activity, using crutches or a walker,

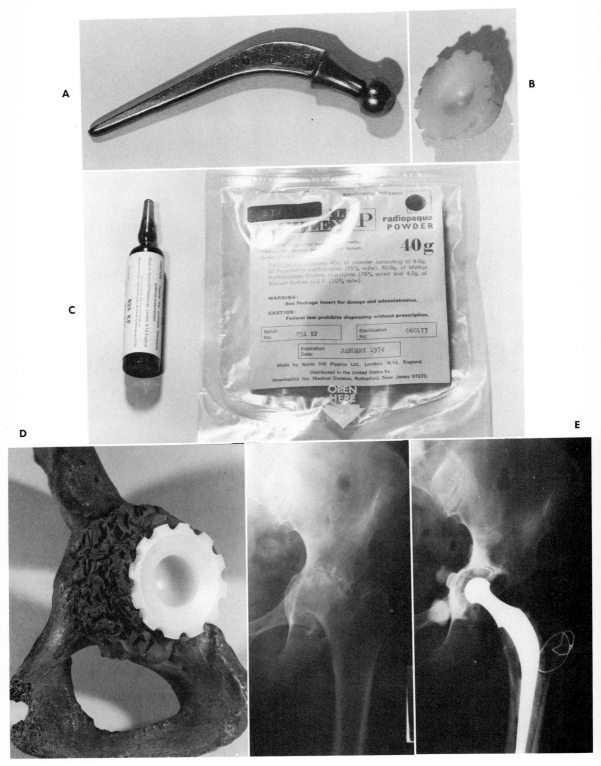

Fig. 375 For legend, see opposite page.

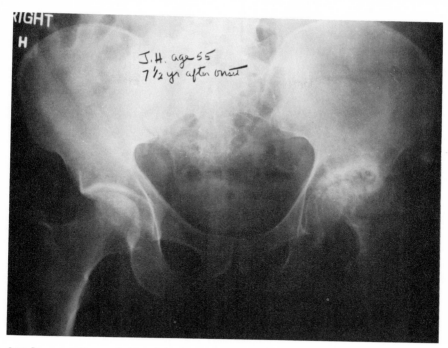

Fig. 376 Degenerative arthritis of the left hip after seven and one-half years of pain. Note that the articular joint space has disappeared and that nature's attempt to repair has changed the shape of the head of the femur.

taking analgesics, and receiving physical therapy treatments in an attempt to relieve pain and to maintain mobility. Conservative treatment has not been successful in preventing progressive functional disability or in eliminating pain. Roentgenograms of the involved joint show marked thinning of the joint cartilage, and the joint surfaces appear irregular. As the joint cartilage wears thin or disappears, bone rubbing against bone causes the patient a very disabling kind of pain. With total hip replace-

ment, as described earlier, the diseased structures of the joint are removed and replaced with smooth artificial surfaces.

Preoperative teaching is essential for the patient who is going to have total hip replacement. Preparation of the patient and his family includes an explanation of the surgical procedure and information concerning the necessary postoperative care. Helping the patient understand what to expect, such as type of apparatus to be used, positions maintained, and exercises he will

Fig. 375 Component parts of Charnley type of total hip replacement. **A,** The femoral component is constructed of surgical stainless steel, and various lengths are available. The diameter of the head is small to reduce frictional wear. Other types such as the Müller utilize a larger sized head to spread the weight-bearing load over a larger surface area. **B,** Acetabular component is constructed of high-density polyethylene to reduce friction and better withstand impact loading with each step. **C,** Bone cement consisting of a powder (polymer) and a liquid (monomer), mixed as needed during the operation by the scrub nurse. **D,** After six to ten minutes the mixture at a "dough" stage is ready to be placed in the bone bed. The component part is immediately inserted into the dough, which then sets and firmly fixes the component part to the bone in three to five minutes. **E,** The preoperative and postoperative roentgenograms show the intrapelvic protrusion of the hip and the total hip replacement, respectively. Both the amount and distribution of the bone cement can be seen in the postoperative film since a radiopaque material is present in the mixture.

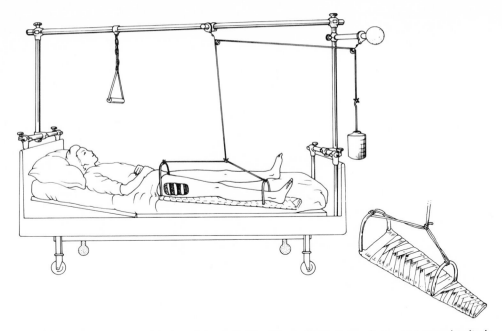

Fig. 377 Traction for total hip replacement (Hodgen splint). The splint maintains the limb in abduction and adds to the patient's comfort by providing some immobilization. (From the Orthopedic nursing procedure manual, University of Iowa Hospitals and Clinics, The University of Iowa, Iowa City, Iowa.)

need to perform, will help prevent some of the anxiety and fear he and his family might otherwise experience.

The operation is a relatively major one, and the blood loss, because of the exposed vascular bone, can be rather large. Much of the loss may occur during the early postoperative period. Blood replacement can vary from none to 10 units, but usually 3 units of blood are required. Much of the blood loss can go unnoticed because it takes place in the deep soft tissues in the upper thigh and buttock. In some instances, drainage is established by securing a wound tube(s) in the operated area prior to surgical closure. This tube is attached to a Hemovac or a Porto-Vac, and a vacuum is established that provides for gentle suctioning of the drainage material. The tube remains in place for twenty-four to forty-eight hours, is checked carefully for excessive amounts of bleeding, and is emptied at regular intervals. This is a closed system of drainage, and sterility is imperative. Hematocrit evaluations are done routinely the first or second day following surgery.

Antiembolic stockings are worn postop-

eratively. These are removed for bathing the extremities and need to be reapplied carefully to avoid injury and discomfort. Continued use of the stockings, following discharge, should be encouraged. In some instances, to prevent phlebitis, prophylactic doses of an anticoagulant drug also are prescribed.

Following surgery, coughing and deep breathing should be encouraged at least every hour while the patient is awake. However this, in itself is not always enough to prevent pulmonary complications of bed rest. Intermittent positive pressure breathing frequently is prescribed for the elderly patient.

The patient is confined to bed rest the first four to seven postoperative days. During this time, maintaining the extremity in the correct position is a precautionary measure against dislocation of the prosthetic head. The nurse should seek specific instructions from the surgeon regarding this matter. The desired position varies from patient to patient depending on the surgical approach and stability of the hip joint. Some abduction of the limb is usually desirable and can be maintained with an abduction splint or traction (Fig. 377). If the side-lying position is permitted following removal of the traction, pillows or a splint should be used to maintain the abducted position. Flexion of the hip to a 90° angle seldom is permitted during the first few postoperative days. However, alternate raising and lowering of the headrest to provide for 30° to 45° of flexion and full extension of the hip joint is usually desirable. When sitting is permitted, marked flexion of the hip joint should be avoided. The use of a toilet seat elevator is helpful and should be used in the home as well as in the hospital for a prescribed period of time. In the sitting position, abduction of the hip joint is maintained by placing a pillow between the thighs and knees, and patients must be discouraged from crossing their legs during this early postoperative period.

If the patient remains active, serious skin problems usually do not occur. Those areas needing frequent observation and massage are the coccyx, heels, and elbows. A trapeze is helpful in that it permits the patient to lift himself from the bed, position himself correctly, and assist in the daily nursing care activities. It is important that the patient and the nurse understand that active use of the hip may be painful but will not damage the hip joint.

Exercises of the lower extremities (as prescribed) should be stressed. These are important in maintaining muscle strength and range of motion and in preventing phlebitis. Commonly used exercises are (1) quadriceps setting, (2) plantar flexion and dorsiflexion of the foot, (3) internal and external rotation of the hip, and (4) gluteal setting.

Four to seven days postoperatively, standing is usually permitted. Some patients in the older age group will experience vertigo. If this occurs, use of the tilt table several times daily will help overcome the problem. Ambulation is started in the parallel bars with weight bearing on the involved limb as tolerated. The patient progresses from the parallel bars to a walker or to crutches. The three-point crutch gait is taught. After about ten days, instruction and assistance in ascending and descending stairsteps is started, and such exercises as straight leg–raising, hip flexion, and knee flexion are instituted and encouraged.

Temporary discouragement is common as the patient begins to get out of bed, learn to walk again, and take care of himself. Frequent reassurance and encouragement are essential to help the patient remain motivated and cooperative. Learning to walk with crutches can be difficult at first. If the patient believes that there will be improvement and gets daily encouragement, this phase will progress more quickly. The patient should be encouraged to use his hip as normally as possible and not to be overprotective of it. He should be helped, not just told, to do everything for himself. A positive attitude by all concerned is very important.

Throughout the hospitalization, the nurse should be alert for symptoms or complications that can occur after any major operation. These include shock, pulmonary emboli, pneumonia, phlebitis, paralytic ileus, urinary retention, wound infection, and fecal impaction.

Dislocation of the prosthetic parts can occur after total hip replacement. Symptoms include inability to rotate the hip internally or externally, inability to bear weight, shortening of the affected leg, and usually increased pain. If dislocation is suspected, the physician should be notified immediately.

Another serious complication of joint replacement is wound infection. Infection of the prosthetic hip may necessitate removal of the prosthesis to control or eradicate the infection. Following removal, the patient will have an unstable hip joint and a shortened extremity. Also, due to the diminished function of the abductor muscle, the gait is altered, and the use of a crutch is necessary for ambulation. Elevation of the shoe on the involved side helps to overcome the problems associated with the shortened extremity.

Occasionally, the acetabular or stem components loosen because of excessive absorption of bone at the interface with the acrylic cement, and the resultant pain can be sufficient to warrant operative reseating of the loosened component.

The length of the hospitalization postoperatively is usually between two and three weeks. The patient will walk with crutches

WRITTEN INSTRUCTIONS FOR PATIENTS HAVING TOTAL HIP REPLACEMENT*

Because many people have questions that are common and recurring after total hip replacement surgery, we have prepared this sheet of "do's and don'ts" to assist you. This information is by no means intended to take the place of our conversations regarding your individual situation but merely covers the "routine activities" after this surgery. We will, of course, endeavor to answer any of your questions or amplify any of the information given here.

1 The usual time required in the hospital following surgery is two and one-half to three weeks barring any complications and depending upon how well and how quickly you progress with crutch walking. When both hips are operated upon, the average stay is about five weeks. We would like you to be fairly independent as far as walking and climbing three to four steps before leaving the hospital.

2 When you are discharged from the hospital, we will give you a definite appointment date to return for an outpatient visit. This appointment is generally arranged for about two months following the date of surgery (or about five weeks following discharge). At this clinic visit, we will examine you and obtain x-ray films of the hip. We will ask you to return at six months and at one year following surgery.

3 You should *continue to use the crutches or walker,* according to the manner in which you were instructed while in the hospital, at least until the clinic visit at two months. We will advise you further at that time.

You may bear as much weight on the operated leg *(using crutches)* as is comfortable. Muscle aching indicates you are bearing too much weight or walking too much, and your activities should be cut back a bit.

Walking is the best form of physical therapy and muscle strengthening following this operation. However, the simple exercise of flexing the hip and knee in bed ten to twenty times morning and night will increase flexibility and eventually allow you to get to your shoes and stockings.

4 After discharge we advise that you not sit for prolonged periods (not more than thirty minutes at a time if possible). You should *not* sit in a low chair and should keep your knees twelve to eighteen inches apart when sitting. *Do not attempt to cross your legs.* You should sleep on your back with a pillow between your legs.

5 If you develop a bacterial infection such as pneumonia or "strep" throat, you should be promptly placed on antibiotics by your local physician. This also applies if you should have any dental extractions. This measure should prevent the occasional complication of a distant infection localizing in your total hip replacement.

6 We suggest that you not drive a car until we see you at your two-month follow-up visit.

7 Return to work is generally possible within four to six months, but there is considerable latitude in this depending upon your progress and type of employment.

*Courtesy Department of Orthopedic Surgery, The University of Iowa Hospitals and Clinics, Iowa City, Iowa.

for several weeks after the operation and then with a cane for several months.

By six months after the hip replacement, the patient has a 95% chance of having minimal or no pain, walking with minimal or no limp, and having enough motion to sit and stand normally and probably to bend down to tie his shoelaces. He should be able to do almost anything he wants to do. Many patients are working at their occupations full time after the operation.

Prior to discharge, it is the nurse's responsibility to see that the patient and his family are prepared for the posthospital phase. The surgeon should explain his regimen to the patient. A list of important activities, restrictions, and exercises can be a helpful guide. Reviewing such a list with the patient and his family can prepare them more fully for the weeks and months ahead. Written instructions can also serve as a reference for the patient if a question

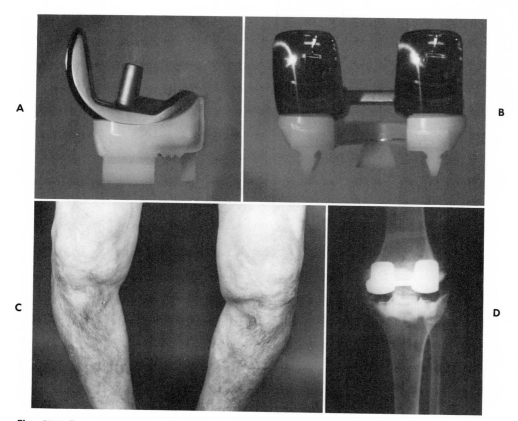

Fig. 378 Component parts of the geomedic design for total knee replacement. **A,** Side view. The upper metallic portion substitutes for the femoral condyles, while the lower high-polymer plastic portion substitutes for the tibial joint surfaces. **B,** Front view. Each of the upper components is convex to fit a similar concave groove in the tibia component. Bone cement (methyl methacrylate) is used to fix both components to bone. **C,** A marked varus deformity of both knees, which could be corrected by osteotomy if a good joint surface is present on the tibia. In this case, no cartilage remained in the joint, and bone had already eroded on the medial tibial plateau. **D,** Component parts of the total knee replacement inserted and aligned to correct the deformity and provide a joint surface for motion and weight bearing. Note that the tibial component is radiolucent and has markers present to aid in interpretation of position.

arises after he is home (see sample on op-posite page).

Knee joint

Unlike the hip joint, the knee is not a simple ball-and-socket type of joint. Consequently, there are more variables in the design of implants for knee replacement. Analysis of the mechanics of knee functions indicates that the femoral condyles do not form perfect spheres but rather are shaped in compound arcs that cause a degree of forward sliding as well as surface-to-surface gliding in contact motion with the tibia.

Some of this slide can be observed best when the knee is extended in the standing position. The kneecap can be observed to point inward as the medial femoral condyle moves backward on the fixed tibia. This position provides stability by tightening the ligaments and requires very little muscle energy to sustain it and has been referred to as the "screwed home" mechanism of the knee.

The implants for total knee replacement (Fig. 378) now in use do provide motion in flexion and extension that is satisfactory for the ordinary activities of daily living but do not provide a mechanism to withstand the stresses and stability required in competitive sports.

The indication for total knee joint replacement is destruction of the normal joint cartilage by disease or injury with impairment of joint function by limitation of motion, contractural deformity, and pain, with or without knee deformity.

The postoperative management consists of some form of external support such as a plaster splint to hold the knee in a nearly extended position to protect the soft tissues for a few days. Gentle quadriceps control exercises are begun as soon as tolerated and, when knee extension is under muscle control, the patient is ready for instruction in walking. Ordinarily, walking is assisted with crutches, and with appropriate progress, the patient may walk unassisted in six to twelve weeks.

In the postoperative period, it is customary to maintain the leg in some elevation to control swelling. In addition to the complications of infection and thrombophlebitis, the nurse should be aware of the potential complications secondary to swelling, which are obstruction to blood flow distal to the knee and interference with nerve function, particularly the peroneal nerve. The warning signals may be pain and paresthesia or inability to dorsiflex the big toe and should be reported to the surgeon promptly.

Nursing intervention. Arthritic changes in the knee joint are not an uncommon problem in the aging individual. If severe, the person has pain and limitation of motion, both of which are caused by changes that have taken place within the joint. The cartilage covering the ends of the bones wears thin and along with this decreased amount of cartilage, there is also loss of joint space and the joint surfaces become rough and irregular. These changes help to produce laxity of the ligaments, and joint instability develops. Gross deformity (varus or valgus) of the arthritic knee is not uncommon (Fig. 378). As these changes take place, the individual is forced to be less active and, with less activity, atrophy and loss of strength in the muscles surrounding the joint will occur. These arthritic changes may be the result of the "wear-and-tear" process of life (osteoarthritis) or an inflammatory process (rheumatoid arthritis), or

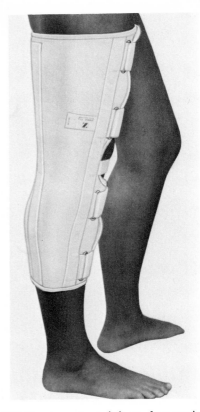

Fig. 379 The knee immobilizer, frequently used following total knee replacement, is made of heavy canvas material, reinforced with heavy metal stays, and fastened with Velcro straps and buckles. (Courtesy Zimmer, Warsaw, Ind.)

they can occur secondary to an injury to the joint (traumatic arthritis).

Total knee replacement, as the name implies, means removal of the diseased bone ends (distal femur and proximal tibia) and their replacement with artificial parts. Prior to surgery, a thorough medical examination of the individual is essential and includes respiratory, cardiovascular, and renal status evaluations. Assessment of the patient's physical abilities, including gait, range of motion, and muscle strength, are also made prior to the surgical procedure. Preoperative exercises to strengthen the quadriceps muscle may be prescribed and usually include quadriceps-setting and straight leg–raising exercises. Preoperative teaching also will help allay some of the patient's anxiety by helping him to understand what to expect following the operation.

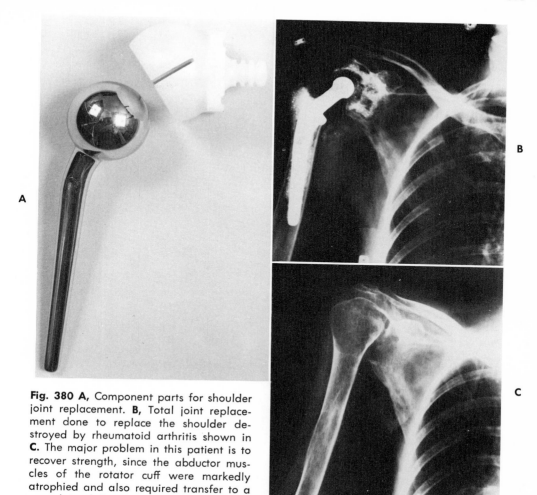

Fig. 380 A, Component parts for shoulder joint replacement. **B,** Total joint replacement done to replace the shoulder destroyed by rheumatoid arthritis shown in **C.** The major problem in this patient is to recover strength, since the abductor muscles of the rotator cuff were markedly atrophied and also required transfer to a new lateral insertion into bone at the base of the prosthetic neck.

Postoperatively, some form of immobilization will be utilized to maintain the knee joint in a position of extension. A knee immobilizer (Fig. 379) is commonly used. However, in some instances, a cylinder cast may be applied. Elevation of the extremity postoperatively is important. Sitting in a chair with the involved limb elevated and standing at the bedside with no weight bearing are permitted as soon as the patient's condition is stable, usually on the first or second postoperative day. The length of time the knee immobilizer or cast is worn may vary, depending on the surgical procedure done and the knee problems encountered. In some instances, a week or ten days postoperatively the knee

immobilizer is removed for short periods to permit gentle flexion exercises of the knee joint. Ambulation, with weight bearing as tolerated (with the immobilizer in place), may be started two to three weeks postoperatively. A walker or crutches are utilized, depending on the needs of the individual. Exercises to strengthen the knee extensors are continued. Since maintaining joint stability is one of the problems associated with the prosthetic knee joint, improving the strength of the muscles about the joint is essential.

Total knee replacement, as with all joint replacement procedures, is designed to provide the patient with relief from the chronic pain he has experienced for a number of

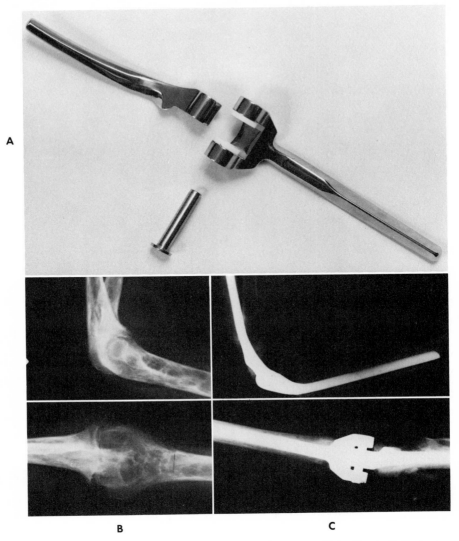

Fig. 381 A, Component parts for elbow joint replacement. Note the bolt that serves as an axle to join the two parts after their insertion into bone. **B,** Preoperative roentgenograms of the elbow showing marked destruction of the joint. **C,** Component parts in situ postoperatively to correct original loss of joint surface. The head of the radius has been removed to permit pronation and supination while the joint replacement permits only flexion and extension.

years and to maintain sufficient range of motion (full extension and approximately 60° of flexion or more) to accomplish the normal activities of daily living.

The postoperative nursing care of the patient with a total knee replacement is similar to that needed by any postsurgical patient. The prevention of postsurgical complications and providing the kind of

care needed by the older individual are of prime concern to the nurse.

• • •

Total joint replacements, other than the hip and knee, are being designed and tried. Examples of the shoulder, elbow, wrist, and ankle replacements are illustrated only to acquaint the nurse with the direction of

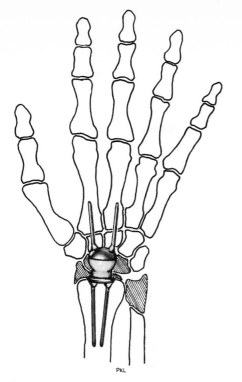

Fig. 382 Replacement for the wrist requires a ball-and-socket type of joint with built-in restraints to the range of motion. Fixation into the metacarpals and radius is accomplished by projecting prongs and can be secure without bone glue. Note that the distal portion of the ulna has been removed or osteotomized to permit pronation and supination.

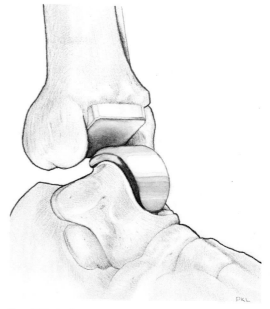

Fig. 383 A diagrammatic view of the component parts for ankle joint replacement. The mechanics of this type of replacement does not allow for motion in a lateral plane but does permit flexion and extension. Future ankle joint replacement parts will be improved as the mechanics become better understood.

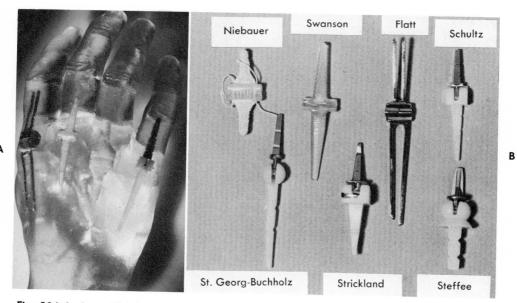

Fig. 384 A, An artificial transparent hand showing a different design of metacarpophalangeal joint replacement in each finger. **B,** Commonly used designs for replacement of small joints of the fingers.

surgical intervention that may become commonplace (Figs. 380 to 384).

Arthroplasty

Unlike total joint replacement, arthroplasty is a form of joint reconstruction in which the diseased or damaged joint surfaces (Fig. 385) are trimmed away and the remaining bone sculptured so as to resemble the shape of the normal joint. To be successful, the repair of new joint surfaces is dependent on the normal body reparative process to regenerate a fibrocartilage covering of the bone ends. Reconstructed joints can function very well and painlessly. However, the predictability is not so good as in total joint replacement and the convalescent period is much longer.

The hip joint lends itself to arthroplasty better than most other joints. A metallic cup-shaped mold is placed over the reconstructed head of the femur before it is reduced into the newly constructed acetab-

ulum (Fig. 386). It acts as a barrier to prevent two bony surfaces from healing by fusion and acts as a mold in which the fibrocartilaginous surfaces repair in a shape resembling the normal congruity of the head of the femur and acetabulum. Repair does, in fact, occur (Fig. 387), and the position of the new acetabulum is carefully selected to provide the optimal mechanical advantage to assure a good gait.

Since the indications for cup arthroplasty are the same as for total hip replacement, the selection of cup arthroplasty would most likely be made when reasons to question the outcome of total hip replacement exist. The long-term results of cup arthroplasty are known; therefore, the procedure may be the operation of choice in younger patients. Cup arthroplasty that sacrifices very little bone stock may be the choice for those patients who fear complication that may necessitate removal of the total hip implants, in which case the result will be the equivalent of a joint excision.

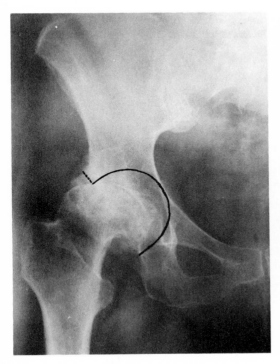

Fig. 385 An arthritic hip joint. Note the lack of joint space and the deformed femoral head. Prior to placement of a Vitallium cup, the femoral head and acetabulum must be surgically reshaped.

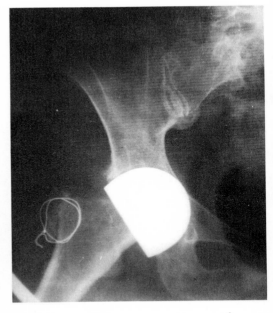

Fig. 386 Postoperative roentgenogram of a cup arthroplasty. The metallic cup is freely movable between the reshaped bony head of the femur, which fits inside the cup, and the acetabulum. It acts as a guide for the fibrocartilage repair and thereafter serves no purpose. The trochanter has been transferred and fixed with wire loops. The new position gives better muscle leverage.

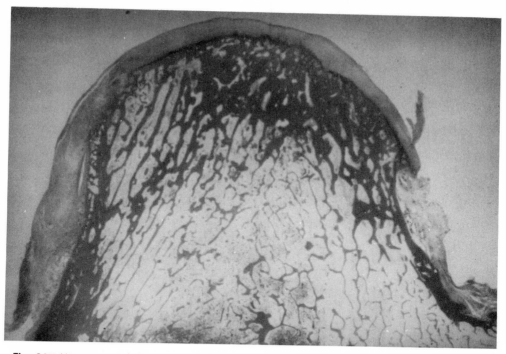

Fig. 387 Microscopic slide to show the repair of fibrocartilage and dense subchondral bone that occurs on the head of the newly constructed femoral head one and one-half years after cup arthroplasty. These have maintained good repair for twenty-five years after operation.

The postoperative management in arthroplasty requires more effort and time on the part of the patient than does total joint replacement. A minimum of six months on crutches and then a cane for a year are common.

Nursing intervention. Postoperatively, the patient who has had a cup arthroplasty is placed in suspension traction (Fig. 126). The purposes of such traction are (1) to provide support for the limb, (2) to maintain the extremity in a position of abduction, (3) to provide increased comfort for the patient, and (4) to facilitate nursing care. Bed position and posture are extremely important. The affected limb is maintained in a position of abduction and internal rotation. To help the patient maintain this position, the nurse will not only need to teach him what constitutes good position, but also to help him attain it in many instances. A sandbag placed against the medial aspect of the unaffected limb will remind the patient that he must not recline so that his body lies diagonally on the bed.

If this position is permitted, abduction of the extremity is lost. A sandbag placed against the chest wall on the unaffected side will help him to keep the iliac crests level. A footboard or bolster for the unaffected extremity will help maintain good position, and when the backrest is elevated, there will be flexion of the hip joints and not flexion of the lumbar spine. A small pad placed beneath the lumbar region will add greatly to the patient's comfort. It must be remembered, however, that extension of the hip joint without increased lumbar lordosis is desirable. Several days after surgery the patient should be doing things for himself. He may need to be encouraged to use the trapeze for shifting his position and to assist with nursing care procedures (Fig. 388). Exercise and use of the unaffected extremity will help maintain muscle strength and prevent generalized weakness.

The exercises that promote flexion and extension of the hip joint and that increase muscle strength are illustrated in Figs. 389 and 390. These exercises are a very impor-

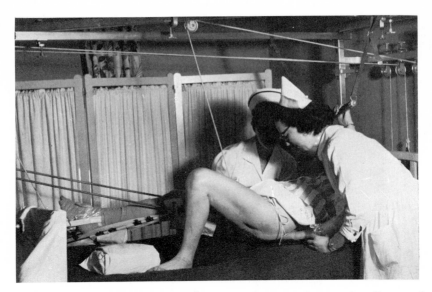

Fig. 388 Method of giving back care to the patient in suspension traction. By grasping the trapeze and pushing with the normal extremity, with the knee and hip flexed, the patient is able to lift the buttocks off the bed. Because of the balanced weights, the splint supporting the affected extremity elevates as the patient's body is lifted. When linen beneath a patient is being changed, the soiled linen is loosened on the patient's uninvolved side and moved toward the center of the bed. The clean sheet is then placed on this portion of the bed beneath the uninvolved foot. As illustrated, the patient raises his shoulders and hips off the bed, and both the soiled and the clean linen are pushed beneath him toward the involved side. The nurse then goes to the opposite side of the bed and completes the bedmaking process.

tant part of the treatment and care of the patient with a cup arthroplasty, and they are ordered specifically by the surgeon for the individual patient. The patient undertakes gradually one exercise after another to keep motion and to build muscle until further gain cannot be made. After a year or so, the new joint will have reached its optimal function, although small gains may still be made year after year.

Tendon transplantation

Several principles of tendon transplantation may be of interest to nurses. It is good to know the reason in a given case for the tendon transplant.

Substitution. In patients with neuromuscular conditions, there is frequently residual paralysis of certain muscle groups that easily can be determined. In any such circumstance, if strong muscles exist in the same extremity, the function of the strong muscle may be transferred by tendon redirection (1) to gain certain function or (2) to eliminate bracing, as in anterior tibial substitution.

Replacement. In crushing hand injuries, certain tendons may be damaged beyond repair. In such instances, a tendon from a less important area may be surgically grafted to replace the damaged tendon; this is known as a free graft.

Realignment. Uncorrected deformities are sometimes increased by the pull of normal muscles in an abnormal direction. Such muscle pull can be redirected by surgical transfer of a tendon so that it tends to correct the deformity. An example is a shift of the anterior tibial tendon to a more lateral position in a patient with clubfoot.

A great deal of the ultimate success of tendon transfers will depend upon prolonged and skillful physical therapy treatments, and nurses should make every effort to see that follow-up treatments are continued until recovery of maximum function has been obtained.

Hip. When there is a flexion contracture of the hip, the muscle attachments, including a shell of bone, can be freed from the anterior and lateral portions of the iliac crest (Speed), thereby releasing the con-

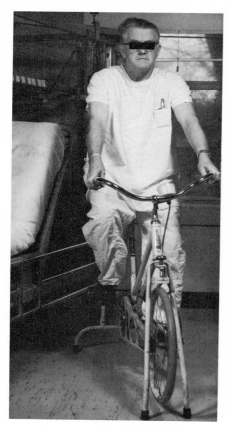

Fig. 389 The stationary bicycle provides flexion and extension exercises of the hip and knee joints. The patient must sit well back on the bicycle seat, with his foot placed squarely on the pedal. The first time he may not be able to make a complete turn with the pedal. However, the nurse must remember that, in the beginning, all of these exercises are for short periods and are gradually increased to periods of ten minutes or more and are performed several times daily. To promote development of the hip muscles, resistance may be applied against the bicycle wheel. To increase flexion of the hip joint, the bicycle seat may be lowered.

tracted muscles and permitting correction of the deformity. A plaster hip spica is used for six to ten weeks to maintain correction.

• • •

There are comparatively few tendon transplants that are permanently successful in the lower extremities, but there is one that gives quite satisfactory results. In pa-

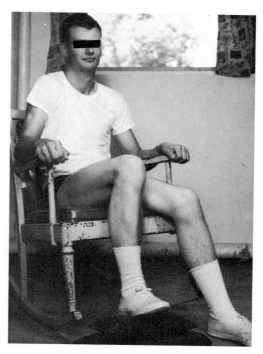

Fig. 390 Rocking chair exercise. Note that the patient sits with his hips well back in the seat of the chair and that the foot of the affected extremity is placed on sandbags. This increases the amount of flexion at the hip joint as he rocks forward.

tients with clawfoot (retraction of the toes), successful results are obtained by the transplantation of the extensors of the toes into the metatarsal bones near the heads. It is usually necessary to fasten these tendons through drill holes in the metatarsal bones so that anchorage will be secure.

A common operation on tendons is a simple release of the tendon sheath or tunnel that has become constricted and interferes with the normal glide of the tendon. Examples of this would be a "snapping" finger, wherein the flexor tendon becomes entrapped as a small enlargement on the tendon is caught by a thickened constriction in the tendon sheath and snaps as it is extended. Another example is stenosing tenovaginitis (drummer's thumb), wherein the sheath of the thumb abductor tendon becomes thickened at the groove in the lower end of the radius and constricts or restrains the tendon.

21 The patient undergoing amputation surgery

Although amputation surgery is as old as surgery itself, the past three decades have brought enormous progress to the field. With the help of antibiotics, vascular surgery, and effective control of diabetes, many limbs are now being saved that would have required amputation in the past. Since World War II, intensive research in the development of artificial limbs, or prostheses, and an excellent educational program have been sponsored by several federal agencies. Greatly improved care for the patient with a threatened or doomed limb is now generally available. The outlook for returning to a nearly normal life is much brighter today for the amputee as a result of these developments.

Amputation is far more common in civilians than in members of the armed services, even during wartime. Nurses will encounter patients with amputations on the general surgical wards as well as on the orthopedic wards. The ultimate goal in the care of each patient is maximum restoration of physical, economic, emotional, and social capacity. This means the amputee must

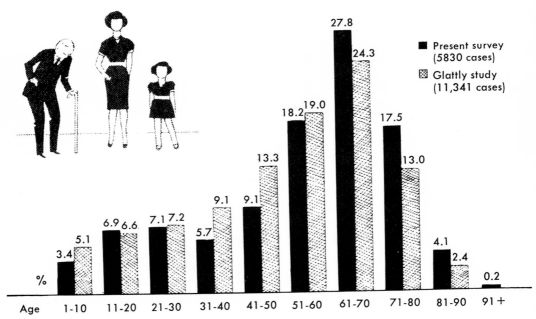

Fig. 391 Relative incidence of amputations by age. (From Kay, H. W., and Newman, J. D.: Relative incidences of new amputations, Orthotics & Prosthetics **29:**3-16, Jun 1975.)

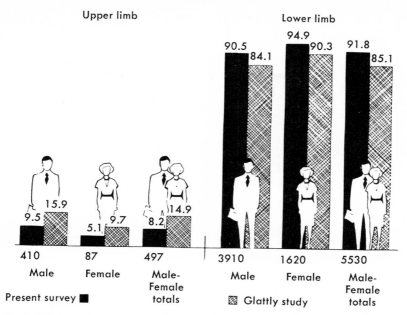

Fig. 392 Relative incidence of amputations by extremity and sex. (From Kay, H. W., and Newman, J. D.: Relative incidences of new amputations, Orthotics & Prosthetics **29**:3-16, Jun 1975.)

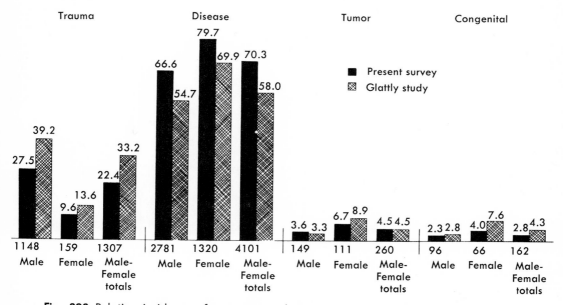

Fig. 393 Relative incidence of amputations by cause and sex. (From Kay, H. W., and Newman, J. D.: Relative incidences of new amputations, Orthotics & Prosthetics **29**:3-16, Jun 1975.)

learn to walk, using his artificial limb, learn to care for his own toilet and dressing, and sometimes learn a new job in keeping with his new abilities. To accomplish this goal requires effective teamwork and meticulous nursing care. Nurses must have a fund of knowledge that will enable them to offer advice or assistance when the occasion arises. Besides the knowledge of the care required immediately after surgery, they must teach stump hygiene and know something of prosthesis construction, fit, and function.

The major causes for amputations are as follows:

1 Injury. Amputation sometimes becomes necessary as a result of severe crushing or extensive lacerations of arteries and nerves.

2 Disease. Vascular disease, especially arteriosclerosis, may result in gangrene of a limb because of inadequate blood supply to the tissues. The elderly patient with an above-knee amputation as a result of arteriosclerosis is by far the most common amputee. Diabetes is often accompanied by severe vascular disease, as well as loss of the skin sensation and marked susceptibility to infections. Extensive osteomyelitis may so damage a limb that the patient prefers amputation and a prosthesis.

3 Tumors. Malignant bone tumors are most common in the second decade of life and in many cases are best treated by amputation.

4 Congenital disorders. Absence of limbs (phocomelia) or severe malformations of a limb present at birth are the result of faulty embryonic development. Thalidomide, a sedative, has caused multiple severe limb malformations in the infants born of mothers who had taken the drug. Amputation may be necessary if a malformed limb will not respond to other corrective treatments.

Figs. 391 through 393 illustrate comparative data of the Glattly study made in 1963 and a study reported in 1975. Findings of the recent study closely parallel the findings of the Glattly study in relation to sex and age of new amputees and the cause and level of amputations.

Amputation surgery

The surgeon attempts as much as possible to perform an amputation with standard techniques at standard sites, saving as much of the limb as feasible. Each level of amputation, therefore, has certain characteristic features and problems with which the nurse should be familiar. For example, the Syme amputation is a removal of the foot at the ankle joint (disarticulation), and

it is done in younger patients with good circulation. It provides an excellent weight-bearing stump that allows the patient to walk with or without a prosthesis. Below-knee (BK), knee-bearing (KB), above-knee (AK), hip disarticulation (HD), and hemipelvectomy (HP) are other standard levels in the lower extremity. Wrist disarticulation, below-elbow (BE), elbow disarticulation, above-elbow (AE), and shoulder disarticulation (SD) are standard upper extremity amputation levels.

The surgeon designs skin flaps to cover the bone stump (Fig. 394). Each tissue is handled carefully and in its own prescribed way to avoid unnecessary damage. The major vessels are doubly secured with suture ligatures before being divided. In closure of the wound, only enough sutures are used to bring the tissues into approximation without undue tension. Drains placed deep within the wound may be brought out through the skin incision line to allow escape of fluid and blood from beneath the skin flaps. Suction tubes to serve the same purpose may be brought out from the skin adjacent to the incision line.

Occasionally, a guillotine amputation is necessary because of uncontrolled infection. In this type of amputation, the tissues and bone are severed at the same level without skin flaps being made. The wound is not closed but usually can be approximated by use of skin traction postoperatively, or it may require secondary closure in the operating room some days later. A snug compression dressing is applied in the operating room. Some surgeons prefer skin traction that can be applied in the operating room or immediately after the patient is conscious. This is necessary in some cases to ensure proper conditions for healing. Methods of applying traction may vary somewhat. Stockinet and skin glue, moleskin straps, and rubber surface traction are in common usage (Fig. 395).

If stockinet is used, the material is rolled doughnut fashion and applied over the dressing. The top of the stockinet is secured to the skin of the leg above the dressing by some kind of skin adherent.

The most commonly used type of traction is made by four strips of adhesive tape, one applied on each of the four aspects of the thigh above the dressing—medial, lateral, posterior, and anterior. Either a circle of

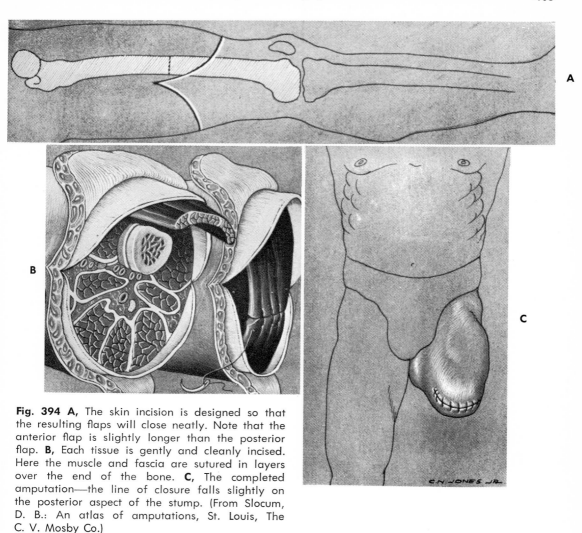

Fig. 394 **A,** The skin incision is designed so that the resulting flaps will close neatly. Note that the anterior flap is slightly longer than the posterior flap. **B,** Each tissue is gently and cleanly incised. Here the muscle and fascia are sutured in layers over the end of the bone. **C,** The completed amputation—the line of closure falls slightly on the posterior aspect of the stump. (From Slocum, D. B.: An atlas of amputations, St. Louis, The C. V. Mosby Co.)

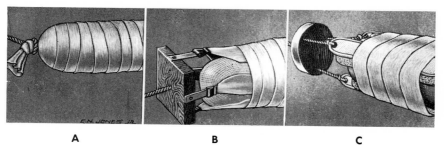

Fig. 395 Skin traction. **A,** Stockinet and skin glue. **B,** Adhesive tape. **C,** Rubber pad. (From Slocum, D. B.: An atlas of amputations, St. Louis, The C. V. Mosby Co.)

heavy wire, stabilized by two crosspieces of wire, or a wooden hexagon may be used as a spreader for the adhesive. Rope is extended from this spreader to a pulley attached to the end of the bed. A five lb weight attached to the traction is usually considered adequate.

Postoperative care. Immediately after surgery, the patient who has had an amputation is subject to complications inherent in the administration of any anesthetic and major surgical procedure. Close observation in a recovery room or another facility where suction appartus, oxygen, infusion packs, and other emergency equipment are at the bedside must be maintained for several hours after surgery. It is not enough to have these facilities in the next room—they must be at the bedside for immediate use. This is the sole responsibility of the nurse who is in charge of the recovery area. Nothing whatsoever must distract attention from the postoperative patient, because this time is nearly as critical for the welfare of the patient as is the actual operation. Frequent observations and recordings of the vital signs are necessary. Restraints may be necessary until the patient is fully alert to prevent disturbing the dressing, the intravenous infusions, and suction tube apparatus. The patient is encouraged to cough and take deep breaths every fifteen minutes. The physician may have him placed temporarily in the side-lying position to prevent aspiration of vomitus into the airway. If elevation of the extremity is necessary because of shock or hemorrhage, it is wiser to raise the end of the bed than to place pillows under the stump. Extensive bleeding from a loosened ligature on a major vessel is fortunately very rare. When it does occur, it is an emergency of the gravest degree. To avert a possible catastrophe, many surgeons order a tourniquet routinely kept at the bedside during the postoperative period.

Curiously enough, the pain after amputation is almost always quite mild. Mild analgesics usually suffice, and often no analgesic at all is necessary after the first twenty-four hours. Pain of great severity may indicate a wound complication, and the physician should be notified at once of the patient's discomfort.

The doctor usually will permit sips of fluids as soon as the patient is fully awake and free of nausea. The following day, a light diet usually is well tolerated. The insulin requirements of diabetic patients undergoing amputation may fluctuate in the postoperative period. This is especially true when infection is a complicating factor.

Amputation usually is accompanied by a more or less profound degree of psychologic shock, which, of course, can be readily understood. This reaction is seen less frequently in patients who have been psychologically well prepared for their surgery. It is most profound in the patient who has an amputation as a result of an injury and has not had time to adjust to the loss. This psychologic shock may be manifested by depression, hostility, denial, and occasionally, feelings of futility. The elderly patient often demonstrates extreme confusion during the postoperative period, and young patients may have feelings of mutilation or emasculation. These reactions in general are seen less often in the patient with a well-balanced, stable personality. The patient will need reassurance—starting even before surgery and continuing during the first few difficult days after surgery. Nurses are in an excellent position to supply reassurance that he is not to become a cripple, unable to walk or look after his own needs. Because nurses are fully aware of the advances made in regard to walking with artificial limbs, they can be a source of great encouragement to the patient at this time. They should supply continual firm, affirmative support and constant reassurance. This type of assistance should be continued throughout the rehabilitation period.

From the outset, nurses should be alert to signs of flexion and abduction contractures at the hip. A position of flexion and abduction is a natural one for the patient to assume in bed, partly because he feels he is protecting the fresh wound from any disturbance. The hip then may become contracted quite insidiously. Strenuous measures must be taken to avoid this complication, because it makes efficient walking with a prosthesis difficult, if not impossible (Fig. 396). Even a slightly sagging bed can contribute to contractures, and bed boards may be necessary to provide a firm support. Pillows under the thigh are almost certain to result in some degree of flexion at the hip level. To prevent these complications, the above-knee amputee should lie prone for half-hour intervals several times during the day (Fig. 397). If the patient uses the backrest or a wheelchair for long periods during the day, he should be encouraged to spend comparable periods in a position of full extension to prevent contracture of the hip flexors. Bed exercises will be started after a day or two, not only to prevent con-

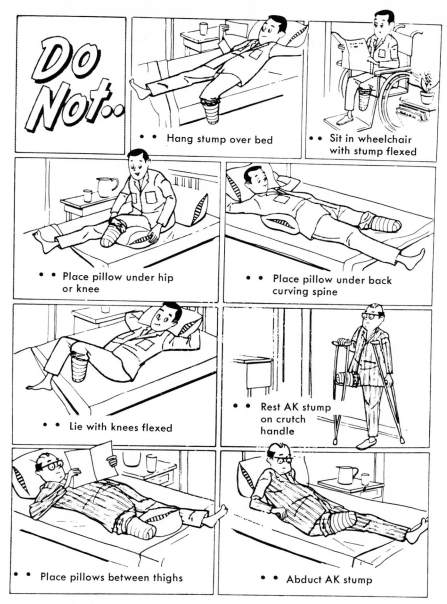

Fig. 396 To avoid contractures and to assure the best conditions for wound healing, the patient should be cautioned to avoid the activities shown. (From Wilson, A. B., Jr.: Limb prosthetics today, Artif Limbs **7**:1-42, Autumn 1963.)

tracture but also to start building needed muscle strength.

A great deal of the patient's future ability to walk will depend on the remaining limb, and care should be taken to keep it in normal muscle tone. Supports should be provided to encourage good anatomic position in bed. A sensitive heel sometimes develops in the remaining foot because of the pa-

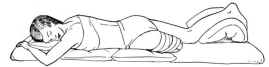

Fig. 397 Prone position. The pillow under the patient's lower trunk protects the wound from pressure on the bed and maintains the hip in extension (From Moskopp, M. E., and Sloan, J.: Nursing care for amputee, Am J Nurs **50**:550-555, Sep 1950.)

tient's inclination to push himself up in bed by digging his heel into the mattress. An overhead trapeze will help him to pull himself up in bed without using his heel.

The patient may be allowed out of bed as early as the day after amputation to reduce the danger of embolism. He should be fitted with a good shoe when he begins to bear any weight on the foot.

These things will not be difficult to encourage in the healthy adult, but the debilitated, elderly patient will need to be encouraged by frequent explanations about the necessity of what he is doing. Otherwise, it seems too much trouble to him to warrant the effort he must put forth.

Physical therapy

Two forms of treatment that are almost universally followed after amputation are bandaging and exercise. It is desirable, although sometimes not possible, that these be given under the direction of a physical therapist. If such service is not available, nurses must request demonstration from the physician. It is not enough in these circumstances that the demonstration be given to the patient alone, since the nurse will need to encourage and guide the patient in the proper application of the bandage.

Exercises

Bed exercises may be started on the first or second postoperative day. These help greatly in preventing contractures as well as in preserving and increasing muscle power for the training to come. While lying in the prone position, the patient is instructed to bring the stump close to the normal leg, to lift it, and to contract the gluteal muscles as he does so. Nurses supervising this bed exercise should see to it that the patient lies with his foot over the edge of the mattress, keeping the normal leg on the mattress while he is extending the stump. Another exercise the surgeon may sometimes suggest is that of squeezing a pillow between the thighs. If the patient has a below-knee amputation, considerable attention may be given to strengthening the quadriceps muscle as well. One commonly used exercise is to tighten the kneecap, using the quadriceps muscle, for ten seconds and then to relax for ten seconds. The exercise is repeated four or more times

several times each day. Patients understand more quickly if they do this in unison with the normal leg and are taught to feel the medial portion contract during the final 10° of full extension.

The stump should be kept dry at all times until healed, and it is not permissible to use hot packs or the whirlpool bath. Heat should be used with extreme care, particularly in patients with diabetes or diseases of the vascular system. For such patients the physician may order a foot cradle and a lamp suspended over the limb area. This type of heat will increase the circulation of the limb without endangering the stump area itself.

When the patient can be out of bed, it is essential that he learn to balance himself properly as he stands on his remaining foot. Parallel bars or crutches will assist him in attaining this balance. In the patient with poor vision, poor balance, or tremors, a walker may be of great benefit. The body should be held straight and the stump should hang straight without flexion or ab-

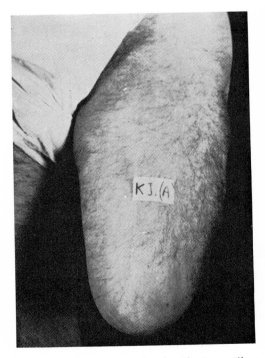

Fig. 398 Proper compression bandaging will result in a well-molded stump that is ready for prosthetic fitting. (From Wilson, A. B., Jr.: Limb prosthetics today, Artif Limbs **7:**1-42, Autumn 1963.)

duction. There should be no distortion of the body because of the missing limb. Drawing in of the abdominal muscles and pinching the gluteal muscles together will help him to avoid shifting his weight to the side of the normal leg.

Compression or shrinker bandaging of stump

As soon as the wound is healing well, the doctor may order some type of shrinker or compression bandage to be applied to the stump. The preferred material for this bandage is usually cotton elastic. Bandages are worn at all times except during physical therapy treatments and until the patient is fitted with a prosthesis. With careful bandaging, the stump can be molded into the desired shape for fitting with a prosthesis. (Fig. 398). Without bandaging, the stump tends to remain boggy, swollen, and flabby —and in this condition a prosthesis cannot be satisfactorily fitted. The chief cause of delay in the fitting of the prosthesis and rehabilitation of the patient is an improperly molded stump as a result of inadequate or incorrect compression bandaging. A poorly applied bandage is probably worse than no bandage at all. If it is properly applied, however, a shrinker bandage may play a most important part in the ultimate rehabilitation of the amputee.

Because the bandage needs to be reapplied several times during the day to be most effective, nurses should be familiar with the correct application. Also, since the patient will be expected to apply the bandage at home, it is desirable that he be taught and supervised in its application.

For the thigh of an average adult, two or three 4-in to 6-in all-cotton elastic bandages will be necessary. For convenience and security, they are sewed together end-to-end. The bandage is started on the front of the thigh at an angle with and over one side of the distal portion of the stump. It may be anchored in place by having the patient hold it with his thumbs, one on either side of the thigh. The bandage is then carried around and up to cover the high adductor skin in the inguinal region (Fig. 399). (Unless the patient is very large, his hands

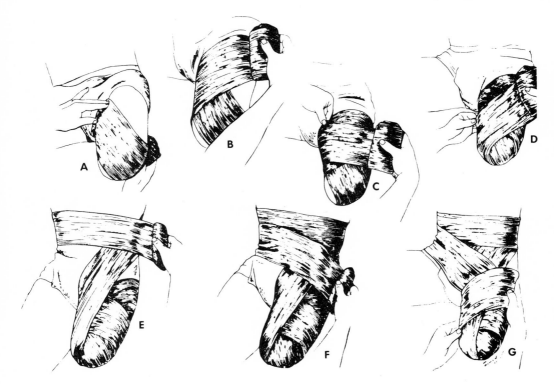

Fig. 399 Application of a modified figure-of-eight style of compression bandage. (After D. Shurr, The University of Iowa Hospitals and Clinics, Iowa City, Iowa.)

should be able to encircle his thigh in this fashion.) Now the bandage is carried down the back of the thigh, going somewhat obliquely this time, over the end of the stump, back up to the groin level, and then down obliquely again, this time over the inner aspect of the stump. Each time the loop is held by the patient's fingers and thumbs and each time the end of the stump must be compressed securely. The maximum force of the bandage should always be at the stump end and should diminish as the bandage ascends.

Two spiral turns of the bandage downward to the end of the stump are now made, and the patient is turned on his normal side. The bandage is then carried spirally upward around the thigh, compressing the soft tissues on the side of the stump in an upward and outward direction, and then over the outerside of the buttock near the iliac crest. It crosses the abdomen and then passes around the hip of the normal side, across the back, and around the amputated leg at the groin level. A spiral to the end of the stump is made and a second spiral is made as before, always working from within outward and always using the bandage to compress soft tissues at the stump end. The bandage is finally brought back to the stump and completed by a few spiral turns as the length of the bandage allows. It may be secured by safety pins or bandage clips.

The finished bandage should be observed to check that the spiral crossings that make the hip spica bandage do not lie on the front of the thigh, a condition that encourages hip flexion. Also, the bandage must cover the inner surface of the thigh as high as possible on the groin. If this is not done, a fleshy roll will likely occur at the top of the bandage, which will be uncomfortable to the patient and also will cause the bandage to slip downward from that level. An unhealed stump must not be bandaged too snugly, and bandages for healed stumps should not be applied so snugly that actual discomfort occurs.

The below-knee bandage is applied in much the same manner as the one for the thigh stump, omiting, of course, the technique for the hip spica. If the bandage extends above the knee, the patella should remain uncovered and the leg should be held in extension. The popliteal area must not be compressed by too snug a bandage.

Because compression bandages must be reapplied several times during the day, it is advisable to have several sets on hand. After each wearing, they should be carefully washed with mild soap and warm water, very thoroughly rinsed, squeezed out, and then laid on a flat surface to dry because they tend to lose their elasticity if hung. When dry, they should be rolled snugly but without stretching.

As soon as the wound is well healed and the patient understands stump wrapping, exercises, and positioning, he will be discharged from the hospital. He is seen at frequent intervals by the physician, and as soon as his stump is well molded and firm, he is ready for prescription of an artificial limb and rehabilitation.

Prostheses

Prosthesis prescription. When the stump is well healed and firmly molded, the patient is ready for a prosthesis. In well-run amputee clinics, experience has shown that the prescription and training in the use of the limb are best carried out jointly by a physician familiar with amputees and prostheses, the prosthetist who will construct and fit the limb, and the physical therapist or occupational therapist who will train the patient in its use. Rehabilitation counselors and social workers usually also are involved. Interested nurses are in an excellent position to contribute to this team through their knowledge of the patient. Many factors must be considered in selecting the proper type of prosthesis and prosthetic component. Some of the more important considerations are the following:

1 Age. Special problems exist at the extremes of life. Children need simpler mechanical devices than adults, and their limited attention span makes special training techniques necessary. They outgrow the prosthesis every two to three years. The elderly amputee may need extra stability to prevent falls.

2 Occupation. Obviously, an active laborer will require heavy-duty components and construction, whereas a weak, elderly nursing home patient will desire a lighter prosthesis.

3 Agility and intelligence. A feeble-

minded patient cannot be expected to master a complicated upper extremity prosthesis, and an obese clumsy patient will require more safeguards and stability than the average patient.

4 Other health problems. Cardiac reserve is seldom an absolute limiting factor in training because the exertion required to walk with an artificial limb is less than that required for crutch walking. Poor vision, poor balance, paralysis, diminished skin sensation, and tolerance are other health considerations.

5 Finances. Artificial limbs are very expensive. Recently developed components—e.g., the commercially available hydraulic knee unit—add greatly to this expense. Charitable or governmental agencies furnish 70% to 80% of all prostheses today. Cost must be kept as low as possible. Luxury components can rarely be used.

6 Motivation. The most important consideration of all is motivation, for without it the patient will not use the prosthesis and all rehabilitation efforts are doomed. The nurse, with knowledge of the patient, can contribute greatly in this evaluation. In general, it is uncommon for a prosthetic prescription team to decide that the patient is not a candidate for an artificial limb of any sort.

After a prescription has been written, the prosthetist takes a mold and certain measurements of the stump to use in construction of the prosthesis. When the mold has been taken, shrinker bandaging should be discontinued because further shrinkage of the stump will result in an ill-fitting prosthetic socket. The construction of artificial limbs requires the highest standards of craftsmanship and technical skill. The prosthetist must have a thorough understanding of the intricate mechanics of body motion that he is attempting to replace. Construction of the socket is critical for the proper fit and distribution of weight. Sometimes the unit is hand carved in basswood or willow wood; otherwise, a plastic laminated socket is constructed from a plaster mold. Only certain definite areas on the stump and buttocks are capable of withstanding the pressures of body weight, and the socket must distribute the weight accordingly. Alignment is equally critical,

since the position of the prosthesis at all times must closely match that of a normal limb. The prosthetist must finish the prosthesis so that it will be pleasing to the eye. carefully matching the patient's own coloring and contour, or else the patient may not wear the limb at all. The prosthetist must be exacting in each detail of construction. This is no mail-order procedure.

Prosthesis components. Familiarity with prostheses can be gained only by seeing several of each type. The nurse should examine the workings and fit of each artificial limb encountered. For the interested nurse whose duty requires working with large numbers of amputees, attendance at any of the large prosthesis centers would be invaluable. The following brief account of the commonest prosthesis components can best

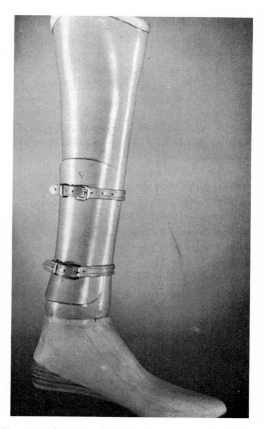

Fig. 400 The Canadian Syme prosthesis. A panel on the medial side permits the bulbous stump to enter the prosthesis. A SACH foot is used in this prosthesis. (Courtesy Prosthetic and Sensory Aids Service of the Veterans Administration, Washington, D. C.)

be understood if actual prostheses also can be seen and investigated.

Lower extremity. The Syme prosthesis is constructed to permit direct weight bearing on the end of the tibia (Fig. 400). A small side or rear opening panel in the shank allows the bulbous stump to enter the prosthesis. The socket is made entirely of plastic laminate. A SACH (Solid Ankle, Cushion Heel) foot is provided, and this has no actual moving ankle joint. Sponge rubber in the heel simulates the ankle function of absorbing the impact of heel strike with each step. With no moving parts, this foot combines a pleasing appearance with trouble-free wear.

For the below-knee amputee, the patellar tendon–bearing (PTB) socket has become widely popular (Fig. 401). This socket is constructed of plastic laminate with a thin leather and sponge rubber liner. The bulk of the weight in this instance is distributed to the patellar tendon, which is admirably suited for the job. Usually a single cuff around the thigh just above the kneecap is

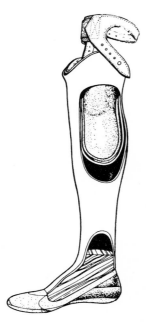

Fig. 401 Cutaway view of the patellar tendon-bearing prosthesis for below-knee amputees. Usually, only a light strap above the knee is necessary for suspension. (From Wilson, A. B., Jr.: Limb prosthetics today, Artif Limbs **7:**1-42, Autumn 1963.)

sufficient for suspension. The SACH foot is generally used in combination with the PTB socket prosthesis. The older hand-carved wooden socket, or so-called soft socket, depends on hinged upright thigh bands and leather lacers to carry much of the weight. The lower end of the socket is left open and is combined either with a SACH foot or with single-axis ankle-foot components. Although it has proved to be a satisfactory prosthesis for years, it has a few disadvantages and is being gradually replaced by the PTB socket.

The above-knee amputee faces additional problems because the prosthesis must have a knee articulation. Many types of knee units are in current use, but nearly all incorporate a design that promotes friction during the swing phase of walking. This is necessary to limit the height of the rise of the heel from the floor and to prevent a jarring impact as the knee is again extended just prior to the time the heel strikes the floor. The knee is so aligned that in standing, with knee fully extended, it is balanced against sudden flexion—a disaster that would send the wearer sprawling on the floor. An automatic knee brake (the Bock safety knee) is useful for elderly or infirm patients because it prevents the knee from buckling whenever weight is borne on the prosthesis, whether the knee is safely extended or not. For the especially active wearer, there are several hydraulic knee units available that produce a marvelously smooth gait. These are expensive and only occasionally troublesome.

The quadrilateral or Berkley socket has virtually replaced the older, round socket or plug socket for the above-knee amputee. As the name implies, its rectangular shape does not conform to the shape of the stump, but it does make use of the remaining muscles of the stump. Weight is distributed principally on the ischial tuberosity and the tough origins of the hamstring muscles. The socket is carved from wood or molded in plastic. In some cases, a total-contact socket is used to alleviate or prevent certain stump skin problems. As the name implies, all portions of the stump are in contact with the socket wall. The suction socket has definite advantages for the active above-knee amputee. It not only reduces the need for harnessing, but also gives improved perception

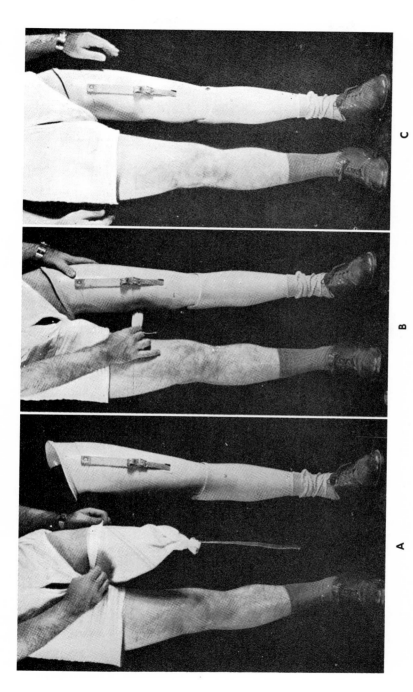

Fig. 402 Application of the suction socket above-knee prosthesis. **A,** A thin cotton sock is placed on the stump. Note that a string is attached to the bottom of the sock. When the stump is placed in the limb, this is threaded out through the valve to facilitate drawing the sock from the stump. **B,** The stump is placed in the limb, and the sock is pulled out through the open valve. **C,** Weight is placed firmly on the limb to evacuate any possible air; the suction valve is closed. The limb is now ready for use and is maintained on the stump through negative pressure and muscle action. No stump sock is worn with this type of suspension. (From Slocum, D. B.: An atlas of amputations, St. Louis, The C. V. Mosby Co.)

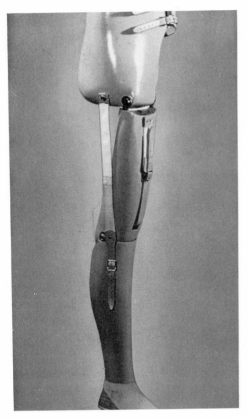

Fig. 403 The hip disarticulation prosthesis. (Courtesy Prosthetic and Sensory Aids Service of the Veterans Administration, Washington, D. C.)

of the movement and location of the prosthesis. The wearer feels that the prosthesis is more a part of his body. When once applied, the stump is pumped up and down to expel all air from the bottom of the socket. A valve is then closed that permits no air to enter, and a suction effect is created.

The hip disarticulation prosthesis is the current standard prescription for patients who have had a hemipelvectomy or hip disarticulation (Fig. 403). The socket is a plastic laminate mold designed to distribute weight on the ischium or other available structures. The hip joint hinge is located toward the front of the socket in a position ahead of the thigh. This alignment eliminates the need for a lock at the hip joint because it cannot buckle suddenly during standing or normal walking. This arrangement also facilitates sitting while wearing the prosthesis. The remaining components

consist of a constant-friction knee and a SACH foot.

With the recent advances in prosthetic systems, the modular endoskeletal system offers the patient an alternative to the wood and plastic conventional prosthesis. The endoskeletal variety (Fig. 404) offers the patient a lighter, more cosmetic, and fully adjustable prosthesis. In addition, parts are interchangeable, allowing repair or replacement of portions of the prosthesis with minimal effort. A foam cover, made to the specifications of the remaining limb, completes the system.

Immediate postsurgical fitting of lower extremity prosthesis. Fig. 405 illustrates the type of prosthesis that is applied to a below-knee amputee when ambulation and weight bearing are advocated two to three weeks postoperatively. Immediately after surgery, a sterile stump sock is applied over the fluffed gauze dressing. This protects the stump from the plaster-of-Paris dressing. In addition, felt pads are placed in position to protect bony prominences from pressure caused by weight bearing. An elastic plaster-of-Paris bandage is then applied to the stump in a specified manner. This dressing is reinforced with the conventional plaster-of-Paris bandage. A suspension strap, as illustrated, is incorporated into the plaster. Later, this suspension belt is fastened to the waist belt. When the cast is dry, additional layers of plaster of Paris are used to attach and hold the adjustable portion of the prosthetic unit in the correct position. This cast is worn for eight to fourteen days unless there are indications for removing it, such as an elevated temperature, discomfort, or a loose-fitting bandage. If the cast is removed or accidentally comes off, it is important that another stump cast be applied very soon to prevent edema of the stump. The first postoperative day, active assistive exercise of the hip joint and weight bearing on the prosthesis are encouraged as tolerated by the patient. During the next three to four weeks, ambulation, with three-point partial weight bearing, is increased as determined by the surgeon and as tolerated by the patient. The rigid dressing tends to prevent severe pain when weight bearing is instituted soon after amputation, and phantom pain has not been a problem. When early ambulation is accomplished,

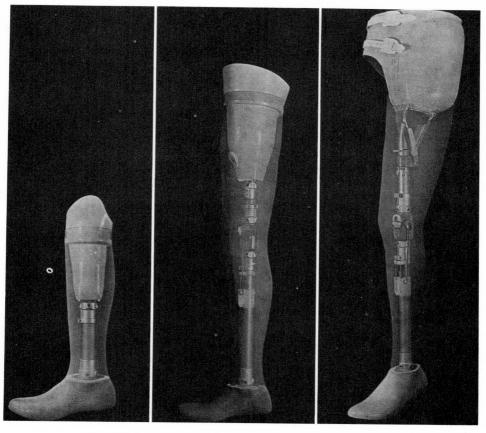

Fig. 404 Otto Bock modular endoskeletal prosthetic system.

the patient feels encouraged and the complications frequently caused by inactivity may be avoided. With this regime for the amputee, the rigid bandage and early ambulation with weight bearing, it appears that the process of stump shrinking and shaping begins much earlier than in treatment by the conventional method.

Upper extremity. For the upper extremity amputee, prosthesis function and fitting present some quite different problems. Replacing the prehensile human hand is clearly an impossibility, and prostheses can make available only a rough approximation of the hand's function. In most cases, the prosthetic hand provides only holding and assistive functions for the intact hand. Placing the hand at a desired position in space away from the body and holding it there becomes an intricate problem in levers, cables, and locks. Cosmetic appearance is of far more concern to the average upper extremity amputee. These many problems lead to a lower rate of success in the number of amputees wearing upper extremity prostheses as compared to those wearing lower extremity prostheses.

For the wrist disarticulation or below-elbow (BE) amputee, the replacement consists of some type of terminal device that is powered by a cable arrangement from the shoulder. Many types of terminal devices are available, but these divide naturally into hooks (Fig. 406) and mechanical hands. The term hook is a misnomer that conjures ugly visions of pirate captains, but it is so entrenched in common usage that we are left little alternative except to refer to it nonspecifically as a terminal device. Actually, it is seldom used as a hook, and it would make a clumsy weapon in combat. Most hooks are of the voluntary opening variety, which means that the wearer actively opens the hook to grasp objects, but

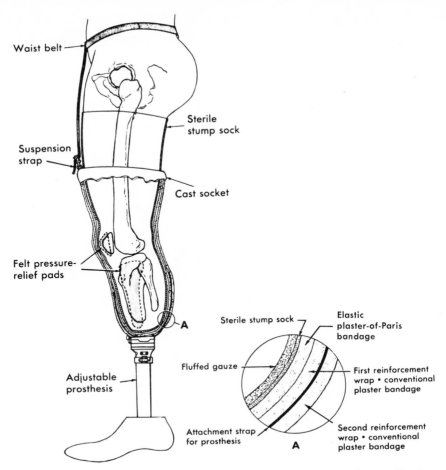

Fig. 405 Schematic cross section showing most of the elements in the application of a prosthesis to a below-knee amputee immediately after surgery. For the sake of clarity, the suture line, silk dressing, and drain are not shown. **A,** An enlarged schematic section of the cast socket, prosthetic unit attachment strap, stump sock, and fluffed gauze at the distal portion of the stump. The fluffed gauze does not extend beyond the area indicated. (From Immediate postsurgical prosthetics, Washington, D. C., 1967, Veterans Administration.)

that closure is powered by stout bands of elastic rubber. Voluntary closing hooks remain open until the wearer activates the mechanism to close or pinch an object. This provides more delicate function, but the device is inclined to malfunction more frequently. A simple voluntary opening hook is the more efficient, functional, and trouble-free terminal device. It is the logical choice for the new amputee.

Mechanical hands are complex pieces of apparatus that are made in answer to the demand for better cosmetic appearance. In this they do quite well, for they do

simulate the form of the hand and a flesh-colored rubber glove adds a reasonable approximation to human skin. They operate on a voluntary closing principle. The dexterity they afford is less than that of the hook, and because they are intricate devices, they are subject to more frequent malfunction. Many amputees prefer the hook for everyday use and the mechanical hand for dress-up occasions.

Just as prosthesis design is more complex for the above-knee amputee than the below-knee amputee, so is it for the above-elbow amputee than for the below-elbow

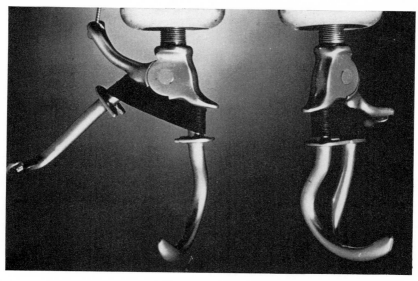

Fig. 406 A common type of voluntary opening hook. Opening is achieved when the wearer applies pull to the cable. Closure is powered by stout bands of elastic rubber. (Courtesy Prosthetic and Sensory Aids Service of the Veterans Administration, Washington, D. C.)

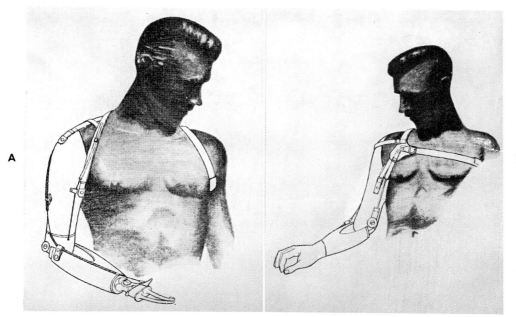

Fig. 407 A, Typical prosthesis for an above-elbow amputee. The voluntary opening hook is powered by a cable arrangement from the shoulder harness. Two cables are required for use of this prosthesis. **B,** The elbow disarticulation amputee requires a slightly different elbow joint. Note the mechanical hand and the harness. (From Wilson, A. B., Jr.: Limb prosthetics today, Artif Limbs **7:**1-42, Autumn 1963.)

amputee (Fig. 407). Elbow joint function must be replaced in order to place the hand at a desired position in space. This requires some kind of cable control to pro-

vide elbow flexion (forearm lift) and the elbow lock. Often the forearm lift is controlled by the same cable and shoulder harness as that which operates the terminal de-

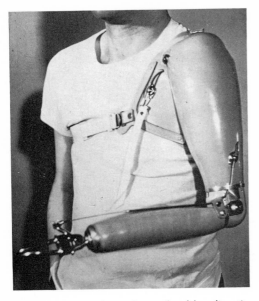

Fig. 408 The prosthesis for a shoulder disarticulation amputee has a larger, wider socket to receive the remaining shoulder. A hinge joint in the shoulder provides some passive motion. (Courtesy Prosthetic and Sensory Aids Service of the Veterans Administration, Washington, D. C.)

vice. The elbow lock control unit usually is operated by a separate control cable.

The shoulder disarticulation prosthesis (Fig. 408) varies from the above-elbow prosthesis in only two ways. A friction joint is provided in the shoulder region, which allows the wearer to preposition the shoulder joint for special uses. There is no mechanical device that activates the shoulder joint, and most of the time the shoulder remains by the side. The second difference is that an excellent power source for operation of control cables (humeral flexion) has been lost. Consequently, less convenient movements at a greater distance from the shoulder must be harnessed to operate the terminal device, the forearm lift, and the elbow lock.

The sockets for all upper extremity prostheses usually are made from plastic laminates that are individually constructed to fit each patient. Terminal devices, elbow joints, and other hardware are available in a variety of sizes. The harness is made of leather and heavy cotton-web belting. The axillary loop is coated with impervious, smooth plastic because of the constant

moisture and friction in the axilla. The control cables are mounted upon the harness in such a way that they derive power from the relative motion between two part of the body.

Training in use of prostheses. Immediately after receiving his prosthesis, the patient should again be seen by the prescription team. The prosthesis should be checked to see that it is satisfactory in every way. The stump should be checked for edema, joint contracture, and muscle strength. If faults exist, the appropriate therapy is instituted. As soon as it is determined that the prosthesis fits properly and consists of the components prescribed, training can begin. The amputee must not be allowed to attempt to put on the limb and begin using it without guidance—faulty habits and pressure sores cannot easily be undone.

The therapist's first job is to teach the amputee to care for the prosthesis and how to put on and to remove the aid himself. The patient should be instructed in the mechanisms of the prosthesis; every effort should be made to give him confidence that it will not collapse. To apply the typical above-knee prosthesis, the amputee places the wool stump sock over his stump. The stump is placed in the limb socket and the wearer settles his weight into it until he feels proper weight distribution on the proper place. The pelvic belt or harness is then buckled securely.

The patient is usually given instructions by the prosthetist in caring for his prosthesis or, if he is an elderly person, some member of the family may be provided with these instructions. With reasonable care, the length of useful wear is greatly increased beyond that of a prosthesis carelessly worn and cared for. The patient is instructed never to allow the limb to become excessively wet because this will do irreparable damage to the appliance.

Most prosthetists recommend that the prosthesis be cleaned at frequent intervals. The socket, at least, should be cleaned daily with mild soap and water. It is especially important that the socket be dried thoroughly after each use. The patient may be allowed to lubricate and to adjust the friction of certain hinges. The shoe worn on the prosthetic foot should not become excessively worn. Stockings may be held up by adhesive tape or by garters; the use of thumb tacks is discouraged. Hooks should not be used as tools to pry or hammer. Anything other than the most minor repairs should be performed by the prosthetist and should be done without delay. Preventive maintenance will greatly prolong wear.

The patient will need a period of intensive practice and learning to balance himself in this new limb before he attempts to walk with it. When he has mastered balance in standing with the new limb, he will be ready to take a few steps using the parallel bars. From this he graduates to crutches or to two canes that will later be discarded, one at a time. In crutch walking, a three-point crutch gait is advised; a four-point crutch gait is rarely prescribed. The patient should not be allowed to consider crutches or canes indispensable. The artificial limb is strong enough to support the patient if he learns to use it properly.

Since a fall may occur, the patient is taught how to fall as gracefully as possible and how to rise from the floor. When level walking has been mastered, ascending and descending stairs can be taught. Throughout the period of gait training, three essential points must be emphasized in teaching the patient to use the artificial limb. He must learn (1) to balance his body in good posture, (2) to use steps of equal length, and (3) to attain normal speed in walking.

One of the commonest errors observed in people who use artificial limbs is the rolling gait caused by abduction of the stump and prosthesis in taking a step. It is extremely difficult to overcome once it is acquired, and nurses should be alert to a tendency to walk in this fashion. The patient should not raise or hike his hip and shoulder on the amputated side as he walks.

Use training for the upper extremity amputee starts with operation of the terminal device. It may be necessary to strengthen the groups of muscles that power the terminal device. This is followed in the above-elbow amputee by learning to manage the elbow lock and forearm lift. One by one, such skills as using a knife and fork, tying shoelaces, and managing a billfold are mastered. Training emphasizes two-handed activities or those that require special techniques.

The patient sometimes becomes discouraged and frustrated during the period of training. The nurse should make every effort at this time to give special encouragement and commendation for his achievements. The major single cause for failure is lack of motivation.

Care of stump. Good care of the amputated stump is essential to continued successful use of a prosthesis. Skin problems of many sorts arise unless positive action is taken to avoid them. Enclosing the stump in an airtight container (the socket) inevitably leads to the accumulation of perspiration, skin waste products, and skin bacteria. Incubation of this mixture at normal body heat all day long produces a noxious brew. The slightest abrasion or ingrown hair quickly becomes a boil.

The stump should be washed thoroughly each night at bedtime with warm water and a mild soap. Thorough rinsing and drying also are essential. The stump should be kept free of irritating substances such as oil, alcohol, and medicated talcum powders. Iodine and strong disinfectants are never allowed. A high-quality, nonmedicated talcum may be used occasionally. During initial use training especially, the stump should be inspected frequently for red spots, blisters, and boils. The patient should be specifically asked whether he has any pinched or painful areas. If the slightest skin irritation is in evidence, wearing of the prosthesis should be discontinued until the stump and the socket are checked by the physician. Neglect of these apparently innocent friction spots can lead to serious problems that may make the fit of any future prosthesis difficult.

A stump sock, which is worn with the lower extremity prosthesis, should be made of pure virgin wool. The patient will need two or three of these because they must be changed at least once daily. In hot weather more changes will be needed. Socks should never be used if they are torn, patched, or roughened, and they should fit snugly except at the end. Wrinkles in the sock will inevitably lead to irritation and discomfort. These socks need special washing care. They should be washed with mild soap in lukewarm water and rinsed several times. Woolite used in cold water is quite satisfactory. The wool sock should be squeezed dry, not wrung, then spread flat or placed on a sock stretcher to dry. A rubber ball of proper size will help maintain shape of the distal end. Three measurements are needed when ordering stump socks; the circumference of the upper rim of the socket, the circumference of the distal end of the stump, and the length of the stump (distal end of stump to the place where the upper rim of the prosthesis strikes the leg, plus a couple of inches to turn back over the socket of the prosthesis).

Some shrinkage may continue in the stump over a period of years, and it is not unusual to find patients attempting to fill the space between the stump and the socket by wearing more and more stump socks. If it is discovered that the patient is wearing three or four of these to raise the stump, he should be advised to contact the prosthetist because a new socket liner or even a new socket may be necessary. The maximum number of stump socks worn at one time should not exceed two.

Phantom limb sensations are experienced by some adult amputees after removal of the limb. These are usually not distressing to the patient, and upon direct questioning he is likely to regard them as a curiosity. Over a period of years, the feelings from the absent limb seem to shrink into the stump gradually until the phantom sensation is gone altogether. Distressing phantom limb pains are fortunately a rather rare occurrence—1% to 2% of all amputations. When present, the amputee often feels that the absent toes are being pinched and squeezed or being burned. The phantom limb pains may not make their appearance until years after amputation. Invariably there is a heavy emotional overlay, and these patients can think and talk of nothing else. The cause of the phantom limb pain is not clear. Many types of operative procedures have been devised, but little seems to benefit the wretched condition of patients suffering from this sensation.

On the other hand, true neuroma formation is a fairly frequent condition. Actually, this is the natural reparative reaction (attempted regrowth) of any peripheral nerve that has been cut. If the neuroma is in a location subject to pressure or trauma, it may become quite sensitive. It is characterized by electric or lightning-like pains that are triggered at one well-localized spot. Surgical removal of the offending neuroma is usually very beneficial.

In children with amputations, bony overgrowth of the amputated limb is a common complication. The explanation for this phenomenon is not clear, but the bone simply outstrips the surrounding soft tissue in its growth. Again, resection of the excessive bone is usually necessary, and this may have to be repeated several times until the growth of the skeleton ceases.

The community health nurse inspecting a prosthesis on a home visit should observe the apparatus for loose or worn joints, for signs of deterioration in rubber, leather, or other fabrics, and for signs of wearing or cracking in the wood or plastic. Any of these are indications that the prosthesis should be seen by the prosthetist at the earliest possible moment. The nurse also should observe the number and condition of the stump socks that the patient is using. The skin of the stump should be inspected for swelling or irritation, and the nurse should inquire about the stump hygiene routine. The patients should be reminded that any abnormality or discomfort (such as swelling, redness, blisters, irritation, or induration) is a danger signal that needs immediate attention. When these things occur, he must stop weight bearing until suitable adjustment can be made in the socket of his prosthesis.

The nurse also may observe the patient's walking habits to see that he is making the best mechanical use of the prosthesis. Poor walking habits acquired early by the wearer of an artificial limb are extremely hard to overcome, but considerable improvement is often possible if the patient understands what is expected of him and if he is given practical suggestions for increasing his ability to use the limb more effectively.

Rehabilitation of amputee

Rehabilitation ideally should start before the patient enters the hospital for amputation. As previously stated, psychologic problems in the well-prepared patient are minimal. The average patient of today is likely to be much more cooperative and less subject to emotional shock if he is provided in advance with a reasonable expectation of what he is to experience. Often the surgeon will give the patient a general explanation of this, including a rough timetable not only of events during hospitalization but also of postoperative office visits up to the time when the stump is ready for limb prescription. The doctor also will tell the patient in a general way what activities he can reasonably expect to do after training with his new limb. It is not within the scope of nurses' training or responsibility to provide this information. They should be prepared, however, to answer the patient's direct questions as honestly as possible. If any doubt exists, the questions should be referred to the doctor, but cheerful reassurance can be a source of great comfort to the patient at this time. On the other hand, unfounded optimism can be extremely cruel.

The young person who has had a single-limb amputation and who has been fitted with a prosthesis and trained in its proper use should be able to carry on an active self-supporting life. His family and friends should recognize that the greatest help they can give him is to treat him as normally as possible. The problem of the person with two amputations is manifestly more com-

plex. It is absolutely necessary that such persons be given the benefit of the specialized therapy—physical, diversional, and vocational—that will enable them to attain the maximum degree of independence.

When amputation has resulted from some systemic disease, vitality is usually lowered and habits of invalidism are easily acquired. The patient may tend to prefer a wheelchair rather than to struggle with the problems associated with the use of an artificial limb. As his general health improves, however, the patient should be encouraged to resume his normal activities insofar as possible. Sensible goals set for him to work toward, accompanied by encouragement and an attitude of hopefulness on the part of the community health nurse, will often pay dividends in the patient's increased capacity and willingness to care for his own needs.

Amputees as a group offer better results in terms of returning to social and economic independence than do patients with many other major maladies—e.g., blindness and paraplegia. The chief cause for failure in rehabilitation of the amputee is lack of motivation. In this regard, the nurse can be of enormous benefit to the patient.

Unit V STUDY QUESTIONS

SPECIAL OPERATIVE PROCEDURES

1 Define the following terms:
  a Arthrotomy
  b Arthrodesis
  c Arthroplasty
  d Arthroscopy
  e Ankylosis
  f Tenotomy
  g Osteotomy
  h Fusion
2 Discuss the pathologic changes within a joint that necessitate total joint replacement.
3 What benefits should a patient expect following total joint replacement?
4 Discuss the complications that may develop following a total hip replacement and the care needed to prevent or minimize the possibility of their occurrence.
5 Describe the procedure for giving back care and changing bed linen for the patient in traction who must remain in the supine position.
6 Discuss nursing intervention measures that may be utilized to prevent the development of:
  a A hip-flexion contracture
  b A knee-flexion contracture
7 The knee immobilizer is frequently used following a total knee replacement. Explain.
8 Quadriceps-setting and gluteal muscle–setting exercises usually are prescribed following surgery of the hip joint, as well as dorsiflexion and plantar flexion of the ankle joint. Describe these exercises and explain why they are necessary.

THE PATIENT UNDERGOING AMPUTATION SURGERY

1 Care of the patient after an amputation includes prevention of contractures in adjacent joints.
  a Describe types of contractures most likely to develop following (1) below-knee amputation and (2) above-knee amputation.
  b Discuss care necessary to prevent each of these contractures.
2 Describe method of applying a compression bandage following a midthigh amputation.
3 Early application of a prosthesis and early ambulation are being advocated for the lower-limb amputee. Discuss advantages the patient may gain from the activity.

Unit V REFERENCES

SPECIAL OPERATIVE PROCEDURES

1 Adkins, E. W. O.: Posterior-lateral fusion of the spine, Physiotherapy 60:34-36, Feb 1974.
2 Amstutz, H. C.: Complications of total hip replacement, Clin Orthop 72:123-137, Sep-Oct 1970.
3 Aufranc, O. E., and Turner, R. H.: Total replacement of the arthritic hip, Hosp Pract 6:66-81, Oct 1971.
4 Auld, M., Craven, R., and West, J.: Wound healing, Nursing (Jenkintown) 2:36-40, Oct 1972.
5 Bain, A. M.: Surgical treatment of osteoarthrosis, Physiotherapy 59:47-52, Feb 1973.
6 Bennage, B., and Cummings, M.: Nursing the patient undergoing total hip arthroplasty, Nurs Clin North Am 8:107-116, Mar 1973.
7 Bowden, S.: New surgery for arthritic hands, Nursing (Jenkintown) 6:46-48, Aug 1976.
8 Bryan, R. S., and Lowell, F. A. P.: The quest for the replacement knee, Orthop Clin North Am 2:715-728, Nov 1971.
9 Buck, B. I.: Total hip replacement, Superv Nurse 3:74-76 passim, May 1972.
10 Casscells, S. W., and Eilert, R. E.: Arthroscopy: an informative way to view the knee, Mod Med 43:41-42, 1 Jun 1975.
11 Clayton, M. L.: Care of the rheumatoid hip, Clin Orthop 90:70-76, Jan-Feb 1973.
12 Cockin, J.: Osteotomy of the hip, Orthop Clin North Am 2:59-74, Mar 1974.
13 Convery, F. R., and Beber, C. A.: Total knee arthroplasty, Clin Orthop 94:42-47, Jul-Aug 1973.
14 Coventry, M. B.: Treatment of infections occurring in total hip surgery, Orthop Clin North Am 6:991-1003, Oct 1975.
15 Dee, R.: Total replacement arthroplasty of the elbow for rheumatoid arthritis, J Bone Joint Surg [Br] 54:88-95, Feb 1972.
16 Demopoulos, J. T., and Selman, L.: Rehabilitation following total hip replacement, Arch Phys Med Rehabil 53:51-59, Feb 1972.
17 Donn, M. C.: Right total hip replacement, Nurs Times 70:1654-1657, 24 Oct 1974.
18 Drain, C. B.: The athletic knee injury, Am J Nurs 71:536-537, Mar 1971.
19 Evarts, C. M., editor: Symposium on interposition and implant arthroplasty, Orthop Clin North Am 4:235-596, Apr 1973.
20 Eyre, M. K.: Total hip replacement, Am J Nurs 71:1384-1387, Jul 1971.
21 Farrell, J.: Pulmonary embolism, ONA J 2:14-16, Jan 1975.

22 Farrell, J.: Fat embolism, ONA J 2:41-42, Feb 1975.

23 Givilliam, S.: Total knee arthroplasty, Can Nurse 70:33-36, Sep 1974.

24 Goodyear, M.: Arthroscopy, ONA J 3:190, Jun 1976.

25 Gossling, H. R., Ellison, L. H., and Degraff, A. C., Jr.: Fat embolism; the role of respiratory failure and its treatment, J Bone Joint Surg [Am] 56:1327-1337, Oct 1974.

26 Graves, S., and Vincent, S.: Total hip replacement is a family affair, RN 34:35-41, Jun 1971.

27 Guy, F. M.: Implants used in orthopaedic surgery. Part 1, Nurs Times 68:463-466, 20 Apr 1972.

28 Guy, F. M.: Implants used in orthopaedic surgery. Part 2, Nurs Times 68:500-503, 27 Apr 1972.

29 Harrold, A. J.: Internal derangements of the knee, Nurs Times 67:1575-1577, Dec 1971.

30 Herbert, J. J., and Alain, H.: A new total knee prosthesis, Clin Orthop 94:202-210, Jul-Aug 1973.

31 Hughes, M., and Neer, C. S.: Glenohumeral joint replacement and postoperative rehabilitation, Phys Ther 55:850-858, Aug 1975.

32 Jackson, J. P.: Internal derangement of the knee, Nurs Times 72:651-654, 29 Apr 1976.

33 Jennings, K.: The cheerful operation: total hip replacement, Nursing (Jenkintown) 6:32-37, Jul 1976.

34 Johnson, C. F., and Convery, F. R.: Preventing emboli after total hip replacement, Am J Nurs 75:804-806, May 1975.

35 Jones, V., and Killian, M.: Pulmonary embolism, ONA J 2:170-172, Jul 1975.

36 Kettlekamp, D. B., and Leach, R. B., guest editors: Symposium: Total knee replacement, Clin Orthop 94:2-256, Jul-Aug 1973.

37 Kluge, L. B.: The Walldius prosthesis; a total treatment program, Phys Ther 52:26-33, Jan 1972.

38 Longton, E. B.: Orthopaedic surgery in arthritic lower-limb joints, Physiotherapy 59:116-119, Apr 1973.

39 McFarland, M. B.: Fat embolism syndrome, Am J Nurs 76:1942-1944, Dec 1976.

40 McKee, G. K.: Development of total prosthetic replacement of the hip, Clin Orthop 72:85-103, Sep-Oct 1970.

41 Morris, J. M.: Biomechanical aspects of the hip joint, Orthop Clin North Am 2:33-54, Mar 1971.

42 Müller, M. E.: Total hip prostheses, Clin Orthop 72:46-68, Sep-Oct 1970.

43 Neufeld, A. J.: Modern metals in orthopedic implant surgery, ONA J 1:59-61, Oct 1974.

44 Nute, L. F., Rhine, P., Mott, C., Shoemaker, A., Noel, K., and Prete, J.: Nursing care of patient undergoing a total hip arthroplasty, ONA J 3:43-54, Feb 1976.

45 Parks, V.: Arthroscopy, Nurs Times 71:2058-2059, 25 Dec 1975.

46 Rockwell, S. M.: Total hip replacement: the OR nurse's role, RN 34:1-9, Jun 1971.

47 Rosenberg, E. F.: Total hip replacement; viewpoint of a rheumatologist, Postgrad Med 51:124-127, Apr 1972.

48 Sculco, C. D., and Sculco, T. P.: Management of the patient with an infected total hip arthroplasty, Am J Nurs 76:584-587, Apr 1976.

49 Shoemaker, R. R.: Total knee replacement, Nurs Clin North Am 8:117-125, Mar 1973.

50 Thomas, B. J.: Total knee: new surgical miracle, RN 36:36-39, Sep 1973.

51 Townley, C., and Hill, L.: Total knee replacement, Am J Nurs 74:1612-1617, Sep 1974.

52 Waters, E. A.: Physical therapy management of patients with total knee replacement, Phys Ther 54:936-942, Sep 1974.

53 Wilde, A. H.: Synovectomy of the knee, Orthop Clin North Am 2:191-205, Mar 1971.

THE PATIENT UNDERGOING AMPUTATION SURGERY

54 Alves, R., and Martin, T.: An overview of orthotics and prosthetics, ONA J 4:231-235, Sep 1977.

55 Arnold, H. M.: Elderly diabetic amputees, Am J Nurs 69:2646-2649, Dec 1969.

56 Baker, W. H., Barnes, R. W., and Shurr, D.: The healing of below-knee amputations, Am J Surg 133:716-718, Jun 1977.

57 Bosanko, L. A.: Immediate postoperative prosthesis, Am J Nurs 71:280-283, 1971.

58 Buck, B., and Lee, A.: Amputation: two views, Nurs Clin North Am 11:641-657, Dec 1976.

59 Burgess, E., Traub, J., and Wilson, A. B.: Immediate postsurgical prosthetics in the management of lower extremity amputees, Washington, D. C., 1967 U. S. Government Printing Office.

60 Cantrell, D.: The child with missing arm or leg, ONA J 3:90-92, Mar 1976.

60a Cheney, R.: Immediate postsurgical prosthetics in the management of below-knee amputees, ONA J 4:260-263, Oct 1977.

61 Compere, C. L.: Early fitting of prostheses following amputation, Surg Clin North Am 48:215-226, Feb 1968.

62 Cummings, G. S., and Girling, J.: A clinical assessment of immediate postoperative fitting of prosthesis for amputee rehabilitation, Phys Ther 51:1007-1012, Sep 1971.

63 Davies, E. J., Friz, B. R., and Clippinger, F. W.: Amputees and their prostheses, Artif Limbs 14:19-48, Autumn 1970.

64 Engstrand, J. L.: Rehabilitation of the patient with a lower extremity amputation, Nurs Clin North Am 11:659-669, Dec 1976.

65 Fansa, M. R., and Helal, B.: A symposium on carpal tunnel syndrome; surgical treatment, Nurs Mirror 142:47-50, 10 June 1976.

66 Fliegel, O., and Feuer, S. G.: Historical development of lower-extremity prostheses, Arch Phys Med Rehabil 47:275-285, May 1966.

67 Friedmann, L. W., and Friedmann, L.: The quality of hope for the amputee, Arch Surg 110:760, Jun 1975.

68 Gerhardt, J. J., King, P. S., Peirson, G. A.,

Fowlks, E. W., and Altman, D. C.: Immediate post-surgical prosthetics: rehabilitation aspects, Am J Phys Med 49:3-105, Feb 1970.

69 Golbranson, F. L., Asbelle, C., and Strand, D.: Immediate postsurgical fitting and early ambulation; a new concept in amputee rehabilitation, Clin Orthop 56:119-131, Jan-Feb 1968.

70 Harding, J. M.: Amputation of the lower limb, Nurs Times 70:1025-1027, 4 Jul 1974.

71 Holt, P. J.: Upper-limb endoprostheses, Physiotherapy 59:112-115, Apr 1973.

72 Jones, C.: Nursing care study; above-knee amputation, Nurs Mirror 138:77-80, 7 Jun 1974.

73 Jordan, H. S., and Cypres, R.: All-around care for the leg amputee, Nursing (Jenkintown) 4:51-55, Apr 1974.

74 Kirkpatrick, S.: Battle casualty: amputee, Am J Nurs 68:998-1005, May 1968.

75 Knapp, M. E.: Lower-extremity amputations and prosthetics; prosthetics, Postgrad Med 44:259-264, Nov 1968.

76 Knapp, M. E.: Lower-extremity amputations and prosthetics; surgical considerations, Postgrad Med 44:259-264, Oct 1968.

77 McClinton, V. S.: Nursing of the upper extremity amputee and preparation for prosthetic training, Nurs Clin North Am 11:671-677, Dec. 1976.

78 Martin, N.: Rehabilitation of the upper extremity amputee, Nurs Outlook 18:50-51, Feb 1970.

79 Pasnau, R., and Pfefferbaum, B.: Psychologic aspects of postamputation pain, Nurs Clin North Am 11:679-685, Dec 1976.

80 Patterson, T., Loche, M., and Flournoy, M.: Traumatic amputation, Nursing (Jenkintown) 2:40-45, 1972.

81 Plaisted, L. M., and Friz, B. R.: The nurse on the amputee clinic team, Nurs Outlook 16:34-37, Oct 1968.

82 Sarmiento, A.: Recent trends in lower extremity amputation, Nurs Clin North Am 2:399-408, Sep 1967.

83 Sarmiento, A., editor: Symposium on amputation surgery and prosthetics, Orthop Clin North Am 3:265-494, Jul 1972.

84 Soules, B. J.: Thalidomide victims in a rehabilitation center, Am J Nurs 66:2023-2026, Sep 1966.

85 Staros, A., and Gardner, H. F.: Direct forming of below-knee PTB sockets with a thermoplastic material, Artif Limbs 14:57-54, Spring 1970.

86 Stolov, W. C., Burgess, E. M., and Romano, R. L.: Progression of weight bearing after immediate prosthesis fitting following below-knee amputation, Arch Phys Med Rehabil 52:491-502, Nov 1971.

87 Thompson, A.: An early walking aid for geriatric amputees, Physiotherapy 57:585-588, Dec 1971.

88 Tooms, R. E.: Amputations. In Crenshaw, A. H., editor: Campbell's Operative orthopaedics, ed. 5, St. Louis, 1971, The C. V. Mosby Co.

89 Warren, R.: Early rehabilitation of the elderly lower extremity amputee, Surg Clin North Am 48:807-816, Aug 1968.

90 Wiley, L., editor: Traumatic amputation, Nursing (Jenkintown) 2:40-45, Nov 1972.

91 Wilson, A. B., Jr.: Limb prosthetics—1970, Artif Limbs 14:1-52, Spring 1970.

92 Wilson, A. B., Jr.: A material for direct forming of prosthetic sockets, Artif Limbs 14:53-56, Spring 1970.

93 Zalewski, N., Geronemus, D., Siegel, H.: Hemipelvectomy: the triumph of Ms. A., Am J Nurs 73:2073-2077, Dec 1973.

Unit VI
REHABILITATIVE ASPECTS OF ORTHOPEDIC NURSING

22 General considerations in rehabilitation

Rehabilitation as we know it envisions a total effort directed at restoration of the abilities of a physically handicapped person to lead a happy and useful life. Total effort means surgical correction, functional restoration through exercise, special education, vocational training, and, finally, employment (Fig. 409). Rehabilitative aspects of patient care must begin as soon as the patient enters the hospital. A team of health workers combine their efforts to meet this responsibility. Rehabilitation, for the sake of discussion here, will refer to the medical segment of the total effort. Obviously, not all handicapped persons are equally capable of complete rehabilitation.

Many of the hospitals have established rehabilitation units where efforts on the purely physical elements of restoration can be concentrated. This includes medical direction of physical therapy, occupational therapy, speech therapy, brace-fitting, rehabilitative nursing, psychologic evaluation, and on-the-spot work training. A pat-

tern of treatment that will help achieve maximum rehabilitation is available for patients with many physical defects, such as those resulting from paraplegia, amputation, hemiplegia, and cerebral palsy. The Army rehabilitation centers in World War II showed how special exercises after acute trauma can hasten recovery. Graduated exercise programs, including heavy resistance exercises, are now commonplace therapy after surgical operations on bones and joints. The field is so broad that it would be impossible to outline all the details here, but discussions throughout this book have included rehabilitation as applied to specific conditions.

Development of healthy attitudes toward handicapped persons

Irresponsible sentimentality and excessive sympathy are not conducive to rehabilitation. Nurses should avoid such shallow responses to the handicapped person. They must recognize and control their

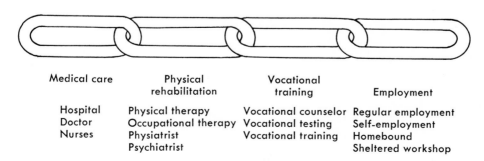

Medical care	Physical rehabilitation	Vocational training	Employment
Hospital	Physical therapy	Vocational counselor	Regular employment
Doctor	Occupational therapy	Vocational testing	Self-employment
Nurses	Physiatrist	Vocational training	Homebound
	Psychiatrist		Sheltered workshop

Fig. 409 Concept of total rehabilitation.

emotional reactions to physical disabilities. It is paramount that they avoid doing too much for the person. Rather, they should work with the handicapped individual to encourage and help him to master doing things for himself. Threaded through orthopedic nursing is the need not only for helping the person with a handicap to become capable of functioning independently but also for helping him to develop the desire and motivation to help himself. This thread must run through all nursing care for the handicapped and through teaching the patient's family. A nurse may feel a desire to protect and indulge the patient and care for his wants so solicitously that he has no need to do anything for himself. This desire is often even more potent among members of the patient's family and may seem good and natural to them. To the parents, the rehabilitative procedures used for a handicapped child may seem almost cruel, and they may call the nurse heartless and insensitive. On the other hand, parents, in trying to create greater self-reliance in their crippled child by showing a little healthy neglect, may be criticized by their neighbors.

To avoid overprotection of the handicapped person, one must teach him not only to care for his own needs insofar as he is able, but also to take responsibility for his mistakes and misdeeds. If the patient has had such training at home, the nurse should recognize the importance of doing nothing to undermine it in spite of personal feelings. In many cases, the individual has not been taught these things at home. Occasionally, tyrannical traits in the patient will be observed when his family visits him. The nurse should be aware that the incomparable experience in communal living that is given this overprotected person in an orthopedic unit is not the least of the benefits he may receive in the hospital. Sharing his pleasures with the other patients and, in turn, sharing theirs and assuming his share of responsibility for misdemeanors will perhaps be new to him, but the nurse should recognize the opportunity to use these experiences as first steps in his long fight for social and emotional maturity. The wise nurse points out and makes purposeful these problems in everyday living. Properly directed, the experi-ence should be highly beneficial to the handicapped person. It should help him adjust to other disabled individuals and to his nonhandicapped companions. It should help to prepare him to live with greater harmony in his own family. It may serve also to help overcome a crippled attitude of mind—a more serious disability, after all, than a crippled spine.

Rehabilitation team

In rehabilitation, the nurse always work as a member of a team. The team includes all those who are in some way contributing toward the total care of the patient, whether it be physical, psychologic, social, spiritual, or vocational. The team, always working under the leadership of the physician, may consist of the hospital nurse and assistants, the community nurse, the psychologist, the physical and occupational therapists, the chaplain, the teacher, the social worker, the speech therapist, the vocational counselor, the parents or family, and, last but not least, the patient himself.

For everyone working with a team, it is extremely important that the common objectives be clearly recognized. It is equally important to learn how to work with people. It often may be necessary to subordinate one's own ego for the good of the whole group. The complete rehabilitation of a patient may require more of one group of workers than it does of another at certain stages of the program, but there are actually no stars on the team except the patient.

Rehabilitation teamwork demands that the nurse, particularly the hospital nurse, have long-range perspectives. The time that the patient being rehabilitated spends in the hospital is, as a rule, only a small period compared with the long years that he may have been or will be disabled. The nurse should look both backward and forward. There was a time, before the disability occurred, when the patient lived as a normal member of a family and a community. Then the illness or accident happened that changed him from a normal person to one with a handicap. There may have been a period before he decided, perhaps with considerable anxiety and dread, to submit himself for treatment. Then there is a brief but intensive period

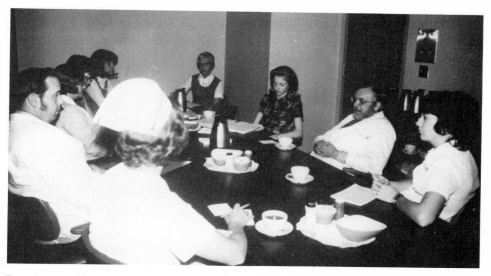

Fig. 410 In a rehabilitation team conference, the physician, nurses, physical and occupational therapists, social worker, and speech therapist discuss the progress of a patient and plans for further care.

of treatment in the hospital where nurses, occupational and physical therapists, and others work with the surgeon on physical restoration or on some reconstructive problem that in itself is only a beginning. He will then return to his home, his family, and his community to continue the treatment begun in the hospital. There may be a new group working with him, including perhaps the social worker, the community nurse, and the visiting physical therapist. Other therapists may help round out his functional recovery. It is a long road on which the patient meets many people working to help him.

The more aware hospital nurses are of the road the patient has traveled beforehand and of the distance he must go before reaching maximum recovery, the more intelligent and unselfish will be their contribution to the rehabilitation team.

It is sometimes difficult to work harmoniously with other groups when one is under pressure. Often it seems that there are endless conflicts in aims and methods, and one may feel that there is a great deal of pulling in opposite directions. It is vital for the efficiency of the program that such conflicts be resolved as soon as they occur. Frequent conferences between groups with opportunities to discuss troublesome problems are bound to pay divi-

dends in easier working relationships. The goal of all team members is the same: to assist the patient in his fight for recovery and rehabilitation (Fig. 410).

What can the nurses do to promote better working relationships with other clinical groups?

First and more important, they can develop a cordial spirit for other people working in the rehabilitation area. Since nurses may feel more at home on the unit, they are able to make other persons who work there feel comfortable and welcome.

Second, nurses must seek to learn as much as possible about the work of other clinical workers, including the aims of treatment of various team members, the problems, and many of the skills and therapeutic techniques that enter into the care of the patient. It will be necessary to encourage the patient to carry out correctly the instructions agreed upon by the team. Without follow-through, the relatively brief periods the patient spends with a therapist may be of little lasting value. The nurse must supervise the patient's practice of the exercises given to him, or he may be slipshod in their performance, knowing that the therapist is not there to observe him. Also, the nurse must work with other team members and with the

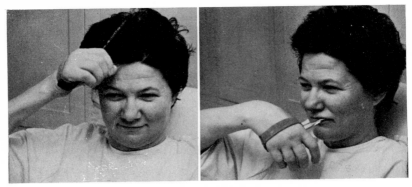

Fig. 411 By using the leather holder, this quadriplegic is able to comb her hair and to brush her teeth.

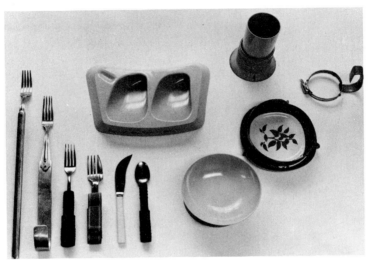

Fig. 412 Mechanical aids that facilitate self-feeding for the person with weakness or paralysis of the muscles of the upper extremity. Suction-cup dishes that adhere to the table and have divided compartments make getting food onto the spoon easier. Padded or enlarged handles may make it possible for the disabled person to grasp the eating utensil.

social worker to plan a coordinated home program to fit the needs and capabilities of the patient. Instructions given to family or patient should be a joint responsibility, and conferences should be held frequently so that no overlapping or omissions occur.

Third, the nurse should help prepare the patient to go to the occupational or physical therapy departments, to the school, or to the speech therapist by caring for his basic needs. He should be clean and dressed, and he should have had an opportunity to use the bedpan or urinal before he goes. If he is scheduled for walking exercises, his braces should be correctly applied and his crutches placed

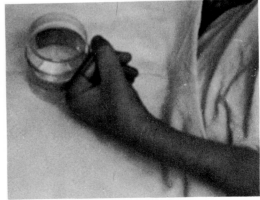

Fig. 413 This glass holder enables the person who is unable to grasp objects with his fingers to drink from a glass.

beside him. He should be sent on time; if some unavoidable emergency makes this impossible, the department should be notified so that the therapist can rearrange his schedule with as little time loss as possible. The attitude of nursing personnel toward the therapy should be positive and cooperative.

It must be assumed that each worker on the rehabilitation team is trying sincerely to aid the patient's full recovery. However, unless one views the recovery process in its entirety, it may resemble a jigsaw puzzle, with each worker concentrating on his own phase of the work to the exclusion of the others. The central theme is always the patient. He is the focal point. The pieces of the puzzle must be fitted together for his benefit with tolerance, understanding, and mutual respect. This will result in a coordinated program for the patient and in more satisfaction and sense of accomplishment for the workers themselves.

The whole truth, Steindler once wrote, cannot come from a solitary voice. Similarly, planned rehabilitation does not come from a solitary pair of hands. The nurse who recognizes and wholeheartedly accepts this will occupy an important role on the rehabilitation team with great benefit to the patient and with a feeling of professional satisfaction.

Various aspects of rehabilitation nursing

The basic principles and practices used in good nursing care are applicable and essential in rehabilitation nursing. In fact, they are the essence of rehabilitation nursing.

Good hygienic care is very important for the handicapped patient. It not only is conducive to good physical health, but also has value in sustaining morale and a sense of well-being. The patient is taught and encouraged to care independently for as many of his personal needs as possible. Longer periods of time must be allowed for him to complete these activities. Considerable patience is required of the nurse who works with an encourages the disabled patient to manipulate his own toothbrush or cup or to manage his own brace. Which mechanical aids can be used? Can the patient with weakness of the upper extremities be taught to feed himself and to

brush his own teeth? One no longer concentrates on doing things to or for the patient but thinks in terms of how the patient might do it for himself (Figs. 411 to 413).

Maintaining good nutrition is important in the care of the patient undergoing rehabilitation. A strenuous exercise program increases his nutritional requirements. The paralyzed patient needs adequate intake of protein to help prevent breakdown of the skin and underlying tissues. The individual with an arm or hand disability may experience fatigue when feeding himself and not consume an adequate diet unless help is offered. The problems of the overweight patient must not be forgotten. Extra pounds may make ambulation impossible. At mealtime, the nurse who understands what the rehabilitee is being taught by the occupational therapist can help him practice self-feeding. If he can learn to feed himself, mealtime can become a sociable hour. This is important for the handicapped person attempting to find his place in family and community life. A dining room equipped with tables that accommodate wheelchairs provides a more normal situation for practicing the activities of daily living.

Prevention of decubitus ulcers is another important aspect of rehabilitation

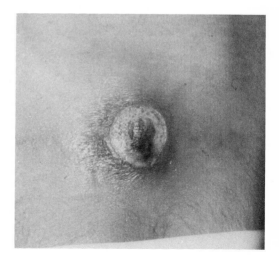

Fig. 414 Decubitus ulcer on the sacrum of a quadriplegic. Muscle paralysis, sensory loss, leakage from a Foley catheter, and failure to turn the patient frequently were factors contributing to this lesion.

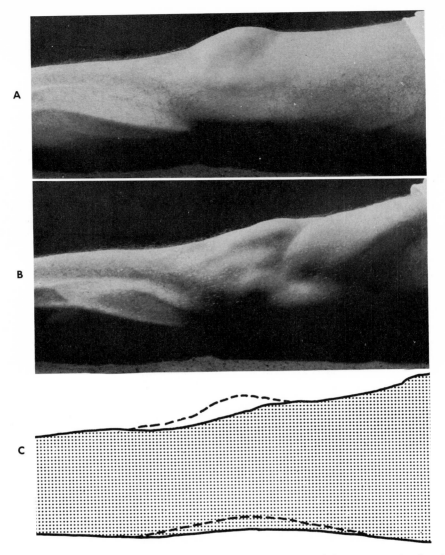

Fig. 415 Quadriceps-setting exercise. **A,** Relaxed thigh and knee joint. **B,** Quadriceps muscle located on the anterior thigh is tightened and shortened, moving the patella proximally. **C,** Movement of the patella proximally and pressing of the popliteal space against the mattress. (**A** and **B,** From Gould, M. L.: Internal derangement of the knee—nursing care, Am J Nurs **56:**577-582, May 1956.)

nursing. Many patients are paralyzed in one or more extremities. Frequently, incontinence is a problem. One or both of these factors make the maintenance of healthy skin a real challenge to nursing personnel (Fig. 414). (See Chapter 4 for details.)

Regardless of the cause of disability, the prevention of deformity is important from the onset. Emphasis is placed on teaching the handicapped individual and

his family how joint deformity can be prevented. "An ounce of prevention is worth a pound of cure" was never more applicable than in the prevention of secondary joint deformity. Those of us who have seen patients spend weeks receiving treatment directed at the correction of contractures, to say nothing of the pain endured, can appreciate the importance of their prevention. Applying knowledge of proper body alignment, providing for fre-

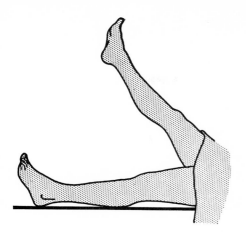

Fig. 416 Performing straight leg-raising exercises develops the strength of the quadriceps muscle. (From Gould, M. L.: Internal derangement of the knee—nursing care, Am J Nurs **56**:577-582, May 1956.)

quent change of position, and maintaining a normal range of joint motion are necessary if deformity is to be prevented.

During the bath, the nurse can easily perform simple passive exercises of the involved extremities to help maintain normal range of motion (see Chapter 3). In addition to exercises of the involved extremities by the nurse or therapist, the disabled patient is taught and encouraged to do simple exercises of the uninvolved extremities himself early in the course of his care. Such exercises are valuable in improving circulation, in maintaining muscle strength, and in preventing tightness of tendons and limitation of joint motion.

While working with the patient, the nurse should observe whether the patient is able to point his foot downward (plantar flexion) and also if he is able to turn his foot inward (inversion) and to pull his foot up (dorsiflexion). These activities are valuable in preventing drop-foot deformity and tightness of the heel cord.

Can the patient tighten the quadriceps muscle? This muscle, located on the anterior portion of the thigh, enables one to extend and stabilize the knee, and it is important in maintaining erect posture. The quadriceps-setting exercise is taught with the patient in the supine position and with the limb in extension. He is instructed to contract the muscles on the anterior

portion of the thigh so that the kneecap is drawn upward toward the thigh. He maintains the muscle contraction for five seconds and then allows the muscle to relax for five seconds. The physician may request that the patient do this exercise for five minutes every hour during the waking day. Straight leg raising is another exercise frequently prescribed to strengthen the quadriceps muscle. In the supine position, with the knee in extension and the foot in a neutral position, the patient lifts the limb off the bed. At first this is difficult, but with practice the limb can be raised to approximately a 45° angle with the body. This position is held for several seconds and then the limb is lowered slowly (Figs. 415 and 416).

If tightness of the hamstrings (flexion contracture) is to be prevented, the knee joint should not be supported continuously in a flexed position. The position of extension must be secured at frequent intervals.

Does the patient lie or sit with his limb in a position of external rotation? A sandbag or tochanter roll placed along the lateral aspect of the thigh will encourage him to maintain the limb in a neutral position. Does he like to have the backrest elevated, or does he sit in a chair for long periods? To avoid flexion contractures of the hips, he needs to lie flat (on a firm mattress) with the hips in full extension. Can he abduct and externally rotate his arms to tie his gown strings and comb his hair, or have his pectoral muscles become too tight?

Is full extension of the cervical spine attained at intervals throughout the day and night, or is the patient lying with marked flexion of the neck? The nurse should remember that maintaining this position for long periods of time promotes poor posture and impairs normal respiratory expansion.

The rehabilitation unit is an ideal place for the patient to practice the activities of daily living. Whether the task is learning to dress, to brush his teeth, to get from the bed to a chair, or to perform exercises in preparation for walking on crutches, the nurse who keeps informed of the plan of treatment and the progress that the patient is making can render valuable

Text continued on p. 436.

EVALUATION OF DAILY LIVING ACTIVITIES
OCCUPATIONAL THERAPY

Name _____ Birth date _____ Age _____ Sex _____

Address/Hospital No. _____

Diagnosis _____ Date onset _____

Vocation _____ Handedness _____

KEY

(Scores indicate skill accomplished within a reasonable time)

0—Cannot be accomplished

1—Can be accomplished with human aid

2—Can be accomplished with adaptation of environment (low bed, special toilet seat, handrails, ramps, etc.)

3—Can be accomplished with use of mechanical aids (splints, braces, prostheses, crutches, wheelchair, etc.)

4—Can be accomplished without aids, adaptation, or assistance

*—Not practical (time, too much supervision required)

N.A.—Not applicable to this patient

Date and √ form on initial test.

Any changes in status from initial test should be dated.

HOME SITUATION

Note suggestions for adaptation next to each line or check when so indicated. In special instances, diagram of layout will be advisable.

Location: City _____ Rural _____

Travel: Own car _____ Hand controls _____ Taxi _____ Bus _____

Apartment: Floor _____ Rooms _____ Elevator _____ Self-service _____ None _____ Walk up _____

Private house: Floors _____ Rooms _____ Stairs _____ Elevator _____ Self-service _____ None _____

Entrance: Door _____ Step _____ Railing: _____ right _____ left _____ none _____ Ramp _____

Bathroom: Door _____ OK for wheelchair _____ Tub _____ Shower over tub _____ Stall shower _____

Note types of floors: Bedroom _____ Living room _____ Kitchen _____ Bath _____

Information unavailable (explain)

Assistive devices

I BED ACTIVITIES	0	1	2	3	4
1 Moving in bed: Roll to right _____ to left _____					
2 Turn onto abdomen _____					
3 Come to sitting position _____					
4 Sit erect in bed (LSP) _____					
5 Sit on edge of bed (SSP) _____					
6 Adjust blanket, sheets, etc. _____					
7 _____					

II WHEELCHAIR SKILLS					
1 Bed to wheelchair; wheelchair to bed _____					
Method _____					
2 Propel chair _____					
Number of feet _____					
3 Lock/unlock brakes _____					
4 Raise/lower footrests _____					
5 Open, close, and pass through door _____					
Type of door _____					
6 Pick up objects off floor _____					
7 Transfer to/from straight chair _____					
At table _____					
Standing free _____					
8 Transfer to/from easy chair/couch _____					
9 Transfer to/from toilet _____					
Method _____					
10 Transfer to/from car _____					
11 Get from wheelchair to floor, from floor to wheelchair _____					
12 _____					

III PERSONAL HYGIENE					
1 Comb/brush hair _____					
2 Set hair _____					
3 Brush teeth or clean dentures _____					
4 Apply toothpaste to brush _____					
5 Shave/put on cosmetics _____					
6 Care for fingernails/toenails _____					
7 Use handkerchief _____					
8 Give self bed bath _____					
Unable to reach _____					
9 Dry thoroughly with towel _____					
10 Use of shower _____					
11 Get into/out of bath _____					
12 Toilet _____					
Method _____					
Flush toilet _____					
Use of toilet paper _____					
Adjust clothing _____					
Use urinal/bedpan _____					
13 Manage catheter:					
Independent care _____					
Clamp off/unclamp _____					
Empty SP bag _____					
14 Feminine hygiene _____					
15 _____					

Continued.

IV DRESSING	0	1	2	3	4
1 Put on/remove bra_____					
How? What method_____					
2 Put on/remove shorts, panties_____					
Method_____standing, on bed, seated					
3 Put on/remove slipover garments_____					
Method_____standing, on bed, seated					
4 Put on/remove button shirt_____					
Method_____standing, on bed, seated					
5 Put on/remove slacks or pants					
Method_____standing, on bed, seated					
6 Put on/remove socks or hose_____					
Method_____standing, on bed, seated					
7 Put on/remove shoes_____					
Method_____standing, on bed, seated					
8 Lace/unlace shoes_____					
9 Tie/untie laces_____					
10 Hook/unhook garters/suspenders_____					
Front_____					
Back_____					
11 Fasten/unfasten buckle_____					
12 Button/unbutton_____					
Little_____					
Big_____					
Circle location—front, side, back_____					
13 Fasten/unfasten snap_____					
14 Fasten/unfasten zipper_____					
Circle location—front, side					
15 Fasten/unfasten hooks and eyes_____					
16 Tie/untie necktie_____					
17 Fasten/unfasten safety pin_____					
Small_____					
Large_____					
18_____					

V APPARATUS	0	1	2	3	4
1 Put on/remove braces_____					
2 Lock/unlock braces_____					
3 Put on/remove splints, feeders, slings_____					
4 Put on/remove corset_____					
Type of lacing_____					
5_____					

VI EATING	0	1	2	3	4
1 Eat with fingers/sandwich_____					
2 Eat liquids with spoon_____					
3 Eat with fork/cut with fork_____					
4 Cut with knife_____					
5 Butter bread_____					
6 Drink from glass, cup, paper cup_____					
7 Pour liquid from milk carton/pour liquid from					
bedside pitcher_____					
8 Open carton of milk_____					
9_____					
10_____					

VII AMBULATION	0	1	2	3	4
1 Walks					
2 Stand and work at table					
Regular table					
Stand-up table					
3 Walks with package					
4 Get up from floor when falls					
With crutches					
Without crutches					
5					

VIII UTILITIES	0	1	2	3	4
1 Write:					
Legibly					
Name and address					
Copy paragraph					
2 Turn pages of book/magazine					
3 Cut with scissors					
4 Open a package of cigarettes					
5 Light a match/lighter					
6 Pick up change					
7 Make correct change					
8 Telephone:					
Standing					
From wheelchair					
Hold receiver					
Dial					
Use coins					
9 Wind watch					
10 Open/close windows					
11 Open/close drawers					
12 A.D.L. Board check-out					
Height of board					

Numbers accomplished

_____ _____
_____ _____
_____ _____

SUMMARY

Therapist's signature_____

assistance to the patient and the other members on the rehabilitation team by carryover of the program to the unit. The use of a daily living activities chart such as the one illustrated on pp. 432-435 is helpful in keeping all members of the rehabilitation team informed of the patient's progress.

It is essential that those on the rehabilitation team have knowledge of local, state, federal, and private resources that may be utilized in rehabilitation. During recent years, many facilities have been made available. The worker who keeps informed of available resources can offer the patient valuable assistance in meeting his complex needs.

Family and job adjustments

Teaching the patient and his family is an important aspect of rehabilitation. The patient is taught that good skin care is essential to prevent pressure areas. He learns that his position must be changed and that wrinkles and crumbs may cause breaks in the skin. He inspects his skin for redness or blisters that may come from shoes or braces. He knows that poor position may result in deformity and that lack of exercise may lead to stiff joints. He recognizes the necessity for adequate intake of fluid for the prevention of kidney stones, and he learns how to care for and prevent bowel and bladder problems. He practices applying his brace, dressing himself, and taking care of his personal needs. To be successful, rehabilitation must be a learning process for the patient and his family. The disabled person must learn to accomplish many of the activities of daily living by new methods.

The nurse on the rehabilitation team has an excellent opportunity to know and understand the patient and his family. She recognizes that the family members, as well as the patient, experience emotional strain and need to make adjustments. How do they react to the situation? Through this period of adjustment, a trained clinical psychologist can help the family and patient in resolving emotional problems and apprehensions. However, the rehabilitation worker recognizes that the patient and his family must be realistic about his disabilities. False hopes must not be fostered.

It must be realized that certain impairments may persist but that remaining abilities and capacities can be defined, guided, and developed. The regime of treatment should give the patient the opportunity and motivation to do as much for himself as possible. This includes the privilege of making his own decisions and taking responsibility for his own acts. Day-by-day improvement may seem very small. Discouragement and an attitude of futility must be combated from the beginning.

To the extent possible, ordinary activities required for independent daily living must be painstakingly relearned by the patient. These will include sitting, bending, turning, getting out of bed, walking, climbing stairs, putting on clothes and braces, and managing all personal care. The program to develop these skills may be complex. Experience and a high degree of skill are required to teach them effectively. Nurses should know what system of rehabilitation is being employed so that they may constantly encourage and instruct the patient in his struggle for physical independence.

As has been indicated, there are other factors in the total rehabilitation of patients, particularly those concerning family, social, and job adjustments, which are also very important. The advancements made since World War II have been heartening. In many types of jobs, it has been discovered that a handicapped person can contribute as much as any other person. Weaving, watch repairing, typing, printing, metal and leather crafts, painting, and wood carving may provide work for patients with severe orthopedic handicaps and have, in many instances, given them a means of earning a livelihood.

Family acceptance of the severely handicapped person, with an understanding of his need to live his own life as much as is possible, is one of the most important factors in the total rehabilitation program. All of the splendid work accomplished in the hospitals and workshops can be nullified in the home if oversolicitousness, rejection, or pity is evident to the patient. Nurses will need the help of social workers and social agencies to work out problems of family adjustment.

The problem of caring for an occasional

disabled patient is indeed a perplexing one for nurses. If they are cognizant of the dangers and armed with knowledge of means to overcome them, they will play an important part in his early physical rehabilitation. Their initial efforts may help keep the patient alive. If they are imbued with a determination to help the handicapped patient become as independent as possible, they should be able to secure

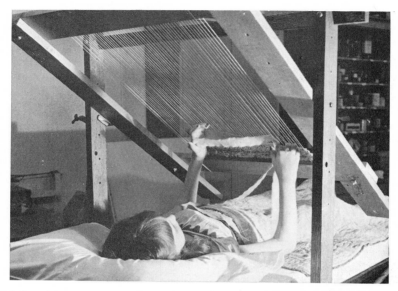

Fig. 417 Adjustable rug-weaving frame for use by the bed patient. This type of activity not only appeals to the patient, but also provides valuable exercise for fingers, wrists, elbows, and shoulders afflicted with arthritis.

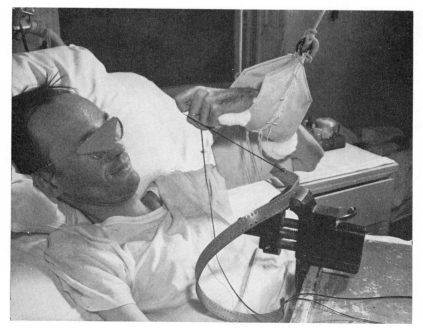

Fig. 418 Arrangement of belt-making equipment for the bed patient. This activity provides muscle-strengthening exercises and joint motion for the fingers and arm.

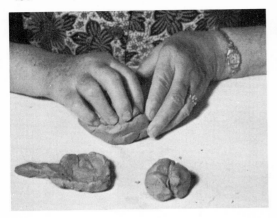

Fig. 419 Using modeling clay for finger mobilization. Sponge rubber also may be used to strengthen finger muscles.

assistance from others to aid the patient at various stages of his progress.

Occupational therapy

By definition, "Occupational therapy is the art and science of directing man's responses to selected activity to promote and maintain health, to prevent disability, to evaluate behavior and to treat or train patients with physical psychosocial dysfunction."[*] The primary goal of an occupational therapist for an orthopedic patient is restoration of physical function. For each patient, this may include restoring joint motion, regaining muscle strength, or improving coordination. The general aims with all patients are the development of work tolerance, socioeconomic adjustment, and prevocational testing (Figs. 417 to 425).

Certainly, psychologic manifestations must not be overlooked in the orthopedic patient. The tendency of a patient to withdraw from society or to dwell on pain and problems suggests he has not made a healthy adjustment. The occupational therapist substitutes an activity for inactivity, thus helping to prevent such regression and promoting a better adjustment.

The methods used in accomplishing these objectives are varied. Frequently, a wrong impression is created when a patient busy with a craft is observed.

_____
[*]Official definition adopted by the Delegate Assembly of the American Occupational Therapy Association. Am J Occup Ther **24:**324, Jul-Aug 1970.

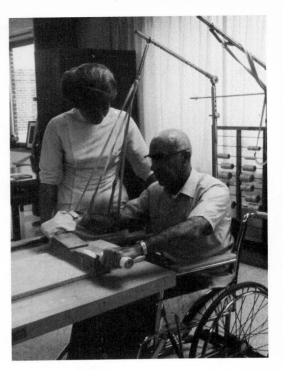

Fig. 420 Bilateral sanding used as reciprocal exercise for the arms. The overhead suspension sling supports the weaker arm.

The craft is noticed, but the activity is not. The _occupational_ of occupational therapy is not the project the patient is working on, nor is it his vocation or avocation outside the hospital; rather, it is the _occupation_ or activity of mind and body. Use of arts and crafts is a valuable method employed by the occupational therapist, but it is only one of many. Adapted recreational activities and self-help training in bathing, dressing, and feeding skills are other important methods. Writing, use of the telephone, manipulation of doors, latches, and dials, and similar activities of daily living are taught to the handicapped patient (Fig. 426). The methods are selected with the specific patient in mind. The referring physician's aim and the patient's impairment, interests, background, age and sex and many other factors must be carefully considered.

Occupational therapy plays a coordinating role in the total rehabilitation of a patient. It bridges the gap from hospitalization to life outside the hospital by enabling the patient to improve his ability to care

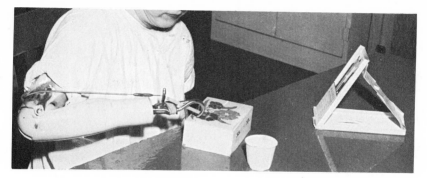

Fig. 421 A patient with amputation of the upper extremity learning to perform fine movements with a prosthetic appliance.

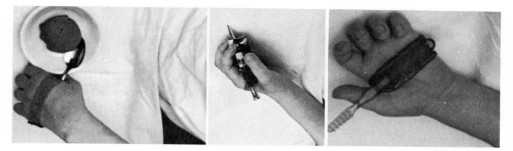

Fig. 422 The leather holder with a pocket for holding a spoon, pencil, or other utensil is helpful for the person who has lost the use of the small muscles of the hand but still has some shoulder and elbow motion.

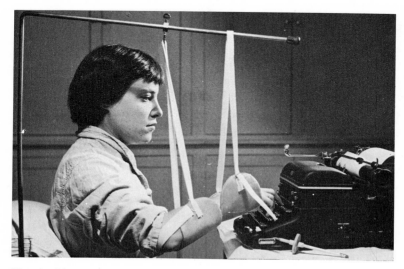

Fig. 423 The disabled person who possesses the use of her fingers but has weakness or paralysis of the arm and shoulder muscles may find this suspension sling helpful in performing activities of daily living.

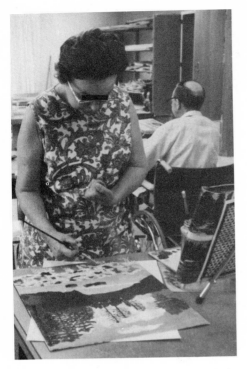

Fig. 424 Painting provides practice in fine finger coordination for this patient with posttraumatic cerebral dysfunction.

for himself and to carry out activities utilizing the movements or action learned in physical therapy. Occupational therapy helps to prevent the disability that often results from disuse, it encourages the development of latent abilities, it trains the patient in prevocational skills, and it develops work tolerance.

Diversional therapy

The importance of diversional treatment in occupational therapy should be appreciated. The nurse should be aware of the hazards of prolonged, enforced idleness. The handicapped person hospitalized for long periods often has too little to do and too much time to think and worry. This often is associated with depression and an excessive number of complaints and demands. Under such circumstances, diversional activity may be invaluable in keeping the individual occupied and partially fulfilling his need to feel productive. Diversional therapy should not be considered only a frill or luxury. It may be much more therapeutic for the patient than many of the daily nursing routines, such as the bath, which occupy so much of the attention of the nurse. In rehabilitation, activi-

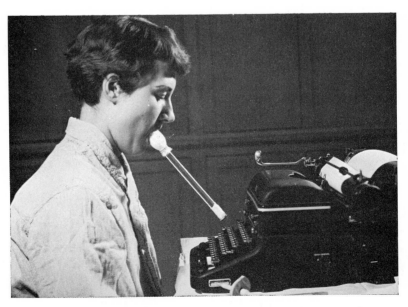

Fig. 425 The handicapped person with paralyzed upper extremities may learn to use the typewriter by utilizing a mouth stick. The stick is made of plastic material and has plastic-covered padding, which facilitates holding it in the mouth and provides protection for the teeth.

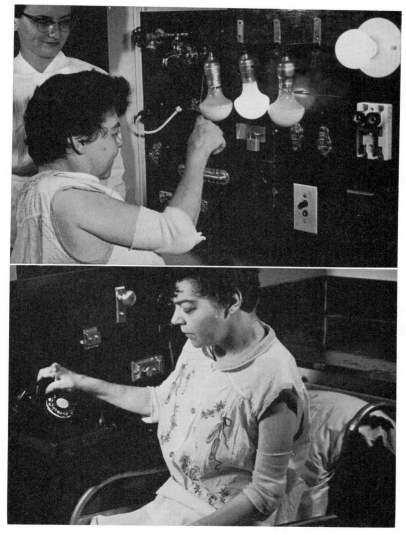

Fig. 426 The person with shoulder, elbow, or hand disability finds these boards most helpful in practicing and mastering activities essential to everyday living. The boards may be raised or lowered and contain such articles as light switches, water faucets, doorknobs, locks, and telephone.

ties performed by the patient himself are usually more important than things done to or for him.

Education for handicapped child

In considering the future of a handicapped youngster, the nurse should understand that education for the disabled child is imperative—perhaps more even than for his nonhandicapped brother. Many means of self-sufficiency and self-support available to the normal person are barred to the handicapped. A handicapped person must be better prepared to fulfill even limited types of occupation. The student nurse should understand that the newest concept of vocational guidance and placement emphasizes the versatility rather than the limitations of crippled individuals. Perhaps the student nurse may one day imbue earnest members of some civic group with an urge to help the handicapped, to take upon themselves responsibility for the higher education of some homebound child. Services are generally available for the home-bound child through two-way radio class communication as well as home teacher service provided by the public school system.

Physical therapy

Physical therapy may be defined as the science that deals with the management of disease by means of physical agents such as light, heat, cold, water, electricity, mechanical agents, and therapeutic exercise.

From ancient times, the principles of physical therapy have been employed but not always on a scientific basis. The practices of lying in the sun, rubbing a bruised muscle, and bathing a wound in a woodland stream have led through the years to the development of present methods of treatment. These have an important function and are well recognized in most hospitals today.

Thermal therapy

Heat. Heat is a commonly employed form of treatment. It often is used before massage and exercise and seems to enhance the other treatment measures. Physiologic effects of the various types of heat that may be used are similar. External application of heat results in increased temperature of the tissues, vasodilatation, and increased blood flow. Local metabolic activity is increased. Heat tends to relieve pain and muscular tension.

Superficial heat. Any object hotter than its surroundings will give off infrared rays. The infrared lamp is a simple way to apply local heat. There are various kinds and sizes of infrared lamps. The energy output that reaches the patient depends on the wattage of the lamp, the distance from the lamp to the patient, the angle at which the rays strike the patient, and the total area irradiated. Infrared radiation includes the light radiation from 7,700 to 120,000 Å. The amount used in physical therapy usually ranges from 1,200 to 1,500 mμ. This includes no bacteriocidal rays. The main effect consists of heating the local area. Smaller infrared lamps are usually placed fourteen to eighteen inches from the skin; larger ones, twenty-four to thirty inches. The patient should feel comfortably warm but not hot.

Infrared radiation is used in the treatment of arthritis, bursitis, fibrositis, muscle strain, and muscle spasm. It is a convenient way to apply heat at home.

Infrared treatment should not be given following large doses of deep irradiation because serious burns sometimes result.

Hot packs. Many types of hot packs are used in hospitals and at home. One of the most convenient is a very heavy Turkish towel—or two Turkish towels sewed together—heated in boiling water and then quickly wrung out so that as little steam as possible escapes. The pack is then wrapped into a forty-inch square of wool blanket. The patient's skin is not touched by the hot towels but only by the dry wool with the steam coming through it. There is no danger of burning the patient if he is carefully dried between the applications of packs. While one set of packs is on the patient, another set should be boiling. The first set is left on for three to four minutes, and then the second is applied. Three or four changes are usually needed. These packs are easily applied to almost any area of the body, either by laying the pack on the area or by wrapping it. They have been found very beneficial in treating muscle spasm, strains, sprains, arthritis, and bursitis. Many hospitals prefer hot packs for heat over any other available method (Fig. 427).

In addition to the conventional moist hot packs, commercially prepared compresses or packs with automatic heating units are available. These retain heat for twenty to thirty minutes and eliminate the task of wringing hot water from packs. Such packs are removed from the unit, wrapped in several layers of terry cloth, and applied to the desired area. These packs can be obtained in several sizes and are well suited for use in the home, as well as the hospital, when there is need for repeated application of moist heat.

Paraffin. Melted paraffin to which light mineral oil has been added is very satisfactory as a method of applying heat. The melted paraffin is kept at a temperature between 124° and 132° F. If the paraffin is completely melted and has a little scum on the surface, the temperature is correct. Paraffin is an especially satisfactory method of heating the hand or arm afflicted with arthritis. The extremity is dipped into the paraffin six to ten times until a thick coat

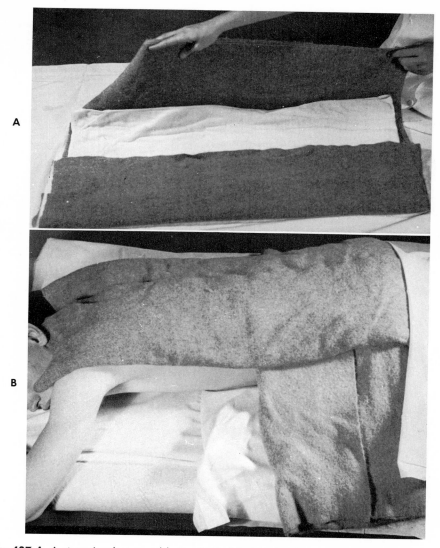

Fig. 427 A, A steaming hot towel being folded inside the dry woolen blanket. **B,** Hot packs applied to the back for pain in the lower portion.

(one-eighth of an inch) is obtained. This, carefully wrapped in a bath towel or bath blanket, will hold the heat twenty to thirty minutes.

Paraffin is used chiefly for arthritis, bursitis, fibrositis, or contractures of the hand. Following the paraffin treatment, the treated area is well prepared for massage and exercise. Paraffin-dip treatment can be carried out easily at home by heating the paraffin in a double boiler and using the scum test as a temperature guide. A candy thermometer should be used to check the temperature (Fig. 428).

Deep heat. Subcutaneous fat is a poor conductor of heat. Superficial heating is inadequate for heating deeper tissues. To obtain deeper tissue heating, certain forms of physical energy are used. They are able to penetrate skin and subcutaneous tissue without damage and are changed into heat in the deeper tissues. Types in common use at present are shortwave and microwave diathermy and ultrasound.

Shortwave diathermy. High frequency current is used for deep heating. The resistance of the tissues to the currents forced through them generates heat. An induction

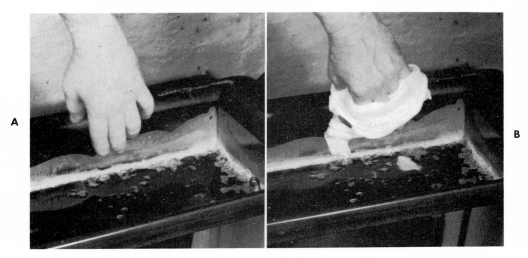

Fig. 428 A, The hand has just been dipped ten times into the melted paraffin. **B,** The paraffin glove is being removed. This may be put back into the paraffin bath and remelted.

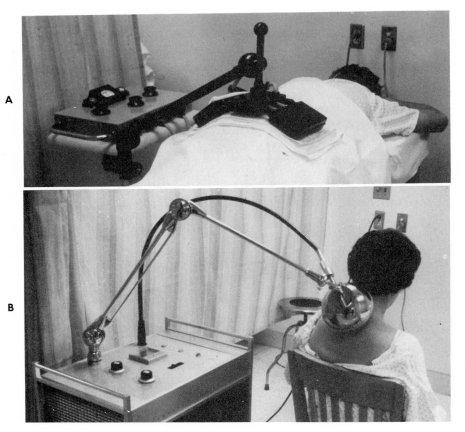

Fig. 429 Shortwave diathermy treatment being administered for low back strain, **A,** and painful neck muscle spasm, **B.**

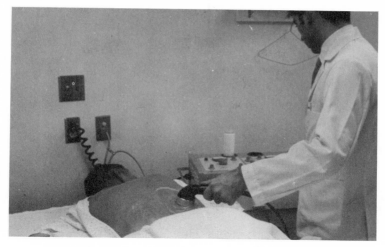

Fig. 430 Ultrasound treatment to relieve muscle pain.

cable is employed to create an electro-magnetic field. The cable can be either wrapped around the part to be treated or coiled to make a flat applicator. Shortwave diathermy is limited to wavelengths of 3 to 30 meters with frequencies of 10 to 100 megacycles. As the high frequency current enters the body, it tends to spread so that a fairly large area is heated. A padding of toweling one-half to two inches thick is used between the skin and electrodes to absorb perspiration and prevent burning. Physiologically, the effects of shortwave diathermy are identical with the effects of other types of heat. The only difference is that the hyperemia produced by shortwave lasts longer and deeper layers of tissues are penetrated.

Diathermy is used for treatment of chronic sinusitis, mild inflammation of bone, joint, and muscle, chronic osteo-myelitis, and various forms of arthritis and bursitis. High-frequency currents also are used surgically. Fulguration and electro-desiccation are used to destroy warts and small skin blemishes. Electrocoagulation is used to remove larger tumors and to stop bleeding (Fig. 429).

Microwave diathermy. Radiated electro-magnetic waves are utilized. Machines pro-vide a wavelength of 12.2 cm at a fre-quency of 2,450 megacycles per second. The director of the machine provides focusing several inches from the skin surface. The heating effect is greater in tissues with high water content.

Ultrasound. The energy for ultrasound therapy consists of mechanical vibrations with frequency from 0.7 to 1 megacycle. These waves do not travel through air, so direct contact with the skin is necessary. A coupling jelly is used between the appli-cator and the skin. Ultrasound may provide heating of tissue at a depth up to 5 cm (Fig. 430).

Cold

Therapeutic cold has been of more limited value than heat. Local applications of cold causes vasoconstriction, decreased blood flow, decreases metabolic activity in local tissue, and decreased local tempera-ture. The response varies depending on the nature and temperature of the coolant ap-plied, duration of the application, and the area treated.

Brief application of cold produces transient vasoconstriction followed by vaso-dilatation, increased blood flow, and local effects that resemble those following heat. Cold sometimes is used to replace heat treatments in patients who tolerate heat poorly.

Ice bags, cold baths, or compresses often are used to minimize the initial reaction of tissues to injury; e.g., sprain. Refrigeration of tissues can induce local anesthesia. In-tense cold (e.g., liquid nitrogen) produces

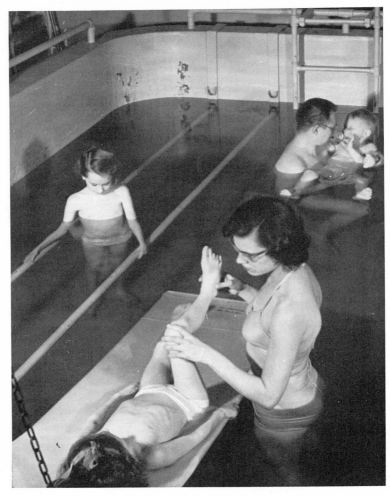

Fig. 431 With the use of this canvas table, routine stretching exercises, as well as underwater exercises and walking practice, can be given in the pool.

tissue destruction and sometimes is used to treat certain skin lesions.

Hydrotherapy

Hydrotherapy consists of the use of therapeutic pools, the Hubbard tank, whirlpools, contrast baths, sprays and douches, and hot packs.

Therapeutic pools. To be most useful, a therapeutic pool should be 12 to 15 ft wide and 20 to 24 ft long. It shouuld have walking bars and proper depth to permit walking practice for the patients. The temperature of the water depends on the amount of activity the patient will perform, his age, the diagnosis, and the length of time he will be in the water. If the program is one

essentially for exercise, the water should be between 80° and 95° F. If a heating effect is desired, the temperature can be as high as 102° F.

Therapeutic pools have proved very valuable in treating children with cerebral palsy. The buoyancy of the water makes it possible for a child to use a weakened muscle through a greater range of motion. Patients can use walking bars in the pool earlier than outside because of the buoyancy of the water. The heat of the water raises the pain threshold so that the patient can tolerate stretching exercises more easily. Both the buoyancy and the heat encourage relaxation of the cerebral palsied patient, and he can perform his exercises with

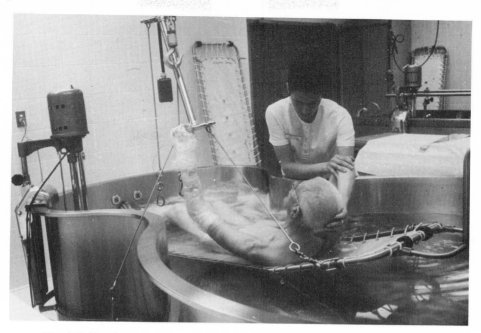

Fig. 432 The therapist is giving exercises to the patient in the Hubbard tank.

more ease. In addition to the physical and physiologic benefits from a therapeutic pool, the psychologic lift to the patient is very valuable (Fig. 431).

Hubbard tank. The shape of the Hubbard tank is such that it permits exercise movements of the arm and legs that are not possible in an ordinary tub (Fig. 432). The temperature of the water usually is kept at about 99° to 100° F. for exercise and 102° F. for heating. Although a Hubbard tank is not so satisfactory as a therapeutic pool for exercise, it is frequently employed. Since it is not necessary for the therapist to be in the pool to treat the patient, as in a therapeutic pool, the Hubbard tank may be more practical as far as the personnel are concerned. Sometimes a whirlpool agitator is placed in the tank.

Whirlpools. The temperature of the water in the whirlpool is maintained between 100° and 110° F, usually 105° F. The air pressure coming into the water gives it a swirling, gentle massaging action. Whirlpools are especially valuable in treating patients with fractures and those who have had tendon or ligament surgery. The whirlpool treatment makes it much easier to clean dry scaly skin from affected areas, increases circulation to the

part, and tends to relieve pain and stiffness. Whirlpools also are used in the treatment of burns and amputations that are not completely healed. In these cases a mild antiseptic solution is often added to the water. Children can be put into the whirlpool tank for general heating of the entire body prior to stretching and exercises. Whirlpool treatment for patients with arthritis has proved very helpful in relieving pain and stiffness (Fig. 433).

Contrast baths. In contrast baths, the patient's feet or hands are moved alternately from hot to cold tubs of water. The temperature in the hot tubs ranges from 100° to 105° F; in the cold tubs, from 65° to 70° F. Immersion should begin and end in hot water—four minutes in hot water and one minute in cold water. Seven to nine immersions usually are given. The treatment generally is used for arthritis and peripheral vascular disease and preceding massage and exercise for sprains and contusions.

Ultraviolet radiation

Ultraviolet radiation is in the range of the light spectrum from 1,800 to 3,900 Å. It can be produced by several artificial sources, including the hot quartz mercury

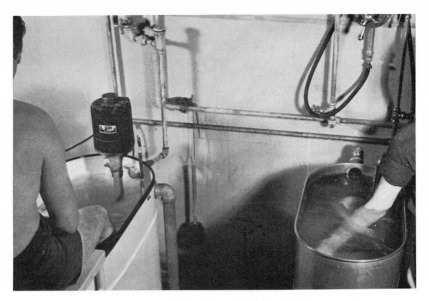

Fig. 433 Leg and arm whirlpools.

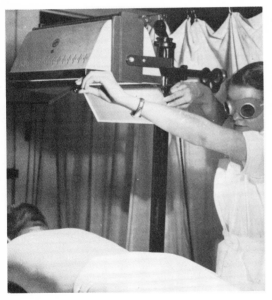

Fig. 434 Ultraviolet lamp being opened for an exposure to the back.

lamp, the cold quartz lamp, or the carbon arc. The dosage is governed by the minimal erythema dose (M.E.D.), which is defined as the shortest exposure at a certain distance that will produce a perceptible reddening of the skin that occurs within six to eight hours after treatment and that

will disappear within twenty-four hours. Care must be taken to cover the eyes of the patient with moistened pledgets of gauze or cotton, and the operator must wear goggles. Conjunctivitis could result from neglect of these precautions (Fig. 434).

The aforementioned erythema with resulting increase in local circulation and the well-known bacteriocidal effect of ultraviolet radiation govern its indications. It is extensively used in the treatment of decubitus ulcers, infected superficial wounds, and many skin diseases. It has been shown to produce antirachitic effects by increasing vitamin D production in the skin.

Electrical stimulation

Each electrical stimulation machine will give a variety of currents or combinations. The main currents used are galvanic and faradic. Galvanic or direct current stimulates the muscle and therefore causes a response even when nerves have been damaged. Faradic or alternating current stimulates the nerve and stimulates the muscle only when it has a normal nerve supply. These currents and their various combinations and derivatives can be used as testing devices to determine whether or not the nerve to the muscle is normal. If it is damaged, the extent of the damage and the rate of nerve regeneration can be determined. Electrical stimulation may cause muscle contractions something like voluntary activity, producing approximately the same metabolic effects. This has proved valuable as a form of exercise to avoid muscle atrophy in denervated muscles.

Massage

Massage is the term applied to the systematic and scientific manipulation of body tissues for remedial and restorative purposes. For effective application of massage, it is essential that one have (1) adequate knowledge of muscle, joint, and nerve anatomy of the affected part, (2) a knowledge of the desired effects, and (3) a skillful technique and understanding of the various strokes.

Physiologic effects of massage on the skin include a sedative effect on the peripheral sensory nerves, reflex stimulation of motor nerves, a temporary hyperemia, and a cleansing of the epidermis. The main effect on the muscles is the hastening of the removal of metabolites from the muscle, which helps relieve fatigue and spasm. Massage will not increase muscle strength. Only active exercise can do that. Depending on the intensity of the stimuli, massage can produce either a sedative or a stimulating effect on the nervous system. It has been shown that massage definitely increases the pain threshold; this is apparently related to the counterirritant phenomenon. Since the lymph circulatory system is entirely dependent upon external pressures (normally, muscle contraction and joint movement), massage has proved valuable in moving lymph fluid in patients with edematous conditions. Massage has a minimal effect on venous or arterial flow; the pumping action of the heart is a much more adequate means of circulating the blood. Massage produces no significant change in red or white blood cell count or in the hemoglobin. Massage cannot rub away excess fatty tissue. Massage is highly effective in stretching excessive fibrous tissue in subcutaneous areas.

The massage technique is generally based on four strokes: effleurage, petrissage, friction, and tapotement.

1 *Effleurage* consists of stroking the surface of the skin. The amount of pressure is varied to make it a light or heavy stroking.
2 *Petrissage* is the kneading of the soft tissues.
3 *Friction* is applied by rotary movements of the skin over underlying tissue. The thumb or fingers are kept in firm contact with the skin, and the movement is between the skin and superficial tissue and the underlying structures.
4 *Tapotement* consists of a percussion type of movement against bodily tissues. This type of massage has very little place in the treatment of pathologic conditions because it is too heavy.

To get the best results from a massage, the patient should be in a comfortable relaxed position. The part to be massaged must be supported and completely uncovered and the rest of the patient's body carefully draped. The operator should be in a comfortable working position. Once the massage is started, the therapist's hands maintain contact with the part being massaged until the massage is completed. The stroking pattern generally follows the muscle groups. The rhythm should be slow and steady, the pressure gentle but firm. The heaviest pressure is on the upward stroke (toward the heart, centripetal in direction), and the return stroke is very light. Massage should never be painful. Pain is the prime contraindication for massage. Cold cream is generally preferred as a lubricant, although cocoa butter is often used for burned or scarred areas, and talcum powder is used over hairy surfaces. Any baby oil, olive oil, or mineral oil may be used.

Massage is used in the treatment of patients with arthritis, fibrositis, edema, and traumatic conditions such as sprains and strains, fractures, burns, amputations, and muscle spasm. Massage should not be given to anyone having any acute inflammatory process, skin eruption, malignancy, or fever.

Therapeutic exercise

One of the principal aims of therapeutic exercise is to maintain or restore the functional activities of the individual at the highest level possible. This can be accomplished through various types of exer-

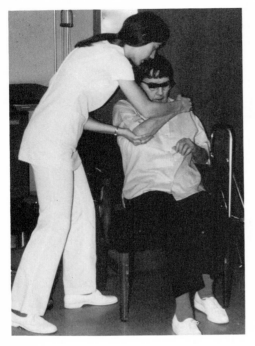

Fig. 435 Passive exercise for a paralyzed arm is administered with some stretching for proprioceptive stimulation to help elict reflex muscle contraction.

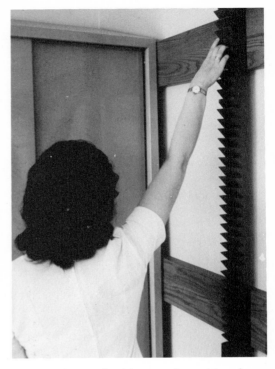

Fig. 436 Active shoulder exercises with a finger ladder.

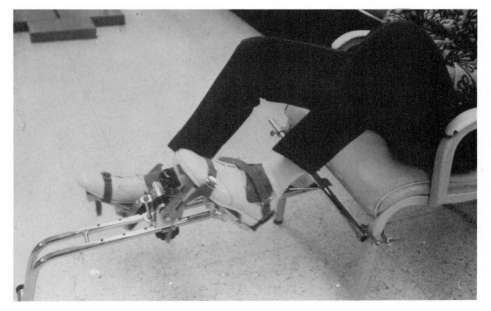

Fig. 437 Active reciprocal motion exercise for the legs using a restorator attached to a chair.

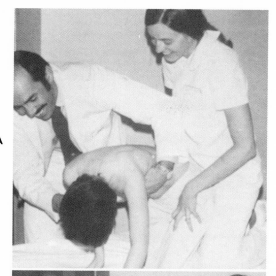

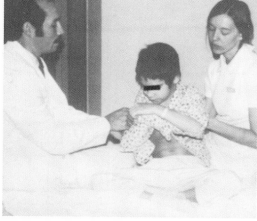

Fig. 438 Youngster with brain damage performing active exercise learning to balance in crawl position, **A,** and sitting position, **B.**

cises. Exercises are classified as passive, active assistive, active, and resistive.

Passive exercise. Passive exercise is the movement of joints and associated tissues (bones, muscles, tendons, and other soft tissues) of various parts of the body by the application of external force, supplied either manually by the therapist or by some kind of mechanical device. This kind of exercise is employed when the patient is unable to perform active exercises. The chief purposes of passive exercise are (1) to promote circulation in the parts being exercised, (2) to maintain or increase range of motion of the joints, and (3) to counteract the development of adhesions and contractures (Fig. 435).

Active assistive exercise. Active assistive exercise is an exercise in which the patient is assisted in the performance of active movement. The assistance may be either manual (provided by the therapist) or mechanical (supplied by pulleys, weights, elastic bands, or slings). Such assistance usually is given to counterbalance the force of gravity acting on the extremity and thus assist the weakened muscles in performing the exercise. The assistance should be minimal so that the muscle is performing at its maximum strength.

Active exercise. Active exercise is executed by the patient himself, using his own muscles without additional resistance. Nurses reinforce active exercises when they have the patient bathe himself, take care of his toilet needs, dress himself, etc. (Figs. 436 to 438).

Resistive exercise. Resistive exercise is active exercise performed by the patient against an external resistive force (Figs. 439 and 440). Resistive exercises are either manual resistive exercise or progressive resistive exercise. In early stages of muscle strengthening, manual resistive exercises are the most useful because they allow the therapist to apply and regulate the resistance given throughout the active movement, direct the movement properly, and eliminate any muscle substitution. Progressive resistive exercises employ maximal contraction of muscles. These exercises enable the patient to increase muscle strength and muscle bulk (hypertrophy), increase efficiency of muscle contraction, and improve muscle coordination through facilitation. Progressive resistive exercises may be done with the use of iron weights, sandbags, elastic bands, or vigorous underwater activity. These exercises should be performed in progression after the therapist has determined the maximum load. The pattern of progression is ten repetitions with 50% maximum load, ten repetitions with 75% maximum load, and then ten repetitions with 100% of maximum load. As strength improves, the resistance used is increased in increments.

To obtain the best results from these exercises, the patient should perform them twice daily for as long as is necessary. In

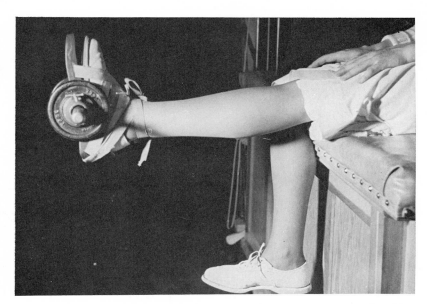

Fig. 439 Resistance exercise for the quadriceps muscle. Starting position for this exercise is sitting with the legs over the edge of the table with a rolled towel placed under the knee for proper support. The leg being exercised is then raised to the position shown, held for a few seconds, and slowly lowered.

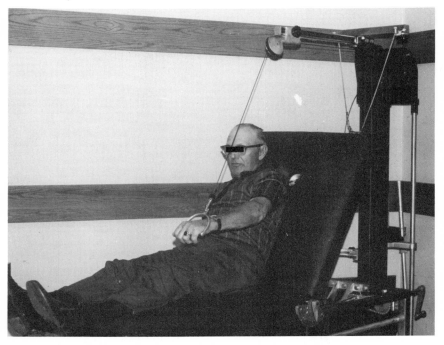

Fig. 440 Resistive exercise for shoulder extension. An exercise table is utilized. Resistance can be increased by adding more weights at the head of the table.

many cases, the exercises must be continued at home after discharge from the hospital. The therapist will instruct the patient and/or the family concerning both the proper technique to use and the length of time to continue the exercises.

The scope of therapeutic exercise is broad. It includes the following:

1 Coordination exercises for patients with multiple sclerosis, cerebral palsy, or cerebellar ataxia
2 Muscle-strengthening exercises for patients with various orthopedic and neurologic disorders
3 Exercises designed to prevent deformity, such as range-of-motion activity for patient with arthritis
4 Exercises to correct deformity, such as heel cord contracture
5 Activities to maintain mobility of joint and muscle, such as stretching for patients with Guillain-Barré syndrome
6 Exercises given for esthetic effect, as in the treatment of patients with postural defects
7 Exercises used to provide relief from pain, as in patients with pain in the lower portion of the back
8 Exercises given to teach patients to relax
9 Respiratory exercises that will increase vital capacity

In England, much work has been done with breathing exercises for patients with asthma. Some patients have been able to increase their breathing during attacks and, in many cases, to prevent attacks. Exercises given for peripheral vascular disease may improve the efficiency of the circulatory system.

Let us briefly follow a patient in his attempt to ambulate after several weeks in traction because of a fracture. During the time the patient has been confined to bed, the therapist has had him perform a series of arm-strengthening exercises and isometric exercises of the involved extremity in preparation for ambulation. The first step may be use of the tilt table where the patient is acclimated to the vertical position. He may be given crutches to take some of the weight off his feet while on the tilt table. When the patient tolerates the tilt table in a vertical position for thirty minutes, he is advanced to parallel bars, where he learns the proper gait and balance. The bars are more stable than crutches, and thus the patient develops confidence in his walking ability. When he can walk several lengths of the parallel bars, he is fitted properly with crutches. Once he learns the proper gait and develops some skill and endurance in handling crutches outside the parallel bars, he is taught how to get into and out of a chair, to go up and down stairs, to walk backward and sideways, and to open and close doors. A person on crutches can learn to be very independent and capable of taking care of himself in almost any circumstance. This pattern of teaching a patient to be ambulatory is in evidence at many stages every day in a physical therapy department.

23 The patient with spinal cord injury

Spinal cord injuries are becoming increasingly common with high-speed automobile accidents and trauma from falls, athletic injuries, and gunshot wounds. With improved techniques of care in the acute phase after the injury, such as better control of shock, tracheostomies to assist breathing and clearing the airway, and treatment of multiple injuries, these patients are surviving to require long-term rehabilitation and ultimately to go home to a new way of life. It is vital that rehabilitative measures be started from the earliest days in the hospital to prevent complicating problems that might severely limit the patient's ultimate functional capacity.

With most spinal cord injuries, it is possible to predict capabilities of individuals with lesions at various levels. However, these general descriptions should be used only as guides, since variations in the patient's ability can occur depending on the specific lesion and motivation. The lesions may be described as complete or incomplete below a certain level, and the amount of involvement may be greater on one side as opposed to the opposite side. If the lesion is at the level of the fourth cervical vertebra, the patient has little or no muscle power in the upper extremities. This patient may learn to use a mouth stick (with dental bite) to accomplish some tasks such as turning book pages, writing, painting, etc. If the lesion is at the level of the fifth/sixth cervical vertebra, the deltoid (shoulder abductor) and biceps (elbow flexor) are usually weakened. Without these muscles, the arm is

of little use, unless special supports are devised. If the lesion is below the sixth cervical vertebra, hand devices which holds a fork, spoon, pencil, or other object may be strapped to the hand or forearm and the individual is able to feed himself, to write, and to have some functional use of the upper extremity. If the patient has use of the intrinsic muscles of the hand, the lesion is usually below the first thoracic vertebra. Injury to the spinal cord in the thoracic region involves the muscles of the back, abdomen, and lower extremities. Intercostal muscles may be involved with high thoracic injury—sixth thoracic vertebra and above. The hip extensors and the quadriceps (knee extensors) will not be involved if the lesion is below the fourth lumbar vertebra (Figs. 326 and 441).

Injury to the spinal cord, depending on the level, results in paraplegia or quadriplegia. Paraplegia is caused by injury to the thoracic or lumbar portions of the spinal cord or to the sacral nerve roots and results in varying degrees of paralysis of the muscles of the lower extremity and trunk. Quadriplegia or tetraplegia means that the muscles of all four extremities and the trunk are involved and is caused by injury to the spinal cord in the cervical or high thoracic regions. Injury in the cervical region, depending on the level, may cause paralysis of the respiratory muscles, leaving only the accessory muscles to perform the function of breathing. The areas of the spine most often involved are the lower cervical, midthoracic, and the thoracolumbar regions.

Spinal cord damage may be caused by

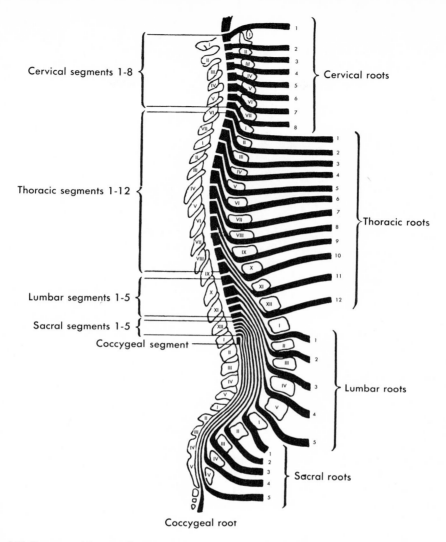

Fig. 441 Topographic correlation between spinal cord segments and vertebral bodies, spinous processes, and intervertebral foramina. (From Haymaker, W.: Bing's Local diagnosis in neurological diseases, ed. 15, St. Louis, The C. V. Mosby Co.)

conditions other than trauma, such as tumors, multiple sclerosis, birth defects, etc. Regardless of the cause, rehabilitation is aimed at helping the individual live as independently as is compatible with the involvement. Most of these patients must learn a new way of moving from place to place and of doing most activities. Some will be able to walk with braces and crutches, others will be confined to a wheelchair, and a few must be dependent on others for help with most of the activities of daily living.

A patient with a fractured spine and with spinal cord involvement presents what may be truly called a major nursing problem. Fractures of the spine may, of course, exist without cord injury, but the patients do not constitute so great a nursing problem as do those with associated cord injury. Attention will therefore be concentrated primarily on the more severe type of injury where cord involvement is present. The following discussion describes measures that make a great difference in the level of function and quality of daily life the person with a spinal cord injury can achieve. These measures are primarily preventive and require a great deal of conscientious thought.

Management of bladder

Injury to the spinal cord is almost invariably accompanied by disturbances in the bowel and bladder function. Nerves located at or below the spinal cord injury no longer function. Messages to and from the brain are lost. Consequently, the cerebrum does not receive sensations indicating need to empty the bladder. Thus, the person with a spinal cord injury is not able to exercise conscious control of voiding. After injury, a state of spinal shock exists, and during this time the bladder is atonic and incapable of emptying itself. As the patient recovers from spinal shock after weeks or months, reflex activity below the level of injury may develop. As this reflex activity returns, some bladder-emptying capacity may be regained. The final result may be a neurogenic bladder that may be spastic or continue to be flaccid. The spastic bladder is very irritable and unable to retain a significant volume of urine; the flaccid bladder retains large volumes of urine and occasionally partially empties by "overflow."

Providing for urinary drainage and preventing urinary tract infection are two of the major problems confronting the patient with a spinal cord injury. Several methods of treatment have been utilized to provide for urinary drainage. If a bladder-training program is prescribed, emptying of the bladder is attempted at regular intervals. Better results may be obtained if the patient can be placed on a commode or a toilet as opposed to the use of a bedpan or urinal. Catheterization to determine the amount of residual urine remaining in the bladder after voiding may be ordered at specified times. A large volume of residual urine increases the possibility of infection, and, if the residual is too great, damage to the kidneys may be caused by vesicoureteral reflux.

The training process to establish an automatic bladder is slow and requires much patience and continuous effort by the patient, physician, and nursing personnel. Provision must be made for emptying the bladder at designated times before the quantity of urine in the bladder induces spontaneous voiding. By trial and error and control of fluid intake, the patient learns how long he can go between voidings and remain dry. He learns to recognize symptoms such as abdominal discomfort, chills, or restlessness as indicative of a need to empty his bladder. Micturition may be induced by such measures as manual pressure on the bladder (Credé's method), by straining, or by other trigger mechanisms the patient may find effective. For some males, a condom catheter may be used if the bladder empties well, but the pattern of voiding remains unpredictable.

When management of the bladder by these procedures is not successful, it may be necessary to resort to continuous catheter drainage. The female frequently will tolerate an indwelling urethral catheter for months or years. Males have much more difficulty because of the high incidence of urethritis. If a urethral catheter is not tolerated, an alternate route of drainage must be provided, such as suprapubic cystostomy or an ileal loop or pouch. With the catheter or with any of these other procedures, there remains an increased incidence of infection. The appearance of chills, fever, or bloody urine or an inability to irrigate the catheter is an indication for the patient to seek medical advice promptly. How frequently a catheter is changed depends upon the kinds of urinary problems the patient is having and the attending physician's orders. The catheter in the suprapubic cystostomy is cared for in a manner similar to that of the urethral indwelling type. Strict asepsis, twice daily irrigations with a bacteriostatic agent such as 0.25% acetic acid, and cleaning around the orifice, followed by the application of a light dressing are required.

The ileal loop or pouch provides for drainage of urine from the ureters through an opening in the abdominal wall. A segment of the small intestine is used to connect the ureters to this abdominal opening. Urine drains into an appliance that is glued to the skin around the orifice and held in place by a strap around the trunk. The bag usually needs to be changed every three to six days, depending on the patient's activity. As with the catheters, the drains may be connected to a leg bag or to bedside drainage. Either of these diversional drainage devices works well in the prone position so long as the tube is not bent acutely.

During recent years, intermittent catheterization has become the method of choice for treating patients with neurogenic bladders. These patients have shown considerable improvement in urinary continence and have had a lower incidence of urinary tract infection. They remain dry and consequently have fewer skin problems, as well as improvement in their mental status. Protection of the urinary tract from infection and prevention of overstretching of the bladder should begin immediately after admission. In some centers, a straight catheter has been utilized every three to four hours. However, if the bladder is not emptied on time, overdistention may produce permanent damage to the muscles of the bladder wall. Overdistention of the bladder results in decreased blood flow to the tissue and lessens its resistance to bacterial infection. If there is reflux from the bladder into the ureters or residual urine left in the bladder, the possibility of bladder infection and the formation of urinary calculi greatly increases. Intermittent catheterization means that the patient is catheterized every three to four hours, and the catheterization schedule must be such that overdistention of the bladder is avoided. This is important in the prevention of bladder infection. As soon as the physical condition of these patients warrants, they are taught self-catheterization. To do self-catheterization, the patient must be able to maintain a sitting balance and must have sufficient function in the upper extremities to position their limbs and to manipulate a catheter. The patient, or a responsible person, is taught how to care for the catheter as well as the procedure technique.

Regardless of the method utilized to provide for urine drainage, a high fluid intake (3,000-5,000 ml) is necessary to help prevent urinary tract infection. Keeping the urine dilute helps to prevent precipitation of the salts that tend to form urinary calculi. Maintenance of an acid urine is also desirable. Acid urine provides a less favorable media for the growth of bacteria and tends to prevent precipitation of calcium. Frequent changing of the patient's position is an aid in preventing stasis of urine in the kidney pelvis. Also, it is well known that weight-bearing stress decreases the amount of calcium lost from the skeletal system. Thus, the early use of the tilt table is valuable in preventing the formation of calculi.

Aseptic technique is important during catheterization procedures and when caring for the bladder. The newer Silastic catheters result in less encrustation and stone formation. In some cases, a three-channel catheter may be utilized so that a closed system of continuous bladder irrigation can be set up. The bladder also may be irrigated intermittently. Sterile solutions of 0.25% acetic acid or other acid mixtures, of dilute aqueous benzalkonium chloride (Zephiran), or of dilute antiinfective agents may be used for bladder irrigation. In addition to these measures, the use of antibacterial agents are frequently a valuable adjunct in the prevention and control of urinary tract infection.

Bowel training

Like bladder training, bowel training is an essential aspect of the care of the paraplegic or quadriplegic. One thing that will help the patient who is on a prescribed bowel-training program is establishing a definite time of day for use of the bedpan, commode, or toilet. The time chosen should take into consideration the patient's work day, his eventual return to gainful employment, and his usual bowel habit. Provision for privacy encourages relaxation, and abdominal massage or pressure downward toward the sigmoid and rectum may be helpful in stimulating peristalsis and defecation. Exercise, as with the nonhandicapped individual, is beneficial.

The diet should include a normal amount of bulky foods; however, it must be remembered that an excessive amount of high-residue food can cause loose stools and disturb a regulated bowel pattern. A fecal moistening agent frequently is prescribed for the patient with a spinal cord injury.

In establishing a pattern, it is frequently found necessary to use suppositories at a regular interval. This can be once daily or at two-day or three-day intervals. Depending on the amount of sensation or reflex established, the use of bisacodyl (Dulcolax) or glycerin suppositories may be required to maintain the habit. With a gloved finger, the suppository should be inserted high in the rectum above the internal sphincter against the bowel wall. As the suppository melts, the rectal mucosa is irritated and peristalsis is stimulated. Twenty minutes to two hours may elapse after the suppository is inserted before bowel evacuation occurs. It is usually important for the patient to establish a routine of exercise and then a relaxed, unhurried period on the bedpan or toilet to develop the habit pattern. Frequently it is found that sitting on the toilet or a bedside commode is more conducive to a good bowel movement than is use of a bedpan or disposable diapers. Teaching the patient the technique of inserting the suppository is important in the learning process. Since sensation is generally lacking, visual check of the volume and consistency of the stool by the nurse and the patient is necessary. Eventually, the bowel evacuation habit may not require the suppository for initiation but may be stimulated by a gloved finger in the rectum, abdominal pressure, or a series of exercises. A bowel movement every second day is usually sufficient. However, impactions are not uncommon among these patients, and at times it may be necessary to gently remove fecal material with a gloved finger. Diarrhea or continuous soiling frequently indicates an impaction. Normal saline enemas may be necessary, but with bowel training the need for enemas is minimized. These should be given with extreme care because the intestine of the paraplegic patient distends easily if too much liquid is given or if it is given too rapidly. On the other hand, some patients may not be able to retain the fluid and it acts more as an irrigation. Since results from the enema frequently continue for several hours after the procedure, protective padding should be provided for the patient. A successful habit without use of enemas is the desired goal.

Body alignment

Special attention to good body alignment, change of position, and range of joint

motion is necessary. If skull traction has been applied, the amount of extension of the cervical region must be carefully controlled according to the attending physician's wishes. In the supine position, the lower extremities are maintained in neutral position. External rotation is prevented by the use of trochanter rolls or sandbags. A padded footboard is used to support the feet at right angles, and the heels must be protected to prevent the development of decubiti. With the quadriplegic, attention must be given to the arms; bony prominences, especially the elbows, are protected. The wrist is slightly dorsiflexed. The metacarpophalangeal joints are positioned in flexion, and the thumb should be kept in a position of opposition, with the web space maintained. In the prone position, the ankles are supported on a pillow. This produces some flexion of the knees and keeps the feet in a functional position.

While involved with maintaining correct body alignment, the nurse must not forget that changing the patient's position at scheduled frequent intervals (insofar as this is possible) is very necessary (see Chapter 3).

The prone position should be used to help relieve pressure on the sides and back. It is also advantageous in improving the oropharyngeal airway, improving drainage and ventilation of posterior lung segments, and improving drainage from the renal pelvis. If a pillow is not placed beneath the abdomen, the abdomen moves freely and breathing is easy.

Preventing joint contractures

For the patient with spinal cord injury, maintaining normal range of joint motion is an important aspect of his care. The individual with paralyzed limbs is dependent on someone else to move his extremities (Fig. 442). Passive exercises to prevent joint contractures are necessary. In some larger hospitals, the physical therapist is assigned this responsibility. However, the nurse not only must be cognizant of the need, but also must know how to move the paralyzed extremities through a normal range of motion. (See Chapter 3.)

Muscle spasms

In patients with spinal cord injury, muscle spasms may produce difficult problems. These may develop as the motor neuron reflex arc returns. Traction, frames, splinting, and even proper bed positioning seems to stimulate reflexes that result in powerful muscle spasms. Apparatus applied to forcibly maintain a desired position frequently causes pressure sores. Pressure sores are also frequently the result of pressure or abrasion of skin against the bedclothes occurring with spasms. As the patient improves, the tendency toward flexion and adduction deformities often becomes a perplexing problem. Even turning the patient in bed may trigger abnormal motor impulses that are almost impossible to control. Side rails or other protective measures must be used to prevent the patient's falling from the bed. Because mass reflexes are so difficult to combat and are so distressing to the patient, surgery sometimes is performed to eliminate them. Intraspinal resection of the nerve roots (rhizotomy) may be performed. This produces a flaccid paralysis that eliminates the mass flexion and adduction spasms. Other procedures to relieve the spasms, which the neurosurgeon may elect to do, are subtotal spinal chordectomy, subarachnoid alcohol block, or peripheral neurectomy. When relief from the muscle spasms has been obtained, it is possible to institute bladder training and to care for pressure sores more adequately

because the bed can be kept dry and the patient can be made comfortable, and deformity can be prevented. Activities of daily living may then be learned, and the previously helpless individual can have a more active and useful life.

Exercise program

It is imperative that a planned active exercise program be carried out for all nonparalyzed muscles and that passive exercises be prescribed for the paralyzed extremities. The patient with cord damage needs not only to maintain normal strength in nonparalyzed muscles, but also to increase the strength in these muscles so they may help substitute for the function of paralyzed muscles. Strong muscles will make it possible for him to change his position in bed, maneuver himself from bed to chair or chair to toilet, and perhaps manipulate crutches and perform other activities of daily living. All of these things are extremely important for the individual adjusting to a new way of life.

An exercise program is aimed primarily at strengthening the muscles of the upper extremities, the shoulders, the back, and abdomen, depending upon the level of cord injury. One of the earliest exercises is getting the patient to reach and to turn himself. Another early exercise prescribed may be weight lifting (Fig. 443). This helps to strengthen the finger flexors, the wrist extensors, and the elbow extensors. These muscles, along with the shoulder de-

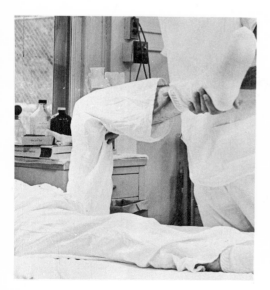

Fig. 442 Passive exercise of paralyzed limbs is an important aspect of the care needed by the patient with spinal cord injury.

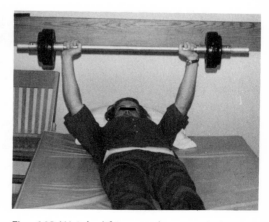

Fig. 443 Weight lifting used as a resistive exercise to strengthen muscles of the upper extremity. This will help the paraplegic master transfer and ambulation techniques.

pressors, are important for transfers and crutch walking. Push-ups also may be recommended (Fig. 444). The bed patient may be taught to do push-ups in the supine position by raising himself to his elbows and then to a sitting position with the

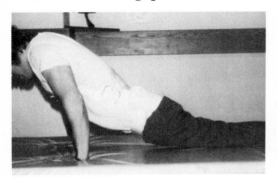

Fig. 444 Push-ups are another type of resistive exercise for arm strengthening in the paraplegic.

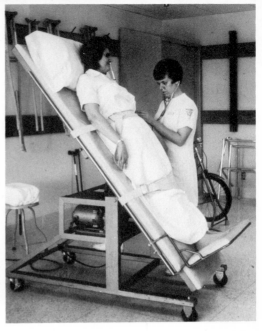

Fig. 445 Early use of the tilt table is helpful to the paraplegic and aids in overcoming postural hypotension. Weight bearing on the long bones helps to slow the development of osteoporosis.

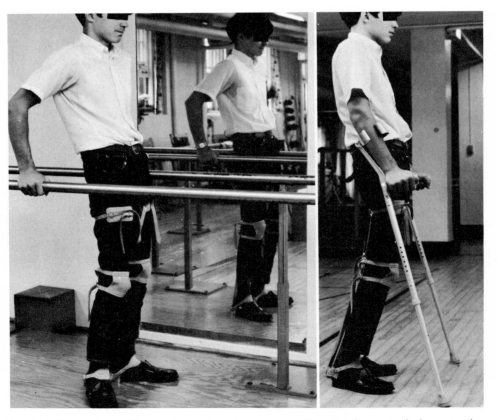

Fig. 446 The patient with paralysis of the lower extremities first learns to balance in the standing position and to walk with the aid of parallel bars and then with crutches.

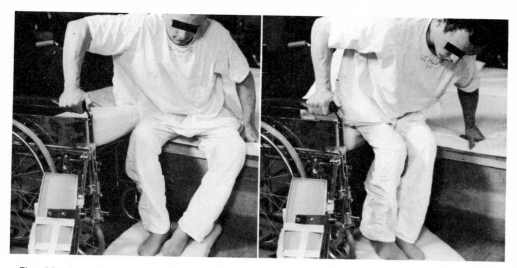

Fig. 447 A patient with paralysis of the lower extremities transfers from the mat (bed) to the wheelchair. The chair is placed parallel to the mat, the wheels are locked, and the armrest nearest the patient is removed. By placing one hand on the chair armrest and the other on the mat, as illustrated, the patient is able to lift and support his body weight as he moves to the chair seat.

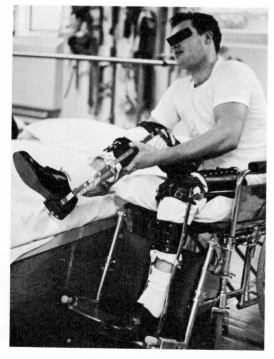

Fig. 448 Transferring from the bed to a wheelchair. With the wheels locked and the armrest nearest the bed removed, the patient uses his arm and shoulder muscles to slide across to the chair seat. Then with his hands, he moves his legs off the bed and places his feet on the wheelchair footrests.

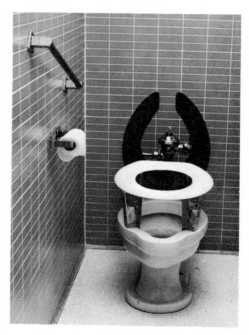

Fig. 449 An elevated toilet seat may be very helpful to the disabled individual, particularly the elderly patient or the patient with a hip problem. Note the handle bar.

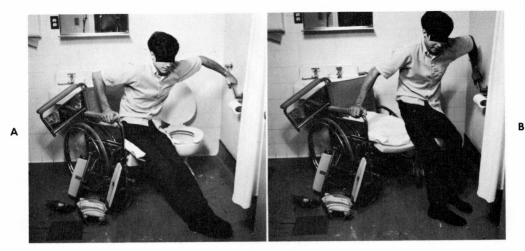

Fig. 450 Transferring from the wheelchair to a toilet seat. **A,** The chair is positioned as illustrated, with the wheels locked and the armrest nearest the stool removed. **B,** By using the chair armrest and the wall handle bar, the patient is able to support his body weight and to transfer from the chair to the toilet seat.

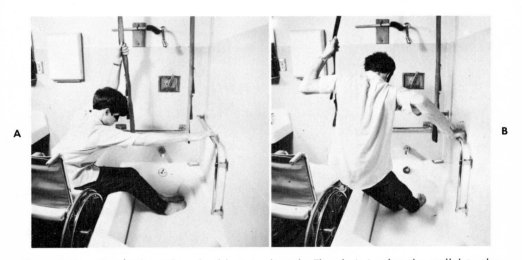

Fig. 451 Transferring from the wheelchair to the tub. The chair is placed parallel to the tub and the armrest nearest the tub is removed. **A,** The patient uses his hands to turn his body and to place his legs over the side of the tub. **B,** Then, by grasping the overhead strap and wall handle bar, he is able to support his weight and lower himself into the tub.

palms of his hands on the bed. In this position, he may use his hands to elevate his body off the bed. Use of the trapeze strengthens the elbow flexor (biceps) primarily and is less valuable. Learning to balance oneself in the sitting position should be practiced.

Early use of the tilt table, mentioned earlier, offers many benefits. The patient may not be able to assume a fully erect position initially. Lightheadedness or faintness may result from postural hypotension. To help prevent pooling of blood in the abdomen and legs, an abdominal binder or elastic stockings may be utilized. Early weight bearing on the tilt table as described previously not only helps prevent osteoporosis, but also serves as a morale booster for the paralyzed individual (Fig. 445).

Wheelchair exercises may include push-

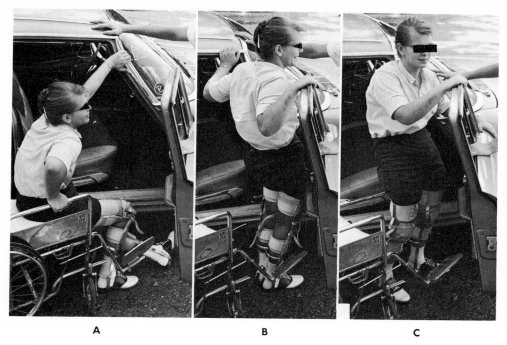

A   **B**   **C**

Fig. 452 Transferring from a wheelchair to a car seat. With the car door open, the chair is placed in the position illustrated. **A,** The patient removes her braced legs from the chair supports and slides forward in the chair. The left leg brace is locked in extension. **B,** By use of the arms as illustrated, the standing position is assumed. **C,** The individual pivots and is in position to lower herself onto the car seat with or without unlocking the braces. She will then use her arms to turn her body and to place her lower extremities in the car. (Courtesy Department of Physical Therapy, University of Iowa Hospitals and Clinics, The University of Iowa, Iowa City, Iowa.)

ups. The patient places his hands on the arms of the chair and raises his buttocks off the seat of the chair. This exercise is desirable for strengthening arm muscles and should be performed at frequent intervals also to relieve and change the pressure on the buttocks area. This can be very helpful in preventing pressure sores. Wheelchair games such as throwing darts or bowling are helpful in strengthening muscles of the upper extremity and provide active recreation.

When the patient has been fitted with braces, parallel bar exercises may be instituted to develop skills in balancing, weight bearing, and walking (Fig. 446). After learning to ambulate in the parallel bars, the patient advances to the use of crutches. He must learn to balance and also to manipulate the crutches. Becoming fully ambulatory with crutches involves more than learning the crutch gait patterns.

To become independent, the individual also must learn to rise from a bed or chair to a standing position, to open and close doors, to go up and down curbs, ramps, and steps, to sit down, to get off and on a toilet seat, to get in and out of a car (Figs. 447 to 452), and many other activities necessary for an active life.

Braces

Many patients with cord injury are fitted with braces. The type of brace prescribed will depend upon the level of the spinal cord lesion and the resulting muscle involvement. Individuals with lesions below the first lumbar vertebra usually are fitted with long leg braces. Patients with a lesion between the tenth thoracic and first lumbar vertebrae will need the long leg braces with a pelvic band or with a lumbosacral corset. If the spinal cord lesion is at the level of the tenth thoracic vertebra or above, the patient may need, in addition, a body brace that is attached to the leg braces. The making and fitting of braces requires considerable time and skill. Consequently, braces are expensive. Helping the paraplegic learn how to care for his braces is a necessary part of his training.

The wearing of braces by the patient with sensory loss is not without hazards. The skin must be checked carefully for reddened areas each time the brace is removed. If the alignment of the brace is not correct or if metal rubs the skin, pressure points will occur. Since the paraplegic does not have pain sensation, he must always be cognizant of his problem. As he learns the skills involved in putting on and removing braces (Fig. 453), he also must learn to visibly check the skin for signs of pressure. Shoes may be a problem for the individual with sensory loss. The heels and toes must be inspected daily for reddened areas or beginning blisters. Furthermore, care must be taken that the shoes worn by the patient fit properly and do not cause blisters.

Prevention and treatment of bedsores and trophic ulcers

One of the chief factors contributing to the development of a pressure sore is impaired circulation. Nerve damage with paralysis and loss of muscle activity results in a diminished blood supply to the part. Also, abnormal sweating in many patients with spinal cord injuries may result in maceration and more skin problems. Eliminating pressure on the affected areas until all signs of redness or inflammation have disappeared is the best and most effective treatment. This may restrict the patient's activities for a few days. The individual who lacks normal sensation must learn to check visually, by use of a hand mirror, all vulnerable spots, and since most patients will not have expensive equipment at home, it is preferable to teach proper skin care without dependence on such major devices as alternating pressure pads. (See Chapter 8.)

Self-help and self-care

As soon as possible, the patient with a spinal cord injury should begin to help with his own care. This will vary greatly among patients, depending upon the level

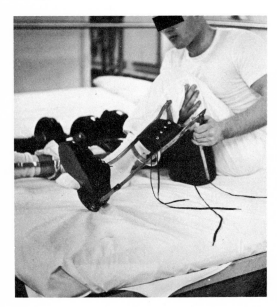

Fig. 453 When the patient is able to maintain his balance in a sitting position, he learns to put on his leg braces. As illustrated, he flexes the knee and lifts his leg with one hand and maneuvers the brace and places his foot in the shoe with the other hand. (Courtesy Department of Physical Therapy, University of Iowa Hospitals and Clinics, The University of Iowa, Iowa City, Iowa.)

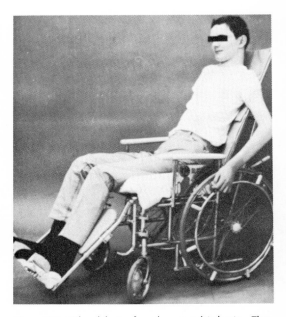

Fig. 454 Wheelchair for the quadriplegic. The high back provides support for the head and shoulders. The wheels are constructed so that the chair can be propelled by the patient who has minimal hand function.

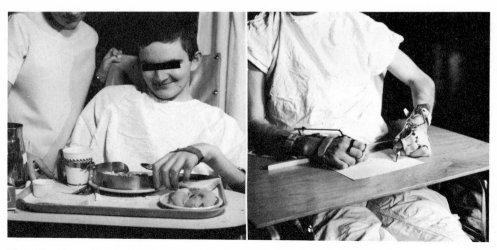

Fig. 455 Use of special equipment that may enable the individual with loss of hand function to feed himself and to grasp a pencil or similar object.

of the lesion, the individual's attitudes and emotional stability, and the nurse working with the patient. The person who is discovering what it means to be disabled from spinal cord injury nearly always has periods of depression. He frequently has little interest in doing very much for himself at this stage. He may be morose, critical, and demanding. Early activity and signs of progress will help the patient begin to regain some self-esteem and help prevent prolonged feelings of discouragement and dependency. A program of graduated activities needs to be planned with the patient and his family. The activities should challenge the patient but at each level should be within his capabilities so that he does not feel constantly frustrated. New interests and skill should be fostered and developed. The most desirable goal for the patient is complete independence and self-sufficiency. If feasible, this should be planned. However, for many of these patients, this is not a realistic goal; some dependency may be necessary. In any case, realistic goals should be established and activities planned to accomplish them (Figs. 454 to 456).

In the rehabilitation unit, group interchange can be fostered. It has been found that the ward situation, where patients can observe and talk about their own and other patients' disabilities, is often helpful. Competition with and encouragement from others can be invaluable. Patients sharing the rehabilitation unit may learn

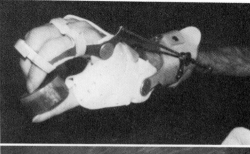

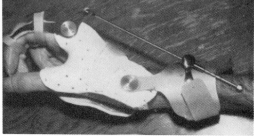

Fig. 456 A wrist-activated dynamic splint may permit certain quadriplegics to use the hand more functionally with stronger pinch and finger extension.

a great deal from each other, from routines for transfer, exercising, and gait training to managing money and sexual and family problems. Recreational activities may be helpful in taking the patient's mind off his disability (Fig. 457).

Emotional and social adjustments

The full impact of the patient's disability may not always become apparent

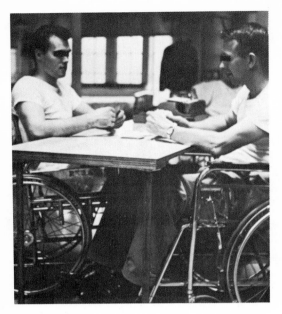

Fig. 457 Diversional activity is important for the paraplegic.

to the individual and to his family during the first few days or weeks. As full awareness of the permanent nature of his handicap becomes evident, major depressions and personality changes can be expected. Indifference, apathy, or self-pity may replace the patient's original attitude of hope, courage, and determination to recover. This is a natural reaction. The individual struggling with physical disabilities and changes in his body image can be expected to go through the process of grieving. The grief reaction as described by Kübler-Ross[47] includes (1) denial and isolation, (2) anger and resentment, (3) bargaining, (4) depression, and (5) acceptance and adjustment. To cope with the problem adequately, the nurse's preparation must be broad, and she must have a deep-seated interest in people and their problems.

The patient's problem is a very real one. Faced in the cold light of day and robbed of the mitigating factors that attend the early illness and the dramatic fight for survival, the outlook may be very bleak indeed. It is a situation that the newly crippled person realizes, however dimly, he has to face alone. The pattern of his life is smashed. He must collect the fragments and make what he can of them, and the task may look hopeless, the effort not worth the while.

Management of these situations demands early recognition of the likelihood of their occurrence. Although the nurse's attitude, like that of the patient, must be based on faith and optimism, statements must be guarded. Acceptance of the patient and his feelings as normal must be communicated by the nurse. His altered body image and loss of self-worth must be dealt with. The patient should very gradually be brought to accept his handicap from the first days of his paralysis and to plan his life in terms of that handicap rather than in terms of a complete functional recovery. This is the only honest course for any of his associates to take. It is kinder than unguarded optimism and cheeriness that break down under the strain of long-deferred hope. It also goes without saying that the principles of mental hygiene that the nurse applies when working with the patient must be discussed with the patient's family to guide them in their understanding of his problems. That this takes ingenuity is an understatement.

To assist these individuals (in addition to providing the nursing care described previously), the nurses should be able to help the family plan for the patient's homecoming. Alterations in the home environment frequently are necessary to make relative independence possible, but certainly no service can be more important. The nurse recognizes that the young individual needs relationships with people his own age and that special efforts by the family are necessary to see that previous friendships are continued and new ones acquired. It is important also for the nurse to be aware of available resources for education and rehabilitation. The patient and family will not know of these, for a few weeks ago the patient was a healthy individual with no need of such services. If ever there was an urgent necessity for broad information on these points, it is at this time when the nurse earnestly accepts the challenge to assist a newly handicapped individual attacked by all the forces of pessimism and personal disintegration.

24 The patient with a cerebrovascular accident

Hemiplegia is a term that literally means "paralysis of one side of the body." The brain is particularly vulnerable to changes in circulation. Interruption in its blood supply, even for as short a time as a few minutes, results in necrosis of the cells and loss of function in the body area innervated by these cells. This is referred to as a "stroke." The area of the brain damaged varies from patient to patient. The loss of blood supply results, in most cases, from a thrombus, an embolism, or a hemorrhage within the brain.

Arteriosclerotic changes in the vessel walls are frequently present in the patient who has suffered a stroke as a result of a thrombus. The etiology of the arteriosclerotic conditions is at present unknown. Today, cerebrovascular accidents rank third as a cause of death in the United States, being exceeded only by heart disease and cancer. Because of the increasing longevity of our population, it is expected that the number of people suffering strokes will increase. The outcome for these patients will depend upon the kind of nursing care they receive from the onset of a cerebrovascular accident. Of course, the extent of the brain damage is paramount with respect to the ultimate functional outcome.

Pathology

The brain is composed of cortical gray matter near its surface, wherein lie cell bodies, and of white matter containing axons or nerve fibers. Cell bodies initiate the functions of the brain, and nerve fibers then carry the massages from the cells out to the rest of the body. The brain not only sends out messages to muscles for movement, balance, speech, respiration, and blood pressure, but also receives information regarding sight, hearing, taste, touch, pain, etc. It must integrate the incoming information, take appropriate action, and carry on the higher thought processes of memory, problem-solving, and personality development. Many functional areas have been identified in the cerebral cortex.

Occlusion in the distribution of the middle cerebral artery is the most common lesion produced by a stroke (Fig. 458). Small vessels that supply fibers in the internal capsule often are occluded. In the internal capsule, fibers from the cortex are grouped together to descend the brainstem and spinal cord. With interruption of these fibers, there may be loss of motor and sensory function to a major part of the body. Hemiplegia or paralysis of one side results. Since most fibers from one side of the brain cross to the other side of the body, a lesion in the right side of the brain results in left hemiplegia and vice versa. A stroke may not result in total loss of function. There may be mild, transient weakness; more persistent partial paralysis or severe hemiplegia occurs in different cases. Also, one may have loss of vision, especially in one visual field, changes in balance, sensory perceptual impairment, or changes in blood pressure or respiration. The areas of the brain concerned with speech and language are located in the dominant cerebral hemisphere. A right-handed person with right hemiplegia caused

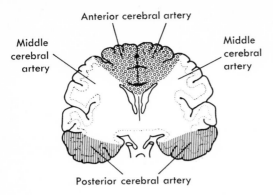

Anterior cerebral artery

Middle cerebral artery

Middle cerebral artery

Posterior cerebral artery

Fig. 458 Coronal section of the brain. Most cerebrovascular accidents produce lesions in the area of the brain supplied by the middle cerebral artery in one hemisphere.

by a left cerebral injury will commonly have trouble with speech (aphasia or dysphasia).

Nursing intervention, including rehabilitative measures

Following a stroke, the more severely involved patient will need intensive nursing care. Safety precautions must be taken to prevent injury should attempts be made to get out of bed. Careful checking of the vital signs is essential. Slowing of the pulse and respiration and elevation of the blood pressure and temperature may indicate rising intracranial pressure affecting vital centers. If swallowing difficulties are present, intravenous therapy may be necessary to help meet the patient's nutritional needs. During the first few days, fluids may be limited and should be given slowly to help prevent cerebral edema. An accurate record of intake and output is an essential part of the care. If the ability to swallow is impaired, aspiration is a great risk if oral feedings are attempted. Stringy foods and foods that are difficult to chew should be avoided. Turning the patient to the unaffected side will help to control liquids and food placed in his mouth. Mouth care should be given at frequent intervals, with particular attention to the paralyzed side. If the patient is accustomed to wearing dentures, he may handle food more easily with the dentures in place. If dysphagia continues to be a problem, a nasogastric tube may be inserted.

If the blink reflex is lost or the patient is unable to close the eyelid, protection for the eye is needed. Irrigation with physiologic saline solution and instillation of eye drops several times daily usually are prescribed to prevent drying and the development of corneal ulcers. If homonymous hemianopsia is present, the patient will have loss of vision in the right or left visual field of both eyes. Therefore, bedside equipment (e.g., eating utensils) should initially be placed within the patient's field of vision. Once the patient becomes oriented to his surroundings and to his problem, however, the center of attention should be shifted so that he is encouraged to look toward the involved side, thus diminishing any tendency toward unilateral neglect of the involved side.

Since many of these patients have limited spontaneous movement, nursing measures aimed at preventing hypostatic pneumonia should be started at the onset of the illness. Early mobilization and encouraging the patient to breathe deeply and to cough will help prevent stasis of secretions in the lungs. For some patients, suctioning may be necessary to remove secretions from the throat. An oropharyngeal airway may be used, and in some cases a tracheostomy is necessary to maintain an open passageway. Frequent changes of body position also are necessary to prevent the development of pressure areas. A planned schedule for turning the patient should be included in the nursing care plan.

Rehabilitation efforts should be started early in the course of the patient's hospital stay. Efforts to prevent deformities should be initiated and correct positioning practiced from the beginning. As the patient's condition improves, more attention can be given to frequent changes of body position, proper alignment of body parts, and range-of-motion exercises to protect the skin and prevent deformities.

The patient may tend to ignore his affected extremities because of changes in his level of consciousness, decreased perception, weakness, and reduced or altered sensation. Attempts should be made to draw the patient's attention to the involved side when positioning. A detailed description of the various positions are included in Chapter 3. The advantages of the prone position include the following:

1 Reduction in the possibilities of acquiring decubitus ulcers from prolonged lying in the supine position
2 Improvement of the airway as a result of the tongue and jaw moving forward
3 Better drainage of mucus from posterior lung areas and upper respiratory tract
4 Decreased possibility of aspiration of gastric contents
5 Decrease in problems with pneumonia and atelectasis

When positioning the patient, keep in mind that the tendency will be for the upper extremity to have a flexor dominant pattern and the lower extremity to have an extensor dominant pattern. In addition, there will be a tendency for the lateral trunk muscles of the involved side to contract or shorten and for the trunk to rotate in a posterior direction. Positioning should be such that this is counteracted.

As a rule, footboards are not recommended, particularly in the patient with spasticity. Pressure placed on the ball of the foot by the hard surface tends to cause the patient to utilize the primitive positive supporting reaction and push down in mass extension with plantar flexion. Increased spasticity and accompanying pain frequently result. The use of soft pillows for propping up the feet and the introduction of early weight-bearing activity are preferred substitutes for the use of the footboard.

The well-meaning use of hard hand splints may have a similar effect on increased spasticity of the hand. Better alternatives include a soft foam hand splint made to go between the patient's fingers or a hard cone placed with the smaller end toward the thumb to give direct tendon pressure. Like the soft hand splint, weaving soft gauze between a patient's toes may, to some degree, alleviate clawing of the toes.

With each change of position, the patient's skin should be checked for redness or blanching, which indicates too much pressure on a given area. Careful attention also must be given to skin hygiene of the axilla, groin, and hands. Dependent limbs, such as hands and feet, also may become

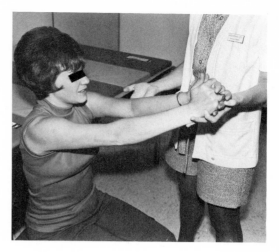

Fig. 459 The hemiplegic should be encouraged to perform symmetrical upper extremity activities with the fingers laced together to promote more appropriate distribution of tone and to draw more attention to the hemiparetic side. This may be initiated while the patient is still confined to bed.

swollen if not properly elevated and exercised through a full range of motion.

As soon as the patient is stabilized, usually within the first twenty-four to forty-eight hours, range-of-motion exercise for all joints should be started to prevent deformities. It should be remembered that on spastic extremities range of motions must be carefully carried out, with emphasis placed on rotational movements rather than force to gain the optimum range of motion. During exercise, pain should be kept to a minimum. Generally, moving each joint through its optimum range of motion two to three times daily will prevent tightness and deformity. In time, members of the patient's family may be taught to help with these passive exercises, or, in some instances, the patient may learn to use his uninvolved arm and leg to move and passively exercise the involved extremities—i.e., lacing fingers together and pushing arms straight out (Fig. 459) and working fingers and wrist.

The patient's motivation may be increased and his self-pity lessened by early indications that plans are being made to assist his recovery. The patient should be encouraged to use all unaffected muscles and joints actively to maintain mobility

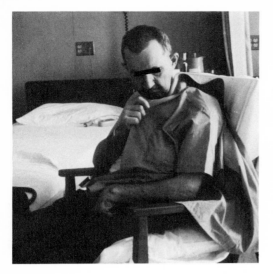

Fig. 460 Man with left hemiplegia practicing dressing himself. He should learn to put his paralyzed arm through the sleeve first.

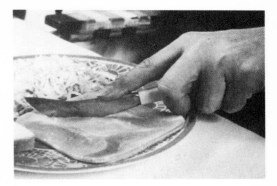

Fig. 461 Using a rounded, sharp, "rocking" knife, this patient with right hemiparesis is able to cut meat with one hand.

and develop motor control. He should be allowed to do as much as he can for himself. Unreasonable requests beyond his capabilities will only be frustrating and should be avoided.

Another major area in rehabilitation that the nurse may help carry out on the unit is training in self-care and the activities of daily living. As soon as the patient's condition permits, he should be encouraged to participate in his own daily care. Bathing, combing his hair, brushing his teeth, shaving, or applying make-up will encourage a sense of well-being and will help improve muscle control and joint function. Initially, these tasks may need to be taught to be performed with one hand. This may be slow and clumsy at first, but the patient should not be hurried because he may become frustrated and discouraged. Desired motor responses on one side in many ways are dependent on normal movement occurring on the opposite side. Thus, the uninvolved normal side of the patient who had a stroke may not respond "normally" when "abnormal" movement is occurring on the involved side.

Nurses should realize that a person who has suffered a stroke may be emotionally labile and frequently may break into tears. Associated factors, such as frustration, speech difficulties, and infections, have an effect on the patient's spasticity and consequently on his performance. When a patient has mastered some of the simpler tasks in self-care, he should be asked to try more difficult and complex activities, such as dressing and writing. In dressing, the affected arm or leg should be placed in the garment first (Fig. 460). In undressing, however, the garment should be removed from the unaffected limb first and then from the paralyzed limb. Often loose-fitting, familiar clothing is easier for the patient to manage and more gratifying than hospital attire.

Gaining independence in feeding is a priority item and may be aided greatly by assistance from a physical or occupational therapist (Fig. 461). (Placing the patient in a sitting position whenever possible may assist him in managing many motor activities with greater ease.) The patient should be up in a chair for meals with the tray at table height. (He should be sitting symmetrically, keeeping the affected arm forward and on the table.) The meal tray should be simplified by having all the main food on one plate rather than in separate small bowls. This is particularly important if visual and perceptual problems exist. Having the patient suck and chew on a Popsicle shortly before and between meals may facilitate lip closure, effective chewing, and removal of food from the pockets between the affected jaw and teeth.

As the patient becomes increasingly able to care for himself, caution must be exercised not to overemphasize compensation with the uninvolved side at the sacrifice of the involved side. For instance, a trapeze and side rails on a bed are sometimes useful. However, if the involved upper extremity possesses a strong dominant pattern, pulling on the trapeze or the side-rail with the uninvolved side, which requires strong biceps muscle contraction, may result in an overflow response to the already hyperactive biceps of the involved side. These compensatory activities may tend to be used long after the need has expired. This is quite frequently seen in the patient lifting the involved leg with the uninvolved leg. Compensation to a point is desirable, but sometimes early extra help on the part of the nurse will yield better long-term results.

Achieving bowel and bladder control may be a frustrating experience for the patient who has suffered a cerebrovascular accident. The bladder is frequently initially flaccid following the stroke, and an indwelling catheter may have to be used. Later, the flaccid bladder may become spastic. At this time, a bladder-training program may be initiated similar to that used for a paraplegic. A bowel-training program also should be initiated. The hemiplegic who remains incontinent after a month of bowel training is usually a poor candidate for independent living.

The patient must be checked for bowel function daily. Disposable diapers are useful for bowel incontinence. Impaction is common, but it is avoidable when close supervision is given. Laxatives and suppositories occasionally are required. Enemas may be useful on occasion but often are expelled incompletely and cause soilage throughout the day. At least 90% of patients will regain bowel and bladder control as sensation improves, consciousness returns, and confusion decreases. Suppositories to establish bowel habits rarely are required for more than a few days. As soon as the patient is well enough, a bedside commode or bathroom privileges will add to his feeling of well-being.

The indwelling catheter is frequently necessary to keep the incontinent patient dry and to protect his skin. Intermittent clamping of the tube and drainage at regular intervals are believed to assist in reestablishing bladder function. It should be noted that there are problems with intermittent clamping, and some physicians do not subscribe to this technique. Because of the irritation and increased chance of infection, it is important to remove the catheter as soon as possible. It is important that the catheter and tubing be cared for in an aseptic manner to prevent bacteria from entering the system. Clean bedside drainage tubes are just as important as clean catheters.

The patient should begin sitting as soon as possible. It should begin in bed and progress to dangling and then to sitting in a chair. As mentioned earlier, maintaining symmetry is important in regaining balanced musculature and proper body image, and this should be kept in mind when helping the patient maintain the upright position. The arm should be supported when necessary to maintain proper alignment. Preferably, the arm should be kept forward and elevated on a table or lapboard to avoid a totally flexed posturing. Perceptual difficulties, particularly prevalent in the patient with left hemiparesis, may complicate the situation. The patient may not want to sit to the involved side nor to the uninvolved side since both positions are unstable for sitting balance. He also may have an impaired perception of the vertical. The nurse should develop a trustful relationship with the patient so he has confidence to use her assistance in finding the proper balance.

The patient may be taught to use a wheelchair until he learns to walk. He usually will need help in learning to propel and guide his chair with his uninvolved arm and leg. If possible, both feet should be used, thus providing an excellent reciprocal activity for the lower extremities. The wheelchair should have a solid seat to enhance body posture. When the patient is simply sitting, a solid standard chair with armrests may have a more favorable psychologic impact on him than a wheelchair. Chairs that are either extremely low or extremely soft should be avoided since they are more difficult from which to rise to a standing position.

The use of forearm slings, once standard with the stroke patient, particularly the one with the flaccid arm, is now of doubtful

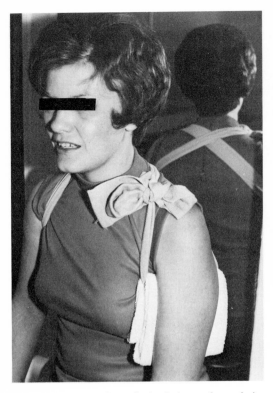

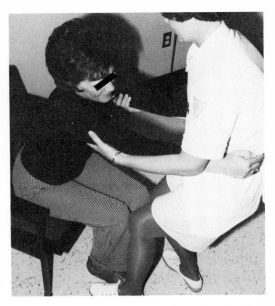

Fig. 463 Demonstrating a preferred method of transferring. Symmetry and weight bearing on both feet are encouraged. Adequate forward bending both on standing up and sitting down enhances the ease of the activity.

Fig. 462 Frequently, relief of discomfort of the upper extremity may be gained through the use of an axillary sling. This may be fashioned using an Ace wrap loosely tied through a towel as demonstrated.

repute. It is questionable how well they control shoulder subluxation. They do eliminate the facilitatory effects of gravity, but their claims to control edema seem dubious in light of the fact that the edema can travel no farther from the hand than the elbow. Slings may interfere with body image and subsequently a coordinate gait pattern. If indications do arise for the use of a sling, there are two more suitable substitutes for the forearm sling: the soft axillary sling held in place by a figure-of-eight wrap (Fig. 462) and the dynamic sling designed with tubing and a cone to help facilitate the extensor mechanism of the arm. If the patient will sit symmetrically, keeping his arm forward and elevated on a table, the need for additional support should be greatly diminished or eliminated.

It is important to properly assist the patient in gaining the standing position once he is ready to transfer (Fig. 463). A physical

therapist can provide valuable assistance in these instances. Whenever possible, it is best for one person to perform the actual transfer, with others spotting for safety. The more people involved in the transfer, the more confused the patient becomes, and consequently the less he does for himself. Allow the patient to contribute what he can. This is better for him and much easier on the person giving the assistance. If more than one person is necessary for the transfer, they should place themselves in such a way that symmetry may be maintained. The patient's knee should be blocked from the front, and the uninvolved side should lead in the direction of movement.

The next area of training involves ambulation (Fig. 464). It is important for all patients, and especially elderly persons, to begin ambulating as soon as possible. Weakness per se may be complicated by perceptual problems, sensory loss, loss of proprioception, or cerebellar injury resulting in balance and coordination difficulties. All these factors must be taken into account when walking is initiated. Symmetry and good weight bearing must be en-

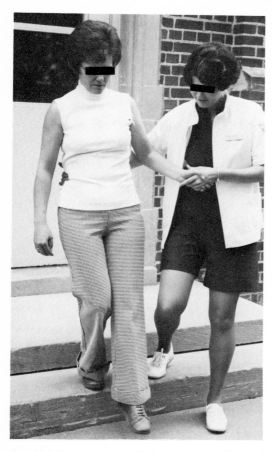

Fig. 464 The patient with hemiparesis is helped down the step so that she leads with her involved leg. The therapist holds the moderately advanced patient in a fashion to best facilitate balance and timing in gait.

couraged. This is crucial to gaining the desired control.

Though bracing is occasionally needed, it is no longer routinely recommended. It usually can be avoided unless the patient has persistent low muscle tone combined with marked sensory deficit, persistent difficulty with supination of the foot, or persistent intellectual difficulties that render extra assistive means necessary. It is believed that in many cases the use of the brace prevents the patient from developing and using his full potential, distorts the already impaired sensory feedback mechanism, and may lead to a less supple foot-ankle complex. It also may accentuate clawing of the toes through a mechanism similar to the tenodesis effect in the hand.

Functional dorsiflexion of the foot may be accomplished even though isolated dorsiflexion is not obtained. The patient should wear a firm pair of low-heeled shoes soon after he begins getting out of bed.

If a brace is indicated, a short leg brace with bilateral uprights and a bichannel ankle joint is most commonly used. The ankle joint usually is set at 90° and allows only a few degrees of dorsiflexion. This setting will provide some stability of the knee as well as the ankle. Metal pins rather than springs are used in the channels of the brace, because the stretch elicited by a spring-controlled brace will increase spasticity. Long leg braces rarely have a place.

Should assistive devices be required, a standard cane with a large flexible crutch tip generally serves the purpose best. This is held in the noninvolved hand and simultaneously moved with the involved leg. When walking up stairs, the uninvolved leg is first placed on the next riser, followed by the cane and involved leg. When going down stairs, the cane is placed on the next step, followed by the involved leg and then the uninvolved leg.

During the first few months following a cerebrovascular accident, various techniques may be used to facilitate or, if necessary, inhibit the function of muscle groups of the affected side (Fig. 465). Biofeedback devices and vibration may aid in gaining muscle reeducation. The patient's body now receives distorted input as to what it is doing, so those assisting him must often act as the patient's feedback. If not informed, the patient may not realize what it is that he is doing incorrectly. The patient should be working for muscle balance and controlled movement, not for bursts of strength. It is far more important for him to work on opening the fingers, straightening the elbow, and controlled extension of the lower extremity with dorsiflexion than on the respective antagonistic movement patterns.

Speech remediation may be helpful for patients with disorders of speech and communication. Some patients are able to speak, but not distinctly, because of limited or poor coordination of the movements of the lip, tongue, and throat muscles. Such dysarthria often improves with regular speech therapy and practice. Others may

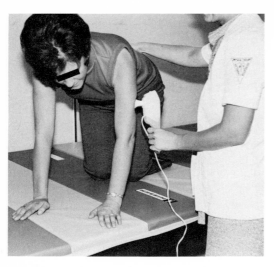

Fig. 465 Facilitation of proper muscle response may be accomplished by weight bearing as gained in the hand-knee position and by vibration to enhance the response of a specific muscle group such as the triceps in this illustration.

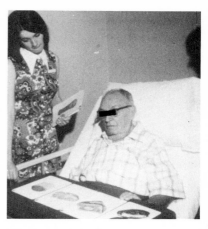

Fig. 466 The speech therapist asks the aphasic patient to identify a common object by pointing to the correct picture and then attempting to repeat the word.

demonstrate an oral apraxia that interferes with the voluntary control of movements. Some patients with lesions of the speech center may have aphasia. Some individuals have expressive aphasia and have problems with speaking, writing, or telling time. Others have trouble understanding the spoken or written word or in recognizing familiar objects and have receptive aphasia. Most patients have a mixed type of aphasia with both receptive and expressive deficits. Some individuals have nonfluent aphasia and say very little. Others have fluent aphasia. They talk in meaningless jargon. It is very important to recognize that the patient's ability to express himself is no index of how well he understands. It is also important to realize that the communication disorder affects only use of language symbols and does not represent a general intellectual deficit. The patient frequently will be responsive to gestures and facial expression and therefore may respond quite appropriately though he does not understand what is said to him. It also should be noted that many older persons have severe hearing impairments that further impair their communication skills. However, ordinarily it is not necessary for persons to speak louder than normal to them. It is

their speech and not their hearing that is the problem. A speech therapist should work with the patient. Repetitive drills may be helpful (Fig. 466). Memory patterns of words or phrases that the patient has retained will be sought by the therapist in an effort to regain some speech function. Much depends on the effort of the patient. This can be encouraged by the nurse on the unit during bathing, bed making, and other periods of patient care. Encourage but do not demand speech. The patient will many times make meaningless or nonsense syllables, but they are attempts. If he lacks functional speech, phrase questions so that a "yes" or "no" answer may be used, for this is at least a start. Realize, however, that the "yes" and "no" may at times be unreliable. Allow him to use speech in any way he can (speaking, writing, reading) as much as possible. Speaking slowly and distinctly with natural intonation will help him understand you. Use relatively short sentences. Provide him with a way to anticipate the nature of the conversation. Again, do not speak louder than you normally do. If he becomes fatigued or resists help, it is best to drop the activity for a time. Do not let him struggle overly long when trying to say something, but allow him an unhurried period to work at it before assisting him.

When taking care of the individual problems such as the skin, body position, the bowel, and speech, it is important not to forget the patient as a whole. He needs sympathetic and knowledgeable help as an individual. If he is an adult, he should be treated as one and be guided to effective coping mechanisms that will allow him to restructure his self-image and feeling of worth. The family may need guidance in understanding the patient's problems, such as accompanying emotional lability, limited attention span, and the need for various activities. If feasible, they should be included in the patient's care while at the same time being discouraged from being overly solicitous or overly demanding. They should be included in discussions of long-term planning or realistic goals. Plans should, of course, include careful consideration of the patient's own desires and priorities. The patient, whenever possible, needs to feel he has some control in the situation.

Muscle strength, coordination, and balance can be achieved through exercises as well as activities. The patient also must become involved in relearning homemaking activities, using new methods of travel, and exploring possible vocational and avocational avenues. He should be referred to local or state public health, social welfare, and vocational rehabilitation agencies when appropriate. These agencies can often assist in the transition from hospital to home. The community nurse can be of invaluable assistance in helping the patient and his family make adjustments in the home, which will help the patient maintain his independence and still provide him with needed assistance and understanding. Members of the family may need continued support and reassurance to help them cope with the many problems that arise. It is important to consider age, the severity of the disability, and the patient's interests, as well as social and cultural factors, when planning rehabilitative self-care and vocational goals. It is also important to be realistic and neither excessively optimistic nor pessimistic with the patient. The patient's hope should be preserved. It may take six to eighteen months for the patient to achieve his maximum gain. (It may also take much less time than this.) Also, it is not rare for patients who remain mentally alert several years after a stroke to make gains with appropriate training. Cooperation of all disciplines is essential for best results.

Unit VI STUDY QUESTIONS

THE PATIENT WITH SPINAL CORD INJURY

A 21-year-old man has been admitted to the rehabilitation area with a fracture of the tenth thoracic vertebra, resulting in cord injury and paralysis of the lower extremities (paraplegia). Review the following aspects of his care.

1 Nursing care will include changing the patient's position at relatively frequent intervals. Describe or demonstrate good body alignment in the prone, supine, and side-lying positions. Explain reasons for frequent turning of the patient.
2 Describe the nursing care that will help to prevent the development of pressure sores. Why is the paraplegic patient prone to develop decubiti?
3 What urinary problems may be anticipated?
4 Passive exercises will be prescribed to help maintain joint motion of the lower extremities. Describe or illustrate range of motion for the ankle, knee, and hip joints.
5 Describe the secondary contractures that may be anticipated when the muscles of the lower extremity are paralyzed.
6 Review some of the physiologic changes that may take place because of the patient's inactivity. Be prepared to substantiate your answers.
7 Use of the tilt table is frequently prescribed early in the care of the paraplegic. Why is this beneficial?
8 Active exercises will be prescribed to strengthen the muscles of the upper extremities. Explain.
9 It will be necessary for this patient to learn to do many things in a new way. Explain some of the activities of daily living that the rehabilitation team will encourage and help him to master.
10 The patient's morale will greatly influence the success of his rehabilitation. Discuss factors that may influence how the patient feels about what has happened to him and his adjustment to a new way of life.

THE PATIENT WITH A CEREBROVASCULAR ACCIDENT

Mr. A. has been admitted to the rehabilitation service with the diagnosis of a cerebrovascular accident. The left side of his body is paralyzed.

1 Describe or demonstrate various bed positions you would utilize for this patient.
2 Is the development of pressure sores a problem?
3 Describe joint contractures that are most likely to develop when a hemiplegic condition is present.
4 What is meant by a functional position of the hand?
5 Why has Mr. A. been admitted to the rehabilitation service? What do you think should be gained by a period of treatment and care in this particular unit?

Unit VI REFERENCES

GENERAL CONSIDERATIONS IN REHABILITATION

1 Anderson, N.: Rehabilitative nursing practice, Nurs Clin North Am 6:303-309, Jun 1971.
2 Bedford, J. B.: Beds and tables. In Licht, S. H., and Kamenetz, H. L., editors: Orthotics etcetera, New Haven, 1966, Elizabeth Licht, Publisher.
3 Boroch, R. M.: Elements of rehabilitation in nursing, St. Louis, 1976, The C. V. Mosby Co.
4 Brown, M. E.: Self-help clothing. In Licht, S. H., and Kamenetz, H. L., editors: Orthotics etcetera, New Haven, 1966, Elizabeth Licht, Publisher.
5 Campbell, E. B.: Nursing problems associated with prolonged recovery following trauma, Nurs Clin North Am 5:551-562, Dec 1970.
6 Christopherson, V. A.: Role modifications of the disabled male, Am J Nurs 68:290-293, Feb 1968.
7 Chronic disease and rehabilitation, Nurs Clin North Am 1:355-519, Sep 1966.
8 Cooper, S. B.: Motivation of the immobilized orthopedic patient, ONA J 3:191-193, Jun 1976.
9 Deaver, G. G.: Crutches, canes and walkers. In Licht, S. H., and Kamenetz, H. L., editors: Orthotics etcetera, New Haven, 1966, Elizabeth Licht, Publisher.
10 Hallburg, J. C.: Teaching patients self care, Nurs Clin North Am 5:223-231, Jun 1970.
11 Halverson, E. A.: Taking rehabilitation to the patient, Can Nurse 67:49-51, Sep 1971.
12 Holmes, J. E.: The physical therapist and team care, Nurs Outlook 20:182-184, Mar 1972.
13 Hopkins, H. L.: Self-help aids. In Licht, S. H., and Kamenetz, H. L., editors: Orthotics etcetera, New Haven, 1966, Elizabeth Licht, Publisher.
14 Kamenetz, H. L.: Selecting a wheelchair, Am J Nurs 72:100-101, Jan 1972.
15 Krusen, F. H., Kottke, F., and Ellwood, P., editors: Handbook of physical medicine and

rehabilitation, ed. 2, Philadelphia, 1971, W. B. Saunders Co.

16 Martin, N., King, R., and Suchinski, J.: The nurse therapist in a rehabilitation setting, Am J Nurs 70:1694-1697, Aug 1970.

17 Moolten, S. E.: Bedsores in the chronically ill patient, Arch Phys Med Rehabil 53:430-438, Sep 1972.

18 Peszczynski, M.: Housing for the disabled. In Licht, S. H., and Kamenetz, H. L., editors: Orthotics etcetera, New Haven, 1966, Elizabeth Licht, Publisher.

19 Plaisted, L. M.: The clinical specialist in rehabilitation nursing, Am J Nurs 69:562-564, Mar 1969.

20 Rosillo, R. H., Fogel, M. L., and Freedman, K.: Affect levels and improvement in physical rehabilitation, J Chronic Dis 24:651-660, Nov 1971.

21 Rothberg, J. S.: The challenge for rehabilitative nursing, Nurs Outlook 17:37-39, Nov 1969.

22 Rusk, H. A.: Rehabilitation medicine, ed. 4, St. Louis, 1977, The C. V. Mosby Co.

23 Schwartz, D.: Problems of self-care and travel among elderly ambulatory patients, Am J Nurs 66:2678-2681, Dec 1966.

24 Sine, R. D., Liss, S. E., Roush, R. E., and Holcomb, J. D., editors: Basic rehabilitation techniques—a self instructional guide, Germantown, Md., 1977, Aspens System Corporation.

25 Smolock, M. A.: The nurse's role in rehabilitation of the handicapped child, Nurs Clin North Am 5:411-420, Sep 1970.

26 Stryker, R. P.: Rehabilitative aspects of acute and chronic nursing care, ed. 2, Philadelphia, 1977, W. B. Saunders Co.

27 Welch, S. R.: Tilt-table therapy in rehabilitation of the trauma patient with brain damage and spinal injury, Nurs Clin North Am 5:621-630, Dec 1970.

THE PATIENT WITH SPINAL CORD INJURY

28 Altshuler, A., Meyer, J., and Butz, M. K.: Even children can learn to do clean self-catheterization, Am J Nurs 77:97-101, Jan 1977.

29 Augustine, R. W., and Dowden, B.: Traction treatment, Nursing (Jenkintown) 4:72-73, May 1974.

30 Boone, E. T., and Self, L. H.: Nursing care of the paraplegic using an experimental electronic spinal neuroprosthesis to activate voiding, J Neurosurg Nurs 4:61-74, Jul 1972.

31 Bromley, I.: Tetraplegia and paraplegia, 1976, Edinburgh, Churchill Livingstone.

32 Carini, E., and Owens, G.: Neurological and neurosurgical nursing, ed. 6, St. Louis, 1974, The C. V. Mosby Co.

33 Champion, V. L.: Clean technique for intermittent self-catheterization, Nurs Res 25:13-18, Jan-Feb 1976.

34 Comarr, A. E., and Gunderson, B. B.: Sexual function in traumatic paraplegia and quadriplegia, Am J Nurs 75:250-255, Feb 1975.

35 Culp, P.: Nursing care of the patient with spinal cord injury, Nurs Clin North Am 2:447-457, Sep 1967.

36 Decker, R.: What to tell a twenty-year-old quad, Phys Ther 51:1299, Dec 1971.

37 Degroot, J., and Kunin, C.: Indwelling catheters, Am J Nurs 75:448-449, Mar 1975.

38 Delehanty, L., and Stravino, V.: Achieving bladder control, Am J Nurs 70:312-316, Feb 1970.

39 Ford, J. R., and Cooke, T. D.: Rehabilitation of the quadriplegic, Can Nurse 67:37-38, Aug 1971.

40 Freeman, L. W., and Perkins, L. C.: Care of the paraplegic patient, Bedside Nurse 3:11-18, Aug 1970.

41 Garner, J. S.: Urinary catheter care, Nursing (Jenkintown) 4:54-56, Feb 1974.

42 Hamric, A., Allen, V., Yoon, R., and Windsor, N.: Caring for the totally dependent patient, Nursing (Jenkintown) 6:38-43, Jul 1976.

43 Hanlon, K.: Maintaining sexuality after spinal cord injury, Nursing (Jenkintown) 5:58-62, May 1975.

44 Henderson, G. M.: Teaching-learning for rehabilitation of the spinal cord-disabled individual, Nurs Clin North Am 6:655-668, Dec 1971.

45 Holliday, J.: Bowel programs of patients with spinal cord injury: a clinical study, Nurs Res 16:4-15, Winter 1967.

46 Jordan, H. S., and Kavchak, M. A.: Transfer techniques, Nursing (Jenkintown) 3:19-22, Mar 1973.

47 Kübler-Ross, E.: On death and dying, New York, 1969, Macmillan Publishing Co., Inc.

48 Langford, T. L.: Nursing problem: bacteriuria and the indwelling catheter, Am J Nurs 72:113-115, Jan 1972.

49 Lapides, J., Diokno, A. C., Gould, F. R., and Lowe, B.: Further observations on self-catheterization, J Urol 116:169-171, Aug 1976.

50 Lapides, J., Diokno, A. C., Silber, S. J., and Lowe, B.: Clean, intermittent self-catheterization in the treatment of urinary tract disease, J Urol 107:458-461, Mar 1972.

50a Larrabee, J.: The person with a spinal cord injury—physical care during early recovery, Am J Nurs 77:1320-1329, Aug 1977.

51 Levine, M., moderator: Quadriplegic adolescent, Nursing (Jenkintown) 2:28-32, Jun 1972.

52 Lindan, R., and Bellomy, V.: The use of intermittent catheterization in a bladder training program, J Chronic Dis 24:727-735, Dec 1971.

53 Lindh, K., and Rickerson, G.: Spinal cord injury: you can make a difference, Nursing (Jenkintown) 4:41-45, Feb 1974.

53a McCauley, C.: Eddie: a successful quad, Am J Nurs 77:1336-1338, Aug 1977.

53b Oliveto, M., Wilson, S., and Mackinnon, H.: Sara: her rehabilitation and its cost, Am J Nurs 77:1338-1342, Aug 1977.

54 Pelosof, H. V., David, F. R., and Carter, R. E.: Hydronephrosis: silent hazard of intermittent catheterization, J Urol 110:375-377, Oct 1973.

54a Pepper, G.: The person with a spinal cord

injury—psychological care, Am J Nurs **77:** 1330-1336, Aug 1977.

55 Pratt, R.: The nursing management of acute spinal paraplegia, Nurs Times **67:**499-500, 29 Apr; 537-540, 6 May; 567-569, 13 May; 604-606, 20 May; 638-639, 27 May; 662-663, 3 Jun; 699-700, 10 Jun 1971.

56 Smith, J., and Bullough, B.: Sexuality and the severely disabled person, Am J Nurs **75:** 2194-2197, Dec 1975.

57 Tudor, L. L.: Bladder and bowel retraining, Am J Nurs **70:**2391-2393, Nov 1970.

58 Turgeon, E.: Self-catheterization for female paraplegics, Nursing (Jenkintown) **4:**83, Jul 1974.

59 Vincent, P. J., Smith, J., and Danglassan, E.: Treatment of patients with spinal cord injuries, Can Nurse **71:**26-30, Aug 1975.

60 Viray, P. C.: Nursing care of the patient with a cervical spine injury, ONA J **2:**115-118, May 1975.

THE PATIENT WITH A CEREBROVASCULAR ACCIDENT

61 Bruetman, M. E., and Gordon, E. E.: Rehabilitating the stroke patient at general hospitals, Postgrad Med **49:**211-215, Mar 1971.

62 Burt, M. M.: Perceptual deficits in hemiplegia, Am J Nurs **70:**1026-1029, May 1970.

63 Dayhoff, N.: Soft or hard devices to position hands? Am J Nurs **75:**1142-1144, Jul 1975.

64 Dolan, M.: Rethinking stroke: autumn months, autumn years, Am J Nurs **75:**1145-1147, Jul 1975.

65 Drew, N.: How to cope with speech defects in stroke patients, Nursing (Jenkintown) **4:** 20-21, Feb 1974.

66 Ellis, R.: After stroke; sitting problems, Am J Nurs **73:**1898-1899, Nov 1973.

67 Elwood, E.: Nursing the patient with a cerebrovascular accident, Nurs Clin North Am **5:**47-53, Mar 1970.

68 Fowler, R. S., Jr., and Fordyce, W. E.: Adapting care for the brain-damaged patient. Part I, Am J Nurs **72:**1832-1835, Oct 1972.

69 Fowler, R. S., Jr., and Fordyce, W. E.: Adapting care for the brain-damaged patient. Part II, Am J Nurs **72:**2056-2059, Nov 1972.

70 Graham, L.: Stroke rehabilitation—a creative process, Nurs Digest **5:**64-67, Spring 1977.

71 Guerrieri, B.: Survey of the knowledge of the nurse in direct-care services concerning proper bed positioning of the patient with hemiplegia, Nurs Res **17:**157-159, Mar-Apr 1968.

72 Hyman, M. D.: The stigma of stroke. Its effects on performance during and after rehabilitation, Geriatrics **26:**132-141, May 1971.

73 Jacobansky, A. M.: Stroke. Am J Nurs **72:** 1260-1263, Jul 1972.

74 Kelly, P.: Mr. Quinto . . . a difficult rehab patient, Nursing (Jenkintown) **3:**27-29, Apr 1973.

75 Knapp, M. E.: Practical physical medicine and rehabilitation. 2. The hemiplegic patient —physical rehabilitation, Postgrad Med **39:** A143-A149, Mar 1966.

76 Knapp, M. E.: Practical physical medicine and rehabilitation. 3. The hemiplegic patient —physical problems, Postgrad Med **39:**A125-132, Apr 1966.

77 Large, H., Tuthill, J. E., Kennedy, F. B., and Pozen, T.: In the first stroke intensive care unit, Am J Nurs **69:**76-80, Jan 1969.

78 Nickel, V. L., editor: Symposium: Orthopedic management of stroke, Clin. Orthop. **63:**3-161, Mar-Apr 1969.

79 Perry, J.: Orthopedic management of the lower extremity in the hemiplegic patient, Phys Ther **46:**345-356, Apr 1966.

80 Pfaudler, M.: After stroke; motor skill rehabilitation for patients, Am J Nurs **73:**1892-1896, Nov 1973.

81 Riehl, J., and Chambers, J.: Better salvage for the stroke patient, Nursing (Jenkintown) **6:**24-31, Jul 1976.

82 Shaw, B. L.: Revolution in stroke care, RN **33:** 56-61, Jan 1970.

83 Stanton, J. H.: Rehabilitation nursing related to stroke, Clin Orthop **63:**39-53, Mar-Apr 1969.

84 Stohl, D. J.: Preserving home life for the disabled, Am J Nurs **72:**1645-1650, Sep 1972.

85 Zankel, H. T.: Stroke rehabilitation, Springfield, Ill., 1971, Charles C Thomas, Publisher.

Index